Optum

Expert

HCPCS Level II

A resourceful compilation of HCPCS codes

Supports HIPAA compliance

2023

optumcoding.com

Publisher's Notice

The Optum *2023 HCPCS Level II* is designed to be an accurate and authoritative source of information about this government coding system. Every effort has been made to verify the accuracy of the listings, and all information is believed reliable at the time of publication. Absolute accuracy cannot be guaranteed, however. This publication is made available with the understanding that the publisher is not engaged in rendering legal or other services that require a professional license.

Our Commitment to Accuracy

Optum is committed to producing accurate and reliable materials.

To report corrections, please email customerassistance@optum.com. You can also reach customer service by calling 1.800.464.3649, option 1.

To view Optum updates/correction notices, please visit http://www.optumcoding.com/ProductUpdates/

Acknowledgments

Denise M. Smith, RN, BSN, *Senior Product Manager*

Stacy Perry, *Manager, Desktop Publishing*

Elizabeth Leibold, RHIT, *Subject Matter Expert*

Jacqueline Petersen, RHIA, CHDA, CPC, *Subject Matter Expert*

Tracy Betzler, *Senior Desktop Publishing Specialist*

Hope M. Dunn, *Senior Desktop Publishing Specialist*

Katie Russell, *Desktop Publishing Specialist*

Lynn Speirs, *Editor*

Copyright

Property of Optum, Inc. Optum, Inc. and the Optum logo are trademarks of Optum, Inc. All other brand or product names are trademarks or registered trademarks of their respective owner.

© 2022 Optum, Inc. All rights reserved.

HS   ISBN 978-1-62254-820-0

Subject Matter Experts

Elizabeth Leibold, RHIT

Ms. Leibold has more than 30 years of experience in the health care profession. She has served in a variety of roles, ranging from patient registration to billing and collections, and has an extensive background in both physician and hospital outpatient coding and compliance. She has worked for large health care systems and health information management services companies, and has wide-ranging experience in facility and professional component coding, along with CPT expertise in interventional procedures, infusion services, emergency department, observation, and ambulatory surgery coding. Her areas of expertise include chart-to-claim coding audits and providing staff education to both tenured and new coding staff. She is an active member of the American Health Information Management Association (AHIMA) and Tennessee Health Information Management Association (THIMA).

Jacqueline Petersen, RHIA, CHDA, CPC

Ms. Petersen is a Clinical/Technical editor with Optum. She has served as Senior Clinical Product Research Analyst with Optum developing business requirements for edits to support correct coding and reimbursement for claims processing applications. Her experience includes development of data-driven and system rules for both professional and facility claims and in-depth analysis of claims data inclusive of ICD-10-CM, CPT, HCPCS, and modifiers. Her background also includes consulting work for Optum, serving as a SME, providing coding and reimbursement education to internal and external clients. Ms. Petersen is a member of the American Academy of Professional Coders (AAPC), and the American Health Information Management Association (AHIMA).

Welcome to over 25 years of coding expertise

Every medical organization knows that medical documentation and coding accuracy are vital to the revenue cycle. As a leading health services business, Optum has proudly created industry-leading coding, billing and reimbursement solutions for more than 25 years. Serving the broad health market, including physicians, health care organizations, payers and government, we help health systems reduce costs and achieve timely and accurate revenue.

You'll find ICD-10-CM/PCS, CPT®, HCPCS, DRG, specialty and reference content across our full suite of medical coding, billing and reimbursement products. And to ensure you have expert insight and the right information at your fingertips, our subject matter experts have incorporated proprietary features into these resources. These include supplementary edits and notations, coding tips and tools, and appendixes — making each product comprehensive and easy to use. Think of it as coding resources built by coders, for coders like you.

Your coding, billing and reimbursement product team,

Ryan
Anita
Jacquie
Ken
Marianne
Denise
Elizabeth
LaJuana
Leanne
Nann

Put Optum medical coding, billing and reimbursement content at your fingertips today. Choose what works for you.

- Publications (print and eBook)
- Online coding tools
- Data files
- Web services

Visit us at **optumcoding.com** to browse our products, or call us at 1-800-464-3649, option 1, for more information.

Optum

CPT is a registered trademark of the American Medical Association.

At our core, we're about coding

Essential medical code sets are just that — essential to your revenue cycle. In our ICD-10-CM/PCS, CPT®, HCPCS and DRG coding tools, we apply our collective coding expertise to present these code set resources in a way that is comprehensive, as well as easy to use and apply. Optum publications (print and eBook) are budget-friendly and easily referenced, created with intuitive features and formats, such as visual alerts, color-coding and symbols to identify important coding notes and instructions — plus, great coding tips.

Find the same content, tips and features of our code books in a variety of formats. Choose from print and eBook publications, online coding tools, data files or web services.

Your coding, billing and reimbursement product team,

Put Optum medical coding, billing and reimbursement content at your fingertips today. Choose what works for you.

- Publications (print and eBook)
- Online coding tools
- Data files
- Web services

Ryan
Anita   Ken   LaJuana
Jacquie   Marianne   Denise   Leanne
                   Elizabeth   Nann

Visit us at **optumcoding.com** to browse our products, or call us at 1-800-464-3649, option 1, for more information.

CPT is a registered trademark of the American Medical Association.

Our specialty coding tools put time on your side

How much time do you think you spend researching elusive codes? Too much, probably. Time you would like to have back. We can't give time back, but we can help you save it. Our all-in-one coding solutions consolidate specialty coding processes so you can find information more easily and quickly. Each specialty-specific procedure code includes its official and lay descriptions, coding tips, cross-coding to common ICD-10-CM codes, relative value units, Medicare edit guidance, *CPT® Assistant* references, CCI edits and, when relevant, specific reimbursement and documentation tips.

With tools available for 33 specialties, we're sure you'll find the right resource to meet your organization's unique needs, even if those needs are allergy, anesthesia/pain management, behavioral health, cardiology, cardiothoracic surgery, critical care, dental, dermatology, emergency medicine, endocrinology, ENT, family care, gastroenterology, general surgery, hematology, infectious disease, internal medicine, laboratory/pathology, nephrology, neurology, neurosurgery, OB/GYN, OMS, oncology, ophthalmology, orthopaedics, pediatrics, physical therapy, plastics, podiatry, primary care, pulmonology, radiology, rheumatology, urology or vascular surgery.

Say good-bye to time wasted digging for those elusive codes.

Your coding, billing and reimbursement product team,

Ryan, Anita, Jacquie, Ken, Marianne, Denise, Elizabeth, LaJuana, Leanne, Nann

Put Optum medical coding, billing and reimbursement content at your fingertips today. Choose what works for you.

- Publications (print and eBook)
- Online coding tools
- Data files
- Web services

Visit us at **optumcoding.com** to browse our products, or call us at 1-800-464-3649, option 1, for more information.

CPT is a registered trademark of the American Medical Association.

A lot goes into coding resources. We know.

Most think that coding, billing and reimbursement includes only your essential code sets, but that leaves out reference products. An important part of the revenue cycle, reference tools provide clarity — along with coding and billing tips — to deepen medical coding knowledge, make the coding process more efficient and help reduce errors on claims. Optum offers reference tools for facility, physician and post-acute markets, in addition to physicians-only fee products that inform the best business decisions possible for practices.

There's a lot that goes into coding, billing and reimbursement. Make sure your organization isn't leaving anything to chance.

Your coding, billing and reimbursement product team,

Ryan, Amita, Jacquie, Ken, Marianne, Denise, Elizabeth, LaJuana, Leanne, Nann

Put Optum medical coding, billing and reimbursement content at your fingertips today. Choose what works for you.

- Publications (print and eBook)
- Online coding tools
- Data files
- Web services

Visit us at **optumcoding.com** to browse our products, or call us at 1-800-464-3649, option 1, for more information.

CPT is a registered trademark of the American Medical Association.

Optum

Ready to renew?

We make it easy

Optum offers many convenient ways to renew your coding resources — so you always have the most up-to-date code sets when you need them.

For the fastest renewal, place your order on optumcoding.com. It's quick and easy, and for every $500 you spend with us online, you earn a $50 coupon toward your next online purchase.* Simply sign in to your optumcoding.com account to view and renew your coding tools today.

Away from your computer? No problem. We also offer the following offline renewal options:

Call: 1-800-464-3649, option 1

Fax: 1-801-982-4033
(include purchase order)

Mail: Optum
PO Box 88050
Chicago, IL 60680-9920
(include payment/purchase order)

Lock in your product price now and avoid rate increases later

Optum offers multi-year contracts for most book resources and online coding tools. Call 1-800-464-3649, option 1, to learn how to lock in your rate.

Optum no longer accepts credit cards by fax or mail.

*Shipping charges and taxes still apply and cannot be used toward your account balance for eRewards coupons. Coupons expire six months after they are earned. Once a coupon expires, it will no longer be available for use. You must be logged in to your online account to have your purchases tracked for reward purposes. Offer valid online only — coupons cannot be earned with orders placed offline and coupons cannot be applied to orders placed offline. Customers who are already part of our Medallion or Reseller programs are not eligible for our eRewards program.

© 2022 Optum, Inc. All rights reserved. WF7452382 06/22

Optum expertise applied to essential medical coding content means quality solutions to meet your needs

Optum can help you drive financial results across your organization with industry-leading resources that cut through the complexity of medical coding challenges.

The Price Match program* is an example of one of the ways in which we can impact your bottom line — to the positive. We're committed to providing you with the best quality product in the market, along with the best price. So if you find a better price on code books, Optum will match it.*

Let us help you find the best coding solution, at the best price, with our Price Match program

Contact your content solutions client manager directly.

Call: 1-800-464-3649, option 1

Visit: optumcoding.com/pricematch

*Some restrictions and exclusions apply. Visit optumcoding.com/pricematch to learn more about the conditions, guidelines and exclusions.

Optum is a registered trademark of Optum, Inc. in the U.S. and other jurisdictions. All other brand or product names are the property of their respective owners. Because we are continuously improving our products and services, Optum reserves the right to change specifications without prior notice. Optum is an equal opportunity employer.

© 2022 Optum, Inc. All rights reserved. WF7452382 05/22

Contents

Introduction .... Introduction—1

Index .... Index — 1

A Codes 1
    Transportation Services Including Ambulance 1
    Medical and Surgical Supplies 2

B Codes 17
    Enternal and Parenteral Therapy 17

C Codes 19
    Outpatient PPS 19

E Codes 31
    Durable Medical Equipment 31

G Codes 45
    Procedures/Professional Services (Temporary) 45

H Codes 87
    Alcohol and Drug Abuse Treatment Services 87

J Codes 89
    J Codes Drugs 89
    J Codes Chemotherapy Drugs 108

K Codes 115
    Temporary Codes 115

L Codes 119
    Orthotic Procedures and Devices 119
    Prosthetic Procedures 131

M Codes 143
    MIPS Value Pathways 143
    Medical Services 143
    Quality Measures 144

P Codes 148
    Pathology and Laboratory Services 148

Q Codes 150
    Q Codes (Temporary) 150

R Codes 160
    Diagnostic Radiology Services 160

S Codes 161
    Temporary National Codes (Non-Medicare) 161

T Codes 173
    National T Codes Established for State Medicaid Agencies 173

U Codes 175
    Coronavirus Services 175

V Codes 176
    Vision Services 176
    Hearing Services 178

Appendixes
    Appendix 1 — Table of Drugs and Biologicals .... Appendixes — 1
    Appendix 2 — Modifiers .... Appendixes — 33
    Appendix 3 — Abbreviations and Acronyms .... Appendixes — 39
    Appendix 4 — Medicare Internet-only Manuals (IOMs) .... Appendixes — 41
    Appendix 5 — New, Revised, and Deleted Codes for 2023 .... Appendixes — 43
    Appendix 6 — Place of Service and Type of Service .... Appendixes — 53
    Appendix 7 — Deleted Code Crosswalk .... Appendixes — 57
    Appendix 8 — Glossary .... Appendixes — 59
    Appendix 9 — Quality Payment Program .... Appendixes — 63

Introduction

Note: All data current as of November 15, 2022.

About HCPCS Codes

HCPCS Level II codes, except for the dental code series, are developed and maintained by a joint editorial panel consisting of the Centers for Medicare and Medicaid Services (CMS), the Blue Cross Blue Shield Association, and the Health Insurance Association of America. HCPCS Level II codes may be used throughout the United States in all Medicare regions. They consist of one alpha character (A through V) followed by four digits. Optum does not change the code descriptions other than correcting typographical errors. There are some codes that appear to be duplicates. CMS has indicated that each of the codes is used to report a specific condition or service. At press time, CMS had not provided further clarification regarding these codes. Additional information may be found on the CMS website, https://www.cms.gov/Medicare/Coding/HCPCSReleaseCodeSets/index.html.

Any supplier or manufacturer can submit a request for coding modification to the HCPCS Level II National codes. A document explaining the HCPCS modification process, as well as a detailed format for submitting a recommendation for a modification to HCPCS Level II codes, is available on the HCPCS website at https://www.cms.gov/Medicare/Coding/MedHCPCSGenInfo/HCPCS_Coding_Questions. Besides the information requested in this format, a requestor should also submit any additional descriptive material, including the manufacturer's product literature and information that is believed would be helpful in furthering CMS's understanding of the medical features of the item for which a coding modification is being recommended. The HCPCS coding review process is an ongoing, continuous process.

The dental (D) codes are not included in the official 2023 HCPCS Level II code set. The American Dental Association (ADA) holds the copyright on those codes and instructed CMS to remove them. As a result, Optum has removed them from this product; however, Optum has additional resources available for customers requiring the dental codes. Please visit www.optumcoding.com or call 1.800.464.3649.

Note: The expanded Medically Unlikely Edit (MUE) tables containing HCPCS/CPT codes, MUE values, MUE adjudication indicators, and MUE rationale are no longer published in this book. The tables are updated quarterly and can be found on the CMS website at https://www.cms.gov/Medicare/Coding/NationalCorrectCodInitEd/MUE.

The table containing the Medicare national average payment (MAP) for services, supplies (DME, orthotics, prosthetics, etc.), drugs, biologicals, and nonphysician procedures using HCPCS Level II codes are available at www.optumcoding.com/2023MedAvgPay.

   Password: OptumMAP23

How to Use HCPCS Level II

Coders should keep in mind that the insurance companies and government do not base payment solely on what was done for the patient. They need to know why the services were performed. In addition to using the HCPCS coding system for procedures and supplies, coders must also use the ICD-10-CM coding system to denote the diagnosis. This book will not discuss ICD-10-CM codes, which can be found in a current ICD-10-CM code book for diagnosis codes. To locate a HCPCS Level II code, follow these steps:

1. Identify the services or procedures that the patient received.

   Example:

   Patient administered PSA exam.

2. Look up the appropriate term in the index.

   Example:

   Screening
      prostate specific antigen test (PSA)

   Coding Tip: Coders who are unable to find the procedure or service in the index can look in the table of contents for the type of procedure or device to narrow the code choices. Also, coders should remember to check the unlisted procedure guidelines for additional choices.

3. Assign a tentative code.

   Example:

   Code G0103

   Coding Tip: To the right of the terminology, there may be a single code or multiple codes, a cross-reference, or an indication that the code has been deleted. Tentatively assign all codes listed.

4. Locate the code or codes in the appropriate section. When multiple codes are listed in the index, be sure to read the narrative of all codes listed to find the appropriate code based on the service performed.

   Example:

   G0103   Prostate cancer screening; prostate specific antigen test (PSA)

5. Check for color bars, symbols, notes, and references.

   G0103   Prostate cancer screening; prostate specific antigen test (PSA)   ♂ A

6. Review the appendixes for the reference definitions and other guidelines for coverage issues that apply.

7. Determine whether any modifiers should be appended.

8. Assign the code.

   Example:

   The code assigned is G0103.

Coding Standards

Levels of Use

Coders may find that the same procedure is coded at two or even three levels. Which code is correct? There are certain rules to follow if this should occur.

When both a CPT and a HCPCS Level II code have virtually identical narratives for a procedure or service, the CPT code should be used. If, however, the narratives are not identical (e.g., the CPT code narrative is generic, whereas the HCPCS Level II code is specific), the Level II code should be used.

Be sure to check for a national code when a CPT code description contains an instruction to include additional information, such as describing a specific medication. For example, when billing Medicare or Medicaid for supplies, avoid using CPT code 99070 Supplies and materials (except spectacles), provided by the physician over and above those usually included with the office visit or other services rendered (list drugs, trays, supplies, or materials provided). There are many HCPCS Level II codes that specify supplies in more detail.

Special Reports

Submit a special report with the claim when a new, unusual, or variable procedure is provided or a modifier is used. Include the following information:

- A copy of the appropriate report (e.g., operative, x-ray), explaining the nature, extent, and need for the procedure
- Documentation of the medical necessity of the procedure
- Documentation of the time and effort necessary to perform the procedure

How To Use Optum HCPCS Level II Books

Organization of Optum HCPCS Level II Expert

The Optum 2023 *HCPCS Level II* contains mandated changes and new codes for use as of January 1, 2023. Deleted codes have also been indicated and cross-referenced to active codes when possible. New codes have been added to the appropriate sections, eliminating the time-consuming step of looking in two places for a code. However, keep in mind that the information in this book is a reproduction of the 2023 HCPCS; additional information on coverage issues may have been provided to Medicare contractors after publication. All contractors periodically update their systems and records throughout the year. If this book does not agree with your contractor, it is either because of a mid-year update or correction, or a specific local or regional coverage policy.

HCPCS Code Index

Because HCPCS is organized by code number rather than by service or supply name, the index enables the coder to locate any code without looking through individual ranges of codes. Just look up the medical or surgical supply, service, orthotic, or prosthetic in question to find the appropriate codes. This index also refers to many of the brand names by which these items are known.

Appendixes

Appendix 1: Table of Drugs and Biologicals
The brand names of drugs and biologicals listed are examples only and may not include all products available for that type. The table lists HCPCS codes from any available section including A codes, C codes, J codes, S codes, and Q codes under brand and generic names with amount, route of administration, and code numbers. While every effort is made to make the table comprehensive, it is not all-inclusive.

Appendix 2: Modifiers
This appendix identifies current modifiers. A modifier is a two-position alpha or numeric code that is appended to a CPT or HCPCS code to clarify the services being reported. Modifiers provide a means by which a service can be altered without changing the procedure code. They add more information, such as anatomical site, to the code. In addition, they help eliminate the appearance of duplicate billing and unbundling. Modifiers are used to increase the accuracy in reimbursement and coding consistency, ease editing, and capture payment data.

Appendix 3: Abbreviations and Acronyms
This appendix contains a list of abbreviations and acronyms found throughout the HCPCS code set that may be helpful. It is not an all-inclusive list.

Appendix 4: Medicare Internet-only Manuals (IOMs)
Previously, this appendix contained a verbatim printout of the Medicare Internet-only Manual references pertaining to specific codes. This appendix now contains a link to the IOMs on the Centers for Medicare and Medicaid Services website. The IOM references to applicable to specific codes can still be found at the code level.

Appendix 5: New, Revised, and Deleted Codes
This appendix is a complete list of all new, revised, and deleted HCPCS codes for the current year. New and revised codes are listed along with their current code descriptors. Deleted codes are provided as a list of codes.

Appendix 6: Place of Service and Type of Service
This appendix contains lists of place-of-service codes that should be used on professional claims and type-of-service codes used by the Medicare Common Working File.

Appendix 7: Crosswalk of Deleted Codes
This appendix is a cross-reference from a deleted code to an active code when one is available. The deleted code cross-reference will also appear under the deleted code description in the tabular section of the book.

Appendix 8: Glossary
This appendix contains general terms and definitions that could be helpful for coding and reimbursement.

Appendix 9: Quality Payment Program (QPP)
Previously, this appendix contained lists of the numerators and denominators applicable to the Medicare PQRS. However, with the implementations of the Quality Payment Program mandated by passage of the Medicare Access and Chip Reauthorization Act (MACRA) of 2015, the PQRS system will be obsolete. This appendix now contains information pertinent to that legislation as well as a brief overview of the proposed changes for the following year as available by date of this publication.

Color-coded Coverage Instructions

The Optum *HCPCS Level II* book provides colored symbols for each coverage and reimbursement instruction. A legend to these symbols is provided on the bottom of each two-page spread.

Green Color Bar—Special Coverage Instructions
A green bar for "special coverage instructions" over a code means that special coverage instructions apply to that code. These special instructions are also typically given in the form of Medicare Internet Only Manuals (IOM) reference numbers.

| A4336 | Incontinence supply, urethral insert, any type, each |

Yellow Color Bar—Carrier Discretion
Issues that are left to "carrier discretion" are covered with a yellow bar. Contact the carrier for specific coverage information on those codes.

| A9581 | Injection, gadoxetate disodium, 1 ml |

Pink Color Bar—Not Covered by or Invalid for Medicare
Codes that are not covered by or are invalid for Medicare are covered by a pink bar. The pertinent Medicare Internet-only Manuals (IOMs) reference numbers are also given explaining why a particular code is not covered. These numbers refer to the appendixes, where the Medicare references are listed.

| A4264 | Permanent implantable contraceptive intratubal occlusion device(s) and delivery system |

Code Icons

Codes in the Optum *HCPCS Level II* follow the AMA CPT book conventions to indicate new, revised, and deleted codes.

A black circle (●) precedes a new code.

| ● Q4262 | Dual Layer Impax Membrane, per sq cm |

A black triangle (▲) precedes a code with revised terminology or rules.

| ▲ J0131 | Injection, acetaminophen, not otherwise specified, 10 mg |

A circle (○) precedes a recycled/reinstated code.

| ○ Q4236 | carePATCH, per sq cm |

Codes deleted from the current active codes appear with a strike-out.

| C1849 | Skin substitute, synthetic, resorbable, per sq cm |

2023 HCPCS LEVEL II — INTRODUCTION

☑ Quantity Alert

Many codes in HCPCS report quantities that may not coincide with quantities available in the marketplace. For instance, a HCPCS code for an ostomy pouch with skin barrier reports each pouch, but the product is generally sold in a package of 10; "10" must be indicated in the quantity box on the CMS claim form to ensure proper reimbursement. This symbol indicates that care should be taken to verify quantities in this code. These quantity alerts do not represent Medicare Unlikely Edits (MUEs) and should not be used for MUEs.

| ☑ J0120 | Injection, tetracycline, up to 250 mg |

♀ Female Only

This icon identifies procedures that some payers may consider female only.

| A4261 | Cervical cap for contraceptive use ♀ |

♂ Male Only

This icon identifies procedures that some payers may consider male only.

| A4326 | Male external catheter with integral collection chamber, anytype, each ♂ |

🅐 Age Edit

This icon denotes codes intended for use with a specific age group, such as neonate, newborn, pediatric, and adult. Carefully review the code description to ensure that the code reported most appropriately reflects the patient's age.

| Q2037 | Influenza virus vaccine, split virus, when administered to individuals 3 years of age and older, for intramuscular use (FLUVIRIN) 🅐 |

🅜 Maternity

This icon identifies procedures that by definition should only be used for maternity patients generally between 12 and 55 years of age.

| H1001 | Prenatal care, at-risk enhanced service; antepartum management 🅜 |

🅐🅩 ASC Payment Indicators

Codes designated as being paid by ASC groupings that were effective at the time of printing are denoted by the group number.

| G0105 | Colorectal cancer screening; colonoscopy on individual at high risk 🅐2 |

♿ DMEPOS

Use this icon to identify when to consult the CMS durable medical equipment, prosthetics, orthotics, and supplies (DMEPOS) for payment of this durable medical item. For modifiers NU, RR, and UE: These modifiers are for use when DME equipment is either new, used, or rented. The RR modifiers must also be used in conjunction with rental modifiers KH, KI, or KJ.

| E0988 | Manual wheelchair accessory, lever-activated, wheel drive, pair ♿ |

🚫 Skilled Nursing Facility (SNF)

Use this icon to identify certain items and services excluded from SNF consolidated billing. These items may be billed directly to the Medicare contractor by the provider or supplier of the service or item.

| A4653 | Peritoneal dialysis catheter anchoring device, belt, each 🚫 |

Drugs commonly reported with a code are listed underneath by brand or generic name.

| C9254 | Injection, lacosamide, 1 mg
Use this code for VIMPAT. |

CMS does not use consistent terminology when a code for a specific procedure is not listed. The code description may include any of the following terms: unlisted, not otherwise classified (NOC), unspecified, unclassified, other, and miscellaneous. If unsure there is no code for the service or supply provided or used, provide adequate documentation to the payer. Check with the payer for more information.

| A0999 | Unlisted ambulance service |

CMS: This notation appears when instruction pertaining to a code appears in a CMS Internet-only Manual (IOM). Previously, appendix 4 contained a verbatim printout of the Medicare Internet-only Manual references pertaining to specific codes. This appendix now contains a link to the IOMs on the Centers for Medicare and Medicaid Services website. The IOM references applicable to specific codes can still be found at the code level.

| A4618 | Breathing circuits
CMS: 100-04, 20, 100.2 |

AHA: American Hospital Association *Coding Clinic® for HCPCS* citations help in finding expanded information about specific codes and their usage. This includes citations for the current year and the preceding five years.

| A2001 | InnovaMatrix AC, per sq cm
AHA: 1Q,22 |

A-Y OPPS Status Indicators

Status indicators identify how individual HCPCS Level II codes are paid or not paid under the OPPS. The same status indicator is assigned to all the codes within an ambulatory payment classification (APC). Consult the payer or resource to learn which HCPCS codes fall within various APCs. **The OPSI contained in this publication were effective as of October 1, 2022. Once released by CMS, the table with data effective January 1, 2023, will be available on our product update page at www.optumcoding.com/ProductUpdates/.**

A	Services furnished to a hospital outpatient that are paid under a fee schedule or payment system other than OPPS, for example: • Ambulance Services • Clinical Diagnostic Laboratory Services • Non-Implantable Prosthetic and Orthotic Devices • Physical, Occupational, and Speech Therapy • Diagnostic Mammography • Screening Mammography
B	Codes that are not recognized by OPPS when submitted on an outpatient hospital Part B bill type (12x and 13x)
C	Inpatient Procedures
E1	Items, Codes, and Services: • Not covered by any Medicare outpatient benefit category • Statutorily excluded by Medicare • Not reasonable and necessary
F	Corneal Tissue Acquisition; Certain CRNA Services and Hepatitis B Vaccines
G	Pass-Through Drugs and Biologicals
H	Pass-Through Device Categories
J1	Hospital Part B services paid through a comprehensive APC
K	Nonpass-Through Drugs and Nonimplantable Biologicals, Including Therapeutic Radiopharmaceuticals
L	Influenza Vaccine; Pneumococcal Pneumonia Vaccine
M	Items and Services Not Billable to the MAC
N	Items and Services Packaged into APC Rates
P	Partial Hospitalization
Q1	STVX-Packaged Codes
Q2	T-Packaged Codes
Q3	Codes That May Be Paid Through a Composite APC
Q4	Conditionally Packaged Laboratory Tests
R	Blood and Blood Products
S	Significant Procedure, Not Discounted when Multiple
T	Significant Procedure, Multiple Procedure Reduction Applies
U	Brachytherapy Sources
V	Clinic or Emergency Department Visit
Y	Nonimplantable Durable Medical Equipment

A	L8440	Prosthetic shrinker, below knee, each
B	Q4005	Cast supplies, long arm cast, adult (11 years +), plaster
C	G0341	Percutaneous islet cell transplant, includes portal vein catheterization and infusion
E1	A0021	Ambulance service, outside state per mile, transport (Medicaid only)
F	V2785	Processing, preserving and transporting corneal tissue
G	C9460	Injection, cangrelor, 1 mg
H	C2613	Lung biopsy plug with delivery system
K	J1750	Injection, iron dextran, 50 mg
L	Q2036	Influenza virus vaccine, split virus, when administered to individuals 3 years of age and older, for intramuscular use (FLULAVAL)
M	G0333	Pharmacy dispensing fee for inhalation drug(s); initial 30-day supply as a beneficiary
N	A4220	Refill kit for implantable infusion pump
P	G0129	Occupational therapy services requiring the skills of a qualified occupational therapist, furnished as a component of a partial hospitalization treatment program, per session (45 minutes or more)
Q3	C8935	Magnetic resonance angiography without contrast, upper extremity
R	P9010	Blood (whole), for transfusion, per unit
S	G0117	Glaucoma screening for high risk patients furnished by an optometrist or ophthalmologist
T	C9727	Insertion of implants into the soft palate; minimum of 3 implants
U	A9527	Iodine I-125, sodium iodide solution, therapeutic, per millicurie
V	G0101	Cervical or vaginal cancer screening; pelvic and clinical breast examination
Y	A5500	For diabetics only, fitting (including follow-up), custom preparation and supply of off-the-shelf depth-inlay shoe manufactured to accommodate multidensity insert(s), per shoe

A2–Z3 ASC Payment Indicators

This icon identifies the ASC status payment indicators. They indicate how the ASC payment rate was derived and/or how the procedure, item, or service is treated under the ASC payment system. For more information about these indicators and how they affect billing, consult Optum's *Revenue Cycle Pro*. **The ASC payment indicators contained in this publication were effective as of October 1, 2022. Once released by CMS, the table with data effective January 1, 2023, will be available on our product update page at www.optumcoding.com/ProductUpdates/.**

Indicator	Description
A2	Surgical procedure on ASC list in CY 2007 or later; payment based on OPPS relative payment weight
C5	Inpatient procedure
F4	Corneal tissue acquisition, hepatitis B vaccine; paid at reasonable cost
G2	Non-office-based surgical procedure added in CY 2008 or later; payment based on OPPS relative payment weight
H2	Brachytherapy source paid separately when provided integral to a surgical procedure on ASC list; payment based on OPPS rate
J7	OPPS pass-through device paid separately when provided integral to a surgical procedure on ASC list; payment based on OPPS rate
J8	Device-intensive procedure paid at adjusted rate
K2	Drugs and biologicals paid separately when provided integral to a surgical procedure on ASC list; payment based on OPPS rate
K7	Unclassified drugs and biologicals; payment contractor-priced
L1	Influenza vaccine; pneumococcal vaccine; packaged item/service; no separate payment made
L6	New Technology Intraocular Lens (NTIOL); special payment
N1	Packaged service/item; no separate payment made
P2	Office-based surgical procedure added to ASC list in CY 2008 or later with MPFS nonfacility PE RVUs; payment based on OPPS relative payment weight
P3	Office-based surgical procedure added to ASC list in CY 2008 or later with MPFS nonfacility PE RVUs; payment based on MPFS nonfacility PE RVUs
R2	Office-based surgical procedure added to ASC list in CY 2008 or later without MPFS nonfacility PE RVUs; payment based on OPPS relative payment weight
Z2	Radiology service paid separately when provided integral to a surgical procedure on ASC list; payment based on OPPS relative payment weight
Z3	Radiology service paid separately when provided integral to a surgical procedure on ASC list; payment based on MPFS nonfacility PE RVUs

Indicator	Code	Description
F4	V2785	Processing, preserving and transporting corneal tissue
H2	A9527	Iodine I-125, sodium iodide solution, therapeutic per millicurie
J7	C1052	Hemostatic agent, gastrointestinal, topical
K2	C9132	Prothrombin complex concentrate (human), Kcentra, per IU of Factor IX activity
K7	C9399	Unclassified drugs or biologicals
L1	Q2037	Influenza virus vaccine, split virus, when administered to individuals 3 years of age and older, for intramuscular use (FLUVIRIN)
N1	C9353	Microporous collagen implantable slit tube (NeuraWrap Nerve Protector), per cm length
Z3	G0130	Single energy x-ray absorptiometry (SEXA) bone density study, one or more sites; appendicular skeleton (peripheral) (e.g., radius, wrist, heel)
Z2	C8911	Magnetic resonance angiography without contrast followed by with contrast, chest (excluding myocardium)

A

Abdomen/abdominal
 dressing holder/binder, A4461, A4463
 pad, low profile, L1270
Abduction
 control, each, L2624
 pillow, E1399
 rotation bar, foot, L3140-L3170
Ablation
 robotic, waterjet, C2596
 transbronchial, C9751
 ultrasound, C9734
Abortion, S0199, S2260-S2267
Absorption dressing, A6251-A6256
Access system, A4301
Accessories
 ambulation devices, E0153-E0159
 artificial kidney and machine (*see also* ES-RD), E1510-E1699
 beds, E0271-E0280
 Medicare IVIG demonstration, Q2052
 oxygen, E1352, E1354-E1358
 retinal prosthesis, L8608
 total artificial heart, L8698
 ventricular assist device, Q0477, Q0501-Q0509
 wheelchairs, E0950-E1012, E1050-E1298, E2201-E2231, E2295, E2300-E2367, K0001-K0108
AccuChek
 blood glucose meter, E0607
 test strips, box of 50, A4253
Accurate
 prosthetic sock, L8420-L8435
 stump sock, L8470-L8485
Acetate concentrate for hemodialysis, A4708
Acid concentrate for hemodialysis, A4709
ACO Model, G9868-G9870
Action Patriot manual wheelchair, K0004
Action Xtra, Action MVP, Action Pro-T, manual wheelchair, K0005
Active Life
 convex one-piece urostomy pouch, A4421
 flush away, A5051
 one-piece
  drainable custom pouch, A5061
  pre-cut closed-end pouch, A5051
  stoma cap, A5055
Activity therapy, G0176
Adaptor
 electric/pneumatic ventricular assist device, Q0478
 neurostimulator, C1883
 pacing lead, C1883
Addition
 cushion AK, L5648
 cushion BK, L5646
 harness upper extremity, L6675-L6676
 to halo procedure, L0861
 to lower extremity orthotic, K0672, L2750-L2760, L2780-L2861
 to lower extremity prosthesis, L5970-L5990
 to upper extremity orthotic, L3891
 wrist, flexion, extension, L6620
Adhesive
 barrier, C1765
 catheter, A4364
 disc or foam pad, A5126
 medical, A4364
 Nu-Hope
  1 oz bottle with applicator, A4364
  3 oz bottle with applicator, A4364
 ostomy, A4364
 pads, A6203-A6205, A6212-A6214, A6219-A6221, A6237-A6239, A6245-A6247, A6254-A6256
 remover, A4455, A4456
 support, breast prosthesis, A4280
 tape, A4450, A4452
 tissue, G0168
Adjunctive blue light cystoscopy, C7554, C9738
 with biopsy(ies), C7550
Adjustabrace 3, L2999
Adjustment
 bariatric band, S2083

Administration
 aerosolized drug therapy, home, S9061
 chemotherapy infusion
  continued in community, G0498
 COVID-19 vaccine, in home administration, M0201
 hepatitis B vaccine, G0010
 influenza virus vaccine, G0008
 medication, T1502-T1503
  direct observation, H0033
 monoclonal anitbody therapy, M0220, M0221, M0222, M0223, M0240, M0241, M0243, M0244, M0245, M0246, M0247, M0248, M0249, M0250
 pneumococcal vaccine, G0009
Adoptive immunotherapy, S2107
Adrenal transplant, S2103
AdvantaJet, A4210
Affinity, Q4159
AFO, E1815, E1830, L1900-L1990, L4392, L4396
Aimsco Ultra Thin syringe, 1 cc or 1/2 cc, each, A4206
Air bubble detector, dialysis, E1530
Air fluidized bed, E0194
Air pressure pad/mattress, E0186, E0197
Air travel and nonemergency transportation, A0140
Aircast air stirrup ankle brace, L1906
Airlife Brand Misty-Neb nebulizer, E0580
AirSep, E0601
Airway device, E0485-E0486
Alarm
 device, A9280
 enuresis, S8270
 pressure, dialysis, E1540
Albumarc, P9041
Albumin, human, P9041, P9045-P9047
Alcohol
 abuse service, H0047
 assessment, G0396-G0397, G2011, H0001
 pint, A4244
 testing, H0048
 wipes, A4245
Alert device, A9280
Algiderm, alginate dressing, A6196-A6199
Alginate dressing, A6196-A6199
Algosteril, alginate dressing, A6196-A6199
Alkaline battery for blood glucose monitor, A4233-A4236
Allergen particle barrier/inhalation filter
 nasal, topical, K1026
AlloDerm, Q4116
AlloGen, Q4212
Allogenic cord blood harvest, S2140
Allograft
 small intestine and liver, S2053
AlloPatch HD, Q4128
AlloSkin, Q4115
AlloSkin AC, Q4141
AlloSkin RT, Q4123
AlloWrap DS, Q4150
Alternating pressure mattress/pad, E0181, E0277
 pump, E0182
Alternative communication device, i.e., communication board, E1902
AltiPly, Q4235
Ambulance, A0021-A0999
 air, A0436
 disposable supplies, A0382-A0398
 non-emergency, S9960-S9961
 oxygen, A0422
 response, treatment, no transport, A0998
Ambulation device, E0100-E0159
Ambulation stimulator
 spinal cord injured, E0762
Aminaid, enteral nutrition, B4154
Amirosyn-RF, parenteral nutrition, B5000
Ammonia test paper, A4774
Amnio Bio, Q4211
AmnioAmp-MP, Q4250
AmnioArmor, Q4168
AmnioBand, Q4151, Q4168
AmnioBind, Q4225
AmnioCore, Q4227

AmnioCyte Plus, Q4242
AmnioExcel, AmnioExcel Plus, Q4137
AmnioMatrix, Q4139
Amnio-Maxx, Q4239
Amnio-Maxx Lite, Q4239
AmnioPro, Q4163
AmnioPro Flow, Q4162
AMNIOREPAIR, Q4235
AmnioText, Q4245
Amniotext patch, Q4247
AmnioWound, Q4181
AmnioWrap2, Q4221
AMNIPLY, Q4249
Amputee
 adapter, wheelchair, E0959
 prosthesis, L5000-L7510, L7520, L8400-L8465
 stump sock, L8470
 wheelchair, E1170-E1190, E1200
Analysis
 dose optimization, S3722
 gene sequence
  hypertrophic cardiomyopathy, S3865, S3866
 semen, G0027
Anchor, screw, C1713
Anesthesia
 dialysis, A4736-A4737
 monitored (MAC), G9654
Angiography
 catheter placement, C7516-C7529, C7552-C7553
 dialysis circuit, C7513-C7515, C7530
 fluorescent
  nonocular, C9733
  iliac artery, G0278
 magnetic resonance, C8901-C8914, C8918-C8920
 reconstruction, G0288
Angioplasty
 coronary, C7532
  placement radiation delivery device, C7533
 dialysis circuit, C7532
 intracranial, C7532
 pulmonary, C7532
Ankle foot system, L5973
Ankle orthosis, L1902, L1904, L1907
Ankle–foot orthotic (AFO), L1900, L1906, L1910-L1940, L2106-L2116
 Dorsiwedge Night Splint, A4570, L2999, L4398
 Specialist
  Ankle Foot Orthotic, L1930
  Tibial Pre-formed Fracture Brace, L2116
 Surround Ankle Stirrup Braces with Foam, L1906
Annual wellness visit, G0438-G0439
Antenna
 replacement
  diaphragmatic/phrenic nerve stimulator, L8696
Anterior-posterior orthotic
 lateral orthotic, L0700, L0710
Antibiotic home infusion therapy, S9494-S9504
Antibiotic regimen, G9286-G9287
Antibody testing, HIV-1, S3645
Anticoagulation clinic, S9401
Antifungal home infusion therapy, S9494-S9504
Antiseptic
 chlorhexidine, A4248
Antisperm antibodies, S3655
Antiviral home infusion therapy, S9494-S9504
Apheresis
 low density lipid, S2120
Apis, A2010
Apligraf, Q4101
Apnea monitor, E0618-E0619
 electrodes, A4556
 lead wires, A4557
 with recording feature, E0619
Appliance
 cleaner, A5131

Appliance — *continued*
 oral
  airway collapse reduction, K1027
  pneumatic, E0655-E0673
Application
 skin substitute, C5271-C5278
 tantalum rings, S8030
Appropriate Use Criteria
 Clinic Decision Support Mechanism, G1001-G1023
AquaPedic sectional gel flotation, E0196
Aqueous
 shunt, L8612
Arch support, L3040-L3100
Architect, Architect PX, or Architect FX, Q4147
Arm
 sling
  deluxe, A4565
  mesh cradle, A4565
  universal
   arm, A4565
   elevator, A4565
 wheelchair, E0973
Arrow, power wheelchair, K0014
Artacent AC (fluid), Q4189
Artacent AC, Q4190
Artacent Cord, Q4216
Artacent Wound, Q4169
Arthodesis
 interphalangeal joint(s), C7506
Arthroereisis
 subtalar, S2117
ArthroFlex, Q4125
Arthroscopy
 knee
  harvest of cartilage, S2112
  removal loose body, FB, G0289
 shoulder
  with capsulorrhaphy, S2300
  with subacromial spacer, C9781
Artificial
 kidney machines and accessories (*see also* Dialysis), E1510-E1699
 larynx, L8500
 saliva, A9155
Ascent, Q4213
Assertive community treatment, H0039-H0040
Assessment
 alcohol and/or substance, G0396-G0397, G2011, H0001
 audiologic, V5008-V5020
 chaplain services, Q9001-Q9003
 chronic care management services
  comprehensive, G0506
 family, H1011
 functional outcome, G9227
 geriatric, S0250
 mental health, H0031
  remote diagnosis, evaluation, treatment, C7900-C7902
  remote, recorded video/images, G2250
 speech, V5362-V5364
 wellness, S5190
Assisted living, T2030-T2031
Assistive listening device, V5268-V5274
 alerting device, V5269
 cochlear implant assistive device, V5273
 FM/DM, V5281
  accessories, V5283-V5290
  system, V5281-V5282
 supplies and accessories, V5267
 TDD, V5272
 telephone amplifier, V5268
 television caption decoder, V5271
Asthma
 education, S9441
 kit, S8097
Attendant care, S5125-S5126
Attends, adult diapers, A4335
Audiologic assessment, V5008-V5020
Audiometry, S0618
Auditory osseointegrated device, L8690, L8691, L8692-L8693
Augmentation
 intervertebral body fracture, C1062
 vertebral, C7507-C7508

Autoclix lancet device, A4258
Auto-Glide folding walker, E0143
Autograft suspension, C1832
Autolance lancet device, A4258
Autolet lancet device, A4258
Autolet Lite lancet device, A4258
Autolet Mark II lancet device, A4258
AxoBioMembrane, Q4211
Axolotl Ambient, Axolotl Cryo, Q4215
Axolotl Graft, Axolotl DualGraft, Q4210

B

Babysitter, child of parents in treatment, T1009
Back school, S9117
Back supports, L0450-L0710
Bacterial sensitivity study, P7001
Bag
 drainage, A4357
 irrigation supply, A4398
 resuscitation bag, S8999
 spacer, for metered dose inhaler, A4627
 urinary, A4358, A5112
Balken, fracture frame, E0946
Ballistocardiogram, S3902
Bandage
 adhesive, A6413
 compression
  high, A6452
  light, A6448-A6450
  medium, A6451
  padding, S8430
  roll, S8431
 conforming, A6442-A6447
 Orthoflex elastic plastic bandages, A4580
 padding, A6441
 self-adherent, A6413, A6453-A6455
 specialist plaster bandages, A4580
 zinc paste impregnated, A6456
Bariatric
 bed, E0302-E0304
 brief/diaper, T4543
 surgery, S2083
Barium enema, G0106
 cancer screening, G0120
Barrier
 4 x 4, A4372
 adhesion, C1765
 with flange, A4373
Baseball finger splint, A4570
Bath chair, E0240
Bathtub
 chair, E0240
 heat unit, E0249
 stool or bench, E0245
 transfer bench, E0247, E0248
 transfer rail, E0246
 wall rail, E0241, E0242
Battery, L7360, L7364
 blood glucose monitor, A4233-A4236
 charger, L7362, L7366, L7368, L8695, L8699, Q0495
 cochlear implant device
  alkaline, L8622
  lithium, L8623-L8624
  zinc, L8621
 hearing device, V5266
 infusion pump, external, A4602, K0601-K0605
 lithium, A4601-A4602, L7367, Q0506
  charger, L7368
 replacement
  charger, L7368
  ear pulse generator, A4638
  external defibrillator, K0607
  external infusion pump, A4602, K0601-K0605
 six volt battery, L7360
 TENS, A4630
 twelve volt battery, L7364
 ventilator, A4611-A4613
 ventricular assist device, Q0496, Q0503
 wheelchair, E2358-E2359, E2397, K0733
Bayer chemical reagent strips, box of 100 glucose/ketone urine test strips, A4250
BCPI home visit, G9187

BCW 600, manual wheelchair, K0007
BCW Power, power wheelchair, K0014
BCW recliner, manual wheelchair, K0007
B-D alcohol swabs, box, A4245
B-D disposable insulin syringes, up to 1 cc, per syringe, A4206
B-D lancets, per box of 100, A4258
Bebax, foot orthotic, L3160
Bed
 accessory, E0315
 air fluidized, E0194
 cradle, any type, E0280
 drainage bag, bottle, A4357, A5102
 extra size for bariatric patients, E0302-E0304
 hospital, E0250-E0270
  full electric, home care, without mattress, E0297
  manual, without mattress, E0293
  pediatric, E0328-E0329
  safety enclosure frame/canopy, E0316
  semi-electric, without mattress, E0295
 pan, E0275, E0276
  Moore, E0275
 rail, E0305, E0310
 safety enclosure frame/canopy, hospital bed, E0316
Behavioral health, H0002-H0030
 day treatment, H2013
 Medicaid certified health clinic services, T1040-T1041
 per hour, H2012
 prescription digital therapy, A9291
 residential treatment program, T2048
BellaCell HD, Q4220
Bell-Horn
 prosthetic shrinker, L8440-L8465
Belt
 adapter, A4421
 exsufflation, K1021
 extremity, E0945
 Little Ones Sur-Fit pediatric, A4367
 ostomy, A4367
 pelvic, E0944
 ventricular assist device, Q0499
 wheelchair, E0978, K0098
Bench, bathtub — see also Bathtub, E0245
Benesch boot, L3212-L3214
Berkeley shell, foot orthotic, L3000
Beta-blocker therapy, G9188-G9192
Betadine, A4246
 swabs/wipes, A4247
Bicarbonate concentration for hemodialysis, A4706-A4707
Bifocal, glass or plastic, V2200-V2299
Bile duct(s)
 exchange drainage catheter
  percutaneous, C7545
 extrahepatic
  intraoperative near-infrared fluorescence imaging, C9776
Bilirubin (phototherapy) light, E0202
Binder
 extremity, nonelastic, A4465
Bio Flote alternating air pressure pump, pad system, E0181, E0182
bio-ConneKt Wound Matrix, Q4161
BioDExcel, Q4137
BioDFence, Q4140
BioDFence DryFlex, Q4138
BioDMatrix, Q4139
Biofeedback device, E0746
BioNextPATCH, Q4228
Biopsy
 bladder
  with cystourethroscopy and adjunctive blue light cystoscopy, C7550
 bone marrow
  biopsy needle, C1830
 lung
  bronchoscopy, C7511-C7512
  non small cell, G9282-G9285, G9288-G9290

Biopsy — continued
 lung — continued
  plug, C2613
  non-lung, G9285, G9291
  open
   cervical node(s), C7503
  other, G9292-G9295
  percutaneous
   bone
    vertebra, C7504-C7505
   breast, C7501-C7502
BioSkin, Q4163
BioSkin Flow, Q4162
BIOVANCE, Q4154
BioWound, BioWound Plus, BioWound Xplus, Q4217
Birth control pills, S4993
Birthing classes, S9436-S9439, S9442
Bite disposable jaw locks, E0700
Blinded procedure
 interatrial shunt/placebo control, C9758
Blood
 Congo red, P2029
 cryoprecipitate, P9012
 glucose monitor
  adjunctive/nonimplanted, E2102
  continuous
   invasive/nondurable
    receiver, A9278
    sensor, A9276
    transmitter, A9277
   nonadjunctive
    nonimplanted, A4239, E2103
   noninvasive, E0607, S1030-S1031
  lancet, A4258
  supply allowance, 1 month, A4238
  test strips, A4253, A4772
 disposable, A9275
 with integrated lancing system, E2101
 with voice synthesizer, E2100
 glucose test strips, A4253
 granulocytes, pheresis, P9050
 ketone test strips, A4252
 leak detector, dialysis, E1560
 leukocyte reduced, P9016, P9040, P9050, P9054, P9056-P9058
 mucoprotein, P2038
 not otherwise specified, P9099
 pressure equipment, A4660, A4663, A4670
 pump, dialysis, E1620
 red blood cells, P9016, P9021-P9022, P9038, P9040, P9057-P9058
 split unit, P9011
 strips
  blood glucose test or reagent strips, A4253
  blood ketone test or reagent strip, A4252
 testing supplies, A4770
 transfusion, home, S9538
 tubing, A4750, A4755
 whole, P9010, P9051, P9056
Bock Dynamic, foot prosthesis, L5972
Body jacket
 scoliosis, L1300, L1310
Body sock, L0984
Body wrap
 foam positioners, E0191
 therapeutic overlay, E0199
Bond or cement, ostomy, skin, A4364
Bone
 debridement with insertion drug delivery device, C7500
Boot
 pelvic, E0944
 surgical, ambulatory, L3260
 walking
  nonpneumatic, L4386-L4387
  pneumatic, L4360-L4361
Boston type spinal orthotic, L1200

Brachytherapy
 cesium 131, C2642-C2643
 cesium-131 chloride solution, C2644
 gold 198, C1716
 iodine 125, A9527
 iridium 192
  high dose, C1717
  nonhigh dose, C1719
 low dose rate (LDR), prostate, G0458
 needle, C1715
 nonhigh dose rate iridium 192, C1719
 nonstranded
  cesium-131, C2643
  gold-198, C1716
  iodine-125, C2634, C2639
  iridium-192, C1717, C1719
  NOS, C2699
  palladium-103, C2635-C2636, C2641
  ytterbium-169, C2637
  yttrium-90, C2616
 palladium-103, C2640
 placement of endorectal intracavitary applicator, C9725
 radioelements, Q3001
 stranded
  cesium-131, C2642
  iodine-125, C2638
  NOS, C2698
  palladium-103, C2640
Brake attachment, wheeled walker, E0159
Breast
 biopsies
  magnetic resonance guidance, C7502
  stereotactic guidance, C7501
 exam (with pelvic exam), G0101
 exam (without pelvic exam), S0613
 milk collection, K1005
 milk processing, T2101
 placement/removal applicator, C9726
 prosthesis, L8000-L8035, L8031, L8600
  adhesive skin support, A4280
  nipple, L2006
 pump, E0602-E0604
  supplies, A4281-A4286
 reconstruction, S2066-S2068
Breathing circuit, A4618
Brief
 adult, T4521-T4524
 bariatric, T4543
 pediatric, T4529-T4530
Brief communication
 technology based service, G2251-G2252
Broncho-Cath endobronchial tubes, with CPAP system, E0601
Bronchoscopy
 ablation, lesion, C9751
 biopsy(ies), C7511-C7512
 diagnostic, C7509
 lavage, C7510
Buck's, traction
 frame, E0870
 stand, E0880
Bulb for therapeutic light box, A4634
Bulking agent
 anal, L8605
 vocal cord, L8607
Burn
 garment, A6501, A6512-A6513
 matrix, Q4103
Bus, nonemergency, A0110

C

Cage
 anterior/lateral, personalized, C1831
Calibrator solution, A4256
Camisole, post mastectomy, S8460
Camping therapy, T2036-T2037
Cancer screening
 barium enema, G0106, G0120, G0122
 breast exam, G0101
 cervical
  exam, G0101
  HPV infectious agent detection by DNA/RNA, G0476

Cancer screening — continued
  colorectal, G0104-G0106, G0120-G0122, G0327-G0328
  prostate, G0102-G0103
Cane, E0100, E0105
  accessory, A4636, A4637
  Easy-Care quad, E0105
  quad canes, E0105
  Quadri-Poise, E0105
  wooden, E0100
Canister
  disposable, used with suction pump, A7000
  non-disposable, used with suction pump, A7001
Cannula
  fistula, set (for dialysis), A4730
  nasal, A4615
  tracheostomy, A4623
Carbon filter, A4680
Cardiac
  monitor
    implantable, C1833
    tranesophageal doppler, G9157
Cardiac contractility modulation generator, C1824
  external recharging system, K1030
Cardiac event, recorder implantable, C1764, E0616
Cardiac rehabilitation, G0422-G0423
  program, S9472
Cardiointegram, S9025
Cardiokymography, Q0035
Cardiovascular services, M0300-M0301
Cardioverter-defibrillator, C1721, C1722, C1882
Care
  attendant, S5125-S5126
  companion, S5135-S5136
  coordination
    cancer treatment, S0353-S0354
  day care, S5100-S5105
  foster, S5140-S5141, S5145-S5146
  home infusion catheter, S5497-S5502
  personal care item, S5199
  planning
    chronic care management services, G0506
  respite, S5150-S5151
Care management
  behavioral health conditions, G0323
  CMMI Model, G0076-G0087
Carelet safety lancet, A4258
carePATCH, Q4236
Carex
  adjustable bath/shower stool, E0245
  aluminum crutches, E0114
  cane, E0100
  folding walker, E0135
  shower bench, E0245
Cartridge
  digestive enzyme(s), B4105
Case management, G9012, T1016-T1017
  per month, T2022
  targeted, T2023
Casec, enteral nutrition, B4155
Cast
  body cast, Q4001-Q4002
  gauntlet, Q4013-Q4016
  hand restoration, L6900-L6915
  hip spica, Q4025-Q4028
  long arm, Q4005-Q4008
  long leg, Q4029-Q4036
  materials, special, A4590
  plaster, A4580
  short arm, Q4009-Q4012
  short leg, Q4037-Q4040
  shoulder, Q4003-Q4004
  supplies, A4580, A4590, Q4050
    body cast, Q4001-Q4002
    Delta-Cast Elite Casting Material, A4590
    Delta-Lite Conformable Casting Tape, A4590
    Delta-Lite C-Splint Fibreglass Immobilizer, A4590
    Delta-Lite "S" Fibreglass Casting Tape, A4590

Cast — continued
  supplies — continued
    Flashcast Elite Casting Material, A4590
    Orthoflex Elastic Plaster Bandages, A4580
    Orthoplast Splints (and Orthoplast II Splints), A4590
    Specialist Plaster Bandages, A4580
    Specialist Plaster Roll Immobilizer, A4580
    Specialist Plaster Splints, A4580
  thermoplastic, L2106, L2126
Caster, wheelchair, E2214, E2219, E2395-E2396
Catheter, A4300-A4364
  anchoring device, A4333, A4334
    percutaneous, A5200
  balloon, C1727
  brachytherapy, C1728
  cap, disposable (dialysis), A4860
  diagnostic, C1730, C1731
    ablation, C1732, C1733
  drainage, C1729
  electrophysiology, C2630
  exchange
    biliary drainage, C7545
  external collection device, A4326-A4330
  extravascular tissue ablation, C1886
  guiding, C1887
  hemodialysis, C1750, C1752
  implantable access, A4301
  implantable intraspinal, E0785
  indwelling, A4338-A4346
  infusion, C1752
  insertion
    centrally inserted infusion, C1751
      inside-out technique, C9780
    midline, infusion, C1751
    midline venous, home health, S5523
    peripherally inserted infusion, C1751
    tray, A4354
  intermittent, with insertion supplies, A4353
  intracardiac echocardiography, C1759
  intradiscal, C1754
  intraspinal, C1755
  intravascular ultrasound, C1753
  irrigation supplies, A4355
  lubricant, A4332
  male, A4326, A4349
  nephrostomy
    convert to nephroureteral, C7547
  nephroureteral
    convert from nephrostomy catheter, C7547
    removal and replacement, C7546
  noncardiac ablation, C1888
  nonvascular balloon dilatation, C1726
  occlusion, C2628
    intermittent, C1982
  oropharyngeal suction, A4628
  pacing, transesophageal, C1756
  placement
    coronary artery(ies), C7516-C7529, C7552-C7553
  pressure generating, C1982
  rectal
    for manual enema system, A4453
  specimen collection, P9612, P9615
  suprapubic, cystoscopic, C2627
  thrombectomy, embolectomy, C1757
  tracheal suction, A4605, A4624
  translumial
    angioplasty
      laser, C1885
      nonlaser, C1725, C2623
    atherectomy
      directional, C1714
      rotational, C1724
    intravascular lithotripsy
      coronary, C1761
  ureteral, C1758
CBC, G0306-G0307
Celera Dual Layer, Dual Membrane, Q4259
Cellesta, Cellesta Duo, Q4184
Cellesta Cord, Q4214
Cellesta Flowable Amnion, Q4185

Cellular therapy, M0075
Cement, ostomy, A4364
Centrifuge, for dialysis, E1500
Cephalin flocculation, blood, P2028
Certified nurse assistant, S9122
Cerumen removal, G0268
Cervical
  collar, L0120, L0130, L0140, L0150, L0170
  halo, L0810-L0830
  head harness/halter, E0942
  helmet, A8000-A8004
  node(s)
    biopsy or excision, C7503
  orthotic, L0180-L0200
  traction equipment, not requiring frame, E0855
Cervical cap contraceptive, A4261
Cervical-thoracic-lumbar-sacral orthotic (CTLSO), L0700, L0710, L1000, L1001
Cesium-131, C2642-C2643
Chair
  adjustable, dialysis, E1570
  bathtub, E0240
  commode, E0163-E0165
  lift, E0627, E0629
  rollabout, E1031
  shower or bath, E0240
  sitz bath, E0160-E0162
Challenger manual wheelchair, K0009
Champion 1000 manual wheelchair, K0004
Champion 30000, manual wheelchair, K0005
Change
  ureteral stent, C7549
  ureterostomy tube, C7549
Chaplain services, Q9001-Q9003
CheckMate Plus blood glucose monitor, E0607
Chelation therapy, M0300
  home infusion, administration, S9355
Chemical endarterectomy, M0300
Chemistry and toxicology tests, P2028-P3001
Chemodenervation
  vocal cord, S2340-S2341
Chemotherapy
  administration
    both infusion and other technique, Q0085
    home infusion, continuous, S9325-S9379, S9494-S9497
    infusion, Q0084
      continued in community, G0498
    other than infusion, Q0083
Chemstrip bG, box of 50 blood glucose test strips, A4253
Chemstrip K, box of 100 ketone urine test strips, A4250
Chemstrip UGK, box of 100 glucose/ketone urine test strips, A4250
Chest shell (cuirass), E0457
Chest wall oscillation system, E0483
Chest wrap, E0459
Childbirth, S9442
  cesarean birth, S9438
  class, S9442
  early induction, G9355-G9356
  elective delivery, G9355-G9356
  Lamaze, S9436
  postpartum education, G9357-G9358
  postpartum evaluation, G9357-G9358
  postpartum screening, G9357-G9358
  preparation, S9436
  refresher, S9437
  VBAC (vaginal birth after cesarean), S9439
Childcare, T2026-T2027
  parents in treatment, T1009
Chin
  cup, cervical, L0150
  strap (for CPAP device), A7036
Chlorhexidine, A4248
Chondrocyte cell harvest, arthroscopic, S2112
Chopart prosthetic
  ankle, L5050, L5060
  below knee, L5100
Chore services, S5130-S5131
Christian Science provider services, S9900
Chromic phosphate, A9564

Chronic pain management, G3002-G3003
Chux, A4554
Circuit
  dialysis, C7513-C7515, C7530
Clamp
  external urethral, A4356
Clarix 100, Q4156
Clarix Cord, Q4148
Clarix Flo,, Q4155
Classes, S9441-S9446
  asthma, S9441
  birthing, S9442
  exercise, S9451
  infant safety, S9447
  lactation, S9443
  nutrition, S9452
  parenting, S9444
  smoking cessation, S9453
  stress management, S9454
  weight management, S9449
Clavicle
  splint, L3650
Cleaning solvent, Nu-Hope
  16 oz bottle, A4455
  4 oz bottle, A4455
Cleanser, wound, A6260
Cleft palate, feeder, S8265
Clevis, hip orthotic, L2570, L2600, L2610
Clinic visit/encounter, T1015
  hospital outpatient, G0463
  multidisciplinary, child services, T1025
Clinical Decision Support Mechanism, G1001-G1024
Clinical trials
  lodging costs, S9994
  meals, S9996
  phase II, S9990
  phase III, S9991
  service, S9988
  transportation costs, S9992
Closure device, vascular, C1760
Clotting time tube, A4771
Clubfoot wedge, L3380
CMMI Model, G0076-G0087, G2001-G2009, G2013-G2015
CMS Innovation Center Model
  assessment, G9490
  care management, G0076-G0087
  in-home visit, G2001-G2009, G2013-G2015
  remote in-home visit, G9481-G9489, G9978-G9987
Cochlear implant, L8614
  battery
    alkaline, L8622
    lithium, L8623-L8624
    zinc, L8621
  external recharging system, L8625
  external sound processor, L8691
  headset, L8615
  microphone, L8616
  replacement, L8619
  transducer/actuator, replacement, L8625
  transmitter cable, L8618
  transmitting coil, L8617
  zinc, L8621
Cocoon Membrane, Q4264
Cogenex Amniotic Membrane, Q4229
Cogenex Flowable Amnion, Q4230
Coil, imaging, C1770
Cold fluid bottle/wrap, A9273
Collagen
  implant, urinary tract, L8603
  microporous nonhuman origin, C9352-C9353
  skin test, Q3031
  wound dressing, A6021-A6024, Q4164
Collar
  cervical
    contour (low, standard), L0120
    multiple post, L0180-L0200
    nonadjustable foam, L0120
    Philadelphia tracheotomy, L0172
    Philly one-piece extraction, L0150
    tracheotomy, L0172
    traction, E0856
    turtle neck safety, E0942

Collection

Collection
  physiologic data
    via remote patient monitoring, G0322
  specimen
    COVID-19, C9803, G2023-G2024
      self-administered, nonprescription, K1034
Coll-e-Derm, Q4193
Colonoscopy, G9659-G9661
  cancer screening
    patient at high risk, G0105
    patient not at high risk, G0121
  consultation, prescreening, S0285
Coloplast
  closed pouch, A5051
  drainable pouch, A5061
    closed, A5054
    small, A5063
  skin barrier
    4 x 4, A4362
    6 x 6, A5121
    8 x 8, A5122
  stoma cap, A5055
Colpopexy, vaginal, C9778
Coma stimulation, S9056
Combo-Seat universal raised toilet seat, E0244
Commode, E0160-E0171
  chair, E0163-E0165, E0170-E0171
  lift, E0172, E0625
  pail, E0167
  seat, wheelchair, E0968
Communication board, E1902
Companion care, S5135-S5136
Composite
  dressing, A6203-A6205
Compressed gas system, E0424-E0480
Compression
  bandage
    high, A6452
    light, A6448
    medium, A6451
  burn garment, A6501-A6512
  burn mask, A6513
  nonpneumatic garment
    full arm, K1025
      controller, K1024
    full leg, K1032
      controller, K1031
    half leg, K1033
  stockings, A6530-A6549
  wrap, A6545
Compressogrip prosthetic shrinker, L8440-L8465
Compressor, E0565, E0570, E0650-E0652, E0670, K0738
Computer aided detection
  breast MRI image, C8937
Concentrator
  oxygen, E1390-E1392
    rental, E1392
Condom
  female, A4268
  male, A4267
Conductive
  garment (for TENS), E0731
  paste or gel, A4558
Conductivity meter (for dialysis), E1550
Conference
  interdisciplinary team, G0175
Conforming bandage, A6442-A6447
Congenital torticollis orthotic, L0112
Congo red, blood, P2029
Consultation
  telehealth, G0406-G0408, G0425-G0427, G0508-G0509
Contact layer, A6206-A6208
Contact lens, S0500, S0512-S0514, V2500-V2599
Continent device, A5081, A5082
Continuous intraoperative neurophysiology monitoring, G0453
Continuous, monitor
  blood glucose
    adjunctive/nonimplanted, E2102
    invasive/nondurable
      receiver, A9278

Continuous, monitor — *continued*
  blood glucose — *continued*
    invasive/nondurable — *continued*
      sensor, A9276
      transmitter, A9277
    nonadjunctive
      nonimplanted, A4239, E2103
      noninvasive, E0607, S1030-S1031
      lancet, A4258
      supply allowance, 1 month, A4238
      test strips, A4253, A4772
Continuous passive motion exercise device, E0936
Continuous positive airway pressure (CPAP) device, E0601
  chin strap, A7036
  face mask, A7030-A7031
  filter, A7038-A7039
  headgear, A7035
  nasal application accessories, A7032-A7034
  oral interface, A7044
  tubing, A7037
Contraceptive
  cervical cap, A4261
  condom
    female, A4268
    male, A4267
  diaphragm, A4266
  etonogestrel, implant, J7307
  foam, A4269
  gel, A4269
  hormone patch, J7304
  implant, A4264, J7306-J7307
  intratubal occlusion device, A4264
  intrauterine
    copper contraceptive, J7300
    etonogestrel, J7307
    levonorgestrel-releasing, J7296-J7298, S4981
    other, S4989
    Progestacert, S4989
  Levonorgestrel, implants and supplies, J7296-J7298, J7301, J7306
  pills, S4993
  spermicide, A4269
  vaginal ring, J7294, J7295
Contracts, maintenance, ESRD, A4890
Contrast material
  high osmolar, Q9958-Q9964
  injection during MRI, A9575-A9579, Q9953
  low osmolar, Q9951, Q9965-Q9967
  nonradioactive NOC, A9698
  oral MRI, Q9954
Controlyte, enteral nutrition, B4155
Convalescent
  platelet rich plasma, C9507
Convulsive therapy, G2000
Coordinated care fee
  home monitoring, G9006
  initial rate, G9001
  maintenance rate, G9002
  physician oversight, G9008
  risk adjusted, G9003-G9005
  scheduled team conference, G9007
Copying fee, medical records, S9981-S9982
CoreCyte, Q4240
CoreText, Q4246
Corn, trim or remove, S0390
Corneal tissue processing, V2785
Coronary artery bypass surgery, direct
  with coronary arterial and venous grafts
    single, each, S2208
    two arterial and single venous, S2209
  with coronary arterial grafts, only
    single, S2205
    two grafts, S2206
  with coronary venous grafts, only
    single, S2207
Coronavirus (2019-nCoV) diagnostic panel, U0001-U0002
  High throughput technologies, U0003-U0005
Corplex, Q4232

Corplex P, Q4231
Corset, spinal orthotic, L0970-L0976
Cough stimulation device, E0482
Counseling
  alcohol, G0443
  cardiovascular disease risk, G0446
  chaplain services, Q9001-Q9003
  end of life, S0257
  genetic, S0265
  lung cancer screening, G0296
  obesity, G0447
    group (2-10), G0473
  prevention
    sexually transmitted infection, G0445
  vaccine, G0310-G0313
    COVID-19, G0314-G0315
Coupling gel/paste, A4559
Cover, shower
  ventricular assist device, Q0501
Cover, wound
  alginate dressing, A6196-A6198
  foam dressing, A6209-A6214
  hydrocolloid dressing, A6234-A6239
  hydrogel dressing, A6242-A6248
  specialty absorptive dressing, A6251-A6256
COVID-19
  specimen collection, C9803, G2023-G2024
    self-administered, nonprescription, K1034
  vaccination administration, M0201
CPAP (continuous positive airway pressure) device, E0601
  chin strap, A7036
  exhalation port, A7045
  face mask, A7030-A7031
  headgear, A7035
  humidifier, E0561-E0562
  nasal application accessories, A7032-A7034
  oral interface, A7044
  supplies, E0470-E0472, E0561-E0562
  tubing, A7037
Cradle, bed, E0280
Cranial
  electrotherapy stimulation, K1002
  supplies/accessories, A4596
Crisis intervention, H2011, S9484-S9485, T2034
Criticare HN, enteral nutrition, B4153
Crutch
  substitute
    lower leg platform, E0118
Crutches, E0110-E0116
  accessories, A4635-A4637, E2207
  aluminum, E0114
  articulating, spring assisted, E0117
  forearm, E0111
    Ortho-Ease, E0111
  underarm, other than wood, pair, E0114
    Quikfit Custom Pack, E0114
    Red Dot, E0114
  underarm, wood, single, E0113
    Ready-for-use, E0113
  wooden, E0112
Cryo-Cord, Q4237
Cryoprecipitate, each unit, P9012
  plasma, pathogen reduced, P9025
Cryoprecipitated fibrinogen complex
  pathogen reduced, P9026
CTLSO, L0700, L0710, L1000-L1120
Cuirass, E0457
Culture sensitivity study, P7001
Culture, urine, bacterial, P7001
Curasorb, alginate dressing, A6196-A6199
Cushion
  decubitus care, E0190
  Oral/Nasal, A7029
  positioning, E0190
  wheelchair
    AK addition, L5648
    BK addition, L5646
Custom
  DME, K0900
  wheelchair/base, K0008, K0013
Custom Masterhinge Hip Hinge 3, L2999
Customized item (in addition to code for basic item), S1002
Cyanocobalamin cobalt, A9546, A9559

Cycler
  disposable set, A4671
Cycler dialysis machine, E1594
Cygnus, Q4170, Q4199
Cylinder tank carrier, E2208
Cymetra, Q4112
Cystoscopy, blue light, C7554, C9738
  with biopsy(ies), C7550
Cystourethroscopy
  for ureteral calculi, S2070
  with adjunctive blue light cystoscopy, C7554
    with biopsy(ies), C7550
  with insertion of transprostatic implant; 1 to 3 implants, C9739
  with insertion of transprostatic implant; 4 or more implants, C9740
  with insertion temporary prostatic implant or stent, C9769
  with lithotripsy, C9761
Cytal, Q4166
Cytopathology, screening, G0123, G0124, G0141, G0143-G0148

D

Day care services, S5100-S5102, S5105
Debridement, bone
  with insertion drug delivery device, C7500
Decompression
  disc, S2348
  hip core, S2325
  lumbar
    percutaneous image guided (pild), G0276
  vertebral axial, S9090
Decubitus care equipment, E0181
  cushion or pillow, E0190
  mattress
    AquaPedic Sectional Gel Flotation, E0196
    Iris Pressure Reduction/Relief, dry, E0184
    PressureGuard II, air, E0186
    TenderFlo II, E0187
    TenderGel II, E0196
  pressure pads, overlays, E0197-E0199
    Body Wrap, E0199
    Geo-Matt, E0199
    Iris, E0199
    PressureKair, E0197
    Richfoam Convoluted and Flat, E0199
  pressure pads, with pumps, E0181
    Bio Flote, E0181
    KoalaKair, E0181
  protectors
    heel or elbow, E0191
      Body Wrap Foam Positioners, E0191
      Pre-Vent, E0191
  pump, E0182
    Bio Flote, E0182
    Pillo, E0182
    TenderCloud, E0182
Deionizer, water purification system, E1615
Delivery system
  kidney, E1510
  oxygen, topical, E0446
Delivery to high risk area requiring escort, S9381
Delivery/set-up/dispensing, A9901
Delta-Cast Elite Casting Material, A4590
Delta-Lite Conformable Casting Tape, A4590
Delta-Lite C-Splint Fiberglass Immobilizer, A4590
Delta-Lite "S" Fiberglass Casting Tape, A4590
Deluxe item, S1001
Demonstration project
  clinic, extended stay, G9140
    CMS Innovation Center Model, G0076-G0087, G2001-G2009, G2013-G2015, G9481-G9490, G9978-G9987
    ESRD, G9013-G9014
    Medicare Care Choice Model (MCCM), G9480
    oncology, G9050-G9139

Demonstration project — *continued*
   radiation oncology, M1072-M1105
   smoking, G9016
Dennis Browne, foot orthotic, L3140, L3150
Department of Veterans Affairs
   Whole Health Partner Services, Q9004
Depression, G9212-G9213
Derata injection device, A4210
DermACELL, DermACELL AWM, DermACELL AWM Porous, Q4122
Dermacyte Amniotic Membrane Allograft, Q4248
Derma-Gide, Q4203
Dermagraft, Q4106
DermaPure, Q4152
DermaSpan, Q4126
Dermavest, Q4153
Derm-Maxx, Q4238
Destruction
   lesion, G0186
   tumor, S2095
Detector, blood leak, dialysis, E1560
Device
   auditory osseointegrated, L8691, L8695
   continuous passive motion, E0936
   drug delivery
      with debridement, bone, C7500
   drug matrix, C1734
   electrical stimulation device for cancer treatment, E0766
   endoscope
      colonoscope, implantable, C1749
      upper GI, insertable, C1748
      urinary, insertable, C1747
   eversion/inversion, A9285
   hygienic, any type, A9286
   implantable/insertable, C1889-C1890
   intermittent limb compression, E0676
   joint, C1776
   medication management, T1505
   occlusive device placement, G0269
   ocular, C1784
   oral
      airway collapse reduction, K1027
   orthopedic, C1734
      bilateral hip, knee, ankle, foot (KAF), K1007
      elbow, wrist, hand, finger (EWHFO), L8701-L8702
   range of motion, E1841
   reaching/grabbing, A9281
   retrieval, C1773
   speech generating, E2500
   tissue localization and excision, C1819
   urinary incontinence repair, C1771, C2631
   ventricular assist device
      supply, Q0477, Q0507-Q0509
Dextrostick, A4772
Diabetes
   alcohol swabs, per box, A4245
   battery for blood glucose monitor, A4233-A4236
   bent needle set for insulin pump infusion, A4231
   blood glucose monitor
      continuous
         adjunctive/nonimplanted, E2102
         invasive/nondurable
            receiver, A9278
            sensor, A9276
            transmitter, A9277
         nonadjunctive
            nonimplanted, A4239, E2103
            noninvasive, E0607, S1030-S1031
      lancet, A4258
      supply allowance, 1 month, A4328
      test strips, A4253, A4772
      with integrated lancer, E2101
      with voice synthesizer, E2100
   blood glucose test strips, box of 50, A4253

Diabetes — *continued*
   drugs
      Humalin, J1815, J1817
      Humalog, J1817, S5551
      insulin, J1815, J1817, S5551
      Novolin, J1815, J1817
   evaluation and management LOPS, G0245
   injection device, needle-free, A4210
   insulin pump, external, E0784, E0787
      infusion set, A4231
      supplies, maintenance, A4226
      syringe with needle, A4232
   lancet device, A4258
   lancets, box of 100, A4259
   MDPP, G9873-G9891
   non-needle cannula for insulin infusion, A4232
   retinal exam, S3000
   self management training
      group, G0109
      individual, G0108
   shoe
      fitting, A5500
      inlay, A5508
      insert, A5512-A5514
      modification, A5503-A5507
   syringe, disposable
      box of 100, S8490
      each, A4206
   urine glucose/ketone test strips, box of 100, A4250
Diabetic management program
   dietitian visit, S9465
   E/M of sensory neuropathy, G0246-G0247
   follow-up visit to MD provider, S9141
   follow-up visit to non-MD provider, S9140
   foot care, G0247
   group session, S9455
   insulin pump initiation, S9145
   MDPP, G9873-G9891
   nurse visit, S9460
Diagnostic
   bronchoscopy, C7509
   panel
      Coronavirus (2019-nCoV), U0001-U0002
      High throughput technologies, U0003-U0004
Dialet lancet device, A4258
Dialysate
   concentrate additives, A4765
   peritoneal dialysis solution, A4720-A4726, A4766
   solution, A4728
   testing solution, A4760
Dialysis
   access system, C1881
   acetate concentrate, A4708
   acid solution, A4709
   air bubble detector, E1530
   anesthetic, A4736-A4737
   bath conductivity, meter, E1550
   bicarbonate concentrate, A4706-A4707
   blood leak detector, E1560
   catheter, C1750, C1752
   centrifuge, E1500
   circuit, C7513-C7514, C7530
      angioplasty, C7533
   cleaning solution, A4674
   concentrate
      acetate, A4708
      acid, A4709
      bicarbonate, A4706-A4707
   Cycler machine, E1594
   documentation, G9231
   drain bag/bottle, A4911
   emergency treatment, G0257
   equipment, E1510-E1699
   ESRD facility
      acute kidney injury without ESRD, G0491-G0492
   extension line, A4672-A4673
   filter, A4680
   fluid barrier, E1575
   heating pad, E0210
   hemostats, E1637

Dialysis — *continued*
   home equipment repair, A4890
   infusion pump, E1520
   machine, E1590
   mask, surgical, A4928
   peritoneal
      clamps, E1634
   pressure alarm, E1540
   protamine sulfate, A4802
   scale, E1639
   shunt accessory, A4740
   supplies, A4671-A4918
   surgical mask, A4928
   syringe, A4657
   Tablo system, E1629
   tourniquet, A4929
   transducer protector, E1575
   unipuncture control system, E1580
   Y set tubing, peritoneal, A4719
Dialyzer, artificial kidney, A4690
Diaper service, T4538
Diaphragm, contraceptive, A4266
Diathermy, home use, K1004
Dietary education, S9449, S9452
Disarticulation
   lower extremities, prosthesis, K1022, L5000-L5999
   upper extremities, prosthesis, L6000-L6692
Discharge, patient, G9254-G9255
Disease management program, S0315, S0317, S0320
Disetronic
   glass cartridge syringe for insulin pump, each, A4232
   H-Tron insulin pump, E0784
   insulin infusion set with bent needle, with or without wings, each, A4231
Disk decompression, lumbar, S2348
Diskard head halter, E0940
Diskectomy, lumbar, S2350, S2351
   single interspace, S2350
Dispensing fee
   BICROS, V5240
   binaural, V5160
   CROS, V5200
   monaural hearing aid, V5241
   new spectacle lenses, S0595
   pharmacy
      inhalation drugs, G0333, Q0513-Q0514
Disposable
   diapers, A4335
   glucose monitor, A9275
   supplies, ambulance, A0382-A0398
   underpads, A4554
DNA analysis, S3840
Dome
   and mouthpiece (for nebulizer), A7016
Don-Joy
   cervical support collar, L0150
   deluxe knee immobilizer, L1830
   wrist forearm splint, L3984
Donor cadaver
   harvesting multivisceral organs, with allografts, S2055
Doppler, transesophageal, G9157
Dornix Plus, E0601
Dorsiwedge Night Splint, A4570, L2999, L4398
Dose optimization, for infusion, S3722
Dosimeter, implantable radiation, ea, A4650
Double bar
   AK, knee-ankle-foot orthotic, L2020, L2030
   BK, ankle-foot orthotic, L1990
Doula services, T1032-T1033
Drainage
   bag, A4357, A4358, A4911
   board, postural, E0606
   bottle, A4911, A5102
   vacuum, A7048
Dressing — *see also* Bandage, A6021-A6404
   absorptive, for use with suction pump, K0744-K0746
   alginate, A6196-A6199
   composite, A6203-A6205
   contact layer, A6206-A6208
   film, A6257-A6259

Dressing — *see also* Bandage — *continued*
   foam, A6209-A6215
   gauze, A6216-A6230, A6402-A6404
   holder/binder, A4461, A4463
   hydrocolloid, A6234-A6241
   hydrogel, A6242-A6248
   resorbable, A6460-A6461
   specialty absorptive, A6251-A6256
   tape, A4450, A4452
   transparent film, A6257-A6259
   tubular, A6457
Dropper, A4649
Drug confirmation, G0480-G0483
Drug delivery device/implant
   deep, C7500
   non-biodegradable
      insertion, G0516
      removal, G0517-G0518
Drug delivery system
   controlled dose delivery system, K0730
   disposable, A4306
Drug testing, G0480-G0483, G0659
Drugs — *see* Table of Drugs
   administered through a metered dose inhaler, J3535
   disposable delivery system, 5 ml or less per hour, A4306
   disposable delivery system, 50 ml or greater per hour, A4305
   infusion supplies, A4221, A4222, A4230-A4232
   not otherwise classified, J3490, J7599, J7699, J7799, J8499, J8999, J9999
   Part B drug CAP NOC, Q4082
Dry pressure pad/mattress, E0184, E0199
DSM IV criteria major depressive disorder, G9212-G9213
Dual Layer Impax Membrane, Q4262
Dunlap
   heating pad, E0210
Duolock curved tail closures, A4421
Durable medical equipment (DME), E0100-E8002
Durr-Fillauer
   cervical collar, L0140
   Pavlik harness, L1620

E

Ear wax removal, G0268
Easy Care
   folding walker, E0143
   quad cane, E0105
ECG
   initial Medicare ECG, G0403-G0405
Echocardiogram
   transesophageal, C8925-C8928
   transthoracic, C8921-C8924, C8929-C8930
Echosclerotherapy, S2202
Economy knee splint, L1830
Edetate
   calcium disodium, J0600
   edetate disodium, J3520
Education
   asthma, S9441
   birthing, S9436-S9439, S9442
   chronic kidney disease, G0420-G0421
   diabetes, S9145
   exercise, S9451
   family planning
      individualized programs, school based, T1018
      nonmedical, H1010
   infant safety, S9447
   lactation, S9443
   Lamaze, S9436
   mental health problems, G0177
   parenting, S9444
   smoking cessation, S9453
   stress management, S9454
   weight management, S9449
Eggcrate dry pressure pad/mattress, E0184, E0199
Elastic support, A6530-A6549
Elbow
   brace, universal rehabilitation, L3720
   disarticulation, endoskeletal, L6450

Elbow — continued
  Masterhinge Elbow Brace 3, L3999
  orthotic
    EO, E1800, L3702-L3740, L3760-L3762
    EWHO, L3764-L3766
  protector, E0191
Elbow, wrist, hand, finger orthotic (EWHFO), L8702
Elbow, wrist, hand orthotic (EWHO), L8701
Electric hand
  adult, L7007
  independently articulating digits, L6880
  pediatric, L7008
Electric heat pad for peritoneal dialysis, E0210
Electric hook, L7009
Electric stimulator supplies, A4595, K1017, K1019
Electrical impedance
  esophageal mucosal integrity testing, C9777
Electrical stimulation, S8930
Electrical stimulation device for cancer treatment, E0766
Electrical work, dialysis equipment, A4870
Electrode
  Electrodes, per pair, A4556
  Electrode/transducer, A4555
Electrodes, per pair, A4556
Electromagnetic therapy, G0295, G0329
Electron beam computed tomography, S8092
Electrotherapy stimulation, cranial, K1002
  supplies/accessories, A4596
Elevating leg rest, K0195
Elevator, air pressure, heel, E0370
Embolization, protection system, C1884
  for tumor destruction, S2095
Embryo
  cryopreserved transferred, S4037
  monitor/store cryopreserved, S4040
  storage, S4027
Emergency response system, S5160-S5162
EMG
  biofeedback device, E0746
  surface, S3900
Encounter, clinic, T1015
End of life care planning, S0257
Endarterectomy, chemical, M0300
Endoscope
  colonoscope device (implantable), C1749
  sheath, A4270
  upper GI, insertable, C1748
  urinary, insertable, C1747
Endoscopic retrograde cholangiopancreatography (ERCP)
  biopsy, C7542
  calculi/debris removal, C7544
  diagnostic, C7541
  sphincterotomy/papillotomy, C7543
Endoscopy
  nasal, C9771, S2342
  submucosal dissection (ESD), C9779
Endoskeletal system, addition, K1022, L5610-L5999
Endovascular, revascularization
  femoral, popliteal artery(ies), C7531, C7534-C7535
  intravascular lithotripsy, C9764, C9772
  catheter, transluminal, C1761
  with atherectomy, C9766, C9774
  with atherectomy and stent placement, C9767, C9775
  with stent placement, C9765, C9773
Enema
  bag, reusable, A4458
  barium, G0106
  cancer screening, G0120
  manual pump system, A4459
  tube
    replacement, any type, K1013
Enrich, enteral nutrition, B4150
Ensure, enteral nutrition, B4150
  HN, B4150
  Plus, B4152
  Plus HN, B4152
  powder, B4150

Enteral
  administration services, feeding, S9340-S9343
  digestive enzyme(s), B4105
  feeding supply kit (syringe) (pump) (gravity), B4034-B4036
  fiber or additive, B4104
  formulae, B4150-B4162
    electrolytes, B4102, B4103
    for metabolic disease, B4157
    intact nutrients, B4149, B4150, B4152
    pediatric, B4158-B4162
  gastronomy tube, B4087-B4088
  nutrition infusion pump, any type, B9002
  supplies, not otherwise classified, B9998
Enterostomal therapy, S9474
Enverse, Q4258
Enzyme(s)
  enteral feeding, B4105
Eosinophil count, S3630
EpiCord, Q4187
EpiFix (injectable), Q4145
EpiFix, Q4186
Equestrian/hippotherapy, S8940
ERCP, C7541-C7544
ESD (endoscopic submucosal dissection), C9779
Esophageal mucosal integrity testing, C9777
ESRD End Stage Renal Disease — see also Dialysis
  bundle demo/basic, G9013
    expanded, G9014
  documentation, G9231
  ESRD facility
    acute kidney injury without ESRD, G0491-G0492
  machines and accessories, E1510-E1699
  plumbing, A4870
  supplies, A4651-A4913
Evaluation
  comprehensive, multi-discipline, H2000
  E/M, prolonged, G0316-G0318, G2212
  for power mobility device, G0372
  ocularist, S9150
  remote, images/video, G2010
  risk factors, G9298-G9299
  self assessment, depression, S3005
  team for handicapped, T1024
Evaluation device, remote
  cardiovascular, G2066
Eversion device, A9285
Exactech lancet device, A4258
Examination
  breast, S0613
  breast and pelvic, G0101
  diabetic for LOPS, G0245-G0246
  for college, S0622
  initial Medicare, G0402
  related to surgical procedure, S0260
Excellagen, Q4149
Exchange
  biliary drainage catheter, C7545
  nephrostomy catheter, C7548
Excision
  deep cervical node(s), C7503
  peripheral nerve neuroma, C7551
  tissue localization, C1819
Exercise
  class, S9451
  continuous passive motion device, E0936
  equipment, A9300
Exo-Static overdoor traction unit, E0860
Exsufflation belt, K1021
External
  ambulatory infusion pump, E0781, E0784
  counterpulsation, G0166
  power, battery components, L7360-L7499
  power, elbow, L7191
External defibrillator
  battery replacement, K0607
  electrode replacement, K0609
  garment replacement, K0608
Extracorporeal shock wave lithotripsy, S0400

Extrahepatic bile duct(s)
  intraoperative
    near-infrared fluorescence imaging, C9776
Extremity belt/harness, E0945
Eye
  lens (contact) (spectacle), S0500-S0514, V2100-V2615
  pad, A6410-A6411
  patch, A6410-A6412
  prosthetic, C1839, V2623-V2629
  service (miscellaneous), V2700-V2799
E-Z Lite wheelchair, E1250
EZ-Derm, Q4136
E-ZJect disposable insulin syringes, up to 1 cc, per syringe, A4206
E-ZJect Lite Angle lancets, box of 100, A4259
E-Z-lets lancet device, A4258

F

Face tent, oxygen, A4619
Facility services
  dental procedure requiring monitored anesthesia, G0330
Family stabilization, S9482
FDG, A9552
Fecal microbiota, preparation/instillation, G0455
Fee, coordinated care
  coordinated care, G9001
Fern test, Q0114
Fertility services
  donor service (sperm or embryo), S4025
  in vitro fertilization, S4013-S4022
  ovulation induction, S4042
  sperm procurement, S4026, S4030-S4031
Fertilization
  in vitro, S4011
Fetal surgery, repair teratoma, S2405
Fetoscopic laser therapy, S2411
Filler
  bone, C9359
  wound
    alginate, A6199
    foam, A6215
    hydrocolloid, A6240-A6241
    hydrogel, A6248
    not elsewhere classified, A6261-A6262
Film
  dressing, A6257-A6259
Filter
  aerosol compressor, A7013
  carbon, A4680
  CPAP device, A7038-A7039
  dialysis carbon, A4680
  ostomy, A4368
  tracheostoma, A4481
  ultrasonic generator, A7013
  vena cava, C1880
  ventricular assist device, Q0500
Financial management, self-directed, T2050
Finasteride, S0138
Finger
  orthotic (FO), L3933-L3935
  splint
    baseball, A4570
    fold-over, A4570
    four-pronged, A4570
    static, Q4049
Fisher&Paykel HC220, E0601
Fistula
  cannulation set, A4730
Fitness club membership, S9970
Flashcast Elite casting material, A4590
Flex HD, Q4128
Flow rate meter, peak, A4614
FlowerAmnioFlo, Q4177
FlowerAmnioPatch, Q4148
FlowerDerm, Q4179
Flowmeter, E0440, E0555, E0580
Fluid barrier, dialysis, E1575
Fluid Flow, Fluid GF, Q4206
Fluorescent imaging
  blue light cystoscopy, C7554, C9738
    with biopsy(ies), C7550

Fluorine-18 fluorodeoxyglucose
  contrast material, A9552
  imaging using dual-head coincidence detection system, S8085
Flutamide, S0175
Flutter device, S8185
Foam
  dressing, A6209-A6215
  pad adhesive, A5126
Folding walker, E0135, E0143
Fold-over finger splint, A4570
Foley catheter, A4312-A4316, A4338-A4346
Follitropin
  beta, S0128
Food supplement, S9434
Food thickener, B4100
Foot care, routine, G0247, S0390
Foot, cast boot
  Specialist Closed-Back Cast Boot, L3260
  Specialist Gaitkeeper Boot, L3260
  Specialist Open-Back Cast Boot, L3260
  Specialist Toe Insert for Specialist Closed-Back Cast Boot and Specialist Health/Post Operative Shoe, A9270
Foot exam, G9225-G9226
Foot impression casting, S0395
Foot insert, L2180, L3000-L3003, L3031, L5000
Foot, insoles/heel cups
  Specialist Heel Cups, L3485
  Specialist Insoles, L3510
Foot, soles
  Masterfoot Walking Cast Sole, L3649
  Solo Cast Sole, L3540
Footdrop splint, L4398
Footplate, E0175, E0970
Footwear, orthopedic, L3201-L3265
Forearm crutches, E0110, E0111
Fortex, alginate dressing, A6196-A6199
Foster care, H0041-H0042, S5140-S5146
Four Poster, fracture frame, E0946
Four-pronged finger splint, A4570
Fracture
  bedpan, E0276
  frame, E0920, E0930, E0946-E0948
  orthotic, L2106-L2136
  orthotic additions, L3995
  pelvic bone, Q0412-Q0415
  specialist pre-formed humeral fracture brace, L3980-L3981
Frame
  meaning spectacles, V2020, V2025
  sales tax, S9999
  safety, for hospital bed, E0316
  sit-to-stand, E0637
  standing system, E0638, E0641-E0642
FreAmine HBC, parenteral nutrition, B5200
Frejka, hip orthotic, L1600
  replacement cover, L1610
Functional outcome assessment, G9227

G

Gait trainer
  pediatric
    anterior, E8002
    posterior, E8000
    upright, E8001
GammaGraft, Q4111
Ganirelix acetate, S0132
Garment breast prosthesis, L8015
Garment covering, A4467
Gas system
  compressed, E0424, E0425
  gaseous, E0430, E0431, E0441, E0443
  liquid, E0434-E0440, E0442, E0444
Gasket, prosthetic socket insert, L7700
Gastric
  band adjustment, S2083
Gastric suction pump, E2000
Gastrostomy tube, B4087-B4088
Gauze, A6216-A6230, A6266
  impregnated, A6222-A6230, A6266
  nonimpregnated, A6216, A6221, A6402
  pads, A6216-A6230, A6402-A6404
    Johnson&Johnson, A6402
    Kendall, A6402
    Moore, A6402

Gel
  conductive, A4558
  coupling for ultrasound, A4559
  pressure pad, E0185, E0196
  sheet, dermal or epidermal, A6025
Generator
  cardiac, C1824
  neurostimulator
    nonrechargeable, C1767, C1823, C1825, C1827
    with rechargeable battery/charging system, C1826
      high frequency, C1822
      nonhigh frequency, C1820
Genesis Amniotic Membrane, Q4198
Genetic
  counseling, S0265
  testing, S3800, S3840-S3842, S3844-S3846, S3849-S3850, S3852-S3854, S3861-S3870
    hypertrophic cardiomyopathy, S3865, S3866
Genmould Creamy Plaster, A4580
Geo-Matt
  therapeutic overlay, E0199
Geronimo PR, power wheelchair, K0011
Gerval Protein, enteral nutrition, B4155
Gestational home visit
  for diabetes, S9214
  for hypertension, S9211
  for preeclampsia, S9213
GIFT, S4013
Glasses
  air conduction, V5070
  binaural, V5120-V5150
  bone conduction, V5080
  frames, V2020, V2025
  hearing aid, V5150, V5190, V5230
  lens, V2100-V2499, V2610, V2718, V2730, V2755, V2770, V2780
Glaucoma screening, G0117-G0118
Global fee, urgent care center, S9083
Gloves
  dialysis, A4927
  non-sterile, A4927
  sterile, A4930
Glucometer
  3 blood glucose meter, E0607
  3 blood glucose test strips, box of 50, A4253
  II blood glucose meter, E0607
  II blood glucose test strips, box of 50, A4253
Glucose
  monitor device, continuous
    adjunctive/nonimplanted, E2102
    invasive/nondurable
      receiver, A9278
      sensor, A9276
      transmitter, A9277
    nonadjunctive
      nonimplanted, A4239, E2103
      noninvasive, E0607, S1030-S1031
    lancet, A4258
    supply allowance, 1 month, A4238
    test strips, A4253, A4772
Gluteal pad, L2650
Gold
  sodium thiomalate, J1600
Gomco
  aspirators, E0600
Grab bar, trapeze, E0910, E0940
Grade-aid, wheelchair, E0974
Gradient pressure aids, S8420-S8429
Grafix Core, GrafixPL Core, Q4132
Grafix Prime, GrafixPL Prime, Q4133
Graft
  vascular, C1768
GRAFTJACKET, Q4107
GRAFTJACKET XPRESS, Q4113
Gravity traction device, E0941
Gravlee jet washer, A4470
Greissing, foot prosthesis, L5978
Guardian, Q4151

Guidance
  breast biopsies
    magnetic resonance, C7502
    stereotactic, C7501
  Stereoscopic, radiation therapy delivery, G6002
  Ultrasonic, radiation therapy fields, G6001
Guide wire, C1769
Guilford multiple-post collar, cervical orthotic, L0190

H

Haberman Feeder, S8265
Habilitation, T2012-T2021, T2047
Hair analysis (excluding arsenic), P2031
Hallus-valgus dynamic splint, L3100
Hallux prosthetic implant, L8642
Halo procedures, L0810-L0859, L0861
Halter, cervical head, E0942
Hand
  electric, L6880, L7007-L7008
  mechanical, L6708-L6709
  orthotic (WHFO), E1805, E1825, L3808, L3900-L3923
  partial prosthesis, L6000-L6020
  restoration, L6900-L6915
  rims, wheelchair, E0967
Handgrip (cane, crutch, walker), A4636
Harness, E0942, E0944, E0945
Harvest
  multivisceral organs, cadaver donor, S2055
  peripheral stem cell, S2150
Harvey arm abduction orthotic, L3960
Health club membership, S9970
Hearing devices, L8614, V5030-V5299
  accessories/supplies, V5267
  analog, V5242-V5251
  assistive listening device, V5268-V5274, V5281-V5290
  battery, V5266
  BICROS, V5211-V5215, V5221, V5230
  binaural, V5120-V5150, V5211-V5215, V5221, V5248-V5249
  body worn, V5030, V5040, V5100
  CROS, V5171-V5172, V5181, V5190
  digital, V5250-V5261
  dispensing fee, V5241
    BICROS, V5240
    bilateral, V5110
    binaural, V5160
    CROS, V5200
    monaural, V5241
    unspecified, V5090
  disposable, V5262-V5263
  ear impression, V5275
  ear mold/insert, V5264-V5265
  glasses, V5070-V5080, V5190-V5230
  middle ear prosthesis, V5095
  monaural, V5030-V5060, V5171-V5172
  programmable
    binaural, V5250-V5253
    monaural, V5244-V5247
Heat
  application, E0200-E0239
  lamp, E0200, E0205
  pad, E0210, E0215, E0217, E0249
  units, E0239
    Hydrocollator, mobile, E0239
    Thermalator T-12-M, E0239
Heater (nebulizer), E1372
Heating pad, Dunlap, E0210
  for peritoneal dialysis, E0210
Heel
  elevator, air, E0370
  loop/holder, E0951
  pad, L3480, L3485
  protector, E0191
  shoe, L3430-L3485
  stabilizer, L3170
Helicoll, Q4164
Helicopter, ambulance — see also Ambulance, A0431
Helmet
  cervical, A8000-A8004
  custom, A8002-A8003
  hard, A8001, A8003

Helmet — continued
  interface replacement, A8004
  prefabricated, A8000-A8001
  soft, A8000, A8002
Hemalet lancet device, A4258
Hematopoietic hormone administration, S9537
Hemilaminectomy, C9757
Hemipelvectomy prosthesis, L5280
Hemi-wheelchair, E1083-E1086
Hemodialysis
  See Dialysis
Hemodialyzer, portable, E1635
Hemostats, for dialysis, E1637
Hemostix, A4773
Heparin
  infusion pump (for dialysis), E1520
HepatAmine, parenteral nutrition, B5100
Hepatic portosystemic pressure gradient measurement
  endoscopic, C9768
Hepatic-aid, enteral nutrition, B4154
Hepatitis B screening
  non-pregnant, high-risk individual, G0499
Hexalite, A4590
Hexior power wheelchair, K0014
High frequency
  chest wall oscillation equipment, A7025-A7026, E0483
  neurostimulator generator
    with battery and charging system, C1822
High osmolar contrast
  150-199 mg iodine, Q9959
  200-249 mg iodine, Q9960
  250-299 mg iodine, Q9961
  300-349 mg iodine, Q9962
  350-399 mg iodine, Q9963
  400 or greater mg iodine, Q9964
  up to 149 mg iodine, Q9958
High throughput technologies
  Coronavirus (2019-nCoV) (SARS-CoV-2), U0003-U0004
Hip
  Custom Masterhinge Hip Hinge 3, L2999
  disarticulation prosthesis, L5250, L5270
  Masterhinge Hip Hinge 3, L2999
  orthotic (HO), L1600-L1686
Hip-knee-ankle-foot orthotic (HKAFO), K1007, L2040-L2090
History and physical
  related to surgical procedure, S0260
HIV-1 antibody testing, S3645
HIV-1 or HIV-2 screening, G0432-G0435
HKAFO, L2040-L2090
hMatrix, Q4134
Holder
  heel, E0951
  surgical dressing, A4461, A4463
  toe, E0952
Hole cutter tool, A4421
Hollister
  belt adapter, A4421
  closed pouch, A5051, A5052
  colostomy/ileostomy kit, A5061
  drainable pouches, A5061
    with flange, A5063
  medical adhesive, A4364
  pediatric ostomy belt, A4367
  remover, adhesive, A4455
  skin barrier, A4362, A5122
  skin cleanser, A4335
  skin conditioning cream, A4335
  skin gel protective dressing wipes, A5120
  stoma cap, A5055
  two-piece pediatric ostomy system, A5054, A5063, A5073
  urostomy pouch, A5071, A5072
Home
  delivered meals, S5170
  modifications, S5165
  ventilator, any type
    invasive interface, E0465
    multifunction, E0467
    non-invasive interface, E0466

Home health
  aerosolized drug therapy, S9061
  aide, S9122, T1030-T1031
    home health setting, G0156
  bundled payment, G9187
  care
    attendant care, S5125-S5126
    certified nurse assistant, S9122, T1021
    home health aide, S9122, T1021
    home health care, Q5001-Q5002, Q5009
  management
    episodic, S0272
    hospice, S0271
    standard, S0270
  nursing care, G0299-G0300, S9122-S9124, T1030-T1031
  outside capitation arrangement, S0273-S0274
  re-certification, G0179-G0180
  training, S5108-S5116
  contracted services, T1022
  gestational
    assessment, T1028
    delivery supplies, S8415
    diabetes, S9214
    hypertension, S9211
    pre-eclampsia, S9213
    preterm labor, S9208-S9209
  hydration therapy, S9373-S9379
  infusion therapy, S5035-S5036, S9325-S9379, S9494-S9497, S9537-S9810
    catheter care, S5497-S5498, S5517-S5518
    corticosteroid infusion, S9490
    insertion midline venous catheter, S5523
    insertion PICC line, S5520, S5522
    supplies, S5517-S5521
  nursing services, G0162, G0490, G0493-G0496, S0274, S9212-S9213
  physician services, S0270-S0273
  postpartum hypertension, S9212
  remote patient monitoring, G0322
  respiratory therapy, S5180-S5181
  services of
    clinical social worker, G0155
    occupational therapist, G0152
      assistant, G2169
    physical therapist, G0151
      assistant, G2168
    skilled nurse, G0299-G0300
    speech/language pathologist, G0153
    speech/language pathologist, G0153, G0161
  therapy, G0151-G0152, G0157-G0160
  transfusion, blood products, S9538
  venipuncture, S9529
  via synchronous telemedicine, G0320-G0321
  wound care, S9097
Home uterine monitor, S9001
Hook
  electric, L7009
  mechanical, L6706-L6707
Hospice
  care, Q5001-Q5010, S9126, T2042-T2046
  care coordinator, G9477
  chaplain, G9473
  dietary counselor, G9474
  evaluation and counseling services, G0337
  nursing services, G0162, G0299-G0300, G0493-G0496
  other counselor, G9475
  other qualified pharmacist, G9479
  other qualified therapist, G9478
  referral visit, S0255
  speech/language pathologist, G0153
  therapy, G0151-G0152, G0157-G0158
  volunteer, G9476
Hospital
  observation
    direct admit, G0379
    per hour, G0378
  outpatient clinic visit, G0463

Hospital — *continued*
    readmission, G9309-G9310
Hospitalist services, S0310
Hot fluid bottle/wrap, A9273
Houdini security suit, E0700
Housing, supported, H0043-H0044
Hoyer patient lifts, E0621, E0625, E0630
H-Tron insulin pump, E0784
H-Tron Plus insulin pump, E0784
Hudson
    adult multi-vent venturi style mask, A4620
    nasal cannula, A4615
    oxygen supply tubing, A4616
    UC-BL type shoe insert, L3000
Human amniotic tissue allograft, Q4163
Human Health Factor 10 Amniotic Patch (HHF10-P), Q4224
Human placental tissue matrix, Q4162
Humidifier, E0550-E0560
    water chamber, A7046
Hyalomatrix, Q4117
Hydration therapy, S9373-S9379
Hydraulic patient lift, E0630
Hydrocollator, E0225, E0239
Hydrocolloid dressing, A6234-A6241
Hydrocortisone
    acetate, J1700
    sodium phosphate, J1710
    sodium succinate, J1720
Hydrocortone
    acetate, J1700
    phosphate, J1710
Hydrogel dressing, A6242-A6248
Hydroxyurea, S0176
Hygienic device/item, A9286
Hyperbaric oxygen chamber
    full body, G0277
    topical, A4575
Hypo-Let lancet device, A4258
Hypothermia
    intragastric, M0100

I

Ice cap/collar, A9273
Ilfeld, hip orthotic, L1650
Imaging, C1770
    coil, MRI, C1770
Implant
    access system, A4301
    aqueous shunt, L8612
    auditory device
        brainstem, S2235
        middle ear, S2230
    breast, L8600
    cardiac monitor, C1833
    cochlear, L8614, L8627-L8628
    collagen
        meniscus, knee, G0428
        urinary, L8603
    contraceptive, A4264, J7306
    device, C1734
    dextranomer/hyaluronic acid copolymer, urinary tract, L8604, L8605
    drug delivery, G0516-G0518
    drug matrix, C1734
    endoscope colonoscope device, C1749
    ganciclovir, J7310
    goserelin acetate, J9202
    hallux, L8642
    infusion pump, E0782-E0783
    injectable bulking agent
        anal, L8605
        urinary tract, L8606
        vocal cord, L8607
    interatrial shunt, C9758
        NYHA IDE study, C9760
    interspinous process distraction device, C1821
    intervertebral body, C1062
    joint, L8630
    lacrimal duct, A4262-A4263
    levonorgestrel, J7306
    metacarpophalangeal joint, L8630
    metatarsal joint, L8641
    Mometasone sinus, J7402

Implant — *continued*
    nerve end
        with excision neuroma, C7551
    neurostimulator
        nonrechargeable, C1767, C1823, C1825
        with rechargeable battery/charging sys
            high frequency, C1822
            nonhigh frequency, C1820
    Norplant, J7306
    not otherwise specified, L8699
    NYHA IDE study
        implantation coronary sinus reduction device, C9783
        interatrial shunt implantation, C9760
        intramyocardial transplantation autologous bone marrow cells, C9782
    ocular, L8610
        drainage assist device, C1783
    orthopedic, C1734
    ossicular, L8613
    osteogenesis stimulator, E0749
    percutaneous access system, A4301
    porcine, C9364
    Propel sinus, S1091
    prosthetic device, C9899
    sinus, J7402, S1091
    urinary tract, L8603-L8604
    vascular access portal, A4300
    vascular graft, L8670
    yttrium 90, S2095
    Zoladex, J9202
Implantable radiation dosimeter, ea, A4650
Impregnated gauze dressing, A6222-A6230
In vitro fertilization, S4011
Incontinence
    appliances and supplies, A4310, A4336, A5051-A5093, A5102-A5114, A5120-A5200
    brief or diaper, T4521-T4528, T4543-T4544
    disposable/liner, T4535
    garment, A4520
    pediatric
        brief or diaper, T4529-T4530
        pull-on protection, T4531-T4532
    penile wrap, T4545
    rectal insert, A4337
    reusable
        diaper or brief, T4539
        pull-on protection, T4536
        underpad, A4553
    underpad
        disposable, T4541, T4542
        reusable, A4553, T4537, T4540
    youth
        brief or diaper, T4533
        pull-on protection, T4534
Indium 111
    capromab pendetide, A9507
    ibritumomab tiuxetan, A9542
    labeled
        platelets, A9571
        white blood cells, A9570
    oxyquinoline, A9547
    pentetate, A9548, A9572
    pentetreotide, A9572
    satumomab pendetide, A4642
Infant safety, CPR, training, S9447
Infection, G9311-G9312
Infusion
    catheter, C1751
    dose optimization, for infusion, S3722
    IV, OPPS, C8957
    monoclonal antibody therapy, M0240, M0241, M0243, M0244, M0245, M0246, M0247, M0248, M0249, M0250
    pump, C1772, C2626
        ambulatory, with administrative equipment, E0781
        epoprostenol, K0455
        heparin, dialysis, E1520
        implantable, E0782, E0783
        implantable, refill kit, A4220

Infusion — *continued*
    pump — *continued*
        insulin, E0784
        mechanical, reusable, E0779, E0780
        nonprogrammable, C1891
        supplies, A4221, A4222, A4226, A4230-A4232
        Versa-Pole IV, E0776
    Sipuleucel-T autologous CD54+, Q2043
    supplies, A4222, A4223
        syringe cartridge, non-insulin pump, K0552
    therapy, home, S9347, S9351, S9497-S9504
Inhalation drugs
    acetylcysteine, J7608
    albuterol, J7609, J7610, J7611
    Alupent, J7668-J7669
    atropine, J7635-J7636
    Atrovent, J7644
    Azmacort, J7684
    beclomethasone, J7622
    betamethasone, J7624
    bitolterol mesylate, J7628-J7629
    Brcanyl, J7680-J7681
    Brethine, J7680-J7681
    budesonide, J7626-J7627, J7633-J7634
    colistimethate sodium, S0142
    cromolyn sodium, J7631
    dexamethasone, J7637-J7638
    dornase alpha, J7639
    flunisolide, J7641
    formoterol, J7606, J7640
    Gastrocrom, J7631
    glycopyrrolate, J7642-J7643
    iloprost, Q4074
    Intal, J7631
    ipratropium bromide, J7644-J7645
    isoetharine HCl, J7647-J7650
    isoproterenol HCl, J7657-J7660
    levalbuterol, J7607, J7614, J7615
    metaproterenol sulfate, J7667-J7670
    methacholine chloride, J7674
    Mucomyst, J7608
    Mucosil, J7608
    Nasalcrom, J7631
    NOC, J7699
    pentamidine isethionate, J7676
    Pulmicort Respules, J7627
    terbutaline sulfate, J7680-J7681
    Tobi, J7682
    tobramycin, J7682, J7685
    Tornalate, J7628-J7629
    triamcinolone, J7683-J7684
Initial
    ECG, Medicare, G0403-G0405
    physical exam, Medicare, G0402
Injectable
    bulking agent
        urinary tract, L8603-L8606
        vocal cord, L8607
Injection — *see also* Table of Drugs
    adjustment, bariatric band, S2083
    bulking agent
        urinary tract, L8603-L8606
        vocal cord, L8607
    contrast material, during MRI, A9576-A9579, Q9953
    dermal filler for LDS, G0429
    sacroiliac joint, G0259-G0260
    subretinal, C9770
    supplies for self-administered, A4211, A4224-A4225
InnovaMatrix AC, A2001
InnovaMatrix FS, A2013
Inpatient telehealth pharmacologic management, G0459
Insert
    convex, for ostomy, A5093
    diabetic, for shoe, A5512-A5514
    foot insert/plate, L3031
    implant
        prosthetic socket, gasket or seal, L7700
    soft palate, C9727
Insertion
    cardioverter-defibrillator system, G0448

Insertion — *continued*
    central venous access device
        inside-out technique, C9780
    intrauterine system, S4981
    tray, A4310-A4316
Instillation fecal microbiota, G0455
Integra
    Bilayer Matrix Wound Dressing, Q4104
    Dermal Regeneration Template, Q4105
    Flowable, Q4114
    Matrix, Q4108
    Meshed Bilayer Wound Matrix, C9363
    MOZAIK Osteoconductive Scaffold Putty, C9359
    MOZAIK Osteoconductive Scaffold Strip, C9362
InteguPLY, Q4126
Interbody cage
    anterior/lateral, personalized, C1831
Interface
    cough stimulating device, A7020
    oral with suction pump, A7047
Interfyl, Q4171
Intermittent
    limb compression device, E0676
    peritoneal dialysis system, E1592
    positive pressure breathing (IPPB) machine, E0500
Interphalangeal joint
    arthrodesis, C7506
    prosthetic implant, L8658
Interrogation, remote evaluation
    cardiovascular, G2066
Interscapular thoracic prosthesis
    endoskeletal, L6570
    upper limb, L6350-L6370
Interspinous process distraction device, C1821
Intervention
    alcohol and/or drug, H0050
    leak of endoluminal contents, G9305-G9306
Intrafallopian transfer
    complete cycle, gamete, S4013
    complete cycle, zygote, S4014
    donor egg cycle, S4023
    incomplete cycle, S4017
Intraocular lenses, C1780, C1840, Q1004-Q1005, S0596, V2630-V2632
    new technology
        category 4, Q1004
        category 5, Q1005
    presbyopia correcting function, V2788
    refractive correcting, S0596
    telescopic, C1840
Intraoperative
    near-infrared fluorescence
        lymphatic mapping, C9756
        major extrahepatic bile ducts, C9776
Intratubal occlusion device, A4264
Intrauterine device
    copper contraceptive, J7300
    etonogestrel, J7307
    levonorgestrel-releasing, J7296-J7298, S4981
    other, S4989
    Progestacert, S4989
Introducer sheath
    guiding, C1766, C1892, C1893
    other than guiding, C1894, C2629
Inversion device, A9285
Investigational device exemption (IDE) study
    interatrial shunt, transcatheter, C9760
Iodine 125, A9527, A9532, C2638-C2639
Iodine I-131
    albumin, A9524
    iobenguane sulfate, A9508
    sodium iodide, A9517
Iodine swabs/wipes, A4247
IPD
    system, E1592
IPPB machine, E0500
    delivery device, A9274, E0784, S5560-S5561, S5565-S5571
    home infusion administration, S9353
    intermediate acting, S5552
    long acting, S5553

IPPB machine — *continued*
  NPH, J1815, S5552
  outpatient IV treatment, G9147
  rapid onset, S5550-S5551
Ipratropium bromide
  administered through DME, J7644-J7645
Iris Preventix pressure relief/reduction mattress, E0184
Iris prosthesis, C1839
Iris therapeutic overlays, E0199
IRM ankle-foot orthotic, L1950
Iron
  sucrose, J1756
Irrigation supplies, A4320, A4322, A4355, A4398-A4400, A4436-A4437
  Surfit
    irrigation sleeve, A4436-A4437
    night drainage container set, A5102
  Visi-flow irrigator, A4398, A4399
Irrigation/evacuation system, bowel
  control unit, E0350
  disposable supplies for, E0352
Islet cell transplant
  laparoscopy, G0342
  laparotomy, G0343
  percutaneous, G0341
Isocal, enteral nutrition, B4150
  HCN, B4152
Isoetharine
  inhalation solution
    concentrated, J7647
    unit dose, J7649-J7650
Isolates, B4150, B4152
Isoproterenol HCl
  administered through DME, J7657-J7660
Isosulfan blue, Q9968
Isotein, enteral nutrition, B4153
IV, G0459
  administration set, non-PVC, S1016
  infusion, OPPS, C8957
  pole, E0776, K0105
  solution
    10% LMD, J7100
    5% dextrose/normal saline, J7042
    D-5-W, J7070
    dextran, J7100, J7110
    Gentran, J7100, J7110
    normal saline, A4217, J7030-J7040, J7050
    Rheomacrodex, J7100
    Ringer's lactate, J7120
  tubing extension set, S1015

J

Jace tribrace, L1832
Jacket
  scoliosis, L1300, L1310
J-cell battery, replacement for blood glucose monitor, A4234
Jejunostomy tube, B4087-B4088
Joint device, C1776
  transcutaneous electrical stimulation, E0762

K

Kaltostat, alginate dressing, A6196-A6199
Kartop Patient Lift, toilet or bathroom (*see also* Lift), E0625
Keramatrix, Kerasorb, Q4165
Keratectomy photorefractive, S0810
Keratoprosthesis, C1818
Kerecis Omega3, Q4158
Keroxx, Q4202
Keto-Diastix, box of 100 glucose/ketone urine test strips, A4250
Key-Pred
  -25,-50, J2650
Kidney
  ESRD supply, A4651-A4913
  system, E1510
  wearable artificial, E1632
Kingsley gloves, above hands, L6890
Kits
  asthma, S8097

Kits — *continued*
  enteral feeding supply (syringe) (pump) (gravity), B4034-B4036
  fistula cannulation (set), A4730
  parenteral nutrition, B4220-B4224
  surgical dressing (tray), A4550
  tracheostomy, A4625
Knee
  Adjustabrace 3, L2999
  disarticulation, prosthesis, K1022, L5150-L5160, L5312
  extension/flexion device, E1812
  immobilizer, L1830
  joint, miniature, L5826
  Knee-O-Prene Hinged Wraparound Knee Support, L1810
  locks, L2405-L2425
  Masterbrace 3, L2999
  Masterhinge Adjustabrace 3, L2999
  orthotic (KO), E1810, L1810, L1820, L1830-L1860, L1851-L1852
Knee Support, L2000-L2038, L2126-L2136
Knee-O-Prene Hinged Knee Sleeve, L1810
Knee-O-Prene Hinged Wraparound Knee Support, L1810
KnitRite
  prosthetic
    sheath, L8400-L8415
    sock, L8420-L8435
    stump sock, L8470-L8485
K-Y Lubricating Jelly, A4332, A4402
Kyphosis pad, L1020, L1025

L

Labor care (not resulting in delivery), S4005
Laboratory tests
  chemistry, P2028-P2038
  miscellaneous, Q0111-Q0115
Lacrimal duct implant
  permanent, A4263
  temporary, A4262
Laminotomy, C9757
Lancet, A4258, A4259
Laparoscopy, surgical
  esophagomyotomy, S2079
Laryngectomy
  tube, A7520-A7522
Larynx, artificial, L8500
Laser
  application, S8948
  assisted uvulopalatoplasty (LAUP), S2080
  in situ keratomileusis, S0800
  myringotomy, S2225
Laser skin piercing device, for blood collection, E0620
  replacement lens, A4257
LAUP, S2080
Lavage
  bronchoscopy, C7510
Lead
  adaptor
    neurostimulator, C1883
    pacing, C1883
  cardioverter, defibrillator, C1777, C1895, C1896
  environmental, home evaluation, T1029
  neurostimulator, C1778
  neurostimulator/test kit, C1897
  pacemaker, C1779, C1898, C1899
  ventricular, C1900
Leg
  bag, A4358, A5112
  extensions for walker, E0158
  Nextep Contour Lower Leg Walker, L2999
  Nextep Low Silhouette Lower Leg Walkers, L2999
  rest, elevating, K0195
  rest, wheelchair, E0990
  strap, A5113, A5114, K0038, K0039
Legg Perthes orthotic, A4565, L1700-L1755
Lens
  aniseikonic, V2118, V2318
  contact, V2500-V2599
  deluxe feature, V2702
  eye, S0504-S0508, S0580-S0590, S0596, V2100-V2615, V2700-V2799

Lens — *continued*
  intraocular, C1780, C1840, V2630-V2632
  low vision, V2600-V2615
  mirror coating, V2761
  occupational multifocal, V2786
  polarization, V2762
  polycarbonate, V2784
  progressive, V2781
  skin piercing device, replacement, A4257
  telescopic, C1840
  tint, V2744
    addition, V2745
Lenticular lens
  bifocal, V2221
  single vision, V2121
  trifocal, V2321
Lerman Minerva spinal orthotic, L0174
Lesion
  destruction, G0186
Leukocyte
  poor blood, each unit, P9016
Levine, stomach tube, B4087-B4088
Levonorgestrel, contraceptive implants and supplies, J7296-J7298, J7301, J7306
Lice infestation treatment, A9180
Lifescan lancets, box of 100, A4259
Lifestand manual wheelchair, K0009
Lifestyle modification program, coronary heart disease, S0340-S0342
Lift
  combination, E0637
  patient, and seat, E0621-E0635
    Hoyer
      Home Care, E0621
      Partner All-Purpose, hydraulic, E0630
      Partner Power Multifunction, E0625
  separate seat mechanism, any type, E0627, E0629
  shoe, L3300-L3334
  standing frame system, E0638
Lift-Aid patient lifts, E0621
Light box, E0203
Lispro insulin, S5551
Lithium battery for blood glucose monitor, A4233-A4236
Lithotripsy, gallstones, S9034
Lithotripsy, intravascular
  catheter, transluminal, C1761
  endovascular revascularization, C9764-C9767, C9772-C9775
Little Ones
  drainable pouch, A5063
  mini-pouch, A5054
  one-piece custom drainable pouch, A5061
  one-piece custom urostomy pouch, A5071
  pediatric belt, A4367
  pediatric urine collector, A4335
  urostomy pouch, transparent, A5073
Lively, knee-ankle-foot orthotic, L2038
Lobectomy, lung, donor, S2061
Lodging
  NOS, S9976
  recipient, escort nonemergency transport, A0180, A0200
  transplant-related, S9975
Lomustine, S0178
Lonalac powder, enteral nutrition, B4150
Low cost, application of skin substitute, C5271-C5278
Low osmolar contrast
  100-199 mgs iodine, Q9965
  200-299 mgs iodine, Q9966
  300-399 mgs iodine, Q9967
  400 or greater mgs iodine, Q9951
Lower limb, prosthesis, addition, L5968
LPN services, T1003
Lubricant, A4332, A4402
Lumbar
  orthotic, L0625-L0627
  pad, L1030, L1040
  sacral orthotic (LSO), L0628-L0640
Lung biopsy plug, C2613
Lung volume reduction surgery services, G0302-G0305

LVRS services, G0302-G0305
Lymphatic
  mapping, intraoperative, near-infrared fluorescence, C9756
Lymphedema therapy, S8950

M

Madamist II medication compressor/nebulizer, E0570
Magnacal, enteral nutrition, B4152
Magnetic
  resonance angiography, C8900, C8901-C8914, C8918-C8920, C8931-C8936
  resonance cholangiopancreatography, S8037
  resonance imaging
    cardiac
      strain imaging, C9762
      stress imaging, C9763
    low field, S8042
    source imaging, S8035
Magnetic resonance guidance
  breast biopsies, C7502
Maintenance contract, ESRD, A4890
Male erection system, L7900
Malibu cervical turtleneck safety collar, L0150
Management
  advanced illness, S0311
  chronic pain, G3002-G3003
  disease, S0316-S0317
  financial, self-directed, T2050
Mapping
  topographic brain, S8040
Marker
  tissue, A4648
Mask
  burn compression, A6513
  CPAP, A7027
  oxygen, A4620
  surgical, for dialysis, A4928
Mastectomy
  bra, L8002
  camisole, S8460
  form, L8020
  prosthesis, L8000-L8039, L8600
  sleeve, L8010
Masterbrace 3, L2999
Masterfoot Walking Cast Sole, L3649
Masterhinge Adjustabrace 3, L2999
Masterhinge Elbow Brace 3, L3999
Masterhinge Hip Hinge 3, L2999
Masterhinge Shoulder Brace 3, L3999
Masters 2 step, S3904
Matrion, Q4201
MatriStem, Q4118
Matrix HD, Q4128
Mattress
  air pressure, E0186, E0197
  alternating pressure, E0277
    pad, Bio Flote, E0181
    pad, KoalaKair, E0181
  AquaPedic Sectional, E0196
  decubitus care, E0196
  dry pressure, E0184
  flotation, E0184
  gel pressure, E0196
  hospital bed, E0271, E0272
  non-powered, pressure reducing, E0373
  Iris Preventix pressure relief/reduction, E0184
  Overlay, E0371-E0372
  pressure reducing, E0181
  TenderFlor II, E0187
  TenderGel II, E0196
  water pressure, E0187, E0198
    powered, pressure reducing, E0277
MCCM, G9480
MCP, multi-axial rotation unit, L5986
MCT Oil, enteral nutrition, B4155
MDPP, G9873-G9891
Meals
  adults in treatment, T1010
  per diem NOS, S9977

Measurement

Measurement
   hepatic portosystemic pressure gradient, endoscopic, C9768
Mechanical
   allergen particle barrier/inhalation filter nasal, topical, K1026
   hand, L6708-L6709
   hook, L6706-L6707
   wound suction, A9272
Medialization material for vocal cord, C1878
Medical and surgical supplies, A4206-A6404
Medical conference, S0220-S0221
Medical food, S9435
Medical home program, S0280-S0281
Medical records copying fee, S9981-S9982
Medical visit, G0463, G9246-G9247
Medicare Care Choice Model (MCCM), G9480
Medicare Diabetes Prevention Program (MDPP), G9873-G9891
Medicare "welcome"
   ECG, G0403-G0405
   physical, G0402
Medication management device, T1505
Medication services
   comprehensive, H2010
   reminder, S5185
Medi-Jector injection device, A4210
MediSense 2 Pen blood glucose monitor, E0607
Mediskin, Q4135
Medralone
   40, J1030
   80, J1040
Membrane Graft, Membrane Wrap, Q4205
MemoDerm, A4126
Menotropins, S0122
Mental health
   assessment, H0031
   education, G0177
   hospitalization, H0035
   peer services, H0038
   remote diagnosis, evaluation, treatment, C7900-C7902
   self-help, H0038
   service plan, H0032
   services, NOS, H0046
   supportive treatment, H0026-H0037
   training, G0177
Meritene, enteral nutrition, B4150
   powder, B4150
MESA, S4028
Mesh, C1781
Metabolism error, food supplement, S9434
Metacarpophalangeal joint prosthesis, L8630
Metatarsal joint, prosthetic implant, L8641
Meter, bath conductivity, dialysis, E1550
Methylene blue injection, Q9968
Methylprednisolone
   acetate, J1020-J1040
   oral, J7509
   sodium succinate, J2920, J2930
Meunster Suspension, socket prosthesis, L6110
Microbiology test, P7001
Microcapillary tube, A4651
   sealant, A4652
Micro-Fine
   disposable insulin syringes, up to 1 cc, per syringe, A4206
   lancets, box of 100, A4259
Microinfusion
   transcatheter therapy, C9759
Microlipids, enteral nutrition, B4155
Microlyte, A2005
Mileage, ambulance, A0380, A0390
Milk, breast
   processing, T2101
Milwaukee spinal orthotic, L1000
Minerva, spinal orthotic, L0700, L0710
Mini-bus, nonemergency transportation, A0120
Minimed
   3 cc syringe, A4232
   506 insulin pump, E0784
   insulin infusion set with bent needle wings, each, A4231

Minimed — *continued*
   Sof-Set 24" insulin infusion set, each, A4230
Miroderm Biologic Wound Matrix, Q4175
Mirragen, A2002
Mitotic rate, G9292-G9294
MLG-Complete, Q4256
Mobilite hospital beds, E0293, E0295, E0297
Moderate sedation, G0500
Moducal, enteral nutrition, B4155
Moisture exchanger for use with invasive mechanical ventilation, A4483
Moisturizer, skin, A6250
Monitor
   apnea, E0618
   blood glucose
      device, continuous
         adjunctive/nonimplanted, E2102
         invasive/nondurable
            receiver, A9278
            sensor, A9276
            transmitter, A9277
      nonadjunctive
         nonimplanted, A4239, E2103
         noninvasive, E0607, S1030-S1031
      lancet, A4258
      supply allowance, 1 month, A4238
      - test strips, A4253, A4772
   blood pressure, A4670
   device, NOC, A9279
   pacemaker, E0610, E0615
   ultrafiltration, S9007
Monoclonal antibody therapy adminstration, M0220, M0221, M0222, M0223, M0240, M0241, M0243, M0244, M0245, M0246, M0247, M0248, M0249, M0250
Monoject disposable insulin syringes, up to 1 cc, per syringe, A4206
Monojector lancet device, A4258
Morcellator, C1782
Mouthpiece (for respiratory equipment), A4617
MRCP, S8037
MRI
   cardiac
      strain imaging, C9762
      stress imaging, C9763
   contrast material, A9576-A9579, Q9954
   low field, S8042
Mucoprotein, blood, P2038
Mucus trap, S8210
Multidisciplinary services, children, T1026
Multifetal pregnancy reduction, ultrasound guidance, S8055
Multiple post collar, cervical, L0180-L0200
Multipositional patient support system, E0636
Muscular dystrophy, genetic test, S3853
Myotonic muscular dystrophy, genetic test, S3853
MyOwn Skin, Q4226
Myringotomy, S2225

N

Nail trim, G0127, S0390
Narrowing device, wheelchair, E0969
Nasal
   application device (for CPAP device), A7032-A7034
   endoscopy, C9771, S2342
   vaccine inhalation, J3530
Nasogastric tubing, B4081, B4082
Nebulizer, E0570-E0585
   aerosol mask, A7015
   aerosols, E0580
      Airlife Brand Misty-Neb, E0580
      Power-Mist, E0580
      Up-Draft Neb-U-Mist, E0580
      Up-Mist hand-held nebulizer, E0580
   compressor, with, E0570
      Madamist II medication compressor/nebulizer, E0570

Nebulizer — *continued*
   compressor, with — *continued*
      Pulmo-Aide compressor/nebulizer, E0570
      Schuco Mist nebulizer system, E0570
   corrugated tubing
      disposable, A7010, A7018
   distilled water, A7018
   filter
      disposable, A7013
      non-disposable, A7014
   heater, E1372
   large volume
      disposable, prefilled, A7008
      disposable, unfilled, A7007
   not used with oxygen
      durable glass, A7017
   pneumatic, administration set, A7003, A7005, A7006
   pneumatic, nonfiltered, A7004
   portable, E0570
   small volume, E0574
   spacer or nebulizer, S8100
      with mask, S8101
   ultrasonic, dome and mouthpiece, A7016
   ultrasonic, reservoir bottle nondisposable, A7009
   water, A7018
   water collection device large volume nebulizer, A7012
      distilled water, A7018
Needle, A4215
   biopsy
      bone marrow, C1830
   brachytherapy, C1715
   non-coring, A4212
   with syringe, A4206-A4209
Negative pressure wound therapy
   dressing set, A6550
   pump, E2402
NeoPatch, Q4176
Neox 100, Q4156
Neox 1K, Neox Cord 1K, Neox Cord RT, Q4148
Neox Flo, Q4155
NephrAmine, parenteral nutrition, B5000
Nephrostomy catheter
   convert to nephroureteral catheter, C7547
   exchange, C7548
Nephroureteral catheter
   convert from nephrostomy catheter, C7547
   removal and replacement, C7546
Neuroma
   excision, C7551
Neuromuscular stimulator, E0745
   ambulation of spinal cord injured, E0762
Neurophysiology monitoring, G0453
Neuro-Pulse, E0720
Neurostimulator
   external upper limb tremor wrist, K1018
   functional transcutaneous, E0764
   generator
      nonrechargeable, C1767, C1823, C1825, C1827
      with rechargeable battery/charging system, C1826
         high frequency, C1822
         nonhigh frequency, C1820
   implantable
      electrode, L8680
      generator, C1826-C1827, L8679, L8685-L8688
      receiver, L8682
   lead, C1778
   patient programmer, C1787, L8681
   receiver and/or transmitter, C1816
   transcutaneous
      distal nerve, K1023
      trigeminal nerve, K1016
   transmitter
      external, L8683-L8684
   vagus nerve, noninvasive, K1020
Newington
   Legg Perthes orthotic, L1710
Newport Lite hip orthotic, L1685
Next Generation ACO Model, G9868-G9870

Nextep Contour Lower Leg Walker, L2999
Nextep Low Silhouette Lower Leg Walkers, L2999
Nicotine
   gum, S4995
   patches, S4990-S4991
Niemann-Pick disease, genetic test, S3849
Nipple prosthesis, L2006, L8032
Noncovered services, A9270, G0293-G0294
Nonemergency transportation, A0080-A0210
Nonimpregnated gauze dressing, A6216, A6221, A6402, A6404
Nonprescription drug, A9150
Nonthermal pulsed high frequency radiowaves treatment device, E0761
Northwestern Suspension, socket prosthesis, L6110
Not medically necessary service, S9986
Not otherwise specified supply, T5999
NovaFix, Q4208
NovaFix DL, Q4254
NovoSorb SynPath, A2006
NuDyn, Q4233
NuHope
   adhesive, 1 oz bottle with applicator, A4364
   adhesive, 3 oz bottle with applicator, A4364
   cleaning solvent, 16 oz bottle, A4455
   cleaning solvent, 4 oz bottle, A4455
   hole cutter tool, A4421
Nursing care, in home
   licensed practical nurse, G0494, G0496, S9124
   nursing visit (FQHC, RHC), G0490
   registered nurse, G0493, G0495, S9123
Nursing services, G0493-G0496, S9211-S9212, T1000-T1004
   nursing facility resident
      evaluation and management, G9685
      treatment, G9679-G9684
NuShield, Q4160
Nutri-Source, enteral nutrition, B4155
Nutrition
   counseling
      dietary, S9452
   enteral formulae, B4150-B4162
   enteral infusion pump, B9002
   medical food, S9433
   errors of metabolism
      inborn, S9435
      noninborn, S9432
   parenteral infusion pump, B9004, B9006
   parenteral solution, B4164-B5200
Nutritional counseling, dietitian visit, S9470
NYHA IDE study
   transcatheter
      implantation coronary sinus reduction device, C9783
      interatrial shunt implantation, C9760
      intramyocardial transplantation autologous bone marrow cells, C9782

O

O&P Express
   above knee, L5210
   ankle-foot orthotic with bilateral uprights, L1990
   anterior floor reaction orthotic, L1945
   below knee, L5105
   elbow disarticulation, L6200
   hip disarticulation, L5250
   hip-knee-ankle-foot orthotic, L2080
   interscapular thoracic, L6370
   knee disarticulation, L5150, L5160
   knee-ankle-foot orthotic, L2000, L2010, L2020, L2036
   Legg Perthes orthotic, Patten bottom type, L1755
   Legg Perthes orthotic, Scottish Rite, L1730
   partial foot, L5000, L5020
   plastic foot drop brace, L1960
   supply/accessory/service, L9900
OASIS
   Burn Matrix, Q4103
   Ultra Tri-Layer Matrix, Q4124
   Wound Matrix, Q4102

Observation service
  direct admission, G0379
  per hour, G0378
Occipital/mandibular support, cervical, L0160
Occlusive device placement, G0269
Occupational multifocal lens, V2786
Occupational therapist
  home health setting, G0152
    performed by assistant, G2169
Occupational therapy, G0129, S9129
Octafluoropropae microspheres, Q9956
Ocular device, C1783, C1784
Ocular prosthetic implant, L8610
Offobock cosmetic gloves, L6895
Ofloxacin, S0034
Ohio Willow
  prosthetic sheath
    above knee, L8410
    below knee, L8400
    upper limb, L8415
  prosthetic sock, L8420-L8435
  stump sock, L8470-L8485
OIVIT, G9147
Olanzapine, S0166
Omegaven, B4187
Omeza Collagen Matrix, A2014
Omnicardiogram, S9025
Oncology
  breast cancer, G9071-G9075, G9131
    gene profiling, S3854
  chronic myelogenous leukemia, G9139
  colon cancer, G9083-G9089
  coordination of care, G9054
  demonstration project, G9050-G9139
  esophageal cancer, G9096-G9099
  evaluation, G9050
  expectant management, G9053
  gastric cancer, G9100-G9104
  head and neck, G9109-G9112
  management
    adheres to guidelines, G9056
    differs from guidelines, G9057-G9060, G9062
    not addressed by guidelines, G9061
  management of care, G9054
  multiple myeloma, G9128-G9130
  no directed therapy, G9053
  non-Hodgkin's lymphoma, G9123-G9125, G9134-G9138
  nonsmall cell lung cancer, G9063-G9070
  ovarian cancer, G9113-G9117, G9126
  pancreatic cancer, G9105-G9108
  prostate cancer, G9077-G9083, G9132-G9133
  rectal cancer, G9090-G9095
  staging, G9050
  supervising care, G9054
  surveillance for recurrence, G9052
  treatment decision making, G9051
  unspecified service, G9055
  work up, G9050
Oncoscint, A4642
One Touch
  Basic blood glucose meter, E0607
  Basic test strips, box of 50, A4253
  Profile blood glucose meter, E0607
One-Button foldaway walker, E0143
Opioid treatment, G1028, G2067-G2088, G2213, G2215-G2216
Oral
  cushion replacement, A7028
  interface for respiratory suction pump, A7047
  interpreter or sign language services, T1013
Organ donor procurement, S2152
Oropharyngeal suction catheter, A4628
Ortho-Ease forearm crutches, E0111
Orthoflex Elastic Plaster Bandages, A4580
Orthoguard hip orthotic, L1685
Orthomedics
  ankle-foot orthotic, L1900
  pediatric hip abduction splint, L1640
  plastic foot drop brace, L1960
  single axis shoe insert, L2180
  ultralight airplane arm abduction splint, L3960

Orthomedics — *continued*
  upper extremity fracture orthotic combination, L3763
    humeral, L3980-L3981
    radius/ulnar, L3982
Orthomerica
  below knee test socket, L5620
  pediatric hip abduction splint, L1640
  plastic foot drop brace, L1960
  single axis shoe insert, L2180
  upper extremity fracture orthotic
    humeral, L3980-L3981
    radius/ulnar, L3982
Orthopedic devices, E0910-E0948
  cervical
    Diskard head halters, E0942
    Turtle Neck safety collars, E0942
Orthopedic shoes
  arch support, L3040-L3100
  footwear, L3201-L3265
  insert, L3000-L3030
  lift, L3300-L3334
  miscellaneous additions, L3500-L3595
  positioning device, L3140-L3170
  transfer, L3600-L3649
  wedge, L3340-L3420
Orthoplast Splints (and Orthoplast II Splints), A4590
Orthotic additions
  ankle/foot, L5969
  carbon graphite lamination, L2755
  cervical congenital torticollis, L0112
  electric lock, L6638
  electronic elbow with microprocessor, L7181
  endoskeletal
    knee disarticulation, K1022
    knee-shin system, K1014, L5848
      with microprocessor, L5856, L5857
  fracture, L2180-L2192, L3995
  halo, L0859
  lock mechanism for elbow, L6698
  lower extremity, K0672, L2200-L2999, L5646-L5648, L5781-L5782, L5984
  ratchet lock, L2430
  removable soft interface, K0672
  replacement strap, L4002
  rocker bottom for ankle, L2232
  scoliosis, L1010-L1120, L1210-L1290
  shoe, L3300-L3595, L3649
  shoulder lock, L6646-L6648
  socket insert for elbow, L6694-L6697
  spinal, L0970-L0999
  suspension sleeve for knee, L5685
  upper extremity joint, L3956
  upper limb, E2631-E2633, L3956, L3995
  vacuum pump, L5781-L5782
Orthotic devices
  additions, K1014-K1015, L1005-L1120, L1210-L1290, L5610-L5999, L5961, L5988-L5990, L6611, L6624
  ankle-foot (*see also* Orthopedic shoes), E1815, E1830, L1900-L1990, L2108-L2116, L3160, L4396-L4397, L4631
  anterior-posterior-lateral, L0700, L0710
  cervical, L0112, L0180-L0200
  cervical-thoracic-lumbar-sacral, L0700, L0710, L1000-L1001
  congenital torticollis, L0112
  cranial remolding, S1040
  cranial-cervical, L0113
  elbow, E1800, L3702-L3740, L3761
  finger, L3925, L3927
  foot
    adductus positioning device, K1015
  fracture, L3980-L3984
  halo, L0810-L0830
  hand, E1805, E1825, L3900-L3930
  hip, L1600-L1686
  hip-knee-ankle-foot, K1007, L2040-L2090
  interface material, L1820
  knee, E1810, L1810-L1820, L1830-L1860, L1851-L1852
  knee-ankle-foot, L2000-L2038, L2126-L2136
  Legg Perthes, A4565, L1700-L1755

Orthotic devices — *continued*
  lumbar, L0625-L0627
  lumbar-sacral, L0628-L0651
  lumbar-sacral, hip, femur, L1690
  multiple post collar, L0180-L0200
  not otherwise specified, L0999, L1499, L2999, L3999, L5999, L7499, L8039
  pneumatic splint, L4350-L4370
  preparatory below knee, L5535
  repair or replacement, L4000-L4210
  replace soft interface material, L4392-L4394
  sacroiliac, L0621-L0624
  scoliosis, L1000, L1200, L1300-L1499
  shoulder, L3650-L3671, L3674-L3678
  shoulder-elbow-wrist-hand, L3960-L3962
  spinal, cervical, L0112, L0180-L0200
  thoracic belt, L0220
  thoracic-lumbar-sacral, L0450-L0492, L1200
  toe, E1830
  transfer (shoe orthotic), L3600-L3640
  walking splint, nonpneumatic, L4386
  wrist hand, L3150, L3905-L3908, L3916
  wrist hand finger, L3806-L3809, L3900-L3904, L3931
Osmolite, enteral nutrition, B4150
  HN, B4150
Ossicula prosthetic implant, L8613
Osteogenic stimulator, E0747-E0749, E0760
Osteotomy, periacetabular, S2115
Ostomy
  absorbent material, A4422
  accessories, A5093
  adhesive remover wipes, A4456
  appliance belt, A4367
  clamp, A4363
  cone/catheter, A4399
  filter, A4368
  irrigation supply, A4398, A4399
  pediatric one-piece system, A5061, A5062
  pediatric two-piece drainable pouch, A5063
  pouch, A4416-A4420, A4423-A4434
    drainable, A4412-A4413, A5056-A5057
    pediatric, A5061-A5062
  skin barrier, A4411, A4414-A4415
    extended wear, A4407-A4410
    paste, A4405-A4406
    wipes or swabs, A5120
  vent, A4366
Otto Bock prosthesis
  battery charger, six volt, L7362
  battery, six volt, L7360
  hook adapter, L6628
  lamination collar, L6629
  pincher tool, L6810
  wrist, L6629
Outpatient hospital clinic visit, G0463
Overlay, mattress, E0371-E0373
Ovulation induction, S4042
Owens & Minor
  cervical collar, L0140
  cervical helmet, L0120
Oximeter, O0445
  probe, A4606
Oxi-Uni-Pak, E0430
Oxygen
  accessory, E1352
  ambulance, A0422
  battery
    charger, E1357
    pack, E1356
  chamber, hyperbaric, topical, A4575
  concentrator, E1390, E1391
    portable, rental, E1392
  gaseous, E0738, S8120
  liquid, S8121
  mask, A4620
  medication supplies, A4611-A4627
  portable, E0433, E0443-E0444, E0447, K0738
  power adapter, E1358
  rack/stand, E1355
  regulator, E1353

Oxygen — *continued*
  respiratory equipment/supplies, A4611-A4627, E0424-E0480
  Oxi-Uni-Pak, E0430
  supplies and equipment, E0425-E0444, E0433, E0455, E1353-E1406
  tent, E0455
  tubing, A4616
  water vapor enriching system, E1405, E1406
  wheeled cart, E1354

P

Pacemaker
  dual chamber
    non-rate responsive, C2619
    rate responsive, C1785
  lead, C1779, C1898, C1899
  monitor, E0610, E0615
  other than single or dual chamber, C2621
  single chamber
    non-rate responsive, C2620
    rate responsive, C1786
  upgrade to dual chamber
    new/replacement
      atrial and ventricular, C7539
      atrial transvenous, C7537
      ventricular transvenous, C7537
    removal with replacement, C7540
Pacer manual wheelchair, K0003
Packing strips, A6407
Pad
  abdominal, L1270
  adhesive, A6203-A6205, A6212-A6214, A6219-A6221, A6237-A6239, A6245-A6247, A6254-A6256
  alginate, A6196-A6199
  alternating pressure, E0181
  arm, K0019
  Asis, L1250
  condylar, L2810
  crutch, A4635
  fluid circulating, cold, with pump, E0218
  gel pressure, E0185, E0196
  gluteal, L2650
  gradient pressure pads, S8421-S8429
  heating, E0210, E0215, E0217, E0249
  heel, L3480, L3485
  kyphosis, L1020, L1025
  lumbar, L1030, L1040, L1240
  nonadhesive (dressing), A6209-A6211, A6216-A6218, A6222-A6224, A6228-A6230, A6234-A6236, A6242-A6244
  orthotic device interface, E1820
  pressure, E0181-E0182
  replacement, infrared heat system, A4639
  rib gusset, L1280
  sheepskin, E0188, E0189
  shoe, L3430-L3485
  stabilizer, L3170
  sternal, L1050
  thoracic, L1060, L1260
  triceps, L6100
  trochanteric, L1290
  truss, L8320, L8330
  water circulating, heat, unit, E0249
  water circulating, heat, with pump, E0217
  water pressure, E0198
Pail, for use with commode chair, E0167
PalinGen Flow or ProMatrX (fluid), Q4174
PalinGen or PalinGen XPlus Membrane, Q4173
Palladium, C2640-C2641
Pan, for use with commode chair, E0167
Pancreas, S1034-S1037
  artificial device system, S1034
    replacement external receiver, S1037
    replacement external transmitter, S1036
    replacement invasive disposable subcutaneous sensor, S1035
Pantoprazole sodium, C9113, S0164
Papanicolaou (Pap) screening smear, P3000, P3001, Q0091
Paraffin, A4265

Paraffin — *continued*
  bath unit, E0235
Paramedic intercept, S0207-S0208
Paranasal sinus ultrasound, S9024
Parathyroid autotransplantation
  with thyroidectomy, C7555
Parenteral nutrition
  administration kit, B4224
  home infusion therapy, S9364-S9368
  pump, B9004, B9006
  solution, B4164-B5200
  supplies, not otherwise classified, B9999
  supply kit, B4220, B4222
Parenting class, S9444
  infant safety, S9447
Parking fee, nonemergency transport, A0170
Partial hospitalization, S0201
PASRR, T2010-T2011
Passive motion
  continuous exercise device, E0936
Paste, conductive, A4558
  conductive, A4558
  coupling for ultrasound, A4559
Pathogen(s)
  reduced, platelets, P9073
  test for platelets, P9100
Pathology and laboratory tests
  molecular pathology, G0452
  surgical
    prostate, G0416
Pathology screening tests, P3000-P3001, Q0091
Patient lift, E0625, E0637, E0639, E0640
Patten Bottom, Legg Perthes orthotic, L1755
Pavlik harness, hip orthotic, L1650
Payment, home health bundled care improvement initiative, G9187
Peak flow meter, S8110
  portable, S8096
Pediatric hip abduction splint
  Orthomedics, L1640
  Orthomerica, L1640
Pediculosis treatment, A9180
PEFR, peak expiratory flow rate meter, A4614
Pelvic and breast exam, G0101
Pelvic belt/harness/boot, E0944
Penicillin G
  potassium, J2540
  procaine, aqueous, J2510
Penlet II lancet device, A4258
Penlet lancet device, A4258
Percussor, E0480
Percutaneous
  access system, A4301
  biliary drainage catheter
    exchange, C7545
  biopsy
    bone
      vertebra, C7504-C7505
    breast, C7501-C7502
    cervical node(s), C7503
  image-guided lumbar decompression (PILD), G0276
  spine
    vertebral augmentations, C7507-C7508
    vertebroplasties, C7504-C7505
  transluminal coronary atherectomy, C9602-C9603
  transluminal revascularization, C9604-C9608
Perflexane lipid microspheres, Q9955
Perflutren lipid microsphere, Q9957
Peripheral
  catheter infusion, C1751
Perlstein, ankle-foot orthotic, L1920
Permacol, C9364
PermeaDerm B, A2016
PermeaDerm C, A2018
PermeaDerm glove, A2017
Peroneal strap, L0980
Peroxide, A4244
Personal care item, S5199
Personal care services, T1019-T1020
Personalized
  anterior/lateral interbody cage, C1831
Pessary, A4561-A4562

PET imaging
  any site, NOS, G0235
  breast, G0252
  whole body, G0219
Pharmacy
  compounding and dispensing, S9430
  dispensing fee
    inhalation drugs
      per 30 days, Q0513
      per 90 days, Q0514
    supply fee
      initial immunosuppressive drugs, Q0510
      oral anticancer antiemetic or immunosuppressive drug, Q0511-Q0512
Pharmaplast disposable insulin syringes, per syringe, A4206
Phelps, ankle-foot orthotic, L1920
Pheresis, platelets, P9034-P9037, P9053
  pathogen reduced, P9073
Philadelphia tracheotomy cervical collar, L0172
Philly One-piece Extrication collar, L0150
pHisoHex solution, A4246
Phoenix Wound Matrix, A2015
Photocoagulation, G0186
Phototherapy
  home visit service (Bili-Lite), S9098
  keratectomy (PKT), S0812
  light (bilirubin), E0202
Physical exam
  for college, S0622
  related to surgical procedure, S0260
Physical therapy, S8990
  shoulder stretch device, E1841
Physical therapy/therapist
  home health setting, G0151, S9131
  performed by assistant, G2168
Physician management
  home care
    episodic, S0272
    hospice monthly, S0271
    standard monthly, S0270
Physician quality reporting system (PQRS)
  See Quality payment program (QPP)
Physician review
  home INR testing, G0250
Physician supervision, G0181-G0182
Pillow
  abduction, E1399
  decubitus care, E0190
  nasal, A7029
  positioning, E0190
Pinworm examination, Q0113
Placement
  applicator, breast, C9726
  catheter
    coronary artery(ies), C7516-C7529, C7552-C7553
    interstitial device radiotherapy, other than prostate, C9728
  occlusive, G0269
Plan of care, T2024
Planning
  cancer treatment, S0353-S0354
Plasma
  autologous platelet rich plasma, G0460, G0465
  cryoprecipitate reduced, P9044
    pathogen reduced, P9025
  frozen, P9058-P9060
    convalescent, C9507
  multiple donor, pooled, frozen, P9023, P9070-P9071
  protein fraction, P9043, P9048
  single donor, fresh frozen, P9017
Plastazote, L3002, L3252, L3253, L3265, L5654-L5658
Plaster
  bandages
    Orthoflex Elastic Plaster Bandages, A4580
    Specialist Plaster Bandages, A4580
    Genmould Creamy Plaster, A4580

Plaster — *continued*
  Specialist J-Splint Plaster Roll Immobilizer, A4580
  Specialist Plaster Roll Immobilizer, A4580
  Specialist Plaster Splints, A4580
Platelets, P9019-P9020, P9031-P9037, P9052-P9053, P9055
  apheresis/pheresis, P9052, P9055
  concentrate, each unit, P9019
  pathogen(s)
    reduced, platelets, P9073
    test, P9100
  pheresis, P9034-P9037, P9053
    pathogen reduced, P9073
  rich plasma, each unit, P9020
  convalescent, C9507
Platform attachment
  forearm crutch, E0153
  walker, E0154
Platform, for home blood glucose monitor, A4255
Plumbing, for home ESRD equipment, A4870
Plurivest, Q4153
Pneumatic nebulizer
  administration set
    small volume
      disposable, A7004
      filtered, A7006
      non-disposable, A7005
      non-filtered, A7003
Polaris, E0601
Polaris Lt, E0601
Polycose, enteral nutrition
  liquid, B4155
  powder, B4155
PolyCyte, Q4241
Poor blood, each unit, P9016
Port
  indwelling, C1788
Portable
  equipment transfer, R0070-R0076
  hemodialyzer system, E1635
  home suction pump, K0743
  nebulizer, E0570
  oxygen contents
    gaseous, E0443
    liquid, E0444, E0447
  oxygen system
    gaseous, E0430-E0431
    liquid, E0433-E0435
  x-ray equipment, Q0092
Portagen Powder, enteral nutrition, B4150
Posey restraints, E0700
Positive airway pressure device supply, A7046
Postcoital examination, Q0115
Postdischarge services
  LVRS surgery, G0305
Postural drainage board, E0606
Potassium
  hydroxide (KOH) preparation, Q0112
Pouch
  Active Life convex one-piece urostomy, A4421
  closed, A4387, A5052
  drainable, A4388-A4389, A5056-A5057, A5061
  fecal collection, A4330
  Little Ones Sur-fit mini, A5054
  ostomy, A4375-A4378, A4387-A4391, A4416-A4420, A4423-A4434, A4435, A5051-A5054, A5061-A5063
  pediatric, drainable, A5061
  Pouchkins pediatric ostomy system, A5061, A5062, A5073
  Sur-Fit, drainable, A5063
  urinary, A4379-A4383, A4391, A5071-A5073
  urostomy, A5073
Power
  mist nebulizer, E0580
  mobility device, K0800-K0812, K0899
  wheelchair, K0813-K0898
    pediatric, E1239
Power mobility device
  does not meet criteria, K0899
  group 1, K0800-K0802, K0813-K0816

Power mobility device — *continued*
  group 2, K0806-K0808, K0820-K0843
  group 3, K0849-K0864
  group 4, K0868-K0886
  group 5, K0890-K0891
  not coded by DME PDAC, K0899
  not otherwise classified (NOC), K0812, K0898
Power operated vehicle
  group 1, K0800-K0802
  group 2, K0806-K0808
  not otherwise classified (NOC), K0812
Precision, enteral nutrition
  HN, B4153
  Isotonic, B4153
Prednisolone
  acetate, J2650
  oral, J7510
Pregnancy care, H1000-H1005
Pregnancy documentation, G9231
Premium knee sleeve, L1830
Prenatal care, H1000-H1005
Preoperative Services
  LVRS surgery, G0302-G0304
Preparatory prosthesis, L5510-L5595
Prescription drug
  brand, S5001
  generic, S5000
Pressure
  alarm, dialysis, E1540
  pad, E0181-E0183
  sensor system, C1834
PressureGuard II, E0186
PressureKair mattress overlay, E0197
Prestige blood glucose monitor, E0607
Pre-Vent heel & elbow protector, E0191
Prevention, developmental delay, H2037
Preventive
  foot care, S0390
  health Medicare
    ECG, G0403-G0405
    exam, G0402
  prolonged services, G0513-G0514
PriMatrix, Q4110
Probe
  cryoablation, C2618
  oximeter, A4606
  percutaneous lumbar discectomy, C2614
Procenta, Q4244
Processing
  breast milk, T2101
Procurement, organ donor, S2152
Procuren, S9055
Professional services, G0068-G0070, G0088-G0090
ProgenaMatrix, Q4222
Prolonged services
  E/M, G0316-G0318, G2212
  preventive, G0513-G0514
Prolotherapy, M0076
ProMatrX wound matrix, Q4174
Promix, enteral nutrition, B4155
Pronation/supination device, forearm, E1802
Propac, enteral nutrition, B4155
Prostate
  low dose rate (LDR) brachytherapy, G0458
  specific antigen test (PSA), G0103
  surgical pathology, G0416
Prosthesis
  addition
    lower extremity prosthesis, L5858, L5859
  breast, C1789, L2006, L8000-L8031, L8035-L8039, L8600
  eye, C1839, L8610, V2623-V2629
  finger joint, L8659
  fitting, L5400-L5460, L6380-L6388
  grasper, L6881
  hand, L6000-L6020, L6708-L6709, L7007-L7008
  hemifacial, L8044
  hook, L6703-L6707, L7009
  implants, L8600-L8699
  iris, C1839
  larynx, L8500, L8505
  lower extremity, L5700-L5999, L8642

Prosthesis — *continued*
  maxillofacial, provided by a nonphysician, L8040-L8048
  metacarpal, L8631
  midfacial, L8041
  miscellaneous service, L8499
  nasal
    septal, L8047
  nipple, L2006, L8032
  partial facial, L8046
  penile
    inflatable, C1813
    non-inflatable, C2622
  repair, L7520
  repair or modification, maxillofacial, L8048-L8049
  retinal
    accessory/component/supply, L8608
  socks (shrinker, sheath, stump sock), L8400-L8480
  tracheoesophageal, L8511-L8514
  tracheo-esophageal, L8507-L8509
  tracheoesophageal gelatin capsule, L8515
  tracheostomy speaking, L8501
  unspecified maxillofacial, L8048
  upper extremity, L6000-L6915
  urinary sphincter, C1815
  vacuum erection system, L7900

Prosthetic
  additions
    lower extremity, L5610
  device, implanted, C9899
  donning sleeve, L7600
  hand, L6708-L6709, L6713-L6714, L6722
  hook, L6706-L6707, L6711-L6712, L6721, L6722, L7009
  shrinker, L8440-L8465

Prosthetic shrinker, L8440-L8465
Protectant, skin, A6250
Protector, heel or elbow, E0191
ProText, Q4246
PSA, G0103
Psychiatric care, H0036-H0037, H2013-H2014, S9480
Psychological services
  CORF, G0409
Psychotherapy
  group, G0410-G0411
PTK, S0812
Pulmo-Aide compressor
  nebulizer, E0570
Pulmonary rehabilitation program, S9473
Pulse generator
  ear, E2120
  battery, A4638
Pump
  alternating pressure pad, E0182
  ambulatory infusion, E0781
  ambulatory insulin, E0784
  Bio Flote alternating pressure pad, E0182
  blood, dialysis, E1620
  breast, E0602-E0604
    supplies, A4281-A4286
  Broncho-Cath endobronchial tubes, with CPAP, E0601
  enteral infusion, B9002
    supply, K0552
  fluid/water circulating pad, E0217, E0218, E0236
  gastric suction, E2000
  Gomco lightweight mobile aspirator, E0600
  Gomco portable aspirator, E0600
  heparin infusion, E1520
  implantable infusion, E0782, E0783
  implantable infusion, refill kit, A4220
  infusion
    nonprogrammable, C1891, C2626
    supplies, A4230-A4232
  insulin, external, E0784, E0787
    instruction, S9145
    supplies, A4226
  negative pressure wound therapy, E2402
  parenteral infusion, B9004, B9006, K0455
  Pillo alternating pressure pad, E0182
  portable home suction, K0743

Pump — *continued*
  suction
    CPAP, E0601
    gastric, E2000
    respiratory, E0600
    urine management, K1006
    wound, K0743
  TenderCloud alternating pressure pad, E0182
PuraPly, PuraPly AM, PuraPly XT, Q4195-Q4197
Purification system, E1610, E1615
Pyeloscopy
  for ureteral calculi, S2070

Q

Quad cane, E0105
Quadri-Poise canes, E0105
Quality assurance, G9148-G9153
Quality Payment Program (QPP)
  abdominal imaging, G9547-G9548, G9551
  ACE or ARB therapy, G8473-G8475, G8506, G8935-G8937, M1200-M1203
  adjuvant treatment, G2205-G2208
  admission
    inpatient, G2176
    Medicare care choice model program (MCCM), G9480
  advancing cancer care, M0001
  alcohol use, G2196-G2200, G2202, G9621-G9624
  alteplase, G8601
  amoxicillin with/without clavulanate as first line antibiotic, G9313-G9315
  anaphylaxis, M1155, M1160-M1161, M1163
  androgen deprivation therapy, G9894-G9897
  anesthesia, post procedure body temperature, G9771-G9773
  anesthetic, inhalation
    for induction, G9955
  antibiotic regimen, G8708-G8712, G8916-G8918, G9286-G9287, G9498, G9505, G9703, G9712
  anticoagulation, G8967-G8969, G9724, G9927-G9928
  antiemetic agents, G9775-G9777, G9956-G9958
  antimicrobial
    systemic, G9959-G9961
  antiplatelet/antithrombotic/aspirin therapy, G2128, G8598-G8599, G9277-G9278, G9609-G9611, G9794, M1055-M1057
  antipsychotic prescriptions, G0032
  antirheumatic drug therapy, G2182
  anti-TNF therapy, G8869, G9504, G9912-G9914
  aortic aneurysm, G9598-G9599
  Appropriate Use Criteria
    Clinical Decision Support Mechanism, G1001-G1023
  assessment, patient
    bone loss, G8863
    declined, G0036
    unable to participate, G0037
  asthma, G9432, G9434
  atherosclerotic cardiovascular disease (ASCVD), G9662, G9674
  atrial fibrillation (AF), G9746
  back pain, G2136-G2139, G9943, G9946
  benzodiazepine prescriptions, G0033
  beta-blocker, G8450-G8452, G9188-G9192
  biologic treatment, G9765
  biopsy, G8878, G8880, G8882-G8885, G8946, G9282-G9285, G9288-G9291, G9939
  bipolar disorder, G9717
  bladder injury, G9625-G9627
  blood pressure, G2129, G8476-G8478, G8752-G8756, G8783-G8785, G8950-G8952, G9273-G9274, G9788-G9790
  blunt head trauma, G0047, G9529-G9533, G9593-G9597
  BMI, G2181, G8417-G8421, G9716
  bone loss, G8863

Quality Payment Program (QPP) — *continued*
  bone marrow transplant, M1157
  bowel injury, G9628-G9630
  brain imaging, G9529-G9530, G9533
  breast cancer, G8875-G8877, G8881, G8946, G9911
    AJCC stage, G9704-G9705, G9831-G9832
  breastfeeding, G9779
  bronchitis/bronchiolitis, G2177
  bronchodilator, inhaled, G9695-G9699
  cancer diagnosis (other than basal cell or melanoma), M1018
  cardiac implantable device
    not readmitted, G9411, G9413
    readmission within 180 days, G9410, G9412
  cardiac stress test imaging, G8961-G8966
  cardiac tamponade, G9408-G9409
  care improvement initiative home visit, G9187
  care management, CMMI Model, G0076-G0087
  case management service NEC, G9012
  cataract, G0916-G0918
    postoperative refraction, G9519-G9520
  cataract surgery, G0915-G0916, G0918
    postoperative refraction, G9519-G9520
  cause
    transient or reversible AF, G9929
  CEA, G8838
  cervical cytology, G9806-G9807
  chemotherapy/systemic cancer-directed therapy, G9847-G9848, M1156
  chlamydia screening, G9820-G9821
  chronic kidney disease (CKD), M1188
  clinical indication
    imaging, G2187-G2195
  CMMI Model
    assessment, G9490
    care management, G0076-G0087
    in-home visit, G2001-G2009, G2013-G2015
    remote in-home visit, G9481-G9489, G9978-G9987
  colectomy, total, G9711
  colitis, M1181-M1182
  collaborative care management, G2214
  colonoscopy, G2204, G9612-G9614, G9659-G9661, G9998-G9999
  colorectal cancer, G9711
  comfort care only, G9930
  competing diagnosis, G2097, G2175, G8709
  coordinated care fee
    home monitoring, G9006
    initial rate, G9001
    maintenance rate, G9002
    physician oversight, G9008
    risk adjusted, G9003-G9005, G9009-G9011
    scheduled team conference, G9007
  corticosteroids, G9468-G9470, M1183-M1185
  Crohn's disease, M1182
  current medications, G8427-G8428
  death, nursing home resident, G9394
  dementia, M1164
  demonstration project, G0076-G0087, G2001-G2009, G2013-G2015, G2020, G2172, G9013-G9014, G9016, G9050-G9139, G9140, G9480-G9490, G9978-G9987
  depression, G8431-G8433, G8510-G8511, G9212-G9213, G9717, M1019-M1020
  DEXA, DXA, G8399-G8400, G9471
  diabetes, G9676
  dialysis documentation, G9231
  discharge, patient, G8818, G8825-G8826, G8833-G8834, G8838, G9254-G9255
    follow up, G9402-G9407
  door to puncture time, G9580-G9582
  dose reduction techniques, G9637-G9638

Quality Payment Program (QPP) — *continued*
  durable medical equipment (DME), G0454
  dysthymia, M1019-M1020
  ear drainage, M1019-M1020
  early induction, G9355-G9356
  ED admitted patients, G2176, G9426-G9427
  elder maltreatment, G8535-G8536, G8733-G8735, G8941
  elective delivery, G9355-G9356
  elective surgery, G9643
  embolization, G9962-G9963
  emergency department visits, G0035, G9521-G9522
  emergency surgery, G9752
  emergent cases, M1142
  encephalitis, M1162
  end of life, G9380-G9382
  endometrial
    ablation/sampling, G9822-G9824
  episode of care, M1106, M1111, M1116, M1121, M1126, M1135
  ESRD documentation, G9231, M1187
  evaluation
    footwear, G2180
  exam
    dilated macula, G9892-G9893, G9974-G9977
  fall risk, M1069-M1070
  female unable to bear children, M1016
  filter placement/removal, G9539-G9544
  final treatment and evaluation, M1009-M1014
  follow up
    colon polyp, 10-year interval, G9862
    endovascular stroke intervention, G0045-G0046
    imaging, G9548-G9550, G9554-G9556, G9755
  food insecurity screening, M1207-M1208
  foot exam, G9225-G9226, G9502
  footwear evaluation, G8410, G8415-G8416
  fraility, G2090-G2091, G2098-G2101, G2106-G2107, G2109-G2110, G2115-G2116, G2118, G2125-G2127
  FS PROM, G9726-G9737, M1149
  functional outcome, G8539-G8543, G9227
  functional status, G2142-G2145, G9916-G9918, M1141
    ankle, foot, lower leg, G8655-G8658
    elbow, wrist or hand, G8667-G8670
    hip, G8651-G8654
    knee, G8647-G8650, M1045-M1046
    knee injury and osteoarthritis outcome score for joint replacement (KOOS, JR), M1141
    LEPF PROM, G8650, G8654, G8658, G9727, G9729, G9731
    low back, G8569-G8662
    neck, cranium or mandible, G2152, G2167
    not measured, G2210
    Oswestry Disability Index (ODI) measurement, G2142-G2145, M1043, M1049
    Oxford Knee Score (OKS), M1045, M1046, M1141
    shoulder, G8663-G8666
  gene mutation
    RAS (KRAS, NRAS), G9840-G9843
  HCV infection screening, G9383-G9386, G9451-G9454
  hearing loss, G8565, G8567
  heart transplant, M1150-M1151
  heart valve, mechanical prosthetic, G0043
  hemodialysis, G0049, G0052, G8956
    continuous catheter, G1026-G1027
  hepatitis B (HBV), G8869, G9504, G9912-G9913, G9915
  hepatocellular cancer screening (HCC), G9455-G9457
  HER2, G9830
  herpes zoster vaccination, M1174-M1176
  high intensity clinical services, G2020
  high risk medication, G9637-G9638, M1209-M1210

Quality Payment Program (QPP) — continued

HIV screening
  antigen/antibody combination assay, G0475
HIV-1 or HIV-2, G0432-G0433, G0435
home health agency (HHA) specimen collection, G0471
home health nursing visit, G0490
hospice, G0051, G9687-G9694, G9700, G9702, G9707, G9709-G9710, G9713-G9715, G9720, G9723, G9725, G9740-G9741, G9758, G9760-G9761, G9768, G9805, G9819, G9858-G9861, G9868-G9870, G9930, G9996, M1059, M1067, M1154, M1159, M1165, M1167, M1186, M1191
hospital readmission, G9309-G9310
housing instability screening, M1207-M1208
HPV
  test, G9806-G9807
  vaccine, G9762-G9763
hypercholesterolemia, G9782
hypertension, G8950-G8952, G9744-G9745
hysteroscopy, G9823-G9824
imaging documentation, G9357, G9457, G9550, G9753, M1027-M1029
immune checkpoint inhibitor therapy, M1180, M1183, M1185
immunocompromising conditions, M1158
immunosuppressant treatment, M1183-M1185
incidental findings, G9547, G9552, G9754
induction, G9361
inflammatory bowel disease (IBD), M1182
influenza vaccination, G8482-G8484, M1168-M1170
injection drug use, G9518
intensive care unit, G9853-G9854
interpersonal safety screening, M1207-M1208
interval and modality follow up, G9755
intervention, leak of endoluminal contents, G9305-G9306
intraoperative cystoscopy, G9606-G9608
itch assessment/rating scale, M1196-M1198, M1204-M1206
IV thrombolytic therapy/TPA, G8600-G8602
kidney care, M0002
kidney health evaluation, M1189-M1190
KRAS testing, G9840-G9841, G9843
left ventricular assist device (LVAD), M1151-M1152
left ventricular ejection fraction (LVEF), G8395-G8396, G8450-G8452, G8694, G8923, G8934, M1150
leg pain, G2140-G2141, G2146-G2147, M1052
LEPF PROM, G8650, G8654, G8658, G9727, G9729, G9731
limited life expectancy
  with catheter, G0050
lumbar spine
  related to
    cancer, fracture, infection, G9945
    idiopathic, congenital scoliosis, G9945
lung cancer screening, G0296
lymph node, G8878, G8880, G8882
mastectomy, G9708
mechanical prosthetic heart valve, G0043
medical visit, G0463, G9246-G9247
Medicare Capitated Payment (MCP), G1025
medication assisted treatment, G2067-G2080, G2112-G2113, M1034-M1035
medication list/review, G8427-G8430
melanoma, G8749, G8944
meningococcal vaccine, G9414-G9415
metastatic disease, G9838, G9842
MIPS specialty set, G0060-G0067, G4000-G4038
MIPS value pathways, G0053-G0059, M0001-M0005

Quality Payment Program (QPP) — continued

mitotic rate, G9292-G9294
mitral stenosis, G0044, G9746
modified Rankin scale (MRS), G0045-G0046, G9646-G9648
monitored anesthesia (MAC), G9654
monoclonal antibody therapy, G9839, G9844-G9845
neck impairment, M1143
neurodegenerative conditions, M0004
neurological conditions, G2151, M0003, M1107, M1112, M1117, M1122, M1127, M1131
neurological exam, G2178-G2179, G8404-G8405, G9529-G9533, G9594, G9646-G9648
nonambulatory patient, G9719, G9721, M1008
nonsmall cell lung cancer, G9418-G9425
numeric rating scale (NRS), M1196, M1204
nursing home resident, M1058
nursing services
  Christian science, journal-listed, per hour, S9901
  home health nursing visit, G0490
ongoing care, M1108-M1110, M1113-M1115, M1118-M1120, M1123-M1125, M1128-M1130, M1132-M1134, M1146-M1148
opioid therapy, G2172, M1032-M1036
oral systemic/biologic therapy, G9765
osteoporosis, G8635, G8863, G9769, M1153
otology referrals, G8559, G8561, G8563-G8564, G8566, G8568, G8856-G8858
P2Y12 antagonists, G9609-G9611
pain, G9949
  multimodal, G2148-G2150
palliative care, G0031, G0034, G0048, G9988, G9992-G9996, M1187
paranasal sinus CT
  more than once within 90 days of diagnosis, G9351-G9354
pathology, G9428-G9429, G9431, G9784-G9786, M1166
  performed by same biopsy clinician, G9939
  report, G9428-G9429, G9431, G9784-G9786, M1193-M1195
  second opinion, G9784
patient alive, G9787
patient care survey, G0914, G0917
patient caregiver, G2183-G2186
patient category, G9428-G9429, G9431
patient death, G9751, G9812-G9813, G9846, G9852, M1060
patient decision making, G9296-G9297
patient has at time of procedure
  lumbar spine cancer, M1037, M1041, M1051
  lumbar spine fracture, M1038, M1041, M1051
  lumbar spine infection, M1039, M1041, M1051
  scoliosis, M1040-M1041, M1051
patient health questionnaire (PHQ), G9393, G9395-G9396, G9509-G9511
patient participation, G2209
patient referred to another provider/clinician, G9968-G9970
patient survey score, G9603-G9605
patient-specific risk assessment, G9316-G9317
PCF model, G2020
PECARN prediction, G0047, G9593, G9597
pediatric head trauma, G9593, G9596-G9597
performance, G2150
peripheral nerve block (PNB), G9770
pharmacological therapy, G8633-G8635, M1032-M1036
PHQ-9/PHQ-9M score, G9393, G9395-G9396, G9509-G9511, M1019-M1020
physical therapy, G0040

Quality Payment Program (QPP) — continued

pneumococcal vaccine, G8864-G8867, G9279-G9280, G9991, M1177-M1179
  not administered, G9990
positive airway pressure, G8845, G8849-G8855
postoperative assessment, G9540
postpartum education, G9357-G9358
postpartum evaluation, G9357-G9358
postpartum screening, G9357-G9358
pregnancy documentation, G9231, G9997
pregnancy location, G8806
preoperative assessment, G9497
preoperative order, IV antibiotic, G8916-G8918
prolonged intubation, G8569-G8570
promoting wellness, M0005
proportion of days covered (PDC), G9512-G9513
prostate cancer, G8465, G9706
prosthetic heart valve, G9746
prosthetic implant, G9305
pschotherapy, M1199
psoriasis
  assessment, G9649, G9651
  treatment, G9764-G9765
psychiatric symptoms, G2121-G2122
RA, M1007-M1008
radiation exposure indices, G9500-G9501
recommended guidelines for incidental pulmonary nodule, G9345-G9347
reexploration, G8577-G8578
referral
  declined, G0041
  not referred, G0039
  not required, G0038
  physical, occupational, speech therapy, G0042
refraction, G9519-G9520
remission (PHQ-9 score), G9509-G9511
renal failure, G8575-G8576, G9722
renal transplant documentation, G9231
rendering treatment in place, G2021-G2022
respiratory, G8842-G8846, G8849-G8855
retinopathy, G8397
return to the operating room, G9307-G9308, G9514-G9515
rhabdomyolysis, G9780
risk adjusted functional status, G8648-G8670
risk factor
  evaluation, G8648-G8674
  postoperative vomiting, G9954
risk score
  CHA2DS2-VASc, G9931
RRT, M1199
safety concerns, G9922-G9926
screening, G9919-G9921
  alcohol use, G9624
  colonoscopy, G2204
  delays, children, G9968
  mammography, G8899-G9900
  tobacco use, G0030, G9902-G9905
search for patient prior imaging studies, G9341-G9344
sexual activity, G9818
sexually transmitted disease, G9228-G9230
silicone oil use, surgical procedures, G9756-G9757
sinusitis
  caused by bacterial infection, G9364
skilled nursing facility (SNF) specimen collection, G0471
sleep apnea, G8839-G8855
special needs plans (SNP)
  institutional, G2081, G2105, G2108, G9898, G9901, G9910, G9938
specimen site, G8797-G8798, G9295, G9430
spirometry, G8924
squamous cell carcinoma, M1192
standard nomenclature for imaging study, G9318-G9319

Quality Payment Program (QPP) — continued

statin therapy, G8815-G8817, G9507-G9508, G9663-G9665, G9675-G9676, G9781, G9796-G9797, G9940
stroke/CVA/TIA, G0045-G0046, G9580-G9582, G9766-G9767
surgical site infection, G9311-G9312
TB screening, M1003-M1006
Td vaccination, M1171-M1173
test, gene mutation, G9840-G9841
tetanus, diphtheria, pertussis vaccine (Tdap), G9416-G9417
thromboembolism risk factor, G8970
thyroid, G9552-G9553, G9557
tobacco use, G0030, G9275-G9276, G9458-G9460, G9642, G9644-G9645, G9791-G9792, G9902-G9908
transfer
  anesthetizing location to PACU/non-ICU, G9656
transfer of care protocol, G9655-G9658
transportation needs screening, M1207-M1208
tumor, G8721-G8724
ulcerative colitis, M1182
ultrasound, G8806-G8808
urgent care, M1021, M1054
URI, G2173-G2174
utility difficulties screening, M1207-M1208
vaccination, G9279-G9281, G9762-G9763
viral load, G9242-G9243
visit complexity, G2211
visual acuity, G9516-G9517
visual analog scale (VAS), G2136-G2141, G2146-G2147, G9949, M1052
visual function, G0913, G0915
visual rating scale (VRS), M1196, M1204
volume management, G8955, G8958
well-child visit, G9964-G9965
wheelchair evaluation, G9156

Quick Check blood glucose test strips, box of 50, A4253
Quick release restraints, E0700
Quikfit crutch, E0114
Quik-Fold Walkers, E0141, E0143

R

Rack/stand, oxygen, E1355
Radiation
  compensator based, G6016
  intensity modulated, G6015
  intrafraction, G6017
  treatment delivery
    single area
      11-19mev, G6005
      20mev or greater, G6006
      6-10mev, G6004
      up to 5mev, G6003
    three or more areas
      11-19mev, G6013
      20mev or greater, G6014
      6-10mev, G6012
      up to 5mev, G6011
    two separate areas
      11-19mev, G6009
      20mev or greater, G6010
      6-10mev, G6008
      up to 5mev, G6007
Radiation dosimeter, implantable, ea, A4650
Radiation Oncology Model, M1072-M1105
Radioelements for brachytherapy, Q3001
Radiofrequency
  radiofrequency transmitter, sacral root neurostimulator, replacement, L8684
Radioimmunoscintigraphy, S8080
Radiolabeled product provided during inpatient stay, C9898
Radiology service, R0070-R0076
Radiopharmaceutical
  ammonia N-13, A9526
  chromic phosphate P-32, A9564
  cyanocobalamin cobalt Co-57, A9559
  diagnostic imaging agent, A4641, A4642, A9597-A9598, A9604

Radiopharmaceutical — *continued*
  gallium Ga-67, A9556
  gallium Ga-68, dotatate, A9587
  gallium Ga-68, dotatoc, C9067
  gallium Ga-68 PSMA-11, A9593-A9594
  indium I-111
    ibitumomab tiuxetan, A9542
    pentreotide, A9572
    satumomab pendetide, A4642
  inpatient, C9898
  nontumor identification, A9598
  not otherwise classified, A9597-A9598, A9699
  PET, diagnostic, A9597-A9598
  radium Ra-223 dichloride, A9606
  rubidium Rb-82, A9555
  sodium
    fluoride F-18, diagnostic, A9580
    iodide I-131, A9528-A9531
    phosphate, A9563
  technetium Tc-99m
    arcitumomab, A9568
    bicisate, A9557
    depreotide, A9536
    disofenin, A9510
    exametazime, A9521, A9569
    fanolesomab, A9566
    glucepatate, A9550
    labeled red blood cells, A9560
    macroaggregated albumin, A9540
    mebrofenin, A9537
    medronate, A9503
    mertiatide, A9562
    oxidronate, A9561
    pentetate, A9539, A9567
    pertechnetate, A9512
    sestamibi, A9500
    sulfur colloid, A9541
    teboroxime, A9501
    tetrofosmin, A9502
    tilmanocept, A9520
  therapeutic, A9517, A9543, A9600, A9604
  tumor identification, PET, A9597
  xenon Xe-133, A9558
  yttrium Y-90 ibritumomab tiuxetan, A9543
Rail
  bathtub, E0241, E0242, E0246
  bed, E0305, E0310
  toilet, E0243
Rancho hip action, hip orthotic, L1680
Range of motion device
  elbow, hand, wrist, L8702
  shoulder, E1841
Rascal, power wheelchair, K0010
Ready-For-Use wooden crutches, E0113
Reassessment, nutrition therapy, G0270-G0271
Receiver
  interstitial glucose monitor, A9278
Recombinant
  ankle splints, L4392-L4398
  DNA insulin, J1815, J1817
Reconstruction
  breast, S2066-S2067
Rectal control system, A4563
Rectal enema system
  catheter, A4453
Red blood cells, P9038-P9040
Red blood cells, each unit, P9021, P9022
Red Dot
  crutches, E0114
  folding walkers, E0135, E0143
REGUaRD, Q4255
Regulator, oxygen, E1353
Rehabilitation
  intensive cardiac, G0422-G0423
  program, H2001
  pulmonary program, S9473
  service
    juveniles, H2033
    mental health clubhouse, H2030-H2031
    psychosocial, H2017-H2018
    social work and psychological, G0409
    substance abuse, H2034-H2036
    supported employment, H2023-H2024

Rehabilitation — *continued*
  vestibular, S9476
Relese, Q4257
Remote patient monitoring, G0323
Removal
  applicator, breast, C9726
  corns/calluses, S0390
  impacted cerumen, G0268
  soft interspace, K0672
  sutures, S0630
RemRes, E0601
REMStar, E0601
Renacidin, Q2004
RenAmin, parenteral nutrition, B5000
Renu, enteral nutrition, B4150
Repair
  contract, ERSD, A4890
  DME, K0739
    oxygen, K0740
  fetal
    congenital malformation NOC, S2409
    cystic adenomatoid malformation, S2402
    extralobar pulmonary sequestration, S2403
    myelomeningocele, S2404
    sacrococcygeal teratoma, S2405
    urinary tract, S2401
  hearing aid, V5014, V5336
  hernia
    diaphragmatic
      fetus, S2400
  home dialysis equipment, A4890
  orthotic, L4000-L4130
  prosthetic, L7510, L7520
Replacement
  battery, A4233-A4236, A4630
    ear pulse generator, A4638
    external infusion pump, K0601-K0605
  cardioverter-defibrillator system, G0448
  handgrip for cane, crutch, walker, A4636
  oral cushion, A7028
  ostomy filters, A4421
  sleeve, intermittent limb compression device, A4600
  tip for cane, crutch, walker, A4637
  underarm pad for crutch, A4635
Rep-Pred
  40, J1030
  80, J1040
Repriza, Q4143
ResCap headgear, A7035
Reservoir
  metered dose inhaler, A4627
Residential care, T2032-T2033
ResMed Sb Elite, E0601
Resource-intensive services
  mobility-assistive technology, G0501
Respiratory therapy, G0237-G0238
  home, S5180-S5181
Respite care, T1005
  in home, S9125
  not in home, H0045
Restorative
  injection
    face, G0429
Restorigin (fluid), Q4192
Restorigin, Q4191
Restraint
  any type, E0710
  belts
    Posey, E0700
    Secure-All, E0700
  Bite disposable jaw locks, E0700
  body holders
    Houdini security suit, E0700
    Quick Release, one piece, E0700
    Secure-All, one piece, E0700
    System2 zippered, E0700
    UltraCare vest-style
      with sleeves, E0700
  hand
    Secure-All finger control mitt, E0700
  limb holders
    Posey, E0700

Restraint — *continued*
  limb holders — *continued*
    Quick Release, E0700
    Secure-All, E0700
  pelvic
    Secure-All, E0700
Restrata, A2007
Resurfacing
  total hip, S2118
Retail therapy item, miscellaneous, T1999
Retinal
  device, intraoperative, C1784
  exam for diabetes, S3000
  prosthesis
    accessory/component/supply, L8608
  tamponade, C1814
Retinoblastoma, genetic test, S3841
Retrieval device, insertable, C1773
Revascularization, endovascular
  femoral, popliteal artery(ies), C7531, C7534-C7535
  intravascular lithotripsy, C9764, C9772
    catheter, transluminal, C1761
    with atherectomy, C9766, C9774
    with atherectomy and stent placement, C9767, C9775
    with stent placement, C9765, C9773
Revascularization, percutaneous transluminal, C9604-C9608
Revita, Q4180
Revitalon, Q4157
Rib belt
  thoracic, L0220
Rice ankle splint, L1904
Richfoam convoluted & flat overlays, E0199
Ride Lite 200, Ride Lite 9000, manual wheelchair, K0004
Ring, ostomy, A4404
Riveton, foot orthotic, L3140, L3150
RN services, T1002
Road Savage power wheelchair, K0011
Road Warrior power wheelchair, K0011
Robotic surgical system, S2900
Rocking bed, E0462
Rollabout chair, E1031
Rubidium RB-82, A9555
Rural health clinic (RHC)
  behavioral health integration services, G0511
  chronic care management services, G0511
  psychiatric COCM services, G0512
  technology based services, G0071

S

Sabre power wheelchair, K0011
Sacral nerve stimulation test
  lead, each, A4290
Sacroiliac
  injection, G0259-G0260
  orthotic, L0621-L0624
Safe, hand prosthesis, L5972
Safety
  enclosure frame/canopy, for hospital bed, E0316
  equipment, E0700
  eyeglass frames, S0516
  vest, wheelchair, E0980
Saline, A4216-A4217
  hypertonic, J7131
  solution, J7030-J7050
Saliva
  artificial, A9155
Saliva test, hormone level
  during menopause, S3650
  preterm labor risk, S3652
Sam Brown, Legg Perthes orthotic, A4565
Sansibar Plus, E0601
Saquinavir, S0140
Satumomab pendetide, A4642
Scale, for dialysis, E1639
Schuco
  mist nebulizer system, E0570
  vac aspirator, E0600
Scintimammography, S8080
Scleral application tantalum rings, S8030
Scleral lens bandage, S0515

Scoliosis, L1000, L1200, L1300-L1499
  additions, L1010-L1120, L1210-L1290
Scott ankle splint, canvas, L1904
Scott-Craig, stirrup orthotic, L2260
Scottish-Rite, Legg Perthes orthotic, L1730
Screening
  alcohol and/or drug, G0442, H0049
  cervical or vaginal, G0101, G0476
  Chlamydia, gonorrhea, syphilis, G9228-G9230
  colorectal cancer, G0104-G0106, G0120-G0122, G0327-G0328
  cytopathology, G0123-G0124, G0141, G0143-G0148
  depression, G0444
  early periodic screening diagnosis and treatment (EPSDT), S0302
  glaucoma, G0117-G0118
  gynecological
    established patient, S0612
    new patient, S0610
  hepatitis B
    non-pregnant, high-risk individual, G0499
  hepatitis C antibody, high risk, G0472
  HIV
    antigen/antibody combination assay, G0475
    HIV-1 or HIV-2, G0432-G0433, G0435
  lung cancer
    counseling visit to discuss CT screening, G0296
  newborn metabolic, S3620
  ophthalmological, including refraction
    established patient, S0621
    new patient, S0620
  pneumococcal, G9279
  preadmission, T2010-T2011
  proctoscopy, S0601
  program participation, T1023
  prostate
    digital, rectal, G0102
    prostate specific antigen test (PSA), G0103
    vaccination not given, G9281
Seal, prosthetic socket insert, L7700
Sealant
  pulmonary, liquid, C2615
  skin, A6250
Seat
  attachment, walker, E0156
  insert, wheelchair, E0992
  lift (patient), E0621, E0627-E0629
  positioning, T5001
  power system, wheelchair, E1002-E1012
Seattle Carbon Copy II, foot prosthesis, L5976
Secure-All
  restraints, E0700
  universal pelvic traction belt, E0890
Sedation, moderate, G0500
Sensitivity study, P7001
Sensor
  invasive blood glucose monitor, A9276
  pulmonary artery, wireless, C2624
Sensory nerve conduction test, G0255
Septal defect implant system, C1817
Sermorelin acetate, Q0515
Serum clotting time tube, A4771
Service assessment, T2024
Services
  attendant, S5125-S5126
  behavioral, H2019-H2020
    prescription digital therapy, A9291
    remote diagnosis, evaluation, treatment, C7900-C7902
  by Christian Science practitioner, S9900-S9901
  chore services, S5120-S5121
  community support, H2015-H2016
  community-based wrap-around, H2021-H2022
  facility
    dental procedure requiring monitored anesthesia, G0330
  homemaker services, S5130-S5131
  laundry, S5175
  Medicare IVIG demonstration, Q2052

Services

Services — continued
  medication reminder, S5185
  provided outside USA, S9989
  psychoeducational, H2027
  remote diagnosis, evaluation, treatment
    mental health/substance abuse,
    C7900-C7902
  sexual offender treatment, H2028-H2029
SEWHO, L3960-L3962
Sexa, G0130
Sheath
  introducer
    guiding, C1766, C1892, C1893
    other than guiding, C1894, C2629
Sheepskin pad, E0188, E0189
Shoes
  arch support, L3040-L3100
  for diabetics, A5500-A5508, A5510, A5512-A5513
  insert, L3000-L3030
    for diabetics, A5512-A5513
  lift, L3300-L3334
  miscellaneous additions, L3500-L3595
  orthopedic (see Orthopedic shoes), L3201-L3265
  positioning device, L3140-L3170
  post-operative
    Specialist Health/Post Operative Shoe, A9270
  transfer, L3600-L3649
  wedge, L3340-L3485
Shoulder
  abduction positioner, L3999
  arthroscopy, C9781, S2300
  braces, L3999
    Masterhinge Shoulder Brace 3, L3999
  disarticulation, prosthetic, L6300-L6320, L6550
  orthotic (SO), L3650-L3677
  spinal, cervical, L0112
Shoulder-elbow-wrist-hand orthotic (SEWHO), L3960-L3978
Shower chair, E0240
Shunt accessory for dialysis, A4740
  aqueous, L8612
Shunt, interatrial
  NYHA IDE study, C9760
Sickle cell anemia, genetic test, S3850
Sierra wrist flexion unit, L6805
Sigmoidoscopy, cancer screening, G0104, G0106
Sign language or oral interpreter services, T1013
Signature APatch, Q4260
Sildenafil citrate, S0090
Silenzio Elite, E0601
Single bar "AK," ankle-foot orthotic, L2000, L2010
Single bar "BK," ankle-foot orthotic, L1980
Sinus
  sinus implant
    Mometasone, J7402
    Propel, S1091
Sitz bath, E0160-E0162
Skilled nurse, G0128, G0493-G0496
Skin
  barrier, ostomy, A4362, A4369, A4385
  bond or cement, ostomy, A4364
  gel protective dressing wipes, A5120
  sealant, protectant, moisturizer, A6250
Skin substitute, Q4100-Q4264
  Affinity, Q4159
  AlloDerm, Q4116
  AlloGen, Q4212
  AlloPatch HD, Q4128
  AlloSkin, Q4115
  AlloSkin AC, Q4141
  AlloSkin RT, Q4123
  AlloWrap DS, Q4150
  AltiPly, Q4235
  Amnio Bio, Q4211
  AmnioAmp-MP, Q4250
  AmnioArmor, Q4188
  AmnioBand, Q4151, Q4168
  AmnioBind, Q4225
  AmnioCore, Q4227

Skin substitute — continued
  AmnioCyte Plus, Q4242
  AmnioExcel, AmnioExcel Plus, Q4137
  AmnioMatrix, Q4139
  Amnio-Maxx, Q4239
  Amnio-Maxx Lite, Q4239
  AmnioPro, Q4163
  AmnioPro Flow, Q4162
  AMNIOREPAIR, Q4235
  AmnioText, Q4245
  Amniotext patch, Q4247
  AmnioWound, Q4181
  AmnioWrap2, Q4221
  AMNIPLY, Q4249
  Apis, A2010
  Apligraf, Q4101
  Architect, Architect PX, or Architect FX, Q4147
  Artacent AC (fluid), Q4189
  Artacent AC, Q4190
  Artacent Cord, Q4216
  Artacent Wound, Q4169
  ArthroFlex, Q4125
  Ascent, Q4213
  AxoBioMembrane, Q4211
  Axolotl Ambient, Axolotl Cryo, Q4215
  Axolotl Graft, Axolotl DualGraft, Q4210
  BellaCell HD, Q4220
  bio-ConneKt Wound Matrix, Q4161
  BioDExcel, Q4137
  BioDFence, Q4140
  BioDFence DryFlex, Q4138
  BioDMatrix, Q4139
  BioSkin, Q4163
  BioSkin Flow, Q4162
  Biovance, Q4154
  BioWound, BioWound Plus, BioWound Xplus, Q4217
  Celera Dual Layer, Dual Membrane, Q4259
  Cellesta, Cellesta Duo, Q4184
  Cellesta Cord, Q4214
  Cellesta Flowable Amnion, Q4185
  Clarix 100, Q4156
  Clarix Cord, Q4148
  Clarix Flo, Q4155
  Cocoon Membrane, Q4264
  Cogenex Amniotic Membrane, Q4229
  Cogenex Flowable Amnion, Q4230
  Coll-e-Derm, Q4193
  CoreCyte, Q4240
  CoreText, Q4246
  Corplex, Q4232
  Corplex P, Q4231
  Cryo-Cord, Q4237
  Cygnus, Q4170, Q4199
  Cymetra, Q4112
  Cytal, Q4166
  DermACELL, DermACELL AWM, DermACELL AWM Porous, Q4122
  Dermacyte Amniotic Membrane Allograft, Q4248
  Derma-Gide, Q4203
  Dermagraft, Q4106
  DermaPure, Q4152
  DermaSpan, Q4126
  Dermavest, Q4153
  Derm-Maxx, Q4238
  Dual Layer Impax Membrane, Q4262
  Enverse, Q4258
  EpiCord, Q4187
  EpiFix (injectable), Q4145
  EpiFix, Q4186
  Excellagen, Q4149
  EZ-Derm, Q4136
  Flex HD, Q4128
  FlowerAmnioFlo, Q4177
  FlowerAmnioPatch, Q4178
  FlowerDerm, Q4179
  Fluid Flow, Fluid GF, Q4206
  GammaGraft, Q4111
  Genesis Amniotic Membrane, Q4198
  Grafix Core, GrafixPL Core, Q4132
  Grafix Prime, GrafixPL Prime, Q4133
  GRAFTJACKET, Q4107
  GRAFTJACKET XPRESS, Q4113
  Guardian, Q4151

Skin substitute — continued
  Helicoll, Q4164
  hMatrix, Q4134
  Human Health Factor 10 Amniotic Patch (HHF10-P), Q4224
  Hyalomatrix, Q4117
  InnovaMatrix AC, A2001
  InnovaMatrix FS, A2013
  Integra
    Bilayer Matrix Wound Dressing, Q4104
    Dermal Regeneration Template, Q4105
    Flowable, Q4114
    Matrix, Q4108
    Meshed Bilayer Wound Matrix, C9363
    MOZAIK Osteoconductive Scaffold Putty, C9359
    MOZAIK Osteoconductive Scaffold Strip, C9362
  InteguPLY, Q4126
  Interfyl, Q4171
  Keramatrix, Kerasorb, Q4165
  Kerecis Omega3, Q4158
  Keroxx, Q4202
  low cost, application of, C5271-C5278
  Matrion, Q4201
  MatriStem, Q4118
  Mediskin, Q4135
  Membrane Graft, Membrane Wrap, Q4205
  MemoDerm, Q4126
  Microlyte, A2005
  Miroderm, Q4175
  Mirragen, A2002
  MLG-Complete, Q4256
  MyOwn Skin, Q4226
  NeoPatch, Q4176
  Neox 100, Q4156
  Neox 1K, Neox Cord 1K, Neox Cord RT, Q4148
  Neox Flo, Q4155
  NovaFix, Q4208
  NovaFix DL, Q4254
  NovoSorb SynPath, A2006
  NuDyn, Q4233
  NuShield, Q4160
  Oasis
    Burn Matrix, Q4103
    Ultra Tri-Layer Matrix, Q4124
    Wound Matrix, Q4102
  Omeza Collagen Matrix, A2014
  PalinGen or PalinGen XPlus, Q4173
  PalinGen or ProMatrX (fluid), Q4174
  PermeaDerm B, A2016
  PermeaDerm C, A2018
  PermeaDerm glove, A2017
  Phoenix Wound Matrix, A2015
  Plurivest, Q4153
  PolyCyte, Q4241
  PriMatrix, Q4110
  Procenta, Q4244
  ProgenaMatrix, Q4222
  ProText, Q4246
  PuraPly, PuraPly AM, PuraPly XT, Q4195-Q4197
  REGUaRD, Q4255
  Relese, Q4257
  Repriza, Q4143
  Restorigin (fluid), Q4192
  Restorigin, Q4191
  Restrata, A2007
  Revita, Q4180
  Revitalon, Q4157
  Signature Apatch, Q4260
  Skin substitute, FDA cleared as a device, NOS, A4100
  SkinTE, Q4200
  Strattice, Q4130
  Stravix, StravixPL, Q4133
  Supra SDRM, Q4011
  SUPRATHEL, A2012
  SureDerm, Q4220
  SurFactor, Q4233
  SurgiCORD, Q4218
  SurgiGRAFT, Q4183

Skin substitute — continued
  SurgiGRAFT-Dual, Q4219
  SurgiMend, C9358
  SurGraft, Q4209
  SurGraft TL, Q4263
  Symphony, A2009
  TAG, Q4261
  Talymed, Q4127
  Tensix, Q4146
  TheraGenesis, A2008
  TheraSkin, Q4121
  Therion, Q4176
  TranCyte, Q4182
  TranZgraft, Q4126
  TruSkin, Q4167
  Vendaje, Q4252
  Vim, Q4251
  WoundEx, Q4163
  WoundEx Flow, Q4162
  WoundFix, WoundFix Plus, WoundFix Xplus, Q4217
  XCellerate, Q4234
  XCelliStem, A2004
  XCM Biologic Tissue Matrix, Q4142
  XWRAP, Q4204
  Zenith Amniotic Membrane, Q4253
SkinTE, Q4200
Sleep apnea treatment, K1001
Sleep study
  home, G0398-G0400
Sleeve
  intermittent limb compression device, A4600
  irrigation, A4436-A4437
  mastectomy, L8010
Sling, A4565
  axilla, L1010
  Legg Perthes, A4565
  lumbar, L1090
  patient lift, E0621, E0630, E0635
  pelvic, L2580
  Sam Brown, A4565
  trapezius, L1070
Smoking cessation
  classes, S9453
  counseling, G9016
SNCT, G0255
Social worker
  CORF, G0409
  home health setting, G0155
  nonemergency transport, A0160
  visit in home, S9127
Sock
  body sock, L0984
  prosthetic sock, L8420-L8435, L8480, L8485
  stump sock, L8470-L8485
Sodium
  chromate Cr-51, A9553
  ferric gluconate in sucrose, J2916
  iothalamate I-125, A9554
  sodium iodide I-131
    diagnostic imaging agent, A9528, A9531
    therapeutic agent, A9530
  succinate, J1720
Soft Touch II lancet device, A4258
Soft Touch lancets, box of 100, A4259
Softclix lancet device, A4258
Solo Cast Sole, L3540
Solo LX, E0601
Solution
  calibrator, A4256
  dialysate, A4728, A4760
  enteral formulae, B4150-B4155
  parenteral nutrition, B4164-B5200
S.O.M.I. brace, L0190, L0200
S.O.M.I. multiple-post collar, cervical orthotic, L0190
Sorbent cartridge, ESRD, E1636
Sorbsan, alginate dressing, A6196-A6198
Source
  brachytherapy
    gold 198, C1716
    iodine 125, C2638-C2639
    non-high dose rate iridium 192, C1719

Source — continued
  brachytherapy — continued
    palladium-103, C2640-C2641, C2645
    yttrium 90, C2616
Spacer
  interphalangeal joint, L8658
Specialist Ankle Foot Orthotic, L1930
Specialist Closed-Back Cast Boot, L3260
Specialist Gaitkeeper Boot, L3260
Specialist Health/Post Operative Shoe, A9270
Specialist Heel Cups, L3485
Specialist Insoles, L3510
Specialist J-Splint Plaster Roll Immobilizer, A4580
Specialist Open-Back Cast Boot, L3260
Specialist Plaster Bandages, A4580
Specialist Plaster Roll Immobilizer, A4580
Specialist Plaster Splints, A4580
Specialist Pre-Formed Humeral Fracture Brace, L3980-L3981
Specialist Pre-Formed Ulnar Fracture Brace, L3982
Specialist Tibial Pre-formed Fracture Brace, L2116
Specialist Toe Insert for Specialist Closed-Back Cast Boot and Specialist Health/Post Operative Shoe, A9270
Specialized mobility technology
  resource-intensive services, G0501
Specialty absorptive dressing, A6251-A6256
Specimen, G9291, G9295
  Collection, C9803, G2023-G2024
Spectacles, S0504-S0510, S0516-S0518
  dispensing, S0595
Speech and language pathologist
  home health setting, G0153
Speech assessment, V5362-V5364
  speech generating device
    software, E2511
    supplies, E2500-E2599
Speech generating device, E2500
Speech therapy, S9128, S9152
Speech volume modulation system, K1009
Spenco shoe insert, foot orthotic, L3001
Sperm
  aspiration, S4028
  donor service, S4025
  sperm procurement, S4026, S4030-S4031
Sphygmomanometer/blood pressure, A4660
Spinal orthotic
  Boston type, L1200
  cervical, L0112, L0180-L0200
  cervical-thoracic-lumbar-sacral orthotic (CTLSO), L0700, L0710, L1000
  halo, L0810-L0830
  Milwaukee, L1000
  multiple post collar, L0180-L0200
  scoliosis, L1000, L1200, L1300-L1499
  torso supports, L0970-L0999
Spirometer
  electronic, E0487
  nonelectronic, A9284
Splint
  ankle, L4392-L4398, S8451
  digit, prefabricated, S8450
  dynamic, E1800, E1805, E1810, E1815
  elbow, S8452
  finger, static, Q4049
  footdrop, L4398
  hallus valgus, L3100
  long arm, Q4017-Q4020
  long leg, L4370, Q4041-Q4044
  pneumatic, L4350, L4360, L4370
  short arm, Q4021-Q4024
  short leg, Q4045-Q4048
  Specialist Plaster Splints, A4580
  supplies, Q4051
  Thumb-O-Prene Splint, L3999
  toad finger, A4570
  wrist, S8451
Spoke protectors, each, K0065
Sports supports hinged knee support, L1832
Standing frame system, E0638, E0641-E0642
Star Lumen tubing, A4616
Stat
  laboratory request, S3600-S3601

Sten, foot prosthesis, L5972
Stent
  coated
    with delivery system, C1874
    without delivery system, C1875
    with delivery system, C1876
    without delivery system, C1877
  noncoronary
    temporary, C2617, C2625
    with delivery system, S1091
Stent placement
  intracoronary, C9600-C9601
    with percutaneous transluminal coronary atherectomy, C9602-C9603
Stereotactic guidance
  breast biopsies, C7501
Stereotactic radiosurgery
  therapy, G0339, G0340
Sterile water, A4216-A4218
Stimulated intrauterine insemination, S4035
Stimulation
  electrical, E0740, G0281-G0283
    acupuncture, S8930
    tongue, K1028-K1029
  electromagnetic, G0295
  electrotherapy, K1002
    supplies/accessories, A4596
Stimulators
  cough, device, E0482
  electric, supplies, A4595
  external upper limb tremor
    wrist, K1018-K1019
  interferential current, S8130-S8131
  joint, E0762
  neuromuscular, E0744, E0745, E0764
  osteogenesis, electrical, E0747-E0749
  pelvic floor, E0740
  salivary reflex, E0755
  transcutaneous, E0770
    distal nerve, K1023
    trigeminal nerve, K1016-K1017
  ultrasound, E0760
  vagus nerve, noninvasive, K1020
Stocking
  gradient compression, A6530-A6549
Stoma
  cap, A5055
  catheter, A5082
  cone, A4399
  plug, A5081
Stomach tube, B4083
Stomahesive
  skin barrier, A4362, A5122
  sterile wafer, A4362
  strips, A4362
Storm Arrow power wheelchair, K0014
Storm Torque power wheelchair, K0011
Strattice, Q4130
Stravix, StravixPL, Q4133
Stress management class, S9454
Stretch device, E1801, E1811, E1816, E1818, E1831, E1841
Strip(s)
  blood, A4253
  glucose test, A4253, A4772
  Nu-Hope
    adhesive, 1 oz bottle with applicator, A4364
    adhesive, 3 oz bottle with applicator, A4364
  urine reagent, A4250
Study
  gastrointestinal fat absorption, S3708
  sleep, G0398-G0400
Stump sock, L8470-L8485
Stylet, A4212
Submucosal dissection, endoscopic (ESD), C9779
Substance abuse, misuse
  ambulatory settings, S9475
  assessment, G2011
  other than tobacco, G0396-G0397
  remote diagnosis, evaluation, treatment, C7900-C7902

Substance abuse, misuse — continued
  treatment, T1006-T1012
Suction
  respiratory, E0600
  urine management, K1006
  wound, A9272, K0743
Sulfamethoxazole and trimethoprim, S0039
Sullivan
  CPAP, E0601
Sumacal, enteral nutrition, B4155
Sunbeam moist/dry heat pad, E0215
Sunglass frames, S0518
Supplies
  infection control NOS, S8301
  insulin pump, external, A4226
  Medicare IVIG demonstration, Q2052
  miscellaneous DME, A9999
  ventricular assist device, Q0477, Q0507-Q0509
Supply allowance
  continuous glucose monitor, A4238-A4239, E2103
Supply fee
  pharmacy
    anticancer oral antiemetic or immunosuppressive drug, Q0511-Q0512
    immunosuppressive drugs, Q0510
Supply/accessory/service, A4436-A4437, A9900
Support
  arch, L3040-L3090
  cervical, L0120
  elastic, A6530-A6549
  ongoing to maintain employment, H2025-H2026
  spinal, L0970-L0999
  vaginal, A4561-A4562
Supported housing, H0043-H0044
Supportive device
  foot pressure off loading, A9283
Supports brokerage, self-directed, T2051
Supra SDRM, A2011
SUPRATHEL, A2012
Supreme bG Meter, E0607
SureDerm, Q4220
Sure-Gait folding walker, E0141, E0143
Sure-Safe raised toilet seat, E0244
SureStep blood glucose monitor, E0607
SurFactor, Q4233
Sur-Fit
  closed-end pouch, A5054
  disposable convex inserts, A5093
  drainable pouch, A5063
  flange cap, A5055
  irrigation sleeve, A4436-A4437
  urostomy pouch, A5073
Sur-Fit/Active Life tail closures, A4421
Surgical
  arthroscopy
    knee, G0289, S2112
    shoulder, C9781, S2300
  boot, L3208-L3211
  mask, for dialysis, A4928
  procedure, return/no return to OR, G9307-G9308
  site infection, G9311-G9312
  stocking, A4490-A4510
  supplies, miscellaneous, A4649
  tray, A4550
SurgiCORD, Q4218
SurgiGRAFT, Q4183
SurgiGRAFT-Dual, Q4219
SurgiMend, fetal bovine, C9358
SurgiMend, neonatal bovine, C9360
SurGraft, Q4209
SurGraft TL, Q4263
Suspension
  autograft, C1832
Sustacal, enteral nutrition, B4150
  HC, B4152
Sustagen Powder, enteral nutrition, B4150
Swabs, betadine or iodine, A4247
Swede, ACT, Cross, or Elite manual wheelchair, K0005
Swede Basic F# manual wheelchair, K0004
Swedish knee orthotic, L1850

Swivel adaptor, S8186
Symphony, A2009
Syringe, A4213
  dialysis, A4657
  insulin, box of 100, S8490
  with needle, A4206-A4209
System2 zippered body holder, E0700

T

Table
  bed, E0274, E0315
  sit-to-stand, E0637
  standing, E0637-E0638, E0641-E0642
Tablo dialysis system, E1629
Tachdijan, Legg Perthes orthotic, L1720
TAG, Q4261
Talymed, Q4127
Tamoxifen citrate, S0187
Tamponade
  retinal, C1814
Tantalum rings scleral application, S8030
Tape
  nonwaterproof, A4450
  waterproof, A4452
Taxi, nonemergency transportation, A0100
Tc-99 from non-highly enriched uranium, Q9969
Team conference, G0175, G9007, S0220-S0221
TechneScan, A9512
Technetium Tc 99
  arcitumomab, A9568
  biscate, A9557
  depreotide, A9536
  disofenin, A9510
  exametazime, A9521, A9569
  fanolesomab, A9566
  glucepatate, A9550
  labeled red blood cells, A9560
  macroaggregated albumin, A9540
  mebrofenin, A9537
  medronate, A9503
  mertiatide, A9562
  oxidronate, A9561
  pentetate, A9539, A9567
  pertechnetate, A9512
  pyrophosphate, A9538
  sestamibi, A9500
  succimer, A9551
  sulfur colloid, A9541
  teboroxime, A9501
  tetrofosmin, A9502
  tilmanocept, A9520
Technol
  Colles splint, L3763
  wrist and forearm splint, L3906
Technology based services
  FQHC or RHC, G0071
Telehealth
  brief communication, technology based, G2251-G2252
  consultation
    emergency department, G0425-G0427
    inpatient, G0406-G0408, G0425-G0427
  critical care, G0508-G0509
  facility fee, Q3014
  home health services, G0320-G0321
  inpatient pharmacologic management, G0459
  transmission, T1014
Telemonitoring
  patient in home, includes equipment, S9110
Television
  amplifier, V5270
  caption decoder, V5271
TenderCloud electric air pump, E0182
TenderFlo II, E0187
TenderGel II, E0196
Tenderlet lancet device, A4258
TenoGlide Tendon Protector Sheet, C9356
TENS, A4595, E0720-E0749
  Neuro-Pulse, E0720
Tensix, Q4146
Tent, oxygen, E0455

Terminal devices, L6703-L6715, L6721-L6722
Terumo disposable insulin syringes, up to 1 cc, per syringe, A4206
Test materials, home monitoring, G0249
Testing
  comparative genomic hybridization, S3870
  Coronavirus (2019-nCoV) diagnostic panel, U0001-U0002
    with High throughput technologies, U0003-U0004
  developmental, G0451
  drug, G0480-G0483, G0659
  genetic, S3800, S3840-S3842, S3844-S3846, S3849-S3850, S3852-S3853, S3861
  Warfarin responsiveness, genetic technique, G9143
Thalassemia, genetic test
  alpha, S3845
  hemoglobin E beta, S3846
Thallous chloride TI 201, A9505
TheraGenesis, A2008
Therapeutic
  agent, A4321
  procedures, respiratory, G0239
Therapeutic radiopharmaceutical
  sodium iodide I-131, A9530
Therapy
  activity, G0176, H2032
  beta-blocker, G9188-G9192
  convulsive, G2000
  infusion, Q0081
  lymphedema, S8950
  nutrition, reassessment, G0270-G0271
  prescription digital behavior, A9291
  respiratory, G0237-G0239
  transcatheter microinfusion, C9759
TheraSkin, Q4121
Therion, Q4176
Thermalator T-12-M, E0239
Thermometer
  oral, A4931
  rectal, A4932
Thickener, food, B4100
Thinning solvent, NuHope, 2 oz bottle, A4455
Thomas
  heel wedge, foot orthotic, L3465, L3470
Thoracic-lumbar-sacral orthotic (TLSO)
  flexible with trunk support, L0450-L0457
  sagittal control, L0466-L0467
  sagittal-coronal control, L0468-L0469, L0490-L0492
  scoliosis, L1200-L1290
  triplanar control, L0458-L0464, L0470-L0488
Threshold
  current perception, G0255
Thumb-O-Prene Splint, L3999
Thymol turbidity, blood, P2033
Thyroidectomy
  with parathyroid autotransplantation, C7555
Thyrotropin
  alpha, J3240
Tibia
  Specialist Tibial Pre-formed Fracture Brace, L2116
  Toad finger splint, A4570
Ticarcillin disodium and clavulanate potassium, S0040
Tip (cane, crutch, walker) replacement, A4637
Tire, wheelchair, E2214, E2220
Tissue
  connective
    human, C1762
    non-human, C1763
  localization and excision device, C1819
  marker, A4648
Tissue marker, A4648
TLSO, L0450-L0492, L1200-L1290
Tobramycin
  inhalation solution, J7682, J7685
  sulfate, J3260
  unit dose, J7682
Toe
  holder, E0952

Toe — continued
  Specialist Toe Insert for Specialist Closed-Back Cast Boot and Specialist Health/Post Operative Shoe, A9270
Toilet accessories, E0167-E0175, E0243, E0244, E0625
  raised toilet seat, E0244
    Combo-Seat Universal, E0244
    Moore, E0244
    Sure-Safe, E0244
  seat lift, E0172
  transfer bench, E0247, E0248
Toll, non-emergency transport, A0170
Tomosynthesis, diagnostic, G0279
Tongue stimulation device, K1025-K1029
Topical hyperbaric oxygen chamber, A4575
Topographic brain mapping, S8040
Toronto, Legg Perthes orthotic, L1700
Total hip resurfacing, S2118
Total Universal Buck's Boot, E0870
Tourniquet, for dialysis, A4929
TPN, home infusion therapy, S9364-S9368
Tracer blood glucose
  meter, E0607
  strips, box of 50, A4253
Tracer II Diabetes Care System, E0607
Tracer Wheelchairs, E1240, E1250, E1260, E1270, E1280, E1285, E1290, E1295
Tracheal suction catheter, A4624
Tracheoesophageal prosthesis supplies, L8511-L8514
Tracheostoma
  adhesive disc, A7506
  filter, A7504
  filter holder, A7503, A7507, A7509
  housing, A7505, A7508
  replacement diaphragm, faceplate, A7502
  valve, A7501
Tracheostomy
  care kit, A4629
  filter, A4481
  mask, A7525
  speaking valve, L8501
  supplies, A4623-A4626, A4628, A4629, A7523-A7526, S8189
  tube, A7520-A7522
Traction equipment, E0840-E0948
  cervical equipment
    not requiring frame, E0855
    stand or frame, E0849
  device
    cervical, E0856
    extremity, E0870, E0880
      Total Universal Buck's Boot, E0870
    head harness/halter, cervical, E0942
    occipital-pull head halter, E0942
    overdoor, cervical, E0860
      Exo-Static, E0860
    pelvic, E0890, E0900
      Secure-All universal, belt, E0890
Training
  child development, T1027
  diabetes, G0108, G0109
  home care, S5108-S5116
  INR monitoring device, G0248
  medication, H0034
  skills, H2014, H2038
Tramacal, enteral nutrition, B4154
TranCyte, Q4182
Transbronchial ablation, C9751
Transcatheter
  microinfusion therapy, C9759
  NYHA IDE study
    implantation coronary sinus reduction device, C9783
    interatrial shunt implantation, C9760
    intramyocardial transplantation autologous bone marrow cells, C9782
Transcutaneous electrical nerve stimulator (TENS), E0720-E0749
  distal nerve, K1023
  trigeminal nerve, K1015-K1016
Transducer protector, dialysis, E1575
Transesophageal doppler, G9157
Transfer (shoe orthoses), L3600-L3640

Transfer board or device, E0705
Transfer system, E1036
Transfusion, blood products, at home, S9538
Transmitter
  interstitial glucose monitor, A9277
Transmitting coil/cable, L8629
Transparent film (for dressing), A6257-A6259
Transplant
  autologous chondrocyte, J7330
  bone marrow, allogeneic, S2150
  islet cell, G0341-G0343
  islet cell tissue, allogeneic, S2102
  lobar lung, S2060
  multivisceral organs, S2054
  pancreas/kidney, S2065
  renal, documentation, G9231
  small intestine and liver allografts, S2053
  stem cell, S2142
Transport chair, E1037-E1038
  heavy weight, E1039
Transportation
  ambulance, A0021-A0999
  corneal tissue, V2785
  EKG (portable), R0076
  extra attendant, A0424
  handicapped, A0130
  nonemergency, A0080-A0210, T2001-T2005, T2049
    mileage, S0215
  parking fees, A0170
  service, including ambulance, A0021-A0999
  taxi, nonemergency, A0100
  toll, nonemergency, A0170
  volunteer, nonemergency, A0080, A0090
  waiting time, T2007
  x-ray (portable), R0070, R0075
TranZgraft, Q4126
Trapeze bar, E0910-E0912, E0940
Trauma response team, G0390
Traum-aid, enteral nutrition, B4154
Travasorb, enteral nutrition, B4150
  Hepatic, B4154
  HN, B4153
  MCT, B4154
  Renal, B4154
Travel allowance, P9603-P9604
Traveler manual wheelchair, K0001
Tray
  insertion, A4310-A4316, A4354
  irrigation, A4320
  surgical (see also kits), A4550
  wheelchair, E0950
Treatment
  fracture
    pelvic bone, G0412-G0415
  nursing facility acute care, G9679-G9684
  outpatient IV insulin, G9147
Treatment planning and care coordination
  cancer, S0353-S0354
  comprehensive, advanced illness, S0311
Trifocal, glass or plastic, V2300-V2399
Trim nails, G0127
Truform prosthetic shrinker, L8440-L8465
TruSkin, Q4167
Truss, L8300-L8330
Tub
  transfer bench, E0247-E0248
Tube/Tubing
  anchoring device, A5200
  blood, A4750, A4755
  chest
    drain valve, A7040
    drainage container, A7041
  CPAP device, A7037
  gastrostomy/jejunostomy, B4087-B4088
  irrigation, A4355
  microcapillary, calibrated, A4651
    sealant, A4652
  nasogastric, B4081, B4082
  oxygen, A4616
  serum clotting time, A4771
  stomach, B4083
  suction pump, each, A7002
  tire, E2212-E2213, E2215
  tracheostomy or laryngotomy plug, A7527
  urinary drainage, A4331

Tube/Tubing — continued
  with integrated heating element, A4604
Tumor
  destruction
    embolization, S2095
  infiltrating lymphocyte therapy, S2107
Turtle Neck safety collars, E0942

U

Ulcers
  electromagnetic therapy, G0329
Ultra Blood Glucose
  monitor, E0607
  test strips, box of 50, A4253
UltraCare vest-style body holder, E0700
Ultrafast computed tomography, S8092
Ultrafine disposable insulin syringes, per syringe, A4206
Ultralightweight wheelchair, K0005
Ultrasound
  ablation, C9734
    uterine, C9734
  aerosol generator, E0574
  guidance
    multifetal pregnancy reduction, S8055
    radiation therapy field placement, G6001
  paranasal sinus, S9024
  therapeutic intervention, C9734
Ultraviolet light-therapy
  bulb, A4633
  cabinet, E0691-E0694
  system panel, E0691-E0693
Underpads, disposable, A4554
Unilet lancet device, A4258
Unipuncture control system, dialysis, E1580
Unistik lancet device, A4258
Universal
  remover for adhesives, A4455
  socket insert
    above knee, L5694
    below knee, L5690
  telescoping versarail bed rail, E0310
Up-Draft Neb-U-Mist, E0580
Upper extremity addition, locking elbow, L6693
Upper extremity fracture orthotic, L3980-L3999
Upper limb prosthesis, L6000-L7499
Ureteral
  stent change, C7549
Ureteroscopy
  for ureteral calculi, S2070
Ureterstomy tube change, C7549
Urethral
  clamp/compression device, A4360
  insert, A4336
Urgent care, S9088
  global fee, S9083
Urinal, E0325, E0326
Urinary
  catheter, A4338-A4346, A4351-A4353
  catheter irrigation, A4321
  collection and retention (supplies), A4310-A4358
  incontinence repair device, C1771, C2631
  incontinence supplies, A4310-A4421, A4423-A4434, A5051-A5093, A5102-A5114, A5120-A5200
  leg bag, A5105, A5112
  tract implant, collagen, L8603
Urine
  collector, A4335
  sensitivity study, P7001
  tests, A4250
Urostomy pouch, A5073
USMC
  hinged Swedish knee cage, L1850
  universal knee immobilizer, L1830
U-V lens, V2755
Uvulopalatoplasty, laser assisted, S2080

V

V Elite, E0601

Vabra aspirator, A4480
Vaccination, administration
    COVID-19 vaccination, in home, M0201
    hepatitis B, G0010
    influenza virus, G0008
    pneumococcal, G0009, G9279
        Not Given
            Before Discharge, G9280
            Not Indicated, G9281
            Refused, G9281
Vacuum erection system, L7900
    tension ring replacement, L7902
Vaginal
    colpopexy, C9778
    contraceptive ring, J7294, J7295
Vaporizer, E0605
Vascular
    catheter (appliances and supplies), A4300-A4306
    closure device, C1760
    synthetic, L8670
Venous thromboembolism prophylaxis, G9298-G9299
Vent
    ostomy, A4366
Ventilator
    battery, A4611-A4613
    home
        any type with invasive interface, E0465
        any type with non-invasive interface, E0466
        multifunction, E0467
    moisture exchanger, disposable, A4483
Ventilator tray
    wheelchair, E1029-E1030
Ventricular assist device
    accessory, Q0507-Q0509
    battery, Q0496, Q0503
        charger, Q0495
        clips, Q0497
    belt, Q0499
    driver, Q0480
    emergency
        hand pump, Q0494
        power cable, Q0492-Q0493
        power source, Q0490-Q0491
    filter, Q0500
    holster, Q0498
    leads, Q0487-Q0488
    microprocessor control unit, Q0481-Q0482
    miscellaneous supply, Q0503, Q0507-Q0509
    mobility cart, Q0502
    monitor
        control cable, Q0485-Q0486
        display module, Q0483-Q0484
    power
        back base, Q0489
            adapter, Q0504
        emergency
            power source, Q0490-Q0491
            power supply cable, Q0492-Q0493
        module, cable, Q0477
    power adapter/module, Q0478-Q0479
    shower cover, Q0501
    supply, Q0507-Q0509, Q0507-Q0509
    vest, Q0499
Versa-Pole IV pole, E0776
Vertebra/Vertebral
    augmentation
        percutaneous, C7507-C7508
    axial decompression, S9090
Vertebroplasty
    percutaneous, C7504-C7505
Vest, E0980
    safety, wheelchair, E0980
    ventricular assist device, Q0499
Vestibular rehabilitation, S9476
Viral load, G9242-G9243
Visi wheelchair tray, E0950
Visi-flow
    irrigation, A4367, A4398, A4399, A4402, A4421, A4436, A4437
    stoma cone, A4399

Vision service, S0500-S0592, V2020-V2799
Visit
    emergency department
        established patient, G0467
        type B, G0380-G0384
    FQHC
        behavioral health integration services, G0511
        chronic care management services, G0511
        established patient, G0467
        IPPE or AWV, G0468
        mental health, established patient, G0470
        mental health, new patient, G0469
        new patient, G0466
        psychiatric COCM services, G0512
        technology based services, G0071
    home by nurse practitioner, S0274
    home by physician, S0273
    hospital outpatient clinic, G0463
    medical, G9246-G9247
        FQHC established patient, G0467
        FQHC IPPE or AWV, G0468
        FQHC mental health, established patient, G0470
        FQHC mental health, new patient, G0469
        FQHC new patient, G0466
    nurse home, T1031
    RHC
        behavioral health integration services, G0511
        chronic care management services, G0511
        psychiatric COCM services, G0512
        technology based services, G0071
Vitajet, A4210
Vital HN, enteral nutrition, B4153
Vitamin
    multiple, A9153
    prenatal 30-day supply, S0197
    single, A9152
    supplement in ESRD, S0194
Vitrectomy, C9770
Vivonex, enteral nutrition
    HN, B4153
    T.E.N., B4153
Vocal cord
    chemodenervation, S2341
    injectable bulking agent, L8607
    medialization material, implantable, C1878
Voice amplifier, L8510
Von Hippel-Lindau disease, genetic test, S3842
Von Rosen, hip orthotic, L1630
Vortex power wheelchair, K0014
VPlus, E0601

W

Waiver services, T2024-T2041, T2050-T2051
Walker, E0130-E0144
    accessories, A4636, A4637
    attachments, E0153-E0159
    enclosed with wheels, E0144
    folding
        Auto-Glide, E0143
        Easy Care, E0143
        framed with wheels, E0144
    heavy duty
        with wheels, E0148
        without wheels, E0149
    heavy duty, multiple braking system, E0141
    One-Button, E0143
    Quik-Fold, E0141, E0143
    Red Dot, E0135, E0143
    Sure-Gait, E0141, E0143
Water
    ambulance, A0429
    distilled (for nebulizer), A7018
    for nebulizer, A7018
    pressure pad/mattress, E0187, E0198
    purification system (ESRD), E1610, E1615
    softening system (ESRD), E1625
    treated, A4714

Water chamber
    humidifier, A7046
Wedge, positioning, E0190
Wedges, shoe, L3340-L3420
Weight management class, S9449
Wellness
    annual visit, G0438-G0439
    assessment, S5190
Wet mount, Q0111
Wheel attachment, rigid pickup walker, E0155
Wheelchair, E0950-E1298, K0001-K0108
    accessories, E0950-E1031, E1036-E1295, E2358-E2359, E2398, E2627-E2633
    elevating legrest, E0990, K0046-K0047, K0195
    wheel lock, E2206
    tray, E0950
        Visi, E0950
    amputee, E1170-E1200
    base, E2358-E2359, E2627-E2633, K0008, K0013
    battery, E2358-E2359, E2397, K0733
    bearings, any type, E2210
    braking system and lock, E2228
    component or accessory, NOS, K0108
    control hand or chin, E2373-E2374
    controller, E2375-E2377
    crutch and cane holder, E2207
    cushion
        back, E2291, E2293, E2605, E2606, E2608-E2617, E2620, E2621
        custom, E2609
        seat, E2610, E2622-E2625
        general, E2601, E2602
        positioning, E2605, E2606, E2607
        replacement cover, E2619
        skin protection, E2603, E2604, E2607, E2622-E2625
    cylinder tank carrier, E2208
    elevating proximal arm, E2631
    foot box, E0954
    hand rim, E0967, E2205
    heavy-duty
        shock absorber, E1015-E1016
        Tracer, E1280, E1285, E1290, E1295
    lightweight, E1240-E1270
        EZ Lite, E1250
        Tracer, E1240, E1250, E1260, E1270
    manual, adult, E1161
        accessories, E2201-E2295, E2300-E2392, E2394-E2397
    motorized, E1239, K0010-K0898
    narrowing device, E0969
    pediatric, E1229, E1231-E1238
        back
            contoured, E2293
            planar, E2291
        modification, E1011
        power, E1239
        power, NOS, E1239
        seat
            contoured, E2294
            planar, E2292
    power, accessories, E2300-E2397, E2378, E2394-E2397, K0098
        battery, E2358-E2359
        gear box, E2369
        motor, E2368
        motor and gear box, E2370
    power seating system
        addition to power seating system
            leg elevation system
                center mount, complete, any type, each, E1012
                mechanically linked, including pushrod and legrest, each, E1009
                power, including legrest, pair, E1010
        recline only
            with mechanical shear reduction, E1004

Wheelchair — continued
    power seating system — continued
        recline only — continued
            with power shear reduction, E1005
            without shear reduction, E1003
        tilt and recline
            with mechanical shear reduction, E1007
            with power shear reduction, E1008
            without shear reduction, E1006
        tilt only, E1002
    reclining back, E1014
    residual limb support, E1020
    rocker arm, E2632
    seat or back cushion, K0669
    specially sized, E1220-E1230
    supinator, E2633
    support, E0953-E0954, E1020, E2626-E2633
    tire, E2211, E2214, E2220-E2222, E2381-E2392
    transfer board or device, E0705
    transport chair, E1037-E1038
    van, nonemergency, A0130, S0209
    wheel, E2227, E2394-E2395
    wheel drive, E0988
WHFO, with inflatable air chamber, L3807
Whirlpool equipment, E1300-E1310, K1003
Wig, A9282
Wipes, A4245, A4247
    Adhesive remover, A4456
    Allkare protective barrier, A5120
Wire, guide, C1769
WIZZ-ard manual wheelchair, K0006
Wooden canes, E0100
Wound
    cleanser, A6260
    cover
        alginate dressing, A6196-A6198
        collagen dressing, A6021-A6024
        foam dressing, A6209-A6214
        hydrocolloid dressing, A6234-A6239
        hydrogel dressing, A6242-A6248
        packing strips, A6407
        specialty absorptive dressing, A6251-A6256
        warming card, E0232
        warming device, E0231
        non-contact warming cover, A6000
    electrical stimulation, E0769
    filler
        alginate, A6199
        foam, A6215
        gel/paste, A6011
        hydrocolloid, A6240-A6241
        hydrogel, A6242-A6248
        not elsewhere classified, A6261-A6262
    healing
        other growth factor preparation, S9055
    matrix, A2001-A4100, Q4100-Q4264
    packing strips, A6407
    pouch, A6154
        warming device, E0231
            cover, A6000
            warming card, E0232
    suction, A9272
    suction pump, K0743
    therapy
        negative pressure
            supplies, A6550
Wound matrix, A2001-A4100, Q4100-Q4264
WoundEx, Q4163
WoundEx Flow, Q4162
WoundFix, WoundFix Plus, WoundFix Xplus, Q4217
Wrap
    abdominal aneurysm, M0301
    cold/heat, A9273
    compression, A6545

Wrist
- brace, cock-up, L3908
- disarticulation prosthesis, L6050, L6055
- hand/finger orthotic (WHFO), E1805, E1825, L3806-L3808
- Specialist Pre-Formed Ulnar Fracture Brace, L3982

X

Xcaliber power wheelchair, K0014
XCellerate, Q4234
XCelliStem, A2004
XCM Biologic Tissue Matrix, Q4142
Xenon Xe-133, A9558

X-ray
- equipment
  - portable, Q0092, R0070, R0075

XWRAP, Q4204

Y

Y set tubing for peritoneal dialysis, A4719

Yttrium 90
- ibritumomab tiuxeton, A9543
- microsphere
  - brachytherapy, C2616
  - procedure, S2095

Z

ZIFT, S4014

2023 HCPCS Level II A0420

Transportation Services Including Ambulance A0021-A0999

This code range includes ground and air ambulance, nonemergency transportation (taxi, bus, automobile, wheelchair van), and ancillary transportation-related fees.

HCPCS Level II codes for ambulance services must be reported with modifiers that indicate pick-up origins and destinations. The modifier describing the arrangement (QM, QN) is listed first. The modifiers describing the origin and destination are listed second. Origin and destination modifiers are created by combining two alpha characters from the following list. Each alpha character, with the exception of X, represents either an origin or a destination. Each pair of alpha characters creates one modifier. The first position represents the origin and the second the destination. The modifiers most commonly used are:

D	Diagnostic or therapeutic site other than "P" or "H" when these are used as origin codes
E	Residential, domiciliary, custodial facility (other than 1819 facility)
G	Hospital-based ESRD facility
H	Hospital
I	Site of transfer (e.g., airport or helicopter pad) between modes of ambulance transport
J	Free standing ESRD facility
N	Skilled nursing facility (SNF)
P	Physician's office
R	Residence
S	Scene of accident or acute event
X	Intermediate stop at physician's office on way to hospital (destination code only)

Note: Modifier X can only be used as a destination code in the second position of a modifier. See S0215. For Medicaid, see T codes and T modifiers.

Ambulance Transport and Supplies

A0021 Ambulance service, outside state per mile, transport (Medicaid only)
CMS: 100-04,15,20.4

A0080 Nonemergency transportation, per mile - vehicle provided by volunteer (individual or organization), with no vested interest
CMS: 100-04,15,20.4

A0090 Nonemergency transportation, per mile - vehicle provided by individual (family member, self, neighbor) with vested interest
CMS: 100-04,15,20.4

A0100 Nonemergency transportation; taxi
CMS: 100-04,15,20.4

A0110 Nonemergency transportation and bus, intra- or interstate carrier
CMS: 100-04,15,20.4

A0120 Nonemergency transportation: mini-bus, mountain area transports, or other transportation systems
CMS: 100-04,15,20.4

A0130 Nonemergency transportation: wheelchair van
CMS: 100-04,15,20.4

A0140 Nonemergency transportation and air travel (private or commercial) intra- or interstate
CMS: 100-04,15,20.4

A0160 Nonemergency transportation: per mile - caseworker or social worker
CMS: 100-04,15,20.4

A0170 Transportation ancillary: parking fees, tolls, other
CMS: 100-04,15,20.4

A0180 Nonemergency transportation: ancillary: lodging-recipient
CMS: 100-04,15,20.4

A0190 Nonemergency transportation: ancillary: meals, recipient
CMS: 100-04,15,20.4

A0200 Nonemergency transportation: ancillary: lodging, escort
CMS: 100-04,15,20.4

A0210 Nonemergency transportation: ancillary: meals, escort
CMS: 100-04,15,20.4

A0225 Ambulance service, neonatal transport, base rate, emergency transport, one way
CMS: 100-02,10,10.1.2; 100-02,10,10.2.1; 100-02,10,30.1; 100-02,10,30.1.1; 100-04,15,20.4

A0380 BLS mileage (per mile)
See code(s): A0425
CMS: 100-02,10,10.1.2; 100-02,10,10.2.1; 100-02,10,10.3.3; 100-02,10,30.1; 100-02,10,30.1.1; 100-04,15,20.4; 100-04,15,30.2

A0382 BLS routine disposable supplies
CMS: 100-02,10,10.1.2; 100-02,10,10.2.1; 100-02,10,30.1; 100-02,10,30.1.1; 100-04,15,20.4

A0384 BLS specialized service disposable supplies; defibrillation (used by ALS ambulances and BLS ambulances in jurisdictions where defibrillation is permitted in BLS ambulances)
CMS: 100-02,10,10.1.2; 100-02,10,10.2.1; 100-02,10,30.1; 100-02,10,30.1.1; 100-04,15,20.4

A0390 ALS mileage (per mile)
See code(s): A0425
CMS: 100-02,10,10.1.2; 100-02,10,10.2.1; 100-02,10,10.3.3; 100-02,10,30.1; 100-02,10,30.1.1; 100-04,15,20.4; 100-04,15,30.2

A0392 ALS specialized service disposable supplies; defibrillation (to be used only in jurisdictions where defibrillation cannot be performed in BLS ambulances)
CMS: 100-02,10,10.1.2; 100-02,10,10.2.1; 100-02,10,30.1; 100-02,10,30.1.1; 100-04,15,20.4

A0394 ALS specialized service disposable supplies; IV drug therapy
CMS: 100-02,10,10.1.2; 100-02,10,10.2.1; 100-02,10,30.1; 100-02,10,30.1.1; 100-04,15,20.4

A0396 ALS specialized service disposable supplies; esophageal intubation
CMS: 100-02,10,10.1.2; 100-02,10,10.2.1; 100-02,10,30.1; 100-02,10,30.1.1; 100-04,15,20.4

A0398 ALS routine disposable supplies
CMS: 100-02,10,10.1.2; 100-02,10,10.2.1; 100-02,10,30.1; 100-02,10,30.1.1; 100-04,15,20.4

Waiting Time

Units	Time
1	1/2 to 1 hr.
2	1 to 1-1/2 hrs.
3	1-1/2 to 2 hrs.
4	2 to 2-1/2 hrs.
5	2-1/2 to 3 hrs.
6	3 to 3-1/2 hrs.
7	3-1/2 to 4 hrs.
8	4 to 4-1/2 hrs.
9	4-1/2 to 5 hrs.
10	5 to 5-1/2 hrs.

A0420 Ambulance waiting time (ALS or BLS), one-half (1/2) hour increments
CMS: 100-02,10,10.1.2; 100-02,10,10.2.1; 100-02,10,30.1; 100-02,10,30.1.1; 100-04,15,20.4

Special Coverage Instructions Noncovered by Medicare Carrier Discretion ☑ Quantity Alert ● New Code ○ Recycled/Reinstated ▲ Revised Code

© 2022 Optum, Inc. A2-Z3 ASC Pmt **CMS:** IOM **AHA:** Coding Clinic DMEPOS Paid ⊘ SNF Excluded

A Codes — 1

Other Ambulance Services

A0422 Ambulance (ALS or BLS) oxygen and oxygen supplies, life sustaining situation
CMS: 100-02,10,10.1.2; 100-02,10,10.2.1; 100-02,10,30.1; 100-02,10,30.1.1; 100-04,15,20.4

A0424 Extra ambulance attendant, ground (ALS or BLS) or air (fixed or rotary winged); (requires medical review)
Pertinent documentation to evaluate medical appropriateness should be included when this code is reported.
CMS: 100-02,10,10.1.2; 100-02,10,10.2.1; 100-02,10,30.1; 100-02,10,30.1.1; 100-04,15,20.4; 100-04,15,30.2.1

A0425 Ground mileage, per statute mile
CMS: 100-02,10,10.1.2; 100-02,10,10.2.2; 100-02,10,10.3.3; 100-02,10,20; 100-02,10,30.1; 100-02,10,30.1.1; 100-02,10,20; 100-04,15,10.3; 100-04,15,20.1.4; 100-04,15,20.4; 100-04,15,20.6; 100-04,15,30; 100-04,15,30.1.2; 100-04,15,30.2.1; 100-04,15,40

A0426 Ambulance service, advanced life support, nonemergency transport, level 1 (ALS 1)
CMS: 100-02,10,10.1.2; 100-02,10,10.2.1; 100-02,10,10.2.2; 100-02,10,10.3.3; 100-02,10,20; 100-02,10,30.1; 100-02,10,30.1.1; 100-02,10,20; 100-04,15,10.3; 100-04,15,20.1.4; 100-04,15,20.4; 100-04,15,30; 100-04,15,30.1.2; 100-04,15,30.2; 100-04,15,30.2.1; 100-04,15,40

A0427 Ambulance service, advanced life support, emergency transport, level 1 (ALS 1 - emergency)
CMS: 100-02,10,10.1.2; 100-02,10,10.2.1; 100-02,10,10.2.2; 100-02,10,10.3.3; 100-02,10,20; 100-02,10,30.1; 100-02,10,30.1.1; 100-02,10,20; 100-04,15,10.3; 100-04,15,20.1.4; 100-04,15,20.4; 100-04,15,30; 100-04,15,30.1.2; 100-04,15,30.2; 100-04,15,30.2.1; 100-04,15,40

A0428 Ambulance service, basic life support, nonemergency transport, (BLS)
CMS: 100-02,10,10.1.2; 100-02,10,10.2.1; 100-02,10,10.2.2; 100-02,10,10.3.3; 100-02,10,20; 100-02,10,30.1; 100-02,10,30.1.1; 100-02,10,20; 100-04,15,10.3; 100-04,15,20.1.4; 100-04,15,20.4; 100-04,15,20.6; 100-04,15,30; 100-04,15,30.1.2; 100-04,15,30.2; 100-04,15,30.2.1; 100-04,15,40

A0429 Ambulance service, basic life support, emergency transport (BLS, emergency)
CMS: 100-02,10,10.1.2; 100-02,10,10.2.1; 100-02,10,10.2.2; 100-02,10,10.3.3; 100-02,10,20; 100-02,10,30.1; 100-02,10,30.1.1; 100-02,10,20; 100-04,15,10.3; 100-04,15,20.1.4; 100-04,15,20.4; 100-04,15,30; 100-04,15,30.1.2; 100-04,15,30.2; 100-04,15,30.2.1; 100-04,15,40

A0430 Ambulance service, conventional air services, transport, one way (fixed wing)
CMS: 100-02,10,10.1.2; 100-02,10,10.2.1; 100-02,10,10.2.2; 100-02,10,10.3.3; 100-02,10,20; 100-02,10,30.1; 100-02,10,30.1.1; 100-02,10,20; 100-04,15,10.3; 100-04,15,20.1.4; 100-04,15,20.3; 100-04,15,20.4; 100-04,15,30; 100-04,15,30.1.2; 100-04,15,30.2; 100-04,15,30.2.1; 100-04,15,40

A0431 Ambulance service, conventional air services, transport, one way (rotary wing)
CMS: 100-02,10,10.1.2; 100-02,10,10.2.1; 100-02,10,10.2.2; 100-02,10,10.3.3; 100-02,10,20; 100-02,10,30.1; 100-02,10,30.1.1; 100-02,10,20; 100-04,15,10.3; 100-04,15,20.1.4; 100-04,15,20.3; 100-04,15,20.4; 100-04,15,30; 100-04,15,30.1.2; 100-04,15,30.2; 100-04,15,30.2.1; 100-04,15,40

A0432 Paramedic intercept (PI), rural area, transport furnished by a volunteer ambulance company which is prohibited by state law from billing third-party payers
CMS: 100-02,10,10.1.2; 100-02,10,10.2.1; 100-02,10,10.2.2; 100-02,10,10.3.3; 100-02,10,20; 100-02,10,30.1; 100-02,10,30.1.1; 100-02,10,20; 100-04,15,10.3; 100-04,15,20.1.4; 100-04,15,20.4; 100-04,15,30; 100-04,15,30.1.2; 100-04,15,30.2; 100-04,15,30.2.1; 100-04,15,40

A0433 Advanced life support, level 2 (ALS 2)
CMS: 100-02,10,10.1.2; 100-02,10,10.2.1; 100-02,10,10.2.2; 100-02,10,10.3.3; 100-02,10,20; 100-02,10,30.1; 100-02,10,30.1.1; 100-02,10,20; 100-04,15,10.3; 100-04,15,20.1.4; 100-04,15,20.4; 100-04,15,30; 100-04,15,30.1.2; 100-04,15,30.2; 100-04,15,30.2.1; 100-04,15,40

A0434 Specialty care transport (SCT)
CMS: 100-02,10,10.1.2; 100-02,10,10.2.1; 100-02,10,10.2.2; 100-02,10,10.3.3; 100-02,10,20; 100-02,10,30.1; 100-02,10,30.1.1; 100-02,10,20; 100-04,15,10.3; 100-04,15,20.1.4; 100-04,15,20.4; 100-04,15,30; 100-04,15,30.1.2; 100-04,15,30.2; 100-04,15,30.2.1; 100-04,15,40

A0435 Fixed wing air mileage, per statute mile
CMS: 100-02,10,10.1.2; 100-02,10,10.2.1; 100-02,10,10.2.2; 100-02,10,10.3.3; 100-02,10,20; 100-02,10,30.1; 100-02,10,30.1.1; 100-02,10,20; 100-04,15,10.3; 100-04,15,20.1.4; 100-04,15,20.3; 100-04,15,20.4; 100-04,15,30; 100-04,15,30.1.2; 100-04,15,30.2; 100-04,15,30.2.1; 100-04,15,40

A0436 Rotary wing air mileage, per statute mile
CMS: 100-02,10,10.1.2; 100-02,10,10.2.1; 100-02,10,10.2.2; 100-02,10,10.3.3; 100-02,10,20; 100-02,10,30.1; 100-02,10,30.1.1; 100-02,10,20; 100-04,15,10.3; 100-04,15,20.1.4; 100-04,15,20.3; 100-04,15,20.4; 100-04,15,30; 100-04,15,30.1.2; 100-04,15,30.2; 100-04,15,30.2.1; 100-04,15,40

A0888 Noncovered ambulance mileage, per mile (e.g., for miles traveled beyond closest appropriate facility)
CMS: 100-02,10,10.1.2; 100-02,10,10.2.1; 100-02,10,20; 100-02,10,30.1; 100-02,10,30.1.1; 100-04,15,20.4; 100-04,15,30.1.2; 100-04,15,30.2.4

A0998 Ambulance response and treatment, no transport
CMS: 100-02,10,10.1.2; 100-02,10,10.2.1; 100-02,10,30.1; 100-02,10,30.1.1; 100-04,15,20.4

A0999 Unlisted ambulance service
CMS: 100-02,10,10.1; 100-02,10,10.1.2; 100-02,10,10.2.1; 100-02,10,20; 100-02,10,30.1; 100-02,10,30.1.1; 100-04,15,20.4

Medical and Surgical Supplies A2001-A9999

This section covers a wide variety of medical, surgical, and some durable medical equipment (DME) related supplies and accessories. DME-related supplies, accessories, maintenance, and repair required to ensure the proper functioning of this equipment is generally covered by Medicare under the prosthetic devices provision.

Skin Substitutes

A2001 InnovaMatrix AC, per sq cm
AHA: 1Q,22

A2002 Mirragen Advanced Wound Matrix, per sq cm
AHA: 1Q,22

▲ **A2004** XCelliStem, 1 mg
AHA: 1Q,22

A2005 Microlyte Matrix, per sq cm
AHA: 1Q,22

A2006 NovoSorb SynPath dermal matrix, per sq cm
AHA: 1Q,22

A2007 Restrata, per sq cm
AHA: 1Q,22

A2008 TheraGenesis, per sq cm
AHA: 1Q,22

A2009 Symphony, per sq cm
AHA: 1Q,22

A2010 Apis, per sq cm
AHA: 1Q,22

● **A2011** Supra SDRM, per sq cm
AHA: 2Q,22

2023 HCPCS Level II   A4255

- A2012 SUPRATHEL, per sq cm N1
  AHA: 2Q,22
- A2013 Innovamatrix FS, per sq cm N1
  AHA: 2Q,22
- A2014 Omeza Collagen Matrix, per 100 mg N1
- A2015 Phoenix Wound Matrix, per sq cm N1
- A2016 PermeaDerm B, per sq cm N1
- A2017 PermeaDerm Glove, each N1
- A2018 PermeaDerm C, per sq cm N1
- A4100 Skin substitute, FDA-cleared as a device, not otherwise specified N1
  AHA: 2Q,22

Injection Supplies

A4206 Syringe with needle, sterile, 1 cc or less, each
A4207 Syringe with needle, sterile 2 cc, each
A4208 Syringe with needle, sterile 3 cc, each
A4209 Syringe with needle, sterile 5 cc or greater, each
A4210 Needle-free injection device, each
Sometimes covered by commercial payers with preauthorization and physician letter stating need (e.g., for insulin injection in young children).
A4211 Supplies for self-administered injections
When a drug that is usually injected by the patient (e.g., insulin or calcitonin) is injected by the physician, it is excluded from Medicare coverage unless administered in an emergency situation (e.g., diabetic coma).
A4212 Noncoring needle or stylet with or without catheter
A4213 Syringe, sterile, 20 cc or greater, each
A4215 Needle, sterile, any size, each
A4216 Sterile water, saline and/or dextrose, diluent/flush, 10 ml
A4217 Sterile water/saline, 500 ml (AU)
CMS: 100-04,20,30.9
A4218 Sterile saline or water, metered dose dispenser, 10 ml
A4220 Refill kit for implantable infusion pump
A4221 Supplies for maintenance of noninsulin drug infusion catheter, per week (list drugs separately)
A4222 Infusion supplies for external drug infusion pump, per cassette or bag (list drugs separately)
A4223 Infusion supplies not used with external infusion pump, per cassette or bag (list drugs separately)
A4224 Supplies for maintenance of insulin infusion catheter, per week
A4225 Supplies for external insulin infusion pump, syringe type cartridge, sterile, each
A4226 Supplies for maintenance of insulin infusion pump with dosage rate adjustment using therapeutic continuous glucose sensing, per week
A4230 Infusion set for external insulin pump, nonneedle cannula type
Covered by some commercial payers as ongoing supply to preauthorized pump.
A4231 Infusion set for external insulin pump, needle type
Covered by some commercial payers as ongoing supply to preauthorized pump.
A4232 Syringe with needle for external insulin pump, sterile, 3 cc
Covered by some commercial payers as ongoing supply to preauthorized pump.

Batteries

A4233 Replacement battery, alkaline (other than J cell), for use with medically necessary home blood glucose monitor owned by patient, each (NU)
A4234 Replacement battery, alkaline, J cell, for use with medically necessary home blood glucose monitor owned by patient, each (NU)
A4235 Replacement battery, lithium, for use with medically necessary home blood glucose monitor owned by patient, each (NU)
A4236 Replacement battery, silver oxide, for use with medically necessary home blood glucose monitor owned by patient, each (NU)

Other Supplies

▲ A4238 Supply allowance for adjunctive, nonimplanted continuous glucose monitor (CGM), includes all supplies and accessories, 1 month supply = 1 unit of service (KF)
- A4239 Supply allowance for nonadjunctive, nonimplanted continuous glucose monitor (CGM), includes all supplies and accessories, 1 month supply = 1 unit of service
A4244 Alcohol or peroxide, per pint
A4245 Alcohol wipes, per box
A4246 Betadine or pHisoHex solution, per pint
A4247 Betadine or iodine swabs/wipes, per box
A4248 Chlorhexidine containing antiseptic, 1 ml
A4250 Urine test or reagent strips or tablets (100 tablets or strips)
CMS: 100-02,15,110

Reference chart

Tablet reagents turn specific colors when urine droplets are placed on them
- pH
- Protein
- Glucose
- Ketones
- Bilirubin
- Hemoglobin
- Nitrate

Dipstick urinalysis: The strip is dipped and color-coded squares are read at timed intervals (e.g., pH immediately; ketones at 15 seconds, etc.). Results are compared against a reference chart

A4252 Blood ketone test or reagent strip, each
A4253 Blood glucose test or reagent strips for home blood glucose monitor, per 50 strips (NU)
Medicare covers glucose strips for diabetic patients using home glucose monitoring devices prescribed by their physicians.
A4255 Platforms for home blood glucose monitor, 50 per box
Some Medicare contractors cover monitor platforms for diabetic patients using home glucose monitoring devices prescribed by their physicians. Some commercial payers also provide this coverage to noninsulin dependent diabetics.

A4256 | Normal, low, and high calibrator solution/chips
Some Medicare contractors cover calibration solutions or chips for diabetic patients using home glucose monitoring devices prescribed by their physicians. Some commercial payers also provide this coverage to noninsulin dependent diabetics.

A4257 | Replacement lens shield cartridge for use with laser skin piercing device, each

A4258 | Spring-powered device for lancet, each
Some Medicare contractors cover lancing devices for diabetic patients using home glucose monitoring devices prescribed by their physicians. Medicare jurisdiction: DME regional contractor. Some commercial payers also provide this coverage to noninsulin dependent diabetics.

A4259 | Lancets, per box of 100
Medicare covers lancets for diabetic patients using home glucose monitoring devices prescribed by their physicians. Medicare jurisdiction: DME regional contractor. Some commercial payers also provide this coverage to noninsulin dependent diabetics.

A4261 | Cervical cap for contraceptive use

A4262 | Temporary, absorbable lacrimal duct implant, each
Always report concurrent to the implant procedure.

A4263 | Permanent, long-term, nondissolvable lacrimal duct implant, each
Always report concurrent to the implant procedure.

A4264 | Permanent implantable contraceptive intratubal occlusion device(s) and delivery system

A4265 | Paraffin, per pound

A4266 | Diaphragm for contraceptive use

A4267 | Contraceptive supply, condom, male, each

A4268 | Contraceptive supply, condom, female, each

A4269 | Contraceptive supply, spermicide (e.g., foam, gel), each

A4270 | Disposable endoscope sheath, each

A4280 | Adhesive skin support attachment for use with external breast prosthesis, each

Two part prosthesis — Adhesive skin support (A4280)
Any of several breast prostheses fits over skin support

A4281 | Tubing for breast pump, replacement
A4282 | Adapter for breast pump, replacement
A4283 | Cap for breast pump bottle, replacement
A4284 | Breast shield and splash protector for use with breast pump, replacement

A4285 | Polycarbonate bottle for use with breast pump, replacement
A4286 | Locking ring for breast pump, replacement
A4290 | Sacral nerve stimulation test lead, each
CMS: 100-04,32,40.1; 100-04,32,40.2.1; 100-04,32,40.4

Vascular Catheters and Drug Delivery Systems

A4300 | Implantable access catheter, (e.g., venous, arterial, epidural subarachnoid, or peritoneal, etc.) external access

A4301 — Needle access, Implanted reservoir under refill injection, Body of reservoir and pump, Catheter
A4300 — Swan-Ganz catheter, Monitoring device, Tip with balloon, Detail of tapered tip and balloon, Markings along catheter measure depth of insertion, Ports, Junction divider

A4301 | Implantable access total catheter, port/reservoir (e.g., venous, arterial, epidural, subarachnoid, peritoneal, etc.)

A4305 | Disposable drug delivery system, flow rate of 50 ml or greater per hour

A4306 | Disposable drug delivery system, flow rate of less than 50 ml per hour

Incontinennce Appliances and Care Supplies
Covered by Medicare when the medical record indicates incontinence is permanent, or of long and indefinite duration.

A4310 | Insertion tray without drainage bag and without catheter (accessories only)

A4311 | Insertion tray without drainage bag with indwelling catheter, Foley type, two-way latex with coating (Teflon, silicone, silicone elastomer or hydrophilic, etc.)

A4312 | Insertion tray without drainage bag with indwelling catheter, Foley type, two-way, all silicone

Code	Description
A4313	Insertion tray without drainage bag with indwelling catheter, Foley type, three-way, for continuous irrigation
A4314	Insertion tray with drainage bag with indwelling catheter, Foley type, two-way latex with coating (Teflon, silicone, silicone elastomer or hydrophilic, etc.)
A4315	Insertion tray with drainage bag with indwelling catheter, Foley type, two-way, all silicone
A4316	Insertion tray with drainage bag with indwelling catheter, Foley type, three-way, for continuous irrigation
A4320	Irrigation tray with bulb or piston syringe, any purpose
A4321	Therapeutic agent for urinary catheter irrigation
A4322	Irrigation syringe, bulb or piston, each
A4326	Male external catheter with integral collection chamber, any type, each
A4327	Female external urinary collection device; meatal cup, each
A4328	Female external urinary collection device; pouch, each
A4330	Perianal fecal collection pouch with adhesive, each
A4331	Extension drainage tubing, any type, any length, with connector/adaptor, for use with urinary leg bag or urostomy pouch, each
A4332	Lubricant, individual sterile packet, each
A4333	Urinary catheter anchoring device, adhesive skin attachment, each
A4334	Urinary catheter anchoring device, leg strap, each
A4335	Incontinence supply; miscellaneous
A4336	Incontinence supply, urethral insert, any type, each
A4337	Incontinence supply, rectal insert, any type, each
A4338	Indwelling catheter; Foley type, two-way latex with coating (Teflon, silicone, silicone elastomer, or hydrophilic, etc.), each
A4340	Indwelling catheter; specialty type, (e.g., Coude, mushroom, wing, etc.), each
A4344	Indwelling catheter, Foley type, two-way, all silicone, each
A4346	Indwelling catheter; Foley type, three-way for continuous irrigation, each
A4349	Male external catheter, with or without adhesive, disposable, each
A4351	Intermittent urinary catheter; straight tip, with or without coating (Teflon, silicone, silicone elastomer, or hydrophilic, etc.), each
A4352	Intermittent urinary catheter; Coude (curved) tip, with or without coating (Teflon, silicone, silicone elastomeric, or hydrophilic, etc.), each
A4353	Intermittent urinary catheter, with insertion supplies
A4354	Insertion tray with drainage bag but without catheter
A4355	Irrigation tubing set for continuous bladder irrigation through a three-way indwelling Foley catheter, each
A4356	External urethral clamp or compression device (not to be used for catheter clamp), each
A4357	Bedside drainage bag, day or night, with or without antireflux device, with or without tube, each
A4358	Urinary drainage bag, leg or abdomen, vinyl, with or without tube, with straps, each
A4360	Disposable external urethral clamp or compression device, with pad and/or pouch, each

Ostomy Supplies

A4361	Ostomy faceplate, each
A4362	Skin barrier; solid, 4 x 4 or equivalent; each
A4363	Ostomy clamp, any type, replacement only, each
A4364	Adhesive, liquid or equal, any type, per oz
A4366	Ostomy vent, any type, each
A4367	Ostomy belt, each
A4368	Ostomy filter, any type, each
A4369	Ostomy skin barrier, liquid (spray, brush, etc.), per oz
A4371	Ostomy skin barrier, powder, per oz

Medical and Surgical Supplies

A4372 — A4420

Code	Description
A4372	Ostomy skin barrier, solid 4 x 4 or equivalent, standard wear, with built-in convexity, each
A4373	Ostomy skin barrier, with flange (solid, flexible or accordion), with built-in convexity, any size, each

Faceplate flange and skin barrier combination (A4373)
- Barrier adheres to skin
- Flange attaches to bag
- Waste moves through hole in membrane

Code	Description
A4375	Ostomy pouch, drainable, with faceplate attached, plastic, each
A4376	Ostomy pouch, drainable, with faceplate attached, rubber, each

Colostomy pouch with faceplate and drain (A4376)

Code	Description
A4377	Ostomy pouch, drainable, for use on faceplate, plastic, each
A4378	Ostomy pouch, drainable, for use on faceplate, rubber, each
A4379	Ostomy pouch, urinary, with faceplate attached, plastic, each
A4380	Ostomy pouch, urinary, with faceplate attached, rubber, each
A4381	Ostomy pouch, urinary, for use on faceplate, plastic, each
A4382	Ostomy pouch, urinary, for use on faceplate, heavy plastic, each
A4383	Ostomy pouch, urinary, for use on faceplate, rubber, each
A4384	Ostomy faceplate equivalent, silicone ring, each
A4385	Ostomy skin barrier, solid 4 x 4 or equivalent, extended wear, without built-in convexity, each
A4387	Ostomy pouch, closed, with barrier attached, with built-in convexity (one piece), each
A4388	Ostomy pouch, drainable, with extended wear barrier attached, (one piece), each
A4389	Ostomy pouch, drainable, with barrier attached, with built-in convexity (one piece), each
A4390	Ostomy pouch, drainable, with extended wear barrier attached, with built-in convexity (one piece), each
A4391	Ostomy pouch, urinary, with extended wear barrier attached (one piece), each
A4392	Ostomy pouch, urinary, with standard wear barrier attached, with built-in convexity (one piece), each
A4393	Ostomy pouch, urinary, with extended wear barrier attached, with built-in convexity (one piece), each
A4394	Ostomy deodorant, with or without lubricant, for use in ostomy pouch, per fl oz
A4395	Ostomy deodorant for use in ostomy pouch, solid, per tablet
A4396	Ostomy belt with peristomal hernia support
A4398	Ostomy irrigation supply; bag, each
A4399	Ostomy irrigation supply; cone/catheter, with or without brush
A4400	Ostomy irrigation set
A4402	Lubricant, per oz
A4404	Ostomy ring, each
A4405	Ostomy skin barrier, nonpectin-based, paste, per oz
A4406	Ostomy skin barrier, pectin-based, paste, per oz
A4407	Ostomy skin barrier, with flange (solid, flexible, or accordion), extended wear, with built-in convexity, 4 x 4 in or smaller, each
A4408	Ostomy skin barrier, with flange (solid, flexible or accordion), extended wear, with built-in convexity, larger than 4 x 4 in, each
A4409	Ostomy skin barrier, with flange (solid, flexible or accordion), extended wear, without built-in convexity, 4 x 4 in or smaller, each
A4410	Ostomy skin barrier, with flange (solid, flexible or accordion), extended wear, without built-in convexity, larger than 4 x 4 in, each
A4411	Ostomy skin barrier, solid 4 x 4 or equivalent, extended wear, with built-in convexity, each
A4412	Ostomy pouch, drainable, high output, for use on a barrier with flange (two-piece system), without filter, each
A4413	Ostomy pouch, drainable, high output, for use on a barrier with flange (two-piece system), with filter, each
A4414	Ostomy skin barrier, with flange (solid, flexible or accordion), without built-in convexity, 4 x 4 in or smaller, each
A4415	Ostomy skin barrier, with flange (solid, flexible or accordion), without built-in convexity, larger than 4 x 4 in, each
A4416	Ostomy pouch, closed, with barrier attached, with filter (one piece), each
A4417	Ostomy pouch, closed, with barrier attached, with built-in convexity, with filter (one piece), each
A4418	Ostomy pouch, closed; without barrier attached, with filter (one piece), each
A4419	Ostomy pouch, closed; for use on barrier with nonlocking flange, with filter (two piece), each
A4420	Ostomy pouch, closed; for use on barrier with locking flange (two piece), each

2023 HCPCS Level II

Medical and Surgical Supplies

Code	Description
A4421	Ostomy supply; miscellaneous — Determine if an alternative HCPCS Level II or a CPT code better describes the service being reported. This code should be used only if a more specific code is unavailable.
A4422	Ostomy absorbent material (sheet/pad/crystal packet) for use in ostomy pouch to thicken liquid stomal output, each
A4423	Ostomy pouch, closed; for use on barrier with locking flange, with filter (two piece), each
A4424	Ostomy pouch, drainable, with barrier attached, with filter (one piece), each
A4425	Ostomy pouch, drainable; for use on barrier with nonlocking flange, with filter (two-piece system), each
A4426	Ostomy pouch, drainable; for use on barrier with locking flange (two-piece system), each
A4427	Ostomy pouch, drainable; for use on barrier with locking flange, with filter (two-piece system), each
A4428	Ostomy pouch, urinary, with extended wear barrier attached, with faucet-type tap with valve (one piece), each
A4429	Ostomy pouch, urinary, with barrier attached, with built-in convexity, with faucet-type tap with valve (one piece), each
A4430	Ostomy pouch, urinary, with extended wear barrier attached, with built-in convexity, with faucet-type tap with valve (one piece), each
A4431	Ostomy pouch, urinary; with barrier attached, with faucet-type tap with valve (one piece), each
A4432	Ostomy pouch, urinary; for use on barrier with nonlocking flange, with faucet-type tap with valve (two piece), each
A4433	Ostomy pouch, urinary; for use on barrier with locking flange (two piece), each
A4434	Ostomy pouch, urinary; for use on barrier with locking flange, with faucet-type tap with valve (two piece), each
A4435	Ostomy pouch, drainable, high output, with extended wear barrier (one-piece system), with or without filter, each
A4436	Irrigation supply; sleeve, reusable, per month
A4437	Irrigation supply; sleeve, disposable, per month

Miscellaneous Supplies

Code	Description
A4450	Tape, nonwaterproof, per 18 sq in (AU, AV, AW) — See also code A4452. CMS: 100-04,20,30.9
A4452	Tape, waterproof, per 18 sq in (AU, AV, AW) — See also code A4450. CMS: 100-04,20,30.9
A4453	Rectal catheter for use with the manual pump-operated enema system, replacement only
A4455	Adhesive remover or solvent (for tape, cement or other adhesive), per oz
A4456	Adhesive remover, wipes, any type, each
A4458	Enema bag with tubing, reusable
A4459	Manual pump-operated enema system, includes balloon, catheter and all accessories, reusable, any type
A4461	Surgical dressing holder, nonreusable, each
A4463	Surgical dressing holder, reusable, each
A4465	Nonelastic binder for extremity
A4467	Belt, strap, sleeve, garment, or covering, any type
A4470	Gravlee jet washer
A4480	VABRA aspirator — CMS: 100-03,230.6; 100-03,240.4
A4481	Tracheostoma filter, any type, any size, each
A4483	Moisture exchanger, disposable, for use with invasive mechanical ventilation
A4490	Surgical stockings above knee length, each — CMS: 100-02,15,110
A4495	Surgical stockings thigh length, each — CMS: 100-02,15,110
A4500	Surgical stockings below knee length, each — CMS: 100-02,15,110
A4510	Surgical stockings full-length, each — CMS: 100-02,15,110
A4520	Incontinence garment, any type, (e.g., brief, diaper), each
A4550	Surgical trays — CMS: 100-04,12,40.1
A4553	Nondisposable underpads, all sizes
A4554	Disposable underpads, all sizes
A4555	Electrode/transducer for use with electrical stimulation device used for cancer treatment, replacement only
A4556	Electrodes (e.g., apnea monitor), per pair — If service is not separately payable, or incident to a physician's service, bill through the local carrier. If other, bill the DME MAC. Some payers only cover apnea monitors for newborn or pediatric use. Review specific carrier policy for apnea monitors and supplies.
A4557	Lead wires (e.g., apnea monitor), per pair — If service is not separately payable, or incident to a physician's service, bill through the local carrier. If other, bill the DME MAC. Some payers only cover apnea monitors for newborn or pediatric use. Review specific carrier policy for apnea monitors and supplies.
A4558	Conductive gel or paste, for use with electrical device (e.g., TENS, NMES), per oz
A4559	Coupling gel or paste, for use with ultrasound device, per oz
A4561	Pessary, rubber, any type
A4562	Pessary, nonrubber, any type — Medicare jurisdiction: DME regional contractor.
A4563	Rectal control system for vaginal insertion, for long term use, includes pump and all supplies and accessories, any type each
A4565	Slings
A4566	Shoulder sling or vest design, abduction restrainer, with or without swathe control, prefabricated, includes fitting and adjustment
A4570	Splint — Dressings applied by a physician are included as part of the professional service.
A4575	Topical hyperbaric oxygen chamber, disposable
A4580	Cast supplies (e.g., plaster) — See Q4001-Q4048.
A4590	Special casting material (e.g., fiberglass) — See Q4001-Q4048.
A4595	Electrical stimulator supplies, 2 lead, per month, (e.g., TENS, NMES) — CMS: 100-03,10.2

© 2022 Optum, Inc.

Medical and Surgical Supplies

A4596 — A4714

Code	Description
● A4596	Cranial electrotherapy stimulation (CES) system supplies and accessories, per month
A4600	Sleeve for intermittent limb compression device, replacement only, each [EI]
A4601	Lithium-ion battery, rechargeable, for nonprosthetic use, replacement [EI]
A4602	Replacement battery for external infusion pump owned by patient, lithium, 1.5 volt, each [N] ♿ (NU)
A4604	Tubing with integrated heating element for use with positive airway pressure device [N] ♿ (NU) CMS: 100-04,36,50.14
A4605	Tracheal suction catheter, closed system, each [N] ☑ ♿ (NU)
A4606	Oxygen probe for use with oximeter device, replacement [N]
A4608	Transtracheal oxygen catheter, each [N] ☑ ♿

Supplies for Oxygen and Related Respiratory Equipment

Code	Description
A4611	Battery, heavy-duty; replacement for patient-owned ventilator [EI]
A4612	Battery cables; replacement for patient-owned ventilator [EI]
A4613	Battery charger; replacement for patient-owned ventilator [EI] ☑
A4614	Peak expiratory flow rate meter, hand held [N] ♿
A4615	Cannula, nasal [N] ♿ CMS: 100-04,20,100.2
A4616	Tubing (oxygen), per foot [N] ☑ ♿ CMS: 100-04,20,100.2
A4617	Mouthpiece [N] ♿ CMS: 100-04,20,100.2
A4618	Breathing circuits [N] ♿ (NU, RR, UE) CMS: 100-04,20,100.2
A4619	Face tent [N] ♿ (NU) CMS: 100-04,20,100.2
A4620	Variable concentration mask [N] ♿ CMS: 100-04,20,100.2
A4623	Tracheostomy, inner cannula [N] ♿
A4624	Tracheal suction catheter, any type other than closed system, each [N] ☑ ♿ (NU)
A4625	Tracheostomy care kit for new tracheostomy [N] ♿
A4626	Tracheostomy cleaning brush, each [N] ☑ ♿
A4627	Spacer, bag or reservoir, with or without mask, for use with metered dose inhaler [EI] CMS: 100-02,15,110
A4628	Oropharyngeal suction catheter, each [N] ☑ ♿ (NU)
A4629	Tracheostomy care kit for established tracheostomy [N] ♿

Replacement Supplies for DME

Code	Description
A4630	Replacement batteries, medically necessary, transcutaneous electrical stimulator, owned by patient [EI] ☑ ♿ (NU)
A4633	Replacement bulb/lamp for ultraviolet light therapy system, each [EI] ☑ ♿ (NU)
A4634	Replacement bulb for therapeutic light box, tabletop model [N]
A4635	Underarm pad, crutch, replacement, each [EI] ☑ ♿ (NU, RR, UE)
A4636	Replacement, handgrip, cane, crutch, or walker, each [EI] ☑ ♿ (NU, RR, UE) CMS: 100-04,36,50.15
A4637	Replacement, tip, cane, crutch, walker, each [EI] ☑ ♿ (NU, RR, UE) CMS: 100-04,36,50.15
A4638	Replacement battery for patient-owned ear pulse generator, each [EI] ☑ ♿ (NU, RR, UE)
A4639	Replacement pad for infrared heating pad system, each [EI] ☑ ♿ (RR)
A4640	Replacement pad for use with medically necessary alternating pressure pad owned by patient [EI] ♿ (NU, RR, UE)

Radiopharmaceuticals

Code	Description
A4641	Radiopharmaceutical, diagnostic, not otherwise classified [N] ☑ CMS: 100-04,13,60.3; 100-04,13,60.3.2
A4642	Indium In-111 satumomab pendetide, diagnostic, per study dose, up to 6 mCi [N] ☑ Use this code for Oncoscint.

Miscellaneous Supplies

Code	Description
A4648	Tissue marker, implantable, any type, each [N] ☑ ⊘ AHA: 2Q,18
A4649	Surgical supply; miscellaneous [N] Determine if an alternative HCPCS Level II or a CPT code better describes the service being reported. This code should be used only if a more specific code is unavailable.
A4650	Implantable radiation dosimeter, each [N] ☑ ⊘
A4651	Calibrated microcapillary tube, each [N] ☑ ⊘
A4652	Microcapillary tube sealant [N] ⊘

Dialysis Supplies

Code	Description
A4653	Peritoneal dialysis catheter anchoring device, belt, each [N] ☑ ⊘
A4657	Syringe, with or without needle, each [N] ☑ ⊘ CMS: 100-04,8,60.2.1; 100-04,8,60.4.4; 100-04,8,60.4.6.3
A4660	Sphygmomanometer/blood pressure apparatus with cuff and stethoscope [N] ⊘
A4663	Blood pressure cuff only [N] ⊘
A4670	Automatic blood pressure monitor [EI]
A4671	Disposable cycler set used with cycler dialysis machine, each [B] ☑ ⊘
A4672	Drainage extension line, sterile, for dialysis, each [B] ☑ ⊘
A4673	Extension line with easy lock connectors, used with dialysis [B] ⊘
A4674	Chemicals/antiseptics solution used to clean/sterilize dialysis equipment, per 8 oz [B] ☑ ⊘
A4680	Activated carbon filter for hemodialysis, each [N] ☑ ⊘
A4690	Dialyzer (artificial kidneys), all types, all sizes, for hemodialysis, each [N] ☑ ⊘
A4706	Bicarbonate concentrate, solution, for hemodialysis, per gallon [N] ☑ ⊘
A4707	Bicarbonate concentrate, powder, for hemodialysis, per packet [N] ☑ ⊘
A4708	Acetate concentrate solution, for hemodialysis, per gallon [N] ☑ ⊘
A4709	Acid concentrate, solution, for hemodialysis, per gallon [N] ☑ ⊘
A4714	Treated water (deionized, distilled, or reverse osmosis) for peritoneal dialysis, per gallon [N] ☑ ⊘

Special Coverage Instructions | Noncovered by Medicare | Carrier Discretion | ☑ Quantity Alert | ● New Code | ○ Recycled/Reinstated | ▲ Revised Code

8 — A Codes | **A** Age Edit | **M** Maternity Edit | ♀ Female Only | ♂ Male Only | **A-Y** OPPS Status Indicators | © 2022 Optum, Inc.

2023 HCPCS Level II   A5131

Code	Description
A4719	"Y set" tubing for peritoneal dialysis
A4720	Dialysate solution, any concentration of dextrose, fluid volume greater than 249 cc, but less than or equal to 999 cc, for peritoneal dialysis
A4721	Dialysate solution, any concentration of dextrose, fluid volume greater than 999 cc but less than or equal to 1999 cc, for peritoneal dialysis
A4722	Dialysate solution, any concentration of dextrose, fluid volume greater than 1999 cc but less than or equal to 2999 cc, for peritoneal dialysis
A4723	Dialysate solution, any concentration of dextrose, fluid volume greater than 2999 cc but less than or equal to 3999 cc, for peritoneal dialysis
A4724	Dialysate solution, any concentration of dextrose, fluid volume greater than 3999 cc but less than or equal to 4999 cc, for peritoneal dialysis
A4725	Dialysate solution, any concentration of dextrose, fluid volume greater than 4999 cc but less than or equal to 5999 cc, for peritoneal dialysis
A4726	Dialysate solution, any concentration of dextrose, fluid volume greater than 5999 cc, for peritoneal dialysis
A4728	Dialysate solution, nondextrose containing, 500 ml
A4730	Fistula cannulation set for hemodialysis, each
A4736	Topical anesthetic, for dialysis, per g
A4737	Injectable anesthetic, for dialysis, per 10 ml
A4740	Shunt accessory, for hemodialysis, any type, each
A4750	Blood tubing, arterial or venous, for hemodialysis, each
A4755	Blood tubing, arterial and venous combined, for hemodialysis, each
A4760	Dialysate solution test kit, for peritoneal dialysis, any type, each
A4765	Dialysate concentrate, powder, additive for peritoneal dialysis, per packet
A4766	Dialysate concentrate, solution, additive for peritoneal dialysis, per 10 ml
A4770	Blood collection tube, vacuum, for dialysis, per 50
A4771	Serum clotting time tube, for dialysis, per 50
A4772	Blood glucose test strips, for dialysis, per 50
A4773	Occult blood test strips, for dialysis, per 50
A4774	Ammonia test strips, for dialysis, per 50
A4802	Protamine sulfate, for hemodialysis, per 50 mg
A4860	Disposable catheter tips for peritoneal dialysis, per 10
A4870	Plumbing and/or electrical work for home hemodialysis equipment
A4890	Contracts, repair and maintenance, for hemodialysis equipment
A4911	Drain bag/bottle, for dialysis, each
A4913	Miscellaneous dialysis supplies, not otherwise specified
	Pertinent documentation to evaluate medical appropriateness should be included when this code is reported. Determine if an alternative HCPCS Level II or a CPT code better describes the service being reported. This code should be used only if a more specific code is unavailable.
	CMS: 100-04,8,20; 100-04,8,60.2.1
A4918	Venous pressure clamp, for hemodialysis, each
A4927	Gloves, nonsterile, per 100
A4928	Surgical mask, per 20
A4929	Tourniquet for dialysis, each
A4930	Gloves, sterile, per pair
A4931	Oral thermometer, reusable, any type, each
A4932	Rectal thermometer, reusable, any type, each

Ostomy Pouches and Supplies

Code	Description
A5051	Ostomy pouch, closed; with barrier attached (one piece), each
A5052	Ostomy pouch, closed; without barrier attached (one piece), each
A5053	Ostomy pouch, closed; for use on faceplate, each
A5054	Ostomy pouch, closed; for use on barrier with flange (two piece), each
A5055	Stoma cap
A5056	Ostomy pouch, drainable, with extended wear barrier attached, with filter, (one piece), each
A5057	Ostomy pouch, drainable, with extended wear barrier attached, with built in convexity, with filter, (one piece), each
A5061	Ostomy pouch, drainable; with barrier attached, (one piece), each
A5062	Ostomy pouch, drainable; without barrier attached (one piece), each
A5063	Ostomy pouch, drainable; for use on barrier with flange (two-piece system), each
A5071	Ostomy pouch, urinary; with barrier attached (one piece), each
A5072	Ostomy pouch, urinary; without barrier attached (one piece), each
A5073	Ostomy pouch, urinary; for use on barrier with flange (two piece), each
A5081	Stoma plug or seal, any type
A5082	Continent device; catheter for continent stoma
A5083	Continent device, stoma absorptive cover for continent stoma
A5093	Ostomy accessory; convex insert

Incontinence Supplies

Code	Description
A5102	Bedside drainage bottle with or without tubing, rigid or expandable, each
A5105	Urinary suspensory with leg bag, with or without tube, each
A5112	Urinary drainage bag, leg or abdomen, latex, with or without tube, with straps, each
A5113	Leg strap; latex, replacement only, per set
A5114	Leg strap; foam or fabric, replacement only, per set
A5120	Skin barrier, wipes or swabs, each (AU, AV)
A5121	Skin barrier; solid, 6 x 6 or equivalent, each
A5122	Skin barrier; solid, 8 x 8 or equivalent, each
A5126	Adhesive or nonadhesive; disk or foam pad
A5131	Appliance cleaner, incontinence and ostomy appliances, per 16 oz

A5200 Percutaneous catheter/tube anchoring device, adhesive skin attachment

Diabetic Shoes, Fitting, and Modifications

According to Medicare, documentation from the prescribing physician must certify the diabetic patient has one of the following conditions: peripheral neuropathy with evidence of callus formation; history of preulcerative calluses; history of ulceration; foot deformity; previous amputation; or poor circulation. The footwear must be fitted and furnished by a podiatrist, pedorthist, orthotist, or prosthetist.

A5500 For diabetics only, fitting (including follow-up), custom preparation and supply of off-the-shelf depth-inlay shoe manufactured to accommodate multidensity insert(s), per shoe
CMS: 100-02,15,140

A5501 For diabetics only, fitting (including follow-up), custom preparation and supply of shoe molded from cast(s) of patient's foot (custom molded shoe), per shoe
CMS: 100-02,15,140

A5503 For diabetics only, modification (including fitting) of off-the-shelf depth-inlay shoe or custom molded shoe with roller or rigid rocker bottom, per shoe
CMS: 100-02,15,140

A5504 For diabetics only, modification (including fitting) of off-the-shelf depth-inlay shoe or custom molded shoe with wedge(s), per shoe
CMS: 100-02,15,140

A5505 For diabetics only, modification (including fitting) of off-the-shelf depth-inlay shoe or custom molded shoe with metatarsal bar, per shoe
CMS: 100-02,15,140

A5506 For diabetics only, modification (including fitting) of off-the-shelf depth-inlay shoe or custom molded shoe with off-set heel(s), per shoe
CMS: 100-02,15,140

A5507 For diabetics only, not otherwise specified modification (including fitting) of off-the-shelf depth-inlay shoe or custom molded shoe, per shoe
CMS: 100-02,15,140

A5508 For diabetics only, deluxe feature of off-the-shelf depth-inlay shoe or custom molded shoe, per shoe
CMS: 100-02,15,140

A5510 For diabetics only, direct formed, compression molded to patient's foot without external heat source, multiple-density insert(s) prefabricated, per shoe

A5512 For diabetics only, multiple density insert, direct formed, molded to foot after external heat source of 230 degrees Fahrenheit or higher, total contact with patient's foot, including arch, base layer minimum of 1/4 inch material of Shore A 35 durometer or 3/16 inch material of Shore A 40 durometer (or higher), prefabricated, each

A5513 For diabetics only, multiple density insert, custom molded from model of patient's foot, total contact with patient's foot, including arch, base layer minimum of 3/16 inch material of Shore A 35 durometer (or higher), includes arch filler and other shaping material, custom fabricated, each

A5514 For diabetics only, multiple density insert, made by direct carving with CAM technology from a rectified CAD model created from a digitized scan of the patient, total contact with patient's foot, including arch, base layer minimum of 3/16 inch material of Shore A 35 durometer (or higher), includes arch filler and other shaping material, custom fabricated, each

Dressings

A6000 Noncontact wound-warming wound cover for use with the noncontact wound-warming device and warming card

A6010 Collagen based wound filler, dry form, sterile, per g of collagen

A6011 Collagen based wound filler, gel/paste, per g of collagen

A6021 Collagen dressing, sterile, size 16 sq in or less, each

A6022 Collagen dressing, sterile, size more than 16 sq in but less than or equal to 48 sq in, each

A6023 Collagen dressing, sterile, size more than 48 sq in, each

A6024 Collagen dressing wound filler, sterile, per 6 in

A6025 Gel sheet for dermal or epidermal application, (e.g., silicone, hydrogel, other), each

A6154 Wound pouch, each

A6196 Alginate or other fiber gelling dressing, wound cover, sterile, pad size 16 sq in or less, each dressing

A6197 Alginate or other fiber gelling dressing, wound cover, sterile, pad size more than 16 sq in but less than or equal to 48 sq in, each dressing

A6198 Alginate or other fiber gelling dressing, wound cover, sterile, pad size more than 48 sq in, each dressing

A6199 Alginate or other fiber gelling dressing, wound filler, sterile, per 6 in

A6203 Composite dressing, sterile, pad size 16 sq in or less, with any size adhesive border, each dressing

A6204 Composite dressing, sterile, pad size more than 16 sq in, but less than or equal to 48 sq in, with any size adhesive border, each dressing

A6205 Composite dressing, sterile, pad size more than 48 sq in, with any size adhesive border, each dressing

A6206 Contact layer, sterile, 16 sq in or less, each dressing

A6207 Contact layer, sterile, more than 16 sq in but less than or equal to 48 sq in, each dressing

A6208 Contact layer, sterile, more than 48 sq in, each dressing

A6209 Foam dressing, wound cover, sterile, pad size 16 sq in or less, without adhesive border, each dressing

A6210 Foam dressing, wound cover, sterile, pad size more than 16 sq in but less than or equal to 48 sq in, without adhesive border, each dressing

A6211 Foam dressing, wound cover, sterile, pad size more than 48 sq in, without adhesive border, each dressing

A6212 Foam dressing, wound cover, sterile, pad size 16 sq in or less, with any size adhesive border, each dressing

A6213 Foam dressing, wound cover, sterile, pad size more than 16 sq in but less than or equal to 48 sq in, with any size adhesive border, each dressing

A6214 Foam dressing, wound cover, sterile, pad size more than 48 sq in, with any size adhesive border, each dressing

A6215 Foam dressing, wound filler, sterile, per g

A6216 Gauze, nonimpregnated, nonsterile, pad size 16 sq in or less, without adhesive border, each dressing

2023 HCPCS Level II

Medical and Surgical Supplies

A6217 Gauze, nonimpregnated, nonsterile, pad size more than 16 sq in but less than or equal to 48 sq in, without adhesive border, each dressing

A6218 Gauze, nonimpregnated, nonsterile, pad size more than 48 sq in, without adhesive border, each dressing

A6219 Gauze, nonimpregnated, sterile, pad size 16 sq in or less, with any size adhesive border, each dressing

A6220 Gauze, nonimpregnated, sterile, pad size more than 16 sq in but less than or equal to 48 sq in, with any size adhesive border, each dressing

A6221 Gauze, nonimpregnated, sterile, pad size more than 48 sq in, with any size adhesive border, each dressing

A6222 Gauze, impregnated with other than water, normal saline, or hydrogel, sterile, pad size 16 sq in or less, without adhesive border, each dressing

A6223 Gauze, impregnated with other than water, normal saline, or hydrogel, sterile, pad size more than 16 sq in but less than or equal to 48 sq in, without adhesive border, each dressing

A6224 Gauze, impregnated with other than water, normal saline, or hydrogel, sterile, pad size more than 48 sq in, without adhesive border, each dressing

A6228 Gauze, impregnated, water or normal saline, sterile, pad size 16 sq in or less, without adhesive border, each dressing

A6229 Gauze, impregnated, water or normal saline, sterile, pad size more than 16 sq in but less than or equal to 48 sq in, without adhesive border, each dressing

A6230 Gauze, impregnated, water or normal saline, sterile, pad size more than 48 sq in, without adhesive border, each dressing

A6231 Gauze, impregnated, hydrogel, for direct wound contact, sterile, pad size 16 sq in or less, each dressing

A6232 Gauze, impregnated, hydrogel, for direct wound contact, sterile, pad size greater than 16 sq in but less than or equal to 48 sq in, each dressing

A6233 Gauze, impregnated, hydrogel, for direct wound contact, sterile, pad size more than 48 sq in, each dressing

A6234 Hydrocolloid dressing, wound cover, sterile, pad size 16 sq in or less, without adhesive border, each dressing

A6235 Hydrocolloid dressing, wound cover, sterile, pad size more than 16 sq in but less than or equal to 48 sq in, without adhesive border, each dressing

A6236 Hydrocolloid dressing, wound cover, sterile, pad size more than 48 sq in, without adhesive border, each dressing

A6237 Hydrocolloid dressing, wound cover, sterile, pad size 16 sq in or less, with any size adhesive border, each dressing

A6238 Hydrocolloid dressing, wound cover, sterile, pad size more than 16 sq in but less than or equal to 48 sq in, with any size adhesive border, each dressing

A6239 Hydrocolloid dressing, wound cover, sterile, pad size more than 48 sq in, with any size adhesive border, each dressing

A6240 Hydrocolloid dressing, wound filler, paste, sterile, per oz

A6241 Hydrocolloid dressing, wound filler, dry form, sterile, per g

A6242 Hydrogel dressing, wound cover, sterile, pad size 16 sq in or less, without adhesive border, each dressing

A6243 Hydrogel dressing, wound cover, sterile, pad size more than 16 sq in but less than or equal to 48 sq in, without adhesive border, each dressing

A6244 Hydrogel dressing, wound cover, sterile, pad size more than 48 sq in, without adhesive border, each dressing

A6245 Hydrogel dressing, wound cover, sterile, pad size 16 sq in or less, with any size adhesive border, each dressing

A6246 Hydrogel dressing, wound cover, sterile, pad size more than 16 sq in but less than or equal to 48 sq in, with any size adhesive border, each dressing

A6247 Hydrogel dressing, wound cover, sterile, pad size more than 48 sq in, with any size adhesive border, each dressing

A6248 Hydrogel dressing, wound filler, gel, per fl oz

A6250 Skin sealants, protectants, moisturizers, ointments, any type, any size
Surgical dressings applied by a physician are included as part of the professional service. Surgical dressings obtained by the patient to perform homecare as prescribed by the physician are covered.

A6251 Specialty absorptive dressing, wound cover, sterile, pad size 16 sq in or less, without adhesive border, each dressing

A6252 Specialty absorptive dressing, wound cover, sterile, pad size more than 16 sq in but less than or equal to 48 sq in, without adhesive border, each dressing

A6253 Specialty absorptive dressing, wound cover, sterile, pad size more than 48 sq in, without adhesive border, each dressing

A6254 Specialty absorptive dressing, wound cover, sterile, pad size 16 sq in or less, with any size adhesive border, each dressing

A6255 Specialty absorptive dressing, wound cover, sterile, pad size more than 16 sq in but less than or equal to 48 sq in, with any size adhesive border, each dressing

A6256 Specialty absorptive dressing, wound cover, sterile, pad size more than 48 sq in, with any size adhesive border, each dressing

A6257 Transparent film, sterile, 16 sq in or less, each dressing
Surgical dressings applied by a physician are included as part of the professional service. Surgical dressings obtained by the patient to perform homecare as prescribed by the physician are covered. Use this code for Polyskin, Tegaderm, and Tegaderm HP.

A6258 Transparent film, sterile, more than 16 sq in but less than or equal to 48 sq in, each dressing
Surgical dressings applied by a physician are included as part of the professional service. Surgical dressings obtained by the patient to perform homecare as prescribed by the physician are covered.

A6259 Transparent film, sterile, more than 48 sq in, each dressing
Surgical dressings applied by a physician are included as part of the professional service. Surgical dressings obtained by the patient to perform homecare as prescribed by the physician are covered.

A6260 Wound cleansers, any type, any size
Surgical dressings applied by a physician are included as part of the professional service. Surgical dressings obtained by the patient to perform homecare as prescribed by the physician are covered.

A6261 Wound filler, gel/paste, per fl oz, not otherwise specified
Surgical dressings applied by a physician are included as part of the professional service. Surgical dressings obtained by the patient to perform homecare as prescribed by the physician are covered.

A6262 Wound filler, dry form, per g, not otherwise specified

Medical and Surgical Supplies

A6266 — A6539

Code	Description
A6266	Gauze, impregnated, other than water, normal saline, or zinc paste, sterile, any width, per linear yd
	Surgical dressings applied by a physician are included as part of the professional service. Surgical dressings obtained by the patient to perform homecare as prescribed by the physician are covered.
A6402	Gauze, nonimpregnated, sterile, pad size 16 sq in or less, without adhesive border, each dressing
	Surgical dressings applied by a physician are included as part of the professional service. Surgical dressings obtained by the patient to perform homecare as prescribed by the physician are covered.
A6403	Gauze, nonimpregnated, sterile, pad size more than 16 sq in but less than or equal to 48 sq in, without adhesive border, each dressing
	Surgical dressings applied by a physician are included as part of the professional service. Surgical dressings obtained by the patient to perform homecare as prescribed by the physician are covered.
A6404	Gauze, nonimpregnated, sterile, pad size more than 48 sq in, without adhesive border, each dressing
A6407	Packing strips, nonimpregnated, sterile, up to 2 in in width, per linear yd
A6410	Eye pad, sterile, each
A6411	Eye pad, nonsterile, each
A6412	Eye patch, occlusive, each
A6413	Adhesive bandage, first aid type, any size, each
A6441	Padding bandage, nonelastic, nonwoven/nonknitted, width greater than or equal to 3 in and less than 5 in, per yd
A6442	Conforming bandage, nonelastic, knitted/woven, nonsterile, width less than 3 in, per yd
A6443	Conforming bandage, nonelastic, knitted/woven, nonsterile, width greater than or equal to 3 in and less than 5 in, per yd
A6444	Conforming bandage, nonelastic, knitted/woven, nonsterile, width greater than or equal to 5 in, per yd
A6445	Conforming bandage, nonelastic, knitted/woven, sterile, width less than 3 in, per yd
A6446	Conforming bandage, nonelastic, knitted/woven, sterile, width greater than or equal to 3 in and less than 5 in, per yd
A6447	Conforming bandage, nonelastic, knitted/woven, sterile, width greater than or equal to 5 in, per yd
A6448	Light compression bandage, elastic, knitted/woven, width less than 3 in, per yd
A6449	Light compression bandage, elastic, knitted/woven, width greater than or equal to 3 in and less than 5 in, per yd
A6450	Light compression bandage, elastic, knitted/woven, width greater than or equal to 5 in, per yd
A6451	Moderate compression bandage, elastic, knitted/woven, load resistance of 1.25 to 1.34 ft lbs at 50% maximum stretch, width greater than or equal to 3 in and less than 5 in, per yd
A6452	High compression bandage, elastic, knitted/woven, load resistance greater than or equal to 1.35 ft lbs at 50% maximum stretch, width greater than or equal to 3 in and less than 5 in, per yd
A6453	Self-adherent bandage, elastic, nonknitted/nonwoven, width less than 3 in, per yd
A6454	Self-adherent bandage, elastic, nonknitted/nonwoven, width greater than or equal to 3 in and less than 5 in, per yd
A6455	Self-adherent bandage, elastic, nonknitted/nonwoven, width greater than or equal to 5 in, per yd
A6456	Zinc paste impregnated bandage, nonelastic, knitted/woven, width greater than or equal to 3 in and less than 5 in, per yd
A6457	Tubular dressing with or without elastic, any width, per linear yd
A6460	Synthetic resorbable wound dressing, sterile, pad size 16 sq in or less, without adhesive border, each dressing
A6461	Synthetic resorbable wound dressing, sterile, pad size more than 16 sq in but less than or equal to 48 sq in, without adhesive border, each dressing

Compression Garments

Code	Description
A6501	Compression burn garment, bodysuit (head to foot), custom fabricated
A6502	Compression burn garment, chin strap, custom fabricated
A6503	Compression burn garment, facial hood, custom fabricated
A6504	Compression burn garment, glove to wrist, custom fabricated
A6505	Compression burn garment, glove to elbow, custom fabricated
A6506	Compression burn garment, glove to axilla, custom fabricated
A6507	Compression burn garment, foot to knee length, custom fabricated
A6508	Compression burn garment, foot to thigh length, custom fabricated
A6509	Compression burn garment, upper trunk to waist including arm openings (vest), custom fabricated
A6510	Compression burn garment, trunk, including arms down to leg openings (leotard), custom fabricated
A6511	Compression burn garment, lower trunk including leg openings (panty), custom fabricated
A6512	Compression burn garment, not otherwise classified
A6513	Compression burn mask, face and/or neck, plastic or equal, custom fabricated
A6530	Gradient compression stocking, below knee, 18-30 mm Hg, each
A6531	Gradient compression stocking, below knee, 30-40 mm Hg, each
A6532	Gradient compression stocking, below knee, 40-50 mm Hg, each
A6533	Gradient compression stocking, thigh length, 18-30 mm Hg, each
A6534	Gradient compression stocking, thigh length, 30-40 mm Hg, each
A6535	Gradient compression stocking, thigh length, 40-50 mm Hg, each
A6536	Gradient compression stocking, full-length/chap style, 18-30 mm Hg, each
A6537	Gradient compression stocking, full-length/chap style, 30-40 mm Hg, each
A6538	Gradient compression stocking, full-length/chap style, 40-50 mm Hg, each
A6539	Gradient compression stocking, waist length, 18-30 mm Hg, each

---

Special Coverage Instructions | Noncovered by Medicare | Carrier Discretion | ☑ Quantity Alert | ● New Code | ○ Recycled/Reinstated | ▲ Revised Code

12 — A Codes | Ⓐ Age Edit | Ⓜ Maternity Edit | ♀ Female Only | ♂ Male Only | A–Y OPPS Status Indicators | © 2022 Optum, Inc.

Code	Description
A6540	Gradient compression stocking, waist length, 30-40 mm Hg, each [EI]
A6541	Gradient compression stocking, waist length, 40-50 mm Hg, each [EI]
A6544	Gradient compression stocking, garter belt [EI]
A6545	Gradient compression wrap, nonelastic, below knee, 30-50 mm Hg, each [N] (AW)
A6549	Gradient compression stocking/sleeve, not otherwise specified [EI]
A6550	Wound care set, for negative pressure wound therapy electrical pump, includes all supplies and accessories [N] CMS: 100-02,7,40.1.2.8

Respiratory Supplies

Code	Description
A7000	Canister, disposable, used with suction pump, each [Y] (NU)
A7001	Canister, nondisposable, used with suction pump, each [Y] (NU)
A7002	Tubing, used with suction pump, each [Y] (NU)
A7003	Administration set, with small volume nonfiltered pneumatic nebulizer, disposable [Y] (NU)
A7004	Small volume nonfiltered pneumatic nebulizer, disposable [Y] (NU)
A7005	Administration set, with small volume nonfiltered pneumatic nebulizer, nondisposable [Y] (NU)
A7006	Administration set, with small volume filtered pneumatic nebulizer [Y] (NU)
A7007	Large volume nebulizer, disposable, unfilled, used with aerosol compressor [Y] (NU)
A7008	Large volume nebulizer, disposable, prefilled, used with aerosol compressor [Y] (NU)
A7009	Reservoir bottle, nondisposable, used with large volume ultrasonic nebulizer [Y] (NU)
A7010	Corrugated tubing, disposable, used with large volume nebulizer, 100 ft [Y] (NU)
A7012	Water collection device, used with large volume nebulizer [Y] (NU)
A7013	Filter, disposable, used with aerosol compressor or ultrasonic generator [Y] (NU)
A7014	Filter, nondisposable, used with aerosol compressor or ultrasonic generator [Y] (NU)
A7015	Aerosol mask, used with DME nebulizer [Y] (NU)
A7016	Dome and mouthpiece, used with small volume ultrasonic nebulizer [Y] (NU)
A7017	Nebulizer, durable, glass or autoclavable plastic, bottle type, not used with oxygen [Y] (NU, RR, UE)
A7018	Water, distilled, used with large volume nebulizer, 1000 ml [Y]
A7020	Interface for cough stimulating device, includes all components, replacement only [Y] (NU)
A7025	High frequency chest wall oscillation system vest, replacement for use with patient-owned equipment, each [N] (RR)
A7026	High frequency chest wall oscillation system hose, replacement for use with patient-owned equipment, each [Y] (NU)
A7027	Combination oral/nasal mask, used with continuous positive airway pressure device, each [Y] (NU)
A7028	Oral cushion for combination oral/nasal mask, replacement only, each [Y] (NU)
A7029	Nasal pillows for combination oral/nasal mask, replacement only, pair [Y] (NU)
A7030	Full face mask used with positive airway pressure device, each [Y] (NU) CMS: 100-04,36,50.14
A7031	Face mask interface, replacement for full face mask, each [Y] (NU) CMS: 100-04,36,50.14
A7032	Cushion for use on nasal mask interface, replacement only, each [Y] (NU) CMS: 100-03,240.4; 100-04,36,50.14
A7033	Pillow for use on nasal cannula type interface, replacement only, pair [Y] (NU) CMS: 100-03,240.4; 100-04,36,50.14
A7034	Nasal interface (mask or cannula type) used with positive airway pressure device, with or without head strap [Y] (NU) CMS: 100-03,240.4; 100-04,36,50.14
A7035	Headgear used with positive airway pressure device [Y] (NU) CMS: 100-03,240.4; 100-04,36,50.14
A7036	Chinstrap used with positive airway pressure device [Y] (NU) CMS: 100-03,240.4; 100-04,36,50.14
A7037	Tubing used with positive airway pressure device [Y] (NU) CMS: 100-03,240.4; 100-04,36,50.14
A7038	Filter, disposable, used with positive airway pressure device [Y] (NU) CMS: 100-04,36,50.14
A7039	Filter, nondisposable, used with positive airway pressure device [Y] (NU) CMS: 100-04,36,50.14
A7040	One way chest drain valve [N]
A7041	Water seal drainage container and tubing for use with implanted chest tube [N]
A7044	Oral interface used with positive airway pressure device, each [Y] (NU) CMS: 100-03,240.4; 100-04,36,50.14
A7045	Exhalation port with or without swivel used with accessories for positive airway devices, replacement only [Y] (NU, RR, UE) CMS: 100-03,240.4; 100-04,36,50.14
A7046	Water chamber for humidifier, used with positive airway pressure device, replacement, each [Y] (NU) CMS: 100-04,36,50.14
A7047	Oral interface used with respiratory suction pump, each [N] (NU)
A7048	Vacuum drainage collection unit and tubing kit, including all supplies needed for collection unit change, for use with implanted catheter, each [N]

Tracheostomy Supplies

Code	Description
A7501	Tracheostoma valve, including diaphragm, each [N]
A7502	Replacement diaphragm/faceplate for tracheostoma valve, each [N]
A7503	Filter holder or filter cap, reusable, for use in a tracheostoma heat and moisture exchange system, each [N]
A7504	Filter for use in a tracheostoma heat and moisture exchange system, each [N]

Special Coverage Instructions | Noncovered by Medicare | Carrier Discretion | ☑ Quantity Alert | ● New Code | ○ Recycled/Reinstated | ▲ Revised Code

© 2022 Optum, Inc. | A2-Z3 ASC Pmt | CMS: IOM | AHA: Coding Clinic | DMEPOS Paid | ⊘ SNF Excluded | A Codes — 13

Medical and Surgical Supplies

Code	Description
A7505	Housing, reusable without adhesive, for use in a heat and moisture exchange system and/or with a tracheostoma valve, each
A7506	Adhesive disc for use in a heat and moisture exchange system and/or with tracheostoma valve, any type each
A7507	Filter holder and integrated filter without adhesive, for use in a tracheostoma heat and moisture exchange system, each
A7508	Housing and integrated adhesive, for use in a tracheostoma heat and moisture exchange system and/or with a tracheostoma valve, each
A7509	Filter holder and integrated filter housing, and adhesive, for use as a tracheostoma heat and moisture exchange system, each
A7520	Tracheostomy/laryngectomy tube, noncuffed, polyvinyl chloride (PVC), silicone or equal, each
A7521	Tracheostomy/laryngectomy tube, cuffed, polyvinyl chloride (PVC), silicone or equal, each
A7522	Tracheostomy/laryngectomy tube, stainless steel or equal (sterilizable and reusable), each
A7523	Tracheostomy shower protector, each
A7524	Tracheostoma stent/stud/button, each
A7525	Tracheostomy mask, each
A7526	Tracheostomy tube collar/holder, each
A7527	Tracheostomy/laryngectomy tube plug/stop, each

Protective Helmet

Code	Description
A8000	Helmet, protective, soft, prefabricated, includes all components and accessories (NU, RR, UE)
A8001	Helmet, protective, hard, prefabricated, includes all components and accessories (NU, RR, UE)
A8002	Helmet, protective, soft, custom fabricated, includes all components and accessories (NU, RR, UE)
A8003	Helmet, protective, hard, custom fabricated, includes all components and accessories (NU, RR, UE)
A8004	Soft interface for helmet, replacement only (NU, RR, UE)

Other Supplies and Devices

Code	Description
A9150	Nonprescription drugs
A9152	Single vitamin/mineral/trace element, oral, per dose, not otherwise specified
A9153	Multiple vitamins, with or without minerals and trace elements, oral, per dose, not otherwise specified
A9155	Artificial saliva, 30 ml
A9180	Pediculosis (lice infestation) treatment, topical, for administration by patient/caretaker
A9270	Noncovered item or service CMS: 100-04,11,100.1; 100-04,20,30.9; 100-04,23,20.9.1.1
A9272	Wound suction, disposable, includes dressing, all accessories and components, any type, each
A9273	Cold or hot fluid bottle, ice cap or collar, heat and/or cold wrap, any type
A9274	External ambulatory insulin delivery system, disposable, each, includes all supplies and accessories
A9275	Home glucose disposable monitor, includes test strips
▲ A9276	Sensor; invasive (e.g., subcutaneous), disposable, for use with nondurable medical equipment interstitial continuous glucose monitoring system (CGM), one unit = 1 month supply
▲ A9277	Transmitter; external, for use with nondurable medical equipment interstitial continuous glucose monitoring system (CGM)
▲ A9278	Receiver (monitor); external, for use with nondurable medical equipment interstitial continuous glucose monitoring system (CGM)
A9279	Monitoring feature/device, stand-alone or integrated, any type, includes all accessories, components and electronics, not otherwise classified
A9280	Alert or alarm device, not otherwise classified
A9281	Reaching/grabbing device, any type, any length, each
A9282	Wig, any type, each
A9283	Foot pressure off loading/supportive device, any type, each
A9284	Spirometer, nonelectronic, includes all accessories
A9285	Inversion/eversion correction device
A9286	Hygienic item or device, disposable or nondisposable, any type, each
▲ A9291	Prescription digital cognitive and/or behavioral therapy, FDA-cleared, per course of treatment
A9300	Exercise equipment

Radiopharmaceuticals

Code	Description
A9500	Technetium Tc-99m sestamibi, diagnostic, per study dose Use this code for Cardiolite.
A9501	Technetium Tc-99m teboroxime, diagnostic, per study dose
A9502	Technetium Tc-99m tetrofosmin, diagnostic, per study dose Use this code for Myoview.
A9503	Technetium Tc-99m medronate, diagnostic, per study dose, up to 30 mCi Use this code for CIS-MDP, Draximage MDP-10, Draximage MDP-25, MDP-Bracco, Technetium Tc-99m MPI-MDP.
A9504	Technetium Tc-99m apcitide, diagnostic, per study dose, up to 20 mCi Use this code for Acutect.
A9505	Thallium Tl-201 thallous chloride, diagnostic, per mCi Use this code for MIBG, Thallous Chloride USP.
A9507	Indium In-111 capromab pendetide, diagnostic, per study dose, up to 10 millicuries Use this code for Prostascint.
A9508	Iodine I-131 iobenguane sulfate, diagnostic, per 0.5 mCi Use this code for MIBG.
A9509	Iodine I-123 sodium iodide, diagnostic, per mCi
A9510	Technetium Tc-99m disofenin, diagnostic, per study dose, up to 15 mCi Use this code for Hepatolite.
A9512	Technetium Tc-99m pertechnetate, diagnostic, per mCi Use this code for Technelite, Ultra-Technelow.

Special Coverage Instructions | Noncovered by Medicare | Carrier Discretion | ☑ Quantity Alert | ● New Code | ○ Recycled/Reinstated | ▲ Revised Code

Ⓐ Age Edit | Ⓜ Maternity Edit | ♀ Female Only | ♂ Male Only | Ⓐ-Ⓨ OPPS Status Indicators | © 2022 Optum, Inc.

2023 HCPCS Level II — A9572

Code	Description
A9513	Lutetium Lu 177, dotatate, therapeutic, 1 mCi Use this code for Lutathera. AHA: 1Q,19
A9515	Choline C-11, diagnostic, per study dose up to 20 mCi
A9516	Iodine I-123 sodium iodide, diagnostic, per 100 mcCi, up to 999 mcCi
A9517	Iodine I-131 sodium iodide capsule(s), therapeutic, per mCi
A9520	Technetium Tc-99m, tilmanocept, diagnostic, up to 0.5 mCi
A9521	Technetium Tc-99m exametazime, diagnostic, per study dose, up to 25 mCi Use this code for Ceretec.
A9524	Iodine I-131 iodinated serum albumin, diagnostic, per 5 mcCi
A9526	Nitrogen N-13 ammonia, diagnostic, per study dose, up to 40 mCi CMS: 100-04,13,60.3; 100-04,13,60.3.2 AHA: 1Q,22
A9527	Iodine I-125, sodium iodide solution, therapeutic, per mCi
A9528	Iodine I-131 sodium iodide capsule(s), diagnostic, per mCi
A9529	Iodine I-131 sodium iodide solution, diagnostic, per mCi
A9530	Iodine I-131 sodium iodide solution, therapeutic, per mCi
A9531	Iodine I-131 sodium iodide, diagnostic, per mcCi (up to 100 mcCi)
A9532	Iodine I-125 serum albumin, diagnostic, per 5 mcCi
A9536	Technetium Tc-99m depreotide, diagnostic, per study dose, up to 35 mCi
A9537	Technetium Tc-99m mebrofenin, diagnostic, per study dose, up to 15 mCi
A9538	Technetium Tc-99m pyrophosphate, diagnostic, per study dose, up to 25 mCi Use this code for CIS-PYRO, Phosphostec, Technescan Pyp Kit.
A9539	Technetium Tc-99m pentetate, diagnostic, per study dose, up to 25 mCi Use this code for AN-DTPA, DTPA, MPI-DTPA Kit-Chelate, MPI Indium DTPA IN-111, Pentate Calcium Trisodium, Pentate Zinc Trisodium.
A9540	Technetium Tc-99m macroaggregated albumin, diagnostic, per study dose, up to 10 mCi
A9541	Technetium Tc-99m sulfur colloid, diagnostic, per study dose, up to 20 mCi
A9542	Indium In-111 ibritumomab tiuxetan, diagnostic, per study dose, up to 5 mCi Use this code for Zevalin.
A9543	Yttrium Y-90 ibritumomab tiuxetan, therapeutic, per treatment dose, up to 40 mCi
A9546	Cobalt Co-57/58, cyanocobalamin, diagnostic, per study dose, up to 1 mcCi
A9547	Indium In-111 oxyquinoline, diagnostic, per 0.5 mCi
A9548	Indium In-111 pentetate, diagnostic, per 0.5 mCi
A9550	Technetium Tc-99m sodium gluceptate, diagnostic, per study dose, up to 25 mCi
A9551	Technetium Tc-99m succimer, diagnostic, per study dose, up to 10 mCi Use this code for MPI-DMSA Kidney Reagent.
A9552	Fluorodeoxyglucose F-18 FDG, diagnostic, per study dose, up to 45 mCi CMS: 100-03,220.6.13; 100-03,220.6.17; 100-04,13,60.15; 100-04,13,60.16; 100-04,13,60.3.2 AHA: 1Q,22
A9553	Chromium Cr-51 sodium chromate, diagnostic, per study dose, up to 250 mcCi Use this code for Chromitope Sodium.
A9554	Iodine I-125 sodium iothalamate, diagnostic, per study dose, up to 10 mcCi Use this code for Glofil-125.
A9555	Rubidium Rb-82, diagnostic, per study dose, up to 60 mCi Use this code for Cardiogen 82. CMS: 100-03,220.6.1; 100-04,13,60.3.2 AHA: 1Q,22
A9556	Gallium Ga-67 citrate, diagnostic, per mCi
A9557	Technetium Tc-99m bicisate, diagnostic, per study dose, up to 25 mCi Use this code for Neurolite.
A9558	Xenon Xe-133 gas, diagnostic, per 10 mCi
A9559	Cobalt Co-57 cyanocobalamin, oral, diagnostic, per study dose, up to 1 mcCi
A9560	Technetium Tc-99m labeled red blood cells, diagnostic, per study dose, up to 30 mCi
A9561	Technetium Tc-99m oxidronate, diagnostic, per study dose, up to 30 mCi Use this code for TechneScan.
A9562	Technetium Tc-99m mertiatide, diagnostic, per study dose, up to 15 mCi Use this code for TechneScan MAG-3.
A9563	Sodium phosphate P-32, therapeutic, per mCi
A9564	Chromic phosphate P-32 suspension, therapeutic, per mCi Use this code for Phosphocol (P32).
A9566	Technetium Tc-99m fanolesomab, diagnostic, per study dose, up to 25 mCi
A9567	Technetium Tc-99m pentetate, diagnostic, aerosol, per study dose, up to 75 mCi Use this code for AN-DTPA, DTPA, MPI-DTPA Kit-Chelate, MPI Indium DTPA IN-111, Pentate Calcium Trisodium, Pentate Zinc Trisodium.
A9568	Technetium Tc-99m arcitumomab, diagnostic, per study dose, up to 45 mCi Use this code for CEA Scan.
A9569	Technetium Tc-99m exametazime labeled autologous white blood cells, diagnostic, per study dose
A9570	Indium In-111 labeled autologous white blood cells, diagnostic, per study dose
A9571	Indium In-111 labeled autologous platelets, diagnostic, per study dose
A9572	Indium In-111 pentetreotide, diagnostic, per study dose, up to 6 mCi Use this code for Ostreoscan.

Medical and Surgical Supplies

A9513 — A9572

Special Coverage Instructions   Noncovered by Medicare   Carrier Discretion   ☑ Quantity Alert   ● New Code   ○ Recycled/Reinstated   ▲ Revised Code

© 2022 Optum, Inc.   A2-Z3 ASC Pmt   CMS: IOM   AHA: Coding Clinic   DMEPOS Paid   ⊘ SNF Excluded   A Codes — 15

Medical and Surgical Supplies

A9575 Injection, gadoterate meglumine, 0.1 ml
Use this code for Dotarem.

A9576 Injection, gadoteridol, (ProHance multipack), per ml

A9577 Injection, gadobenate dimeglumine (MultiHance), per ml

A9578 Injection, gadobenate dimeglumine (MultiHance multipack), per ml

A9579 Injection, gadolinium-based magnetic resonance contrast agent, not otherwise specified (NOS), per ml
Use this code for Omniscan, Magnevist.
CMS: 100-03,1,220.2

A9580 Sodium fluoride F-18, diagnostic, per study dose, up to 30 mCi
CMS: 100-03,220.6.19; 100-04,13,60.18; 100-04,13,60.3.2

A9581 Injection, gadoxetate disodium, 1 ml
Use this code for Eovist.

A9582 Iodine I-123 iobenguane, diagnostic, per study dose, up to 15 mCi

A9583 Injection, gadofosveset trisodium, 1 ml
Use this code for Ablavar, Vasovist.

A9584 Iodine I-123 ioflupane, diagnostic, per study dose, up to 5 mCi
Use this code for DaTscan.

A9585 Injection, gadobutrol, 0.1 ml
Use this code for Gadavist.

A9586 Florbetapir F18, diagnostic, per study dose, up to 10 mCi
Use this code for Amyvid.
CMS: 100-04,13,60.12; 100-04,17, 80.12; 100-04,32,60.12

A9587 Gallium Ga-68, dotatate, diagnostic, 0.1 mCi
Use this code for Netspot.
CMS: 100-04,13,60.3.2
AHA: 1Q,17

A9588 Fluciclovine F-18, diagnostic, 1 mCi
Use this code for Axumin.
CMS: 100-04,13,60.3.2
AHA: 1Q,17

A9589 Instillation, hexaminolevulinate HCl, 100 mg
Use this code for Cysview.
CMS: 100-04,13,60.3.2
AHA: 1Q,19

A9590 Iodine I-131, iobenguane, 1 mCi
Use this code for Azedra.
CMS: 100-04,13,60.3.2

A9591 Fluoroestradiol F-18, diagnostic, 1 mCi
Use this code for Cerianna.
CMS: 100-04,13,60.3.2
AHA: 1Q,21

A9592 Copper Cu-64, dotatate, diagnostic, 1 mCi
Use this code for Detectnet.
CMS: 100-04,13,60.3.2
AHA: 1Q,21

A9593 Gallium Ga-68 PSMA-11, diagnostic, (UCSF), 1 mCi
CMS: 100-04,13,60.3.2
AHA: 3Q,21

A9594 Gallium Ga-68 PSMA-11, diagnostic, (UCLA), 1 mCi
CMS: 100-04,13,60.3.2
AHA: 3Q,21

A9595 Piflufolastat F-18, diagnostic, 1 mCi
Use this code for Pylarify.
CMS: 100-04,13,60.3.2
AHA: 1Q,22

● **A9596** Gallium Ga-68 gozetotide, diagnostic, (Illuccix), 1 mCi
CMS: 100-04,13,60.3.2
AHA: 3Q,22

A9597 Positron emission tomography radiopharmaceutical, diagnostic, for tumor identification, not otherwise classified
CMS: 100-04,13,60.3.2
AHA: 1Q,17

A9598 Positron emission tomography radiopharmaceutical, diagnostic, for nontumor identification, not otherwise classified
CMS: 100-04,13,60.3.2
AHA: 1Q,17

A9600 Strontium Sr-89 chloride, therapeutic, per mCi
Use this code for Metastron.

● **A9601** Flortaucipir F 18 injection, diagnostic, 1 mCi
Use this code for Tauvid.
AHA: 3Q,22

● **A9602** Fluorodopa F-18, diagnostic, per mCi

A9604 Samarium Sm-153 lexidronam, therapeutic, per treatment dose, up to 150 mCi
Use this code for Quadramet.

A9606 Radium RA-223 dichloride, therapeutic, per UCI
Use this code for Xofigo.

● **A9607** Lutetium Lu 177 vipivotide tetraxetan, therapeutic, 1 mCi
Use this code for Pluvicto.

A9698 Nonradioactive contrast imaging material, not otherwise classified, per study
AHA: 1Q,17

A9699 Radiopharmaceutical, therapeutic, not otherwise classified

A9700 Supply of injectable contrast material for use in echocardiography, per study
AHA: 1Q,17

● **A9800** Gallium Ga-68 gozetotide, diagnostic, (Locametz), 1 mCi

Miscellaneous

A9900 Miscellaneous DME supply, accessory, and/or service component of another HCPCS code

A9901 DME delivery, set up, and/or dispensing service component of another HCPCS code

A9999 Miscellaneous DME supply or accessory, not otherwise specified

Enteral and Parenteral Therapy B4034-B9999

This section includes codes for supplies, formulae, nutritional solutions, and infusion pumps.

Enteral Formulae and Enteral Medical Supplies

B4034 Enteral feeding supply kit; syringe fed, per day, includes but not limited to feeding/flushing syringe, administration set tubing, dressings, tape
CMS: 100-03,180.2; 100-04,20,160.2

B4035 Enteral feeding supply kit; pump fed, per day, includes but not limited to feeding/flushing syringe, administration set tubing, dressings, tape
CMS: 100-03,180.2; 100-04,20,160.2

B4036 Enteral feeding supply kit; gravity fed, per day, includes but not limited to feeding/flushing syringe, administration set tubing, dressings, tape
CMS: 100-03,180.2; 100-04,20,160.2

B4081 Nasogastric tubing with stylet
CMS: 100-03,180.2; 100-04,20,160.2

Many types of stylets are used. Some may be fitted with lights or optics. Others are used as guides

B4082 Nasogastric tubing without stylet
CMS: 100-03,180.2; 100-04,20,160.2

B4083 Stomach tube - Levine type
CMS: 100-03,180.2; 100-04,20,160.2

B4087 Gastrostomy/jejunostomy tube, standard, any material, any type, each
CMS: 100-03,180.2

B4088 Gastrostomy/jejunostomy tube, low-profile, any material, any type, each
CMS: 100-03,180.2

B4100 Food thickener, administered orally, per oz
CMS: 100-03,180.2

B4102 Enteral formula, for adults, used to replace fluids and electrolytes (e.g., clear liquids), 500 ml = 1 unit
CMS: 100-03,180.2

B4103 Enteral formula, for pediatrics, used to replace fluids and electrolytes (e.g., clear liquids), 500 ml = 1 unit
CMS: 100-03,180.2

B4104 Additive for enteral formula (e.g., fiber)
CMS: 100-03,180.2

B4105 In-line cartridge containing digestive enzyme(s) for enteral feeding, each
CMS: 100-03,180.2

B4149 Enteral formula, manufactured blenderized natural foods with intact nutrients, includes proteins, fats, carbohydrates, vitamins and minerals, may include fiber, administered through an enteral feeding tube, 100 calories = 1 unit
CMS: 100-03,180.2

B4150 Enteral formula, nutritionally complete with intact nutrients, includes proteins, fats, carbohydrates, vitamins and minerals, may include fiber, administered through an enteral feeding tube, 100 calories = 1 unit
Use this code for Enrich, Ensure, Ensure HN, Ensure Powder, Isocal, Lonalac Powder, Meritene, Meritene Powder, Osmolite, Osmolite HN, Portagen Powder, Sustacal, Renu, Sustagen Powder, Travasorb.
CMS: 100-03,180.2; 100-04,20,160.2

B4152 Enteral formula, nutritionally complete, calorically dense (equal to or greater than 1.5 kcal/ml) with intact nutrients, includes proteins, fats, carbohydrates, vitamins and minerals, may include fiber, administered through an enteral feeding tube, 100 calories = 1 unit
Use this code for Magnacal, Isocal HCN, Sustacal HC, Ensure Plus, Ensure Plus HN.
CMS: 100-03,180.2; 100-04,20,160.2

B4153 Enteral formula, nutritionally complete, hydrolyzed proteins (amino acids and peptide chain), includes fats, carbohydrates, vitamins and minerals, may include fiber, administered through an enteral feeding tube, 100 calories = 1 unit
Use this code for Criticare HN, Vivonex t.e.n. (Total Enteral Nutrition), Vivonex HN, Vital (Vital HN), Travasorb HN, Isotein HN, Precision HN, Precision Isotonic.
CMS: 100-03,180.2; 100-04,20,160.2

B4154 Enteral formula, nutritionally complete, for special metabolic needs, excludes inherited disease of metabolism, includes altered composition of proteins, fats, carbohydrates, vitamins and/or minerals, may include fiber, administered through an enteral feeding tube, 100 calories = 1 unit
Use this code for Hepatic-aid, Travasorb Hepatic, Travasorb MCT, Travasorb Renal, Traum-aid, Tramcal, Aminaid.
CMS: 100-03,180.2; 100-04,20,160.2

B4155 Enteral formula, nutritionally incomplete/modular nutrients, includes specific nutrients, carbohydrates (e.g., glucose polymers), proteins/amino acids (e.g., glutamine, arginine), fat (e.g., medium chain triglycerides) or combination, administered through an enteral feeding tube, 100 calories = 1 unit
Use this code for Propac, Gerval Protein, Promix, Casec, Moducal, Controlyte, Polycose Liquid or Powder, Sumacal, Microlipids, MCT Oil, Nutri-source.
CMS: 100-03,180.2; 100-04,20,160.2

B4157 Enteral formula, nutritionally complete, for special metabolic needs for inherited disease of metabolism, includes proteins, fats, carbohydrates, vitamins and minerals, may include fiber, administered through an enteral feeding tube, 100 calories = 1 unit
CMS: 100-03,180.2

B4158 Enteral formula, for pediatrics, nutritionally complete with intact nutrients, includes proteins, fats, carbohydrates, vitamins and minerals, may include fiber and/or iron, administered through an enteral feeding tube, 100 calories = 1 unit
CMS: 100-03,180.2

B4159 Enteral formula, for pediatrics, nutritionally complete soy based with intact nutrients, includes proteins, fats, carbohydrates, vitamins and minerals, may include fiber and/or iron, administered through an enteral feeding tube, 100 calories = 1 unit
CMS: 100-03,180.2

Enteral and Parenteral Therapy

B4160 Enteral formula, for pediatrics, nutritionally complete calorically dense (equal to or greater than 0.7 kcal/ml) with intact nutrients, includes proteins, fats, carbohydrates, vitamins and minerals, may include fiber, administered through an enteral feeding tube, 100 calories = 1 unit
CMS: 100-03,180.2

B4161 Enteral formula, for pediatrics, hydrolyzed/amino acids and peptide chain proteins, includes fats, carbohydrates, vitamins and minerals, may include fiber, administered through an enteral feeding tube, 100 calories = 1 unit
CMS: 100-03,180.2

B4162 Enteral formula, for pediatrics, special metabolic needs for inherited disease of metabolism, includes proteins, fats, carbohydrates, vitamins and minerals, may include fiber, administered through an enteral feeding tube, 100 calories = 1 unit
CMS: 100-03,180.2

Parenteral Nutrition Solutions and Supplies

B4164 Parenteral nutrition solution: carbohydrates (dextrose), 50% or less (500 ml = 1 unit), home mix
CMS: 100-03,180.2; 100-04,20,160.2

B4168 Parenteral nutrition solution; amino acid, 3.5%, (500 ml = 1 unit) - home mix
CMS: 100-03,180.2; 100-04,20,160.2

B4172 Parenteral nutrition solution; amino acid, 5.5% through 7%, (500 ml = 1 unit) - home mix
CMS: 100-03,180.2; 100-04,20,160.2

B4176 Parenteral nutrition solution; amino acid, 7% through 8.5%, (500 ml = 1 unit) - home mix
CMS: 100-03,180.2; 100-04,20,160.2

B4178 Parenteral nutrition solution: amino acid, greater than 8.5% (500 ml = 1 unit) - home mix
CMS: 100-03,180.2; 100-04,20,160.2

B4180 Parenteral nutrition solution: carbohydrates (dextrose), greater than 50% (500 ml = 1 unit), home mix
CMS: 100-03,180.2; 100-04,20,160.2

B4185 Parenteral nutrition solution, not otherwise specified, 10 g lipids
CMS: 100-03,180.2

B4187 Omegaven, 10 g lipids
CMS: 100-03,180.2

B4189 Parenteral nutrition solution: compounded amino acid and carbohydrates with electrolytes, trace elements, and vitamins, including preparation, any strength, 10 to 51 g of protein, premix
CMS: 100-03,180.2; 100-04,20,160.2

B4193 Parenteral nutrition solution: compounded amino acid and carbohydrates with electrolytes, trace elements, and vitamins, including preparation, any strength, 52 to 73 g of protein, premix
CMS: 100-03,180.2; 100-04,20,160.2

B4197 Parenteral nutrition solution; compounded amino acid and carbohydrates with electrolytes, trace elements and vitamins, including preparation, any strength, 74 to 100 g of protein - premix
CMS: 100-03,180.2; 100-04,20,160.2

B4199 Parenteral nutrition solution; compounded amino acid and carbohydrates with electrolytes, trace elements and vitamins, including preparation, any strength, over 100 g of protein - premix
CMS: 100-03,180.2; 100-04,20,160.2

B4216 Parenteral nutrition; additives (vitamins, trace elements, Heparin, electrolytes), home mix, per day
CMS: 100-03,180.2; 100-04,20,160.2

B4220 Parenteral nutrition supply kit; premix, per day
CMS: 100-03,180.2; 100-04,20,160.2

B4222 Parenteral nutrition supply kit; home mix, per day
CMS: 100-03,180.2; 100-04,20,160.2

B4224 Parenteral nutrition administration kit, per day
CMS: 100-03,180.2; 100-04,20,160.2

B5000 Parenteral nutrition solution: compounded amino acid and carbohydrates with electrolytes, trace elements, and vitamins, including preparation, any strength, renal - Amirosyn RF, NephrAmine, RenAmine - premix
Use this code for Amirosyn-RF, NephrAmine, RenAmin.
CMS: 100-03,180.2; 100-04,20,160.2

B5100 Parenteral nutrition solution compounded amino acid and carbohydrates with electrolytes, trace elements, and vitamins, including preparation, any strength, hepatic-HepatAmine-premix
Use this code for FreAmine HBC, HepatAmine.
CMS: 100-03,180.2; 100-04,20,160.2

B5200 Parenteral nutrition solution compounded amino acid and carbohydrates with electrolytes, trace elements, and vitamins, including preparation, any strength, stress-branch chain amino acids-FreAmine-HBC-premix
CMS: 100-03,180.2; 100-04,20,160.2

Enteral and Parenteral Pumps

B9002 Enteral nutrition infusion pump, any type
CMS: 100-03,180.2; 100-04,20,160.2

B9004 Parenteral nutrition infusion pump, portable
CMS: 100-03,180.2; 100-04,20,160.2

B9006 Parenteral nutrition infusion pump, stationary
CMS: 100-03,180.2; 100-04,20,160.2

B9998 NOC for enteral supplies
CMS: 100-03,180.2

B9999 NOC for parenteral supplies
Determine if an alternative HCPCS Level II or a CPT code better describes the service being reported. This code should be used only if a more specific code is unavailable.
CMS: 100-03,180.2

Outpatient PPS C1052-C9899

This section reports drug, biological, and device codes that must be used by OPPS hospitals. Non-OPPS hospitals, Critical Access Hospitals (CAHs), Indian Health Service Hospitals (HIS), hospitals located in American Samoa, Guam, Saipan, or the Virgin Islands, and Maryland waiver hospitals may report these codes at their discretion. The codes can only be reported for facility (technical) services.

The C series of HCPCS may include device categories, new technology procedures, and drugs, biologicals and radiopharmaceuticals that do not have other HCPCS codes assigned. Some of these items and services are eligible for transitional pass-through payments for OPPS hospitals, have separate APC payments, or are items that are packaged. Hospitals are encouraged to report all appropriate C codes regardless of payment status.

C1052 Hemostatic agent, gastrointestinal, topical
CMS: 100-04,4,60.4.2

C1062 Intravertebral body fracture augmentation with implant (e.g., metal, polymer)
CMS: 100-04,4,60.4.2

C1713 Anchor/screw for opposing bone-to-bone or soft tissue-to-bone (implantable)
CMS: 100-04,4,60.4.2; 100-04,4,60.4.3
AHA: 3Q,22; 2Q,21; 1Q,21; 4Q,20; 2Q,18; 1Q,18; 3Q,16

C1714 Catheter, transluminal atherectomy, directional
CMS: 100-04,4,60.4.2

C1715 Brachytherapy needle
CMS: 100-04,4,60.4.2

C1716 Brachytherapy source, nonstranded, gold-198, per source
CMS: 100-04,4,60.4.2

C1717 Brachytherapy source, nonstranded, high dose rate iridium-192, per source
CMS: 100-04,4,60.4.2

C1719 Brachytherapy source, nonstranded, nonhigh dose rate iridium-192, per source
CMS: 100-04,4,60.4.2

C1721 Cardioverter-defibrillator, dual chamber (implantable)
CMS: 100-04,14,40.8; 100-04,4,60.4.2

C1722 Cardioverter-defibrillator, single chamber (implantable)
CMS: 100-04,14,40.8; 100-04,4,60.4.2
AHA: 2Q,17; 3Q,16

C1724 Catheter, transluminal atherectomy, rotational
CMS: 100-04,4,60.4.1; 100-04,4,60.4.2

C1725 Catheter, transluminal angioplasty, nonlaser (may include guidance, infusion/perfusion capability)
To appropriately report drug-coated transluminal angioplasty catheters, use HCPCS code C2623.
CMS: 100-04,4,60.4.2; 100-04,4,60.4.3

C1726 Catheter, balloon dilatation, nonvascular
CMS: 100-04,4,60.4.2; 100-04,4,60.4.3

C1727 Catheter, balloon tissue dissector, nonvascular (insertable)
CMS: 100-04,4,60.4.2; 100-04,4,60.4.3

C1728 Catheter, brachytherapy seed administration
CMS: 100-04,4,60.4.2

C1729 Catheter, drainage
CMS: 100-04,4,60.4.2; 100-04,4,60.4.3

C1730 Catheter, electrophysiology, diagnostic, other than 3D mapping (19 or fewer electrodes)
CMS: 100-04,4,60.4.2; 100-04,4,60.4.3

C1731 Catheter, electrophysiology, diagnostic, other than 3D mapping (20 or more electrodes)
CMS: 100-04,4,60.4.2; 100-04,4,60.4.3

C1732 Catheter, electrophysiology, diagnostic/ablation, 3D or vector mapping
CMS: 100-04,4,60.4.2; 100-04,4,60.4.3

C1733 Catheter, electrophysiology, diagnostic/ablation, other than 3D or vector mapping, other than cool-tip
CMS: 100-04,4,60.4.2; 100-04,4,60.4.3

C1734 Orthopedic/device/drug matrix for opposing bone-to-bone or soft tissue-to bone (implantable)
CMS: 100-04,4,60.4.2
AHA: 1Q,20

● **C1747** Endoscope, single-use (i.e., disposable), urinary tract, imaging/illumination device (insertable)

C1748 Endoscope, single-use (i.e. disposable), upper GI, imaging/illumination device (insertable)
CMS: 100-04,4,60.4.2
AHA: 2Q,20

C1749 Endoscope, retrograde imaging/illumination colonoscope device (implantable)
CMS: 100-04,4,60.4.2

C1750 Catheter, hemodialysis/peritoneal, long-term
CMS: 100-04,4,60.4.2

C1751 Catheter, infusion, inserted peripherally, centrally or midline (other than hemodialysis)
CMS: 100-04,4,60.4.1; 100-04,4,60.4.2
AHA: 2Q,19; 3Q,16

C1752 Catheter, hemodialysis/peritoneal, short-term
CMS: 100-04,4,60.4.2

C1753 Catheter, intravascular ultrasound
CMS: 100-04,4,60.4.2

C1754 Catheter, intradiscal
CMS: 100-04,4,60.4.2

C1755 Catheter, intraspinal
CMS: 100-04,4,60.4.2

C1756 Catheter, pacing, transesophageal
CMS: 100-04,4,60.4.2

C1757 Catheter, thrombectomy/embolectomy
CMS: 100-04,4,60.4.2

C1758 Catheter, ureteral
CMS: 100-04,4,60.4.2

C1759 Catheter, intracardiac echocardiography
CMS: 100-04,4,60.4.2

C1760 Closure device, vascular (implantable/insertable)
CMS: 100-04,4,60.4.2; 100-04,4,60.4.3

C1761 Catheter, transluminal intravascular lithotripsy, coronary
CMS: 100-04,4,60.4.2
AHA: 4Q,21; 3Q,21

C1762 Connective tissue, human (includes fascia lata)
CMS: 100-04,4,60.4.2; 100-04,4,60.4.3

C1763 Connective tissue, nonhuman (includes synthetic)
CMS: 100-04,4,60.4.2; 100-04,4,60.4.3

C1764 Event recorder, cardiac (implantable)
CMS: 100-04,14,40.8; 100-04,4,60.4.2

C1765 Adhesion barrier
CMS: 100-04,4,60.4.2; 100-04,4,60.4.3

Outpatient PPS

C1766 — C1832

C1766 Introducer/sheath, guiding, intracardiac electrophysiological, steerable, other than peel-away N N1
CMS: 100-04,4,60.4.2

C1767 Generator, neurostimulator (implantable), nonrechargeable N N1
CMS: 100-04,14,40.8; 100-04,32,40.1; 100-04,32,40.2.1; 100-04,32,40.2.4; 100-04,32,40.4; 100-04,4,60.4.2
AHA: 1Q,21; 3Q,16

C1768 Graft, vascular N N1
CMS: 100-04,4,60.4.2

C1769 Guide wire N N1
CMS: 100-04,4,60.4.2
AHA: 1Q,22; 3Q,19; 2Q,19; 3Q,16

C1770 Imaging coil, magnetic resonance (insertable) N N1
CMS: 100-04,4,60.4.2

C1771 Repair device, urinary, incontinence, with sling graft N N1
CMS: 100-04,14,40.8; 100-04,4,60.4.2; 100-04,4,60.4.3

C1772 Infusion pump, programmable (implantable) N N1
CMS: 100-04,14,40.8; 100-04,4,60.4.2

C1773 Retrieval device, insertable (used to retrieve fractured medical devices) N N1
CMS: 100-04,4,60.4.2; 100-04,4,60.4.3

C1776 Joint device (implantable) N N1
CMS: 100-04,14,40.8; 100-04,4,60.4.2; 100-04,4,60.4.3
AHA: 3Q,21; 1Q,20; 3Q,18; 3Q,16

C1777 Lead, cardioverter-defibrillator, endocardial single coil (implantable) N N1
CMS: 100-04,4,60.4.2
AHA: 2Q,17; 3Q,16

C1778 Lead, neurostimulator (implantable) N N1
CMS: 100-04,14,40.8; 100-04,32,40.1; 100-04,32,40.2.1; 100-04,32,40.2.4; 100-04,32,40.4; 100-04,4,60.4.2
AHA: 1Q,21; 3Q,19; 1Q,19; 3Q,16

C1779 Lead, pacemaker, transvenous VDD single pass N N1
CMS: 100-04,14,40.8; 100-04,4,60.4.2; 100-04,4,60.4.3

C1780 Lens, intraocular (new technology) N N1
CMS: 100-04,4,60.4.2; 100-04,4,60.4.3

C1781 Mesh (implantable) N N1
Use this code for OrthADAPT Bioimplant.
CMS: 100-04,4,60.4.2; 100-04,4,60.4.3
AHA: 1Q,19; 3Q,16

C1782 Morcellator N N1
CMS: 100-04,4,60.4.2; 100-04,4,60.4.3

C1783 Ocular implant, aqueous drainage assist device N N1
CMS: 100-04,4,60.4.2
AHA: 1Q,17; 3Q,16

C1784 Ocular device, intraoperative, detached retina N N1
CMS: 100-04,4,60.4.2; 100-04,4,60.4.3

C1785 Pacemaker, dual chamber, rate-responsive (implantable) N N1
CMS: 100-04,14,40.8; 100-04,21,320.4.7; 100-04,32,320.4.1; 100-04,32,320.4.2; 100-04,32,320.4.4; 100-04,32,320.4.6; 100-04,32,320.4.7; 100-04,4,60.4.2

C1786 Pacemaker, single chamber, rate-responsive (implantable) N N1
CMS: 100-04,14,40.8; 100-04,21,320.4.7; 100-04,32,320.4.1; 100-04,32,320.4.2; 100-04,32,320.4.4; 100-04,32,320.4.6; 100-04,32,320.4.7; 100-04,4,60.4.2

C1787 Patient programmer, neurostimulator N N1
CMS: 100-04,4,60.4.2; 100-04,4,60.4.3

C1788 Port, indwelling (implantable) N N1
CMS: 100-04,4,60.4.2
AHA: 2Q,19; 3Q,16

C1789 Prosthesis, breast (implantable) N N1
CMS: 100-04,4,60.4.2

C1813 Prosthesis, penile, inflatable N N1
CMS: 100-04,14,40.8; 100-04,4,60.4.2

C1814 Retinal tamponade device, silicone oil N N1
CMS: 100-04,4,60.4.2; 100-04,4,60.4.3

C1815 Prosthesis, urinary sphincter (implantable) N N1
CMS: 100-04,14,40.8; 100-04,4,60.4.2

C1816 Receiver and/or transmitter, neurostimulator (implantable) N N1
CMS: 100-04,4,60.4.2

C1817 Septal defect implant system, intracardiac N N1
CMS: 100-04,4,60.4.2; 100-04,4,60.4.3

C1818 Integrated keratoprosthesis N N1
CMS: 100-04,4,60.4.2; 100-04,4,60.4.3

C1819 Surgical tissue localization and excision device (implantable) N N1
CMS: 100-04,4,60.4.2

C1820 Generator, neurostimulator (implantable), with rechargeable battery and charging system N N1
Use to report neurostimulator generators that are not high frequency.
CMS: 100-04,14,40.8; 100-04,32,40.2.1; 100-04,32,40.2.4; 100-04,32,40.4; 100-04,4,10.12; 100-04,4,60.4.2

C1821 Interspinous process distraction device (implantable) N N1
CMS: 100-04,4,60.4.2

C1822 Generator, neurostimulator (implantable), high frequency, with rechargeable battery and charging system N N1
Use to report neurostimulator generators that are high frequency.
CMS: 100-04,4,60.4.2

C1823 Generator, neurostimulator (implantable), nonrechargeable, with transvenous sensing and stimulation leads J7
CMS: 100-04,4,260.1; 100-04,4,260.1.1; 100-04,4,60.4.2
AHA: 1Q,19

C1824 Generator, cardiac contractility modulation (implantable) J7
CMS: 100-04,4,60.4.2
AHA: 1Q,20

C1825 Generator, neurostimulator (implantable), nonrechargeable with carotid sinus baroreceptor stimulation lead(s) J7
CMS: 100-04,4,60.4.2

● **C1826** Generator, neurostimulator (implantable), includes closed feedback loop leads and all implantable components, with rechargeable battery and charging system

● **C1827** Generator, neurostimulator (implantable), nonrechargeable, with implantable stimulation lead and external paired stimulation controller

C1830 Powered bone marrow biopsy needle N N1
CMS: 100-04,4,60.4.2

▲ **C1831** Interbody cage, anterior, lateral or posterior, personalized (implantable) J7
CMS: 100-04,4,60.4.2
AHA: 1Q,22; 4Q,21

C1832 Autograft suspension, including cell processing and application, and all system components J7
CMS: 100-04,4,60.4.2
AHA: 1Q,22

Special Coverage Instructions | Noncovered by Medicare | Carrier Discretion | ☑ Quantity Alert | ● New Code | ○ Recycled/Reinstated | ▲ Revised Code

20 — C Codes | A Age Edit | M Maternity Edit | ♀ Female Only | ♂ Male Only | A-Y OPPS Status Indicators | © 2022 Optum, Inc.

C1833 Monitor, cardiac, including intracardiac lead and all system components (implantable) [J7]
CMS: 100-04,4,60.4.2
AHA: 1Q,22

● **C1834** Pressure sensor system, includes all components (e.g., introducer, sensor), intramuscular (implantable), excludes mobile (wireless) software application [J7]

C1839 Iris prosthesis [J7]
CMS: 100-04,4,60.4.2
AHA: 1Q,20

C1840 Lens, intraocular (telescopic) [N][N1]
CMS: 100-04,4,60.4.2

C1841 Retinal prosthesis, includes all internal and external components

C1842 Retinal prosthesis, includes all internal and external components; add-on to C1841

C1849 Skin substitute, synthetic, resorbable, per sq cm

C1874 Stent, coated/covered, with delivery system [N][N1]
CMS: 100-04,4,60.4.2; 100-04,4,60.4.3

C1875 Stent, coated/covered, without delivery system [N][N1]
CMS: 100-04,4,60.4.2; 100-04,4,60.4.3
AHA: 2Q,20; 3Q,16

C1876 Stent, noncoated/noncovered, with delivery system [N][N1]
CMS: 100-04,4,60.4.2; 100-04,4,60.4.3

C1877 Stent, noncoated/noncovered, without delivery system [N][N1]
CMS: 100-04,4,60.4.2

C1878 Material for vocal cord medialization, synthetic (implantable) [N][N1]
CMS: 100-04,4,60.4.2; 100-04,4,60.4.3

C1880 Vena cava filter [N][N1]
CMS: 100-04,4,60.4.2

C1881 Dialysis access system (implantable) [N][N1]
CMS: 100-04,14,40.8; 100-04,4,60.4.2

C1882 Cardioverter-defibrillator, other than single or dual chamber (implantable) [N][N1]
CMS: 100-04,14,40.8; 100-04,4,60.4.2; 100-04,4,60.4.3

C1883 Adaptor/extension, pacing lead or neurostimulator lead (implantable) [N][N1]
CMS: 100-04,32,40.1; 100-04,32,40.2.1; 100-04,32,40.2.4; 100-04,32,40.4; 100-04,4,60.4.2; 100-04,4,60.4.3

C1884 Embolization protective system [N][N1]
CMS: 100-04,4,60.4.2; 100-04,4,60.4.3

C1885 Catheter, transluminal angioplasty, laser [N][N1]
CMS: 100-04,4,60.4.2; 100-04,4,60.4.3

C1886 Catheter, extravascular tissue ablation, any modality (insertable) [N][N1]
CMS: 100-04,4,60.4.2

C1887 Catheter, guiding (may include infusion/perfusion capability) [N][N1]
CMS: 100-04,4,60.4.2; 100-04,4,60.4.3

C1888 Catheter, ablation, noncardiac, endovascular (implantable) [N][N1]
CMS: 100-04,4,60.4.2; 100-04,4,60.4.3

C1889 Implantable/insertable device, not otherwise classified [N][N1]

C1890 No implantable/insertable device used with device-intensive procedures [J7]
CMS: 100-04,4,260.1; 100-04,4,260.1.1
AHA: 1Q,19

C1891 Infusion pump, nonprogrammable, permanent (implantable) [N][N1]
CMS: 100-04,14,40.8; 100-04,4,60.4.2

C1892 Introducer/sheath, guiding, intracardiac electrophysiological, fixed-curve, peel-away [N][N1]
CMS: 100-04,4,60.4.2; 100-04,4,60.4.3

C1893 Introducer/sheath, guiding, intracardiac electrophysiological, fixed-curve, other than peel-away [N][N1]
CMS: 100-04,4,60.4.2

C1894 Introducer/sheath, other than guiding, other than intracardiac electrophysiological, nonlaser [N][N1]
CMS: 100-04,4,60.4.1; 100-04,4,60.4.2
AHA: 2Q,19; 3Q,16

C1895 Lead, cardioverter-defibrillator, endocardial dual coil (implantable) [N][N1]
CMS: 100-04,4,60.4.2

C1896 Lead, cardioverter-defibrillator, other than endocardial single or dual coil (implantable) [N][N1]
CMS: 100-04,4,60.4.2

C1897 Lead, neurostimulator test kit (implantable) [N][N1]
CMS: 100-04,14,40.8; 100-04,32,40.1; 100-04,32,40.2.1; 100-04,32,40.2.4; 100-04,32,40.4; 100-04,4,60.4.2

C1898 Lead, pacemaker, other than transvenous VDD single pass [N][N1]
CMS: 100-04,14,40.8; 100-04,4,60.4.2

C1899 Lead, pacemaker/cardioverter-defibrillator combination (implantable) [N][N1]
CMS: 100-04,4,60.4.2

C1900 Lead, left ventricular coronary venous system [N][N1]
CMS: 100-04,14,40.8; 100-04,4,60.4.2; 100-04,4,60.4.3

C1982 Catheter, pressure generating, one-way valve, intermittently occlusive [J7]
CMS: 100-04,4,60.4.2
AHA: 1Q,20

C2596 Probe, image guided, robotic, waterjet ablation [J7]
CMS: 100-04,4,60.4.2
AHA: 1Q,20

C2613 Lung biopsy plug with delivery system [N][N1]
CMS: 100-04,4,60.4.2

C2614 Probe, percutaneous lumbar discectomy [N][N1]
CMS: 100-04,4,60.4.2

C2615 Sealant, pulmonary, liquid [N][N1]
CMS: 100-04,4,60.4.2; 100-04,4,60.4.3

C2616 Brachytherapy source, nonstranded, yttrium-90, per source [U][H2]☑⊘
CMS: 100-04,4,60.4.2

C2617 Stent, noncoronary, temporary, without delivery system [N][N1]
CMS: 100-04,4,60.4.2; 100-04,4,60.4.3
AHA: 1Q,18; 3Q,16

C2618 Probe/needle, cryoablation [N][N1]
CMS: 100-04,4,60.4.2

C2619 Pacemaker, dual chamber, nonrate-responsive (implantable) [N][N1]
CMS: 100-04,14,40.8; 100-04,21,320.4.7; 100-04,32,320.4.1; 100-04,32,320.4.2; 100-04,32,320.4.4; 100-04,32,320.4.6; 100-04,32,320.4.7; 100-04,4,60.4.2

Outpatient PPS — C2620–C7503

Code	Description
C2620	Pacemaker, single chamber, nonrate-responsive (implantable) [N1] CMS: 100-04,14,40.8; 100-04,21,320.4.7; 100-04,32,320.4.1; 100-04,32,320.4.2; 100-04,32,320.4.4; 100-04,32,320.4.6; 100-04,32,320.4.7; 100-04,4,60.4.2
C2621	Pacemaker, other than single or dual chamber (implantable) [N1] CMS: 100-04,14,40.8; 100-04,4,60.4.2; 100-04,4,60.4.3
C2622	Prosthesis, penile, noninflatable [N1] CMS: 100-04,14,40.8; 100-04,4,60.4.2
C2623	Catheter, transluminal angioplasty, drug-coated, nonlaser [N1] CMS: 100-04,4,60.4.2
C2624	Implantable wireless pulmonary artery pressure sensor with delivery catheter, including all system components [N1] CMS: 100-04,4,60.4.2
C2625	Stent, noncoronary, temporary, with delivery system [N1] CMS: 100-04,4,60.4.2; 100-04,4,60.4.3
C2626	Infusion pump, nonprogrammable, temporary (implantable) [N1] CMS: 100-04,14,40.8; 100-04,4,60.4.2; 100-04,4,60.4.3
C2627	Catheter, suprapubic/cystoscopic [N1] CMS: 100-04,4,60.4.2
C2628	Catheter, occlusion [N1] CMS: 100-04,4,60.4.2
C2629	Introducer/sheath, other than guiding, other than intracardiac electrophysiological, laser [N1] CMS: 100-04,4,60.4.2
C2630	Catheter, electrophysiology, diagnostic/ablation, other than 3D or vector mapping, cool-tip [N1] CMS: 100-04,4,60.4.2; 100-04,4,60.4.3
C2631	Repair device, urinary, incontinence, without sling graft [N1] CMS: 100-04,14,40.8; 100-04,4,60.4.2; 100-04,4,60.4.3
C2634	Brachytherapy source, nonstranded, high activity, iodine-125, greater than 1.01 mCi (NIST), per source [U H2]
C2635	Brachytherapy source, nonstranded, high activity, palladium-103, greater than 2.2 mCi (NIST), per source [U H2]
C2636	Brachytherapy linear source, nonstranded, palladium-103, per 1 mm [U H2]
C2637	Brachytherapy source, nonstranded, ytterbium-169, per source [B]
C2638	Brachytherapy source, stranded, iodine-125, per source [U H2]
C2639	Brachytherapy source, nonstranded, iodine-125, per source [U H2]
C2640	Brachytherapy source, stranded, palladium-103, per source [U H2]
C2641	Brachytherapy source, nonstranded, palladium-103, per source [U H2]
C2642	Brachytherapy source, stranded, cesium-131, per source [U H2]
C2643	Brachytherapy source, nonstranded, cesium-131, per source [U H2]
C2644	Brachytherapy source, cesium-131 chloride solution, per mCi [U]
C2645	Brachytherapy planar source, palladium-103, per sq mm [U H2]
C2698	Brachytherapy source, stranded, not otherwise specified, per source [U H2]
C2699	Brachytherapy source, nonstranded, not otherwise specified, per source [U H2]
C5271	Application of low cost skin substitute graft to trunk, arms, legs, total wound surface area up to 100 sq cm; first 25 sq cm or less wound surface area [T G2]
C5272	Application of low cost skin substitute graft to trunk, arms, legs, total wound surface area up to 100 sq cm; each additional 25 sq cm wound surface area, or part thereof (list separately in addition to code for primary procedure) [N N1]
C5273	Application of low cost skin substitute graft to trunk, arms, legs, total wound surface area greater than or equal to 100 sq cm; first 100 sq cm wound surface area, or 1% of body area of infants and children [T G2]
C5274	Application of low cost skin substitute graft to trunk, arms, legs, total wound surface area greater than or equal to 100 sq cm; each additional 100 sq cm wound surface area, or part thereof, or each additional 1% of body area of infants and children, or part thereof (list separately in addition to code for primary procedure) [N N1]
C5275	Application of low cost skin substitute graft to face, scalp, eyelids, mouth, neck, ears, orbits, genitalia, hands, feet, and/or multiple digits, total wound surface area up to 100 sq cm; first 25 sq cm or less wound surface area [T G2]
C5276	Application of low cost skin substitute graft to face, scalp, eyelids, mouth, neck, ears, orbits, genitalia, hands, feet, and/or multiple digits, total wound surface area up to 100 sq cm; each additional 25 sq cm wound surface area, or part thereof (list separately in addition to code for primary procedure) [N N1]
C5277	Application of low cost skin substitute graft to face, scalp, eyelids, mouth, neck, ears, orbits, genitalia, hands, feet, and/or multiple digits, total wound surface area greater than or equal to 100 sq cm; first 100 sq cm wound surface area, or 1% of body area of infants and children [T G2]
C5278	Application of low cost skin substitute graft to face, scalp, eyelids, mouth, neck, ears, orbits, genitalia, hands, feet, and/or multiple digits, total wound surface area greater than or equal to 100 sq cm; each additional 100 sq cm wound surface area, or part thereof, or each additional 1% of body area of infants and children, or part thereof (list separately in addition to code for primary procedure) [N N1]
● C7500	Debridement, bone including epidermis, dermis, subcutaneous tissue, muscle and/or fascia, if performed, first 20 sq cm or less with manual preparation and insertion of deep (e.g., subfascial) drug-delivery device(s)
● C7501	Percutaneous breast biopsies using stereotactic guidance, with placement of breast localization device(s) (e.g., clip, metallic pellet), when performed, and imaging of the biopsy specimen, when performed, all lesions unilateral and bilateral (for single lesion biopsy, use appropriate code)
● C7502	Percutaneous breast biopsies using magnetic resonance guidance, with placement of breast localization device(s) (e.g., clip, metallic pellet), when performed, and imaging of the biopsy specimen, when performed, all lesions unilateral or bilateral (for single lesion biopsy, use appropriate code)
● C7503	Open biopsy or excision of deep cervical node(s) with intraoperative identification (e.g., mapping) of sentinel lymph node(s) including injection of nonradioactive dye when performed

Legend: Special Coverage Instructions · Noncovered by Medicare · Carrier Discretion · ☑ Quantity Alert · ● New Code · ○ Recycled/Reinstated · ▲ Revised Code · [A] Age Edit · [M] Maternity Edit · ♀ Female Only · ♂ Male Only · [A–Y] OPPS Status Indicators

2023 HCPCS Level II

C7504 Percutaneous vertebroplasties (bone biopsies included when performed), first cervicothoracic and any additional cervicothoracic or lumbosacral vertebral bodies, unilateral or bilateral injection, inclusive of all imaging guidance

C7505 Percutaneous vertebroplasties (bone biopsies included when performed), first lumbosacral and any additional cervicothoracic or lumbosacral vertebral bodies, unilateral or bilateral injection, inclusive of all imaging guidance

C7506 Arthrodesis, interphalangeal joints, with or without internal fixation

C7507 Percutaneous vertebral augmentations, first thoracic and any additional thoracic or lumbar vertebral bodies, including cavity creations (fracture reductions and bone biopsies included when performed) using mechanical device (e.g., kyphoplasty), unilateral or bilateral cannulations, inclusive of all imaging guidance

C7508 Percutaneous vertebral augmentations, first lumbar and any additional thoracic or lumbar vertebral bodies, including cavity creations (fracture reductions and bone biopsies included when performed) using mechanical device (e.g., kyphoplasty), unilateral or bilateral cannulations, inclusive of all imaging guidance

C7509 Bronchoscopy, rigid or flexible, diagnostic with cell washing(s) when performed, with computer-assisted image-guided navigation, including fluoroscopic guidance when performed

C7510 Bronchoscopy, rigid or flexible, with bronchial alveolar lavage(s), with computer-assisted image-guided navigation, including fluoroscopic guidance when performed

C7511 Bronchoscopy, rigid or flexible, with single or multiple bronchial or endobronchial biopsy(ies), single or multiple sites, with computer-assisted image-guided navigation, including fluoroscopic guidance when performed

C7512 Bronchoscopy, rigid or flexible, with single or multiple bronchial or endobronchial biopsy(ies), single or multiple sites, with transendoscopic endobronchial ultrasound (EBUS) during bronchoscopic diagnostic or therapeutic intervention(s) for peripheral lesion(s), including fluoroscopic guidance when performed

C7513 Dialysis circuit, introduction of needle(s) and/or catheter(s), with diagnostic angiography of the dialysis circuit, including all direct puncture(s) and catheter placement(s), injection(s) of contrast, all necessary imaging from the arterial anastomosis and adjacent artery through entire venous outflow including the inferior or superior vena cava, fluoroscopic guidance, with transluminal balloon angioplasty of central dialysis segment, performed through dialysis circuit, including all required imaging, radiological supervision and interpretation, image documentation and report

C7514 Dialysis circuit, introduction of needle(s) and/or catheter(s), with diagnostic angiography of the dialysis circuit, including all direct puncture(s) and catheter placement(s), injection(s) of contrast, all necessary imaging from the arterial anastomosis and adjacent artery through entire venous outflow including the inferior or superior vena cava, fluoroscopic guidance, with all angioplasty in the central dialysis segment, and transcatheter placement of intravascular stent(s), central dialysis segment, performed through dialysis circuit, including all required imaging, radiological supervision and interpretation, image documentation and report

C7515 Dialysis circuit, introduction of needle(s) and/or catheter(s), with diagnostic angiography of the dialysis circuit, including all direct puncture(s) and catheter placement(s), injection(s) of contrast, all necessary imaging from the arterial anastomosis and adjacent artery through entire venous outflow including the inferior or superior vena cava, fluoroscopic guidance, with dialysis circuit permanent endovascular embolization or occlusion of main circuit or any accessory veins, including all required imaging, radiological supervision and interpretation, image documentation and report

C7516 Catheter placement in coronary artery(s) for coronary angiography, including intraprocedural injection(s) for coronary angiography, with endoluminal imaging of initial coronary vessel or graft using intravascular ultrasound (IVUS) or optical coherence tomography (OCT) during diagnostic evaluation and/or therapeutic intervention including imaging supervision, interpretation and report

C7517 Catheter placement in coronary artery(s) for coronary angiography, including intraprocedural injection(s) for coronary angiography, with iliac and/or femoral artery angiography, nonselective, bilateral or ipsilateral to catheter insertion, performed at the same time as cardiac catheterization and/or coronary angiography, includes positioning or placement of the catheter in the distal aorta or ipsilateral femoral or iliac artery, injection of dye, production of permanent images, and radiologic supervision and interpretation

C7518 Catheter placement in coronary artery(ies) for coronary angiography, including intraprocedural injection(s) for coronary angiography, imaging supervision and interpretation, with catheter placement(s) in bypass graft(s) (internal mammary, free arterial, venous grafts) including intraprocedural injection(s) for bypass graft angiography with endoluminal imaging of initial coronary vessel or graft using intravascular ultrasound (IVUS) or optical coherence tomography (OCT) during diagnostic evaluation and/or therapeutic intervention including imaging, supervision, interpretation and report

C7519 Catheter placement in coronary artery(ies) for coronary angiography, including intraprocedural injection(s) for coronary angiography, imaging supervision and interpretation, with catheter placement(s) in bypass graft(s) (internal mammary, free arterial, venous grafts) including intraprocedural injection(s) for bypass graft angiography with intravascular doppler velocity and/or pressure derived coronary flow reserve measurement (initial coronary vessel or graft) during coronary angiography including pharmacologically induced stress

C7520 Catheter placement in coronary artery(ies) for coronary angiography, including intraprocedural injection(s) for coronary angiography, imaging supervision and interpretation, with catheter placement(s) in bypass graft(s) (internal mammary, free arterial, venous grafts) includes intraprocedural injection(s) for bypass graft angiography with iliac and/or femoral artery angiography, nonselective, bilateral or ipsilateral to catheter insertion, performed at the same time as cardiac catheterization and/or coronary angiography, includes positioning or placement of the catheter in the distal aorta or ipsilateral femoral or iliac artery, injection of dye, production of permanent images, and radiologic supervision and interpretation

C7521 Catheter placement in coronary artery(ies) for coronary angiography, including intraprocedural injection(s) for coronary angiography with right heart catheterization with endoluminal imaging of initial coronary vessel or graft using intravascular ultrasound (IVUS) or optical coherence tomography (OCT) during diagnostic evaluation and/or therapeutic intervention including imaging supervision, interpretation and report

Outpatient PPS

● **C7522** Catheter placement in coronary artery(ies) for coronary angiography, including intraprocedural injection(s) for coronary angiography, imaging supervision and interpretation with right heart catheterization, with intravascular doppler velocity and/or pressure derived coronary flow reserve measurement (initial coronary vessel or graft) during coronary angiography including pharmacologically induced stress

● **C7523** Catheter placement in coronary artery(ies) for coronary angiography, including intraprocedural injection(s) for coronary angiography, imaging supervision and interpretation, with left heart catheterization including intraprocedural injection(s) for left ventriculography, when performed, with endoluminal imaging of initial coronary vessel or graft using intravascular ultrasound (IVUS) or optical coherence tomography (OCT) during diagnostic evaluation and/or therapeutic intervention including imaging supervision, interpretation and report

● **C7524** Catheter placement in coronary artery(ies) for coronary angiography, including intraprocedural injection(s) for coronary angiography, imaging supervision and interpretation, with left heart catheterization including intraprocedural injection(s) for left ventriculography, when performed, with intravascular doppler velocity and/or pressure derived coronary flow reserve measurement (initial coronary vessel or graft) during coronary angiography including pharmacologically induced stress

● **C7525** Catheter placement in coronary artery(ies) for coronary angiography, including intraprocedural injection(s) for coronary angiography, imaging supervision and interpretation, with left heart catheterization including intraprocedural injection(s) for left ventriculography, when performed, catheter placement(s) in bypass graft(s) (internal mammary, free arterial, venous grafts) with bypass graft angiography with endoluminal imaging of initial coronary vessel or graft using intravascular ultrasound (IVUS) or optical coherence tomography (OCT) during diagnostic evaluation and/or therapeutic intervention including imaging supervision, interpretation and report

● **C7526** Catheter placement in coronary artery(ies) for coronary angiography, including intraprocedural injection(s) for coronary angiography, imaging supervision and interpretation, with left heart catheterization including intraprocedural injection(s) for left ventriculography, when performed, catheter placement(s) in bypass graft(s) (internal mammary, free arterial, venous grafts) with bypass graft angiography with intravascular doppler velocity and/or pressure derived coronary flow reserve measurement (initial coronary vessel or graft) during coronary angiography including pharmacologically induced stress

● **C7527** Catheter placement in coronary artery(ies) for coronary angiography, including intraprocedural injection(s) for coronary angiography, imaging supervision and interpretation, with right and left heart catheterization including intraprocedural injection(s) for left ventriculography, when performed, with endoluminal imaging of initial coronary vessel or graft using intravascular ultrasound (IVUS) or optical coherence tomography (OCT) during diagnostic evaluation and/or therapeutic intervention including imaging supervision, interpretation and report

● **C7528** Catheter placement in coronary artery(ies) for coronary angiography, including intraprocedural injection(s) for coronary angiography, imaging supervision and interpretation, with right and left heart catheterization including intraprocedural injection(s) for left ventriculography, when performed, with intravascular doppler velocity and/or pressure derived coronary flow reserve measurement (initial coronary vessel or graft) during coronary angiography including pharmacologically induced stress

● **C7529** Catheter placement in coronary artery(ies) for coronary angiography, including intraprocedural injection(s) for coronary angiography, imaging supervision and interpretation, with right and left heart catheterization including intraprocedural injection(s) for left ventriculography, when performed, catheter placement(s) in bypass graft(s) (internal mammary, free arterial, venous grafts) with bypass graft angiography with intravascular doppler velocity and/or pressure derived coronary flow reserve measurement (initial coronary vessel or graft) during coronary angiography including pharmacologically induced stress

● **C7530** Dialysis circuit, introduction of needle(s) and/or catheter(s), with diagnostic angiography of the dialysis circuit, including all direct puncture(s) and catheter placement(s), injection(s) of contrast, all necessary imaging from the arterial anastomosis and adjacent artery through entire venous outflow including the inferior or superior vena cava, fluoroscopic guidance, with transluminal balloon angioplasty, peripheral dialysis segment, including all imaging and radiological supervision and interpretation necessary to perform the angioplasty and all angioplasty in the central dialysis segment, with transcatheter placement of intravascular stent(s), central dialysis segment, performed through dialysis circuit, including all imaging, radiological supervision and interpretation, documentation and report

● **C7531** Revascularization, endovascular, open or percutaneous, femoral, popliteal artery(ies), unilateral, with transluminal angioplasty with intravascular ultrasound (initial noncoronary vessel) during diagnostic evaluation and/or therapeutic intervention, including radiological supervision and interpretation

● **C7532** Transluminal balloon angioplasty (except lower extremity artery(ies) for occlusive disease, intracranial, coronary, pulmonary, or dialysis circuit), initial artery, open or percutaneous, including all imaging and radiological supervision and interpretation necessary to perform the angioplasty within the same artery, with intravascular ultrasound (initial noncoronary vessel) during diagnostic evaluation and/or therapeutic intervention, including radiological supervision and interpretation

● **C7533** Percutaneous transluminal coronary angioplasty, single major coronary artery or branch with transcatheter placement of radiation delivery device for subsequent coronary intravascular brachytherapy

● **C7534** Revascularization, endovascular, open or percutaneous, femoral, popliteal artery(ies), unilateral, with atherectomy, includes angioplasty within the same vessel, when performed with intravascular ultrasound (initial noncoronary vessel) during diagnostic evaluation and/or therapeutic intervention, including radiological supervision and interpretation

● **C7535** Revascularization, endovascular, open or percutaneous, femoral, popliteal artery(ies), unilateral, with transluminal stent placement(s), includes angioplasty within the same vessel, when performed, with intravascular ultrasound (initial noncoronary vessel) during diagnostic evaluation and/or therapeutic intervention, including radiological supervision and interpretation

● **C7537** Insertion of new or replacement of permanent pacemaker with atrial transvenous electrode(s), with insertion of pacing electrode, cardiac venous system, for left ventricular pacing, at time of insertion of implantable defibrillator or pacemaker pulse generator (e.g., for upgrade to dual chamber system)

● **C7538** Insertion of new or replacement of permanent pacemaker with ventricular transvenous electrode(s), with insertion of pacing electrode, cardiac venous system, for left ventricular pacing, at time of insertion of implantable defibrillator or pacemaker pulse generator (e.g., for upgrade to dual chamber system)

● C7539	Insertion of new or replacement of permanent pacemaker with atrial and ventricular transvenous electrode(s), with insertion of pacing electrode, cardiac venous system, for left ventricular pacing, at time of insertion of implantable defibrillator or pacemaker pulse generator (e.g., for upgrade to dual chamber system)
● C7540	Removal of permanent pacemaker pulse generator with replacement of pacemaker pulse generator, dual lead system, with insertion of pacing electrode, cardiac venous system, for left ventricular pacing, at time of insertion of implantable defibrillator or pacemaker pulse generator (e.g., for upgrade to dual chamber system)
● C7541	Diagnostic endoscopic retrograde cholangiopancreatography (ERCP), including collection of specimen(s) by brushing or washing, when performed, with endoscopic cannulation of papilla with direct visualization of pancreatic/common bile ducts(s)
● C7542	Endoscopic retrograde cholangiopancreatography (ERCP) with biopsy, single or multiple, with endoscopic cannulation of papilla with direct visualization of pancreatic/common bile ducts(s)
● C7543	Endoscopic retrograde cholangiopancreatography (ERCP) with sphincterotomy/papillotomy, with endoscopic cannulation of papilla with direct visualization of pancreatic/common bile ducts(s)
● C7544	Endoscopic retrograde cholangiopancreatography (ERCP) with removal of calculi/debris from biliary/pancreatic duct(s), with endoscopic cannulation of papilla with direct visualization of pancreatic/common bile ducts(s)
● C7545	Percutaneous exchange of biliary drainage catheter (e.g., external, internal-external, or conversion of internal-external to external only), with removal of calculi/debris from biliary duct(s) and/or gallbladder, including destruction of calculi by any method (e.g., mechanical, electrohydraulic, lithotripsy) when performed, including diagnostic cholangiography(ies) when performed, imaging guidance (e.g., fluoroscopy), and all associated radiological supervision and interpretation
● C7546	Removal and replacement of externally accessible nephroureteral catheter (e.g., external/internal stent) requiring fluoroscopic guidance, with ureteral stricture balloon dilation, including imaging guidance and all associated radiological supervision and interpretation
● C7547	Convert nephrostomy catheter to nephroureteral catheter, percutaneous via pre-existing nephrostomy tract, with ureteral stricture balloon dilation, including diagnostic nephrostogram and/or ureterogram when performed, imaging guidance (e.g., ultrasound and/or fluoroscopy) and all associated radiological supervision and interpretation
● C7548	Exchange nephrostomy catheter, percutaneous, with ureteral stricture balloon dilation, including diagnostic nephrostogram and/or ureterogram when performed, imaging guidance (e.g., ultrasound and/or fluoroscopy) and all associated radiological supervision and interpretation
● C7549	Change of ureterostomy tube or externally accessible ureteral stent via ileal conduit with ureteral stricture balloon dilation, including imaging guidance (e.g., ultrasound and/or fluoroscopy) and all associated radiological supervision and interpretation
● C7550	Cystourethroscopy, with biopsy(ies) with adjunctive blue light cystoscopy with fluorescent imaging agent
● C7551	Excision of major peripheral nerve neuroma, except sciatic, with implantation of nerve end into bone or muscle
● C7552	Catheter placement in coronary artery(s) for coronary angiography, including intraprocedural injection(s) for coronary angiography, imaging supervision and interpretation; with catheter placement(s) in bypass graft(s) (internal mammary, free arterial, venous grafts) including intraprocedural injection(s) for bypass graft angiography and right heart catheterization with intravascular doppler velocity and/or pressure derived coronary flow reserve measurement (coronary vessel or graft) during coronary angiography including pharmacologically induced stress, initial vessel
● C7553	Catheter placement in coronary artery(s) for coronary angiography, including intraprocedural injection(s) for coronary angiography, imaging supervision and interpretation; with right and left heart catheterization including intraprocedural injection(s) for left ventriculography, when performed, catheter placement(s) in bypass graft(s) (internal mammary, free arterial, venous grafts) with bypass graft angiography with pharmacologic agent administration (e.g., inhaled nitric oxide, intravenous infusion of nitroprusside, dobutamine, milrinone, or other agent) including assessing hemodynamic measurements before, during, after and repeat pharmacologic agent administration, when performed
● C7554	Cystourethroscopy with adjunctive blue light cystoscopy with fluorescent imaging agent
● C7555	Thyroidectomy, total or complete with parathyroid autotransplantation
● C7900	Service for diagnosis, evaluation, or treatment of a mental health or substance use disorder, initial 15-29 minutes, provided remotely by hospital staff who are licensed to provide mental health services under applicable state law(s), when the patient is in their home, and there is no associated professional service
● C7901	Service for diagnosis, evaluation, or treatment of a mental health or substance use disorder, initial 30-60 minutes, provided remotely by hospital staff who are licensed to provided mental health services under applicable state law(s), when the patient is in their home, and there is no associated professional service
● C7902	Service for diagnosis, evaluation, or treatment of a mental health or substance use disorder, each additional 15 minutes, provided remotely by hospital staff who are licensed to provide mental health services under applicable state law(s), when the patient is in their home, and there is no associated professional service (list separately in addition to code for primary service)
C8900	Magnetic resonance angiography with contrast, abdomen CMS: 100-04,13,40.1.1; 100-04,13,40.1.2
C8901	Magnetic resonance angiography without contrast, abdomen CMS: 100-04,13,40.1.1; 100-04,13,40.1.2
C8902	Magnetic resonance angiography without contrast followed by with contrast, abdomen CMS: 100-04,13,40.1.1; 100-04,13,40.1.2
C8903	Magnetic resonance imaging with contrast, breast; unilateral
C8905	Magnetic resonance imaging without contrast followed by with contrast, breast; unilateral
C8906	Magnetic resonance imaging with contrast, breast; bilateral
C8908	Magnetic resonance imaging without contrast followed by with contrast, breast; bilateral

Outpatient PPS

C8909 Magnetic resonance angiography with contrast, chest (excluding myocardium)
CMS: 100-04,13,40.1.1; 100-04,13,40.1.2

C8910 Magnetic resonance angiography without contrast, chest (excluding myocardium)
CMS: 100-04,13,40.1.1; 100-04,13,40.1.2

C8911 Magnetic resonance angiography without contrast followed by with contrast, chest (excluding myocardium)
CMS: 100-04,13,40.1.1; 100-04,13,40.1.2

C8912 Magnetic resonance angiography with contrast, lower extremity
CMS: 100-04,13,40.1.1; 100-04,13,40.1.2

C8913 Magnetic resonance angiography without contrast, lower extremity
CMS: 100-04,13,40.1.1; 100-04,13,40.1.2

C8914 Magnetic resonance angiography without contrast followed by with contrast, lower extremity
CMS: 100-04,13,40.1.1; 100-04,13,40.1.2

C8918 Magnetic resonance angiography with contrast, pelvis
CMS: 100-04,13,40.1.1; 100-04,13,40.1.2

C8919 Magnetic resonance angiography without contrast, pelvis
CMS: 100-04,13,40.1.1; 100-04,13,40.1.2

C8920 Magnetic resonance angiography without contrast followed by with contrast, pelvis
CMS: 100-04,13,40.1.1; 100-04,13,40.1.2

C8921 Transthoracic echocardiography (TTE) with contrast, or without contrast followed by with contrast, for congenital cardiac anomalies; complete
CMS: 100-04,4,200.7.2

C8922 Transthoracic echocardiography (TTE) with contrast, or without contrast followed by with contrast, for congenital cardiac anomalies; follow-up or limited study

C8923 Transthoracic echocardiography (TTE) with contrast, or without contrast followed by with contrast, real-time with image documentation (2D), includes M-mode recording, when performed, complete, without spectral or color doppler echocardiography

C8924 Transthoracic echocardiography (TTE) with contrast, or without contrast followed by with contrast, real-time with image documentation (2D), includes M-mode recording when performed, follow-up or limited study

C8925 Transesophageal echocardiography (TEE) with contrast, or without contrast followed by with contrast, real time with image documentation (2D) (with or without M-mode recording); including probe placement, image acquisition, interpretation and report

C8926 Transesophageal echocardiography (TEE) with contrast, or without contrast followed by with contrast, for congenital cardiac anomalies; including probe placement, image acquisition, interpretation and report

C8927 Transesophageal echocardiography (TEE) with contrast, or without contrast followed by with contrast, for monitoring purposes, including probe placement, real time (2D) image acquisition and interpretation leading to ongoing (continuous) assessment of (dynamically changing) cardiac pumping function and to therapeutic measures on an immediate time basis

C8928 Transthoracic echocardiography (TTE) with contrast, or without contrast followed by with contrast, real-time with image documentation (2D), includes M-mode recording, when performed, during rest and cardiovascular stress test using treadmill, bicycle exercise and/or pharmacologically induced stress, with interpretation and report

C8929 Transthoracic echocardiography (TTE) with contrast, or without contrast followed by with contrast, real-time with image documentation (2D), includes M-mode recording, when performed, complete, with spectral doppler echocardiography, and with color flow doppler echocardiography

C8930 Transthoracic echocardiography (TTE) with contrast, or without contrast followed by with contrast, real-time with image documentation (2D), Includes M-mode recording, when performed, during rest and cardiovascular stress test using treadmill, bicycle exercise and/or pharmacologically induced stress, with interpretation and report; including performance of continuous electrocardiographic monitoring, with physician supervision

C8931 Magnetic resonance angiography with contrast, spinal canal and contents

C8932 Magnetic resonance angiography without contrast, spinal canal and contents

C8933 Magnetic resonance angiography without contrast followed by with contrast, spinal canal and contents

C8934 Magnetic resonance angiography with contrast, upper extremity

C8935 Magnetic resonance angiography without contrast, upper extremity

C8936 Magnetic resonance angiography without contrast followed by with contrast, upper extremity

C8937 Computer-aided detection, including computer algorithm analysis of breast MRI image data for lesion detection/characterization, pharmacokinetic analysis, with further physician review for interpretation (list separately in addition to code for primary procedure)

C8957 Intravenous infusion for therapy/diagnosis; initiation of prolonged infusion (more than 8 hours), requiring use of portable or implantable pump
CMS: 100-04,4,230.2

C9046 Cocaine HCl nasal solution for topical administration, 1 mg
Use this code for Goprelto.
AHA: 2Q,19

C9047 Injection, caplacizumab-yhdp, 1 mg
Use this code for Cablivi.
AHA: 3Q,19

C9067 Gallium Ga-68, Dotatoc, diagnostic, 0.01 mCi
AHA: 4Q,20

C9084 Injection, loncastuximab tesirine-lpyl, 0.1 mg
To report, see ~J9359

C9085 Injection, avalglucosidase alfa-ngpt, 4 mg
To report, see ~J0219

C9086 Injection, anifrolumab-fnia, 1 mg
To report, see ~J0491

C9087 Injection, cyclophosphamide, (AuroMedics), 10 mg
To report, see ~J9071

C9088 Instillation, bupivacaine and meloxicam, 1 mg/0.03 mg
Use this code for Zynrelef.
AHA: 1Q,22

Code	Description
C9089	Bupivacaine, collagen-matrix implant, 1 mg K2 Use this code for Xaracoll. **AHA:** 1Q,22
C9090	Injection, plasminogen, human-tvmh, 1 mg To report, see ~J2998
C9091	Injection, sirolimus protein-bound particles, 1 mg To report, see ~J9331
C9092	Injection, triamcinolone acetonide, suprachoroidal (Xipere), 1 mg To report, see ~J3299
C9093	Injection, ranibizumab, via sustained release intravitreal implant (Susvimo), 0.1 mg To report, see ~J2779
C9094	Injection, sutimlimab-jome, 10 mg To report, see ~J1302
C9095	Injection, tebentafusp-tebn, 1 mcg To report, see ~J9274
C9096	Injection, filgrastim-ayow, biosimilar, (Releuko), 1 mcg To report, see ~Q5125
C9097	Injection, faricimab-svoa, 0.1 mg To report, see ~J2777
C9098	Ciltacabtagene autoleucel, up to 100 million autologous B-cell maturation antigen (BCMA) directed CAR-positive T cells, including leukapheresis and dose preparation procedures, per therapeutic dose To report, see ~Q2056
● **C9101**	Injection, oliceridine, 0.1 mg K2 Use this code for Olinvyk.
C9113	Injection, pantoprazole sodium, per vial N N1 ☑ Use this code for Protonix.
C9142	Injection, bevacizumab-maly, biosimilar, (Alymsys), 10 mg To report, see ~Q5126
● **C9143**	Cocaine HCl nasal solution (Numbrino), 1 mg Use this code for cocaine HCl (Numbrino) manufactured by Lannett.
● **C9144**	Injection, bupivacaine (Posimir), 1 mg
C9248	Injection, clevidipine butyrate, 1 mg N N1 ☑ Use this code for Cleviprex.
C9250	Human plasma fibrin sealant, vapor-heated, solvent-detergent (Artiss), 2 ml K K2 ☑
C9254	Injection, lacosamide, 1 mg N N1 ☑ Use this code for VIMPAT.
C9257	Injection, bevacizumab, 0.25 mg K K2 ☑ Use this code for Avastin. **CMS:** 100-03,110.17
C9285	Lidocaine 70 mg/tetracaine 70 mg, per patch N N1 ☑ Use this code for SYNERA.
C9290	Injection, bupivacaine liposome, 1 mg N K2 ☑ Use this code for EXPAREL.
C9293	Injection, glucarpidase, 10 units K ☑ Use this code for Voraxaze.
C9352	Microporous collagen implantable tube (NeuraGen Nerve Guide), per cm length N N1 ☑
C9353	Microporous collagen implantable slit tube (NeuraWrap Nerve Protector), per cm length N N1 ☑
C9354	Acellular pericardial tissue matrix of nonhuman origin (Veritas), per sq cm N N1 ☑
C9355	Collagen nerve cuff (NeuroMatrix), per 0.5 cm length N N1 ☑
C9356	Tendon, porous matrix of cross-linked collagen and glycosaminoglycan matrix (TenoGlide Tendon Protector Sheet), per sq cm N N1 ☑
C9358	Dermal substitute, native, nondenatured collagen, fetal bovine origin (SurgiMend Collagen Matrix), per 0.5 sq cm N N1 ☑
C9359	Porous purified collagen matrix bone void filler (Integra Mozaik Osteoconductive Scaffold Putty, Integra OS Osteoconductive Scaffold Putty), per 0.5 cc N N1 ☑
C9360	Dermal substitute, native, nondenatured collagen, neonatal bovine origin (SurgiMend Collagen Matrix), per 0.5 sq cm N N1 ☑
C9361	Collagen matrix nerve wrap (NeuroMend Collagen Nerve Wrap), per 0.5 cm length N N1 ☑
C9362	Porous purified collagen matrix bone void filler (Integra Mozaik Osteoconductive Scaffold Strip), per 0.5 cc N N1 ☑
C9363	Skin substitute (Integra Meshed Bilayer Wound Matrix), per sq cm N N1 ☑ **CMS:** 100-04,4,260.1; 100-04,4,260.1.1
C9364	Porcine implant, Permacol, per sq cm N N1 ☑

A synthetic "bridge" is affixed to each end of a severed nerve with sutures. This procedure is performed using an operating microscope

C9399

Code	Description
C9399	**Unclassified drugs or biologicals** [A] [K7] **CMS:** 100-02,15,50.5; 100-04,17,90.3; 100-04,32,400; 100-04,32,400.1; 100-04,32,400.2; 100-04,32,400.2.1; 100-04,32,400.2.2; 100-04,32,400.2.3; 100-04,32,400.2.4; 100-04,32,400.3; 100-04,32,400.4; 100-04,32,400.5; 100-04,4,260.1; 100-04,4,260.1.1 **AHA:** 1Q,17; 4Q,16
C9460	**Injection, cangrelor, 1 mg** [G] [K2] [✓] Use this code for Kengreal.
C9462	**Injection, delafloxacin, 1 mg** [G] [N1] Use this code for Baxdela. **AHA:** 2Q,18
C9482	**Injection, sotalol HCl, 1 mg** [G] [K2] [✓]
C9488	**Injection, conivaptan HCl, 1 mg** [G] [K2] [✓] Use this code for Vaprisol.
C9507	**Fresh frozen plasma, high titer COVID-19 convalescent, frozen within 8 hours of collection, each unit** **AHA:** 2Q,22
C9600	**Percutaneous transcatheter placement of drug eluting intracoronary stent(s), with coronary angioplasty when performed; single major coronary artery or branch** [J] [J8] **AHA:** 4Q,21
C9601	**Percutaneous transcatheter placement of drug-eluting intracoronary stent(s), with coronary angioplasty when performed; each additional branch of a major coronary artery (list separately in addition to code for primary procedure)** [N] [N1]
C9602	**Percutaneous transluminal coronary atherectomy, with drug eluting intracoronary stent, with coronary angioplasty when performed; single major coronary artery or branch** [J] **AHA:** 4Q,21
C9603	**Percutaneous transluminal coronary atherectomy, with drug-eluting intracoronary stent, with coronary angioplasty when performed; each additional branch of a major coronary artery (list separately in addition to code for primary procedure)** [N]
C9604	**Percutaneous transluminal revascularization of or through coronary artery bypass graft (internal mammary, free arterial, venous), any combination of drug-eluting intracoronary stent, atherectomy and angioplasty, including distal protection when performed; single vessel** [J]
C9605	**Percutaneous transluminal revascularization of or through coronary artery bypass graft (internal mammary, free arterial, venous), any combination of drug-eluting intracoronary stent, atherectomy and angioplasty, including distal protection when performed; each additional branch subtended by the bypass graft (list separately in addition to code for primary procedure)** [N]
C9606	**Percutaneous transluminal revascularization of acute total/subtotal occlusion during acute myocardial infarction, coronary artery or coronary artery bypass graft, any combination of drug-eluting intracoronary stent, atherectomy and angioplasty, including aspiration thrombectomy when performed, single vessel** [J] **CMS:** 100-04,4,260.1; 100-04,4,260.1.1 **AHA:** 1Q,19
C9607	**Percutaneous transluminal revascularization of chronic total occlusion, coronary artery, coronary artery branch, or coronary artery bypass graft, any combination of drug-eluting intracoronary stent, atherectomy and angioplasty; single vessel** [J] **AHA:** 4Q,21
C9608	**Percutaneous transluminal revascularization of chronic total occlusion, coronary artery, coronary artery branch, or coronary artery bypass graft, any combination of drug-eluting intracoronary stent, atherectomy and angioplasty; each additional coronary artery, coronary artery branch, or bypass graft (list separately in addition to code for primary procedure)** [N]
C9725	**Placement of endorectal intracavitary applicator for high intensity brachytherapy** [T] [G2] [○]
C9726	**Placement and removal (if performed) of applicator into breast for intraoperative radiation therapy, add-on to primary breast procedure** [N] [N1]
C9727	**Insertion of implants into the soft palate; minimum of three implants** [T] [G2] [✓]
C9728	**Placement of interstitial device(s) for radiation therapy/surgery guidance (e.g., fiducial markers, dosimeter), for other than the following sites (any approach): abdomen, pelvis, prostate, retroperitoneum, thorax, single or multiple** [S] [J8] **AHA:** 2Q,18
C9733	**Nonophthalmic fluorescent vascular angiography** [Q2]
C9734	**Focused ultrasound ablation/therapeutic intervention, other than uterine leiomyomata, with magnetic resonance (MR) guidance** [J]
C9738	**Adjunctive blue light cystoscopy with fluorescent imaging agent (list separately in addition to code for primary procedure)** [N] [N1]
C9739	**Cystourethroscopy, with insertion of transprostatic implant; one to three implants** [♂] [J] [J8]
C9740	**Cystourethroscopy, with insertion of transprostatic implant; four or more implants** [♂] [J] [J8]
C9751	**Bronchoscopy, rigid or flexible, transbronchial ablation of lesion(s) by microwave energy, including fluoroscopic guidance, when performed, with computed tomography acquisition(s) and 3D rendering, computer-assisted, image-guided navigation, and endobronchial ultrasound (EBUS) guided transtracheal and/or transbronchial sampling (e.g., aspiration[s]/biopsy[ies]) and all mediastinal and/or hilar lymph node stations or structures and therapeutic intervention(s)** **CMS:** 100-04,4,260.1; 100-04,4,260.1.1 **AHA:** 1Q,19
C9756	**Intraoperative near-infrared fluorescence lymphatic mapping of lymph node(s) (sentinel or tumor draining) with administration of indocyanine green (ICG) (List separately in addition to code for primary procedure)** **AHA:** 1Q,21; 3Q,19
C9757	**Laminotomy (hemilaminectomy), with decompression of nerve root(s), including partial facetectomy, foraminotomy and excision of herniated intervertebral disc, and repair of annular defect with implantation of bone anchored annular closure device, including annular defect measurement, alignment and sizing assessment, and image guidance; 1 interspace, lumbar** [J8] **AHA:** 1Q,20
C9758	**Blind procedure for NYHA Class III/IV heart failure; transcatheter implantation of interatrial shunt including right heart catheterization, transesophageal echocardiography (TEE)/intracardiac echocardiography (ICE), and all imaging with or without guidance (e.g., ultrasound, fluoroscopy), performed in an approved investigational device exemption (IDE) study**

C9759 Transcatheter intraoperative blood vessel microinfusion(s) (e.g., intraluminal, vascular wall and/or perivascular) therapy, any vessel, including radiological supervision and interpretation, when performed
AHA: 2Q,20

C9760 Nonrandomized, nonblinded procedure for NYHA Class II, III, IV heart failure; transcatheter implantation of interatrial shunt, including right and left heart catheterization, transeptal puncture, transesophageal echocardiography (TEE)/intracardiac echocardiography (ICE), and all imaging with or without guidance (e.g., ultrasound, fluoroscopy), performed in an approved investigational device exemption (IDE) study
AHA: 2Q,20

▲ **C9761** Cystourethroscopy, with ureteroscopy and/or pyeloscopy, with lithotripsy, and ureteral catheterization for steerable vacuum aspiration of the kidney, collecting system, ureter, bladder, and urethra if applicable (must use a steerable ureteral catheter)
AHA: 2Q,21; 4Q,20

C9762 Cardiac magnetic resonance imaging for morphology and function, quantification of segmental dysfunction; with strain imaging
AHA: 2Q,20

C9763 Cardiac magnetic resonance imaging for morphology and function, quantification of segmental dysfunction; with stress imaging
AHA: 2Q,20

C9764 Revascularization, endovascular, open or percutaneous, lower extremity artery(ies), except tibial/peroneal; with intravascular lithotripsy, includes angioplasty within the same vessel(s), when performed
AHA: 2Q,20

C9765 Revascularization, endovascular, open or percutaneous, lower extremity artery(ies), except tibial/peroneal; with intravascular lithotripsy, and transluminal stent placement(s), includes angioplasty within the same vessel(s), when performed
AHA: 2Q,20

C9766 Revascularization, endovascular, open or percutaneous, lower extremity artery(ies), except tibial/peroneal; with intravascular lithotripsy and atherectomy, includes angioplasty within the same vessel(s), when performed
AHA: 2Q,20

C9767 Revascularization, endovascular, open or percutaneous, lower extremity artery(ies), except tibial/peroneal; with intravascular lithotripsy and transluminal stent placement(s), and atherectomy, includes angioplasty within the same vessel(s), when performed
AHA: 2Q,20

C9768 Endoscopic ultrasound-guided direct measurement of hepatic portosystemic pressure gradient by any method (list separately in addition to code for primary procedure)
AHA: 4Q,20

C9769 Cystourethroscopy, with insertion of temporary prostatic implant/stent with fixation/anchor and incisional struts
AHA: 4Q,20

C9770 Vitrectomy, mechanical, pars plana approach, with subretinal injection of pharmacologic/biologic agent
AHA: 3Q,21; 1Q,21

C9771 Nasal/sinus endoscopy, cryoablation nasal tissue(s) and/or nerve(s), unilateral or bilateral
AHA: 1Q,21

C9772 Revascularization, endovascular, open or percutaneous, tibial/peroneal artery(ies), with intravascular lithotripsy, includes angioplasty within the same vessel(s), when performed
AHA: 1Q,21

C9773 Revascularization, endovascular, open or percutaneous, tibial/peroneal artery(ies); with intravascular lithotripsy, and transluminal stent placement(s), includes angioplasty within the same vessel(s), when performed
AHA: 1Q,21

C9774 Revascularization, endovascular, open or percutaneous, tibial/peroneal artery(ies); with intravascular lithotripsy and atherectomy, includes angioplasty within the same vessel(s), when performed
AHA: 1Q,21

C9775 Revascularization, endovascular, open or percutaneous, tibial/peroneal artery(ies); with intravascular lithotripsy and transluminal stent placement(s), and atherectomy, includes angioplasty within the same vessel(s), when performed
AHA: 1Q,21

C9776 Intraoperative near-infrared fluorescence imaging of major extra-hepatic bile duct(s) (e.g., cystic duct, common bile duct and common hepatic duct) with intravenous administration of indocyanine green (ICG) (list separately in addition to code for primary procedure)
AHA: 1Q,22; 2Q,21

C9777 Esophageal mucosal integrity testing by electrical impedance, transoral, includes esophagoscopy or esophagogastroduodenoscopy
AHA: 2Q,21

C9778 Colpopexy, vaginal; minimally invasive extraperitoneal approach (sacrospinous)
AHA: 3Q,21

C9779 Endoscopic submucosal dissection (ESD), including endoscopy or colonoscopy, mucosal closure, when performed
AHA: 4Q,21

C9780 Insertion of central venous catheter through central venous occlusion via inferior and superior approaches (e.g., inside-out technique), including imaging guidance
AHA: 4Q,21

● **C9781** Arthroscopy, shoulder, surgical; with implantation of subacromial spacer (e.g., balloon), includes debridement (e.g., limited or extensive), subacromial decompression, acromioplasty, and biceps tenodesis when performed
AHA: 2Q,22

● **C9782** Blinded procedure for New York Heart Association (NYHA) Class II or III heart failure, or Canadian Cardiovascular Society (CCS) Class III or IV chronic refractory angina; transcatheter intramyocardial transplantation of autologous bone marrow cells (e.g., mononuclear) or placebo control, autologous bone marrow harvesting and preparation for transplantation, left heart catheterization including ventriculography, all laboratory services, and all imaging with or without guidance (e.g., transthoracic echocardiography, ultrasound, fluoroscopy), performed in an approved investigational device exemption (IDE) study
AHA: 2Q,22

● **C9783** Blinded procedure for transcatheter implantation of coronary sinus reduction device or placebo control, including vascular access and closure, right heart catherization, venous and coronary sinus angiography, imaging guidance and supervision and interpretation when performed in an approved investigational device exemption (IDE) study
AHA: 2Q,22

C9803 Hospital outpatient clinic visit specimen collection for severe acute respiratory syndrome coronavirus 2 (SARS-CoV-2) (coronavirus disease [COVID-19]), any specimen source M1
AHA: 2Q,20

C9898 Radiolabeled product provided during a hospital inpatient stay N
CMS: 100-04,4,260.1; 100-04,4,260.1.1

C9899 Implanted prosthetic device, payable only for inpatients who do not have inpatient coverage A

2023 HCPCS Level II   E0161

Durable Medical Equipment E0100–E8002

E codes include durable medical equipment such as canes, crutches, walkers, commodes, decubitus care, bath and toilet aids, hospital beds, oxygen and related respiratory equipment, monitoring equipment, pacemakers, patient lifts, safety equipment, restraints, traction equipment, fracture frames, wheelchairs, and artificial kidney machines.

Canes

E0100 Cane, includes canes of all materials, adjustable or fixed, with tip (NU, RR, UE)
White canes for the blind are not covered under Medicare.

E0105 Cane, quad or three-prong, includes canes of all materials, adjustable or fixed, with tips (NU, RR, UE)

Crutches

E0110 Crutches, forearm, includes crutches of various materials, adjustable or fixed, pair, complete with tips and handgrips (NU, RR, UE)

Forearm cuff
Axilla pad
Standard underarm crutch (E0112–E0117)
Hand grip
Hand grip
Adjustment
Standard forearm crutch (E0110–E0111)

E0111 Crutch, forearm, includes crutches of various materials, adjustable or fixed, each, with tip and handgrips (NU, RR, UE)

E0112 Crutches, underarm, wood, adjustable or fixed, pair, with pads, tips, and handgrips (NU, RR, UE)

E0113 Crutch, underarm, wood, adjustable or fixed, each, with pad, tip, and handgrip (NU, RR, UE)

E0114 Crutches, underarm, other than wood, adjustable or fixed, pair, with pads, tips, and handgrips (NU, RR, UE)

E0116 Crutch, underarm, other than wood, adjustable or fixed, with pad, tip, handgrip, with or without shock absorber, each (NU, RR, UE)

E0117 Crutch, underarm, articulating, spring assisted, each (RR)

E0118 Crutch substitute, lower leg platform, with or without wheels, each
Medicare covers walkers if patient's ambulation is impaired.

Walkers

E0130 Walker, rigid (pickup), adjustable or fixed height (NU, RR, UE)
CMS: 100-04,36,50.15

E0135 Walker, folding (pickup), adjustable or fixed height (NU, RR, UE)
Medicare covers walkers if patient's ambulation is impaired.
CMS: 100-04,36,50.15

E0140 Walker, with trunk support, adjustable or fixed height, any type (RR)
CMS: 100-04,36,50.15

E0141 Walker, rigid, wheeled, adjustable or fixed height (NU, RR, UE)
Medicare covers walkers if patient's ambulation is impaired.
CMS: 100-04,36,50.15

E0143 Walker, folding, wheeled, adjustable or fixed height (NU, RR, UE)
Medicare covers walkers if patient's ambulation is impaired.
CMS: 100-04,36,50.15

E0144 Walker, enclosed, four-sided framed, rigid or folding, wheeled with posterior seat (RR)
CMS: 100-04,36,50.15

E0147 Walker, heavy-duty, multiple braking system, variable wheel resistance (NU, RR, UE)
Medicare covers safety roller walkers only in patients with severe neurological disorders or restricted use of one hand. In some cases, coverage will be extended to patients with a weight exceeding the limits of a standard wheeled walker.
CMS: 100-04,36,50.15

E0148 Walker, heavy-duty, without wheels, rigid or folding, any type, each (NU, RR, UE)
CMS: 100-04,36,50.15

E0149 Walker, heavy-duty, wheeled, rigid or folding, any type (RR)
CMS: 100-04,36,50.15

Attachments

E0153 Platform attachment, forearm crutch, each (NU, RR, UE)

E0154 Platform attachment, walker, each (NU, RR, UE)
CMS: 100-04,36,50.14; 100-04,36,50.15

E0155 Wheel attachment, rigid pick-up walker, per pair (NU, RR, UE)
CMS: 100-04,36,50.15

E0156 Seat attachment, walker (NU, RR, UE)
CMS: 100-04,36,50.14; 100-04,36,50.15

E0157 Crutch attachment, walker, each (NU, RR, UE)
CMS: 100-04,36,50.14; 100-04,36,50.15

E0158 Leg extensions for walker, per set of four (NU, RR, UE)
CMS: 100-04,36,50.14; 100-04,36,50.15

E0159 Brake attachment for wheeled walker, replacement, each (NU, RR, UE)
CMS: 100-04,36,50.15

Commodes

E0160 Sitz type bath or equipment, portable, used with or without commode (NU, RR, UE)
Medicare covers sitz baths if medical record indicates that the patient has an infection or injury of the perineal area and the sitz bath is prescribed by the physician.

E0161 Sitz type bath or equipment, portable, used with or without commode, with faucet attachment(s) (NU, RR, UE)
Medicare covers sitz baths if medical record indicates that the patient has an infection or injury of the perineal area and the sitz bath is prescribed by the physician.

Durable Medical Equipment

E0162 — E0240

Code	Description
E0162	**Sitz bath chair** Y & (NU, RR, UE)
	Medicare covers sitz baths if medical record indicates that the patient has an infection or injury of the perineal area and the sitz bath is prescribed by the physician.
E0163	**Commode chair, mobile or stationary, with fixed arms** Y & (NU, RR, UE)
	Medicare covers commodes for patients confined to their beds or rooms, for patients without indoor bathroom facilities, and to patients who cannot climb or descend the stairs necessary to reach the bathrooms in their homes.
E0165	**Commode chair, mobile or stationary, with detachable arms** Y & (RR)
	Medicare covers commodes for patients confined to their beds or rooms, for patients without indoor bathroom facilities, and to patients who cannot climb or descend the stairs necessary to reach the bathrooms in their homes.
E0167	**Pail or pan for use with commode chair, replacement only** Y & (NU, RR, UE)
	Medicare covers commodes for patients confined to their beds or rooms, for patients without indoor bathroom facilities, and to patients who cannot climb or descend the stairs necessary to reach the bathrooms in their homes.
E0168	**Commode chair, extra wide and/or heavy-duty, stationary or mobile, with or without arms, any type, each** Y ☑ & (NU, RR, UE)
E0170	**Commode chair with integrated seat lift mechanism, electric, any type** Y & (RR)
E0171	**Commode chair with integrated seat lift mechanism, nonelectric, any type** Y & (RR)
E0172	**Seat lift mechanism placed over or on top of toilet, any type** EI
E0175	**Footrest, for use with commode chair, each** Y ☑ & (NU, RR, UE)

Decubitus Care Equipment

Code	Description
E0181	**Powered pressure reducing mattress overlay/pad, alternating, with pump, includes heavy-duty** Y & (RR)
	For Medicare coverage, a detailed written order must be received by the supplier before a claim is submitted.
E0182	**Pump for alternating pressure pad, for replacement only** Y & (RR)
	For Medicare coverage, a detailed written order must be received by the supplier before a claim is submitted.
○ **E0183**	**Powered pressure reducing underlay/pad, alternating, with pump, includes heavy duty** (RR)
E0184	**Dry pressure mattress** Y & (NU, RR, UE)
	For Medicare coverage, a detailed written order must be received by the supplier before a claim is submitted.
E0185	**Gel or gel-like pressure pad for mattress, standard mattress length and width** Y & (NU, RR, UE)
	For Medicare coverage, a detailed written order must be received by the supplier before a claim is submitted.
E0186	**Air pressure mattress** Y & (RR)
	For Medicare coverage, a detailed written order must be received by the supplier before a claim is submitted.
E0187	**Water pressure mattress** Y & (RR)
	For Medicare coverage, a detailed written order must be received by the supplier before a claim is submitted.
E0188	**Synthetic sheepskin pad** Y & (NU, RR, UE)
	For Medicare coverage, a detailed written order must be received by the supplier before a claim is submitted.
E0189	**Lambswool sheepskin pad, any size** Y & (NU, RR, UE)
	For Medicare coverage, a detailed written order must be received by the supplier before a claim is submitted.
E0190	**Positioning cushion/pillow/wedge, any shape or size, includes all components and accessories** EI
E0191	**Heel or elbow protector, each** Y ☑ & (NU, RR, UE)
E0193	**Powered air flotation bed (low air loss therapy)** Y & (RR)
E0194	**Air fluidized bed** Y & (RR)
	An air fluidized bed is covered by Medicare if the patient has a stage 3 or stage 4 pressure sore and, without the bed, would require institutionalization. For Medicare coverage, a detailed written order must be received by the supplier before a claim is submitted.
E0196	**Gel pressure mattress** Y & (RR)
	Medicare covers pads if physicians supervise their use in patients who have decubitus ulcers or susceptibility to them. For Medicare coverage, a detailed written order must be received by the supplier before a claim is submitted.
E0197	**Air pressure pad for mattress, standard mattress length and width** Y & (RR)
	Medicare covers pads if physicians supervise their use in patients who have decubitus ulcers or susceptibility to them. For Medicare coverage, a detailed written order must be received by the supplier before a claim is submitted.
E0198	**Water pressure pad for mattress, standard mattress length and width** Y & (RR)
	Medicare covers pads if physicians supervise their use in patients who have decubitus ulcers or susceptibility to them. For Medicare coverage, a detailed written order must be received by the supplier before a claim is submitted.
E0199	**Dry pressure pad for mattress, standard mattress length and width** Y & (NU, RR, UE)
	Medicare covers pads if physicians supervise their use in patients who have decubitus ulcers or susceptibility to them. For Medicare coverage, a detailed written order must be received by the supplier before a claim is submitted.

Heat/Cold Application

Code	Description
E0200	**Heat lamp, without stand (table model), includes bulb, or infrared element** Y & (NU, RR, UE)
E0202	**Phototherapy (bilirubin) light with photometer** Y & (RR)
E0203	**Therapeutic lightbox, minimum 10,000 lux, table top model** EI
E0205	**Heat lamp, with stand, includes bulb, or infrared element** Y & (NU, RR, UE)
E0210	**Electric heat pad, standard** Y & (NU, RR, UE)
E0215	**Electric heat pad, moist** Y & (NU, RR, UE)
E0217	**Water circulating heat pad with pump** Y & (NU, RR, UE)
E0218	**Fluid circulating cold pad with pump, any type** Y
E0221	**Infrared heating pad system** Y
E0225	**Hydrocollator unit, includes pads** Y & (NU, RR, UE)
E0231	**Noncontact wound-warming device (temperature control unit, AC adapter and power cord) for use with warming card and wound cover** EI
E0232	**Warming card for use with the noncontact wound-warming device and noncontact wound-warming wound cover** EI
E0235	**Paraffin bath unit, portable (see medical supply code A4265 for paraffin)** Y & (RR)
E0236	**Pump for water circulating pad** Y & (RR)
E0239	**Hydrocollator unit, portable** Y & (NU, RR, UE)

Bath and Toilet Aids

Code	Description
E0240	**Bath/shower chair, with or without wheels, any size** EI

Special Coverage Instructions | Noncovered by Medicare | Carrier Discretion | ☑ Quantity Alert | ● New Code | ○ Recycled/Reinstated | ▲ Revised Code

32 — E Codes | A Age Edit | M Maternity Edit | ♀ Female Only | ♂ Male Only | A-Y OPPS Status Indicators | © 2022 Optum, Inc.

2023 HCPCS Level II E0373

Code	Description
E0241	Bathtub wall rail, each
E0242	Bathtub rail, floor base
E0243	Toilet rail, each
E0244	Raised toilet seat
E0245	Tub stool or bench
E0246	Transfer tub rail attachment
E0247	Transfer bench for tub or toilet with or without commode opening
E0248	Transfer bench, heavy-duty, for tub or toilet with or without commode opening
E0249	Pad for water circulating heat unit, for replacement only (NU, RR, UE)

Hospital Beds and Accessories

Code	Description
E0250	Hospital bed, fixed height, with any type side rails, with mattress (RR)
E0251	Hospital bed, fixed height, with any type side rails, without mattress (RR)
E0255	Hospital bed, variable height, hi-lo, with any type side rails, with mattress (RR)
E0256	Hospital bed, variable height, hi-lo, with any type side rails, without mattress (RR)
E0260	Hospital bed, semi-electric (head and foot adjustment), with any type side rails, with mattress (RR)
E0261	Hospital bed, semi-electric (head and foot adjustment), with any type side rails, without mattress (RR)
E0265	Hospital bed, total electric (head, foot, and height adjustments), with any type side rails, with mattress (RR)
E0266	Hospital bed, total electric (head, foot, and height adjustments), with any type side rails, without mattress (RR)
E0270	Hospital bed, institutional type includes: oscillating, circulating and Stryker frame, with mattress
E0271	Mattress, innerspring (NU, RR, UE) CMS: 100-04,36,50.14
E0272	Mattress, foam rubber (NU, RR, UE) CMS: 100-04,36,50.14
E0273	Bed board
E0274	Over-bed table
E0275	Bed pan, standard, metal or plastic (NU, RR, UE) Reusable, autoclavable bedpans are covered by Medicare for bed-confined patients.
E0276	Bed pan, fracture, metal or plastic (NU, RR, UE) Reusable, autoclavable bedpans are covered by Medicare for bed-confined patients.
E0277	Powered pressure-reducing air mattress (RR)
E0280	Bed cradle, any type (NU, RR, UE) CMS: 100-04,36,50.14
E0290	Hospital bed, fixed height, without side rails, with mattress (RR)
E0291	Hospital bed, fixed height, without side rails, without mattress (RR)
E0292	Hospital bed, variable height, hi-lo, without side rails, with mattress (RR)
E0293	Hospital bed, variable height, hi-lo, without side rails, without mattress (RR)
E0294	Hospital bed, semi-electric (head and foot adjustment), without side rails, with mattress (RR)
E0295	Hospital bed, semi-electric (head and foot adjustment), without side rails, without mattress (RR)
E0296	Hospital bed, total electric (head, foot, and height adjustments), without side rails, with mattress (RR)
E0297	Hospital bed, total electric (head, foot, and height adjustments), without side rails, without mattress (RR)
E0300	Pediatric crib, hospital grade, fully enclosed, with or without top enclosure (RR)
E0301	Hospital bed, heavy-duty, extra wide, with weight capacity greater than 350 pounds, but less than or equal to 600 pounds, with any type side rails, without mattress (RR)
E0302	Hospital bed, extra heavy-duty, extra wide, with weight capacity greater than 600 pounds, with any type side rails, without mattress (RR)
E0303	Hospital bed, heavy-duty, extra wide, with weight capacity greater than 350 pounds, but less than or equal to 600 pounds, with any type side rails, with mattress (RR)
E0304	Hospital bed, extra heavy-duty, extra wide, with weight capacity greater than 600 pounds, with any type side rails, with mattress (RR)
E0305	Bedside rails, half-length (RR)
E0310	Bedside rails, full-length (NU, RR, UE) CMS: 100-04,36,50.14
E0315	Bed accessory: board, table, or support device, any type
E0316	Safety enclosure frame/canopy for use with hospital bed, any type (RR)
E0325	Urinal; male, jug-type, any material (NU, RR, UE)
E0326	Urinal; female, jug-type, any material (NU, RR, UE)
E0328	Hospital bed, pediatric, manual, 360 degree side enclosures, top of headboard, footboard and side rails up to 24 in above the spring, includes mattress
E0329	Hospital bed, pediatric, electric or semi-electric, 360 degree side enclosures, top of headboard, footboard and side rails up to 24 in above the spring, includes mattress
E0350	Control unit for electronic bowel irrigation/evacuation system
E0352	Disposable pack (water reservoir bag, speculum, valving mechanism, and collection bag/box) for use with the electronic bowel irrigation/evacuation system
E0370	Air pressure elevator for heel
E0371	Nonpowered advanced pressure reducing overlay for mattress, standard mattress length and width (RR)
E0372	Powered air overlay for mattress, standard mattress length and width (RR)
E0373	Nonpowered advanced pressure reducing mattress (RR)

Oxygen and Related Respiratory Equipment

E0424 Stationary compressed gaseous oxygen system, rental; includes container, contents, regulator, flowmeter, humidifier, nebulizer, cannula or mask, and tubing Y ♿ (RR)

For the first claim filed for home oxygen equipment or therapy, submit a certificate of medical necessity that includes the oxygen flow rate, anticipated frequency and duration of oxygen therapy, and physician signature. Medicare accepts oxygen therapy as medically necessary in cases documenting any of the following: erythocythemia with a hematocrit greater than 56 percent; a P pulmonale on EKG; or dependent edema consistent with congestive heart failure.

CMS: 100-04,20,130.6; 100-04,20,30.6

E0425 Stationary compressed gas system, purchase; includes regulator, flowmeter, humidifier, nebulizer, cannula or mask, and tubing EI

E0430 Portable gaseous oxygen system, purchase; includes regulator, flowmeter, humidifier, cannula or mask, and tubing EI

E0431 Portable gaseous oxygen system, rental; includes portable container, regulator, flowmeter, humidifier, cannula or mask, and tubing Y ♿ (RR)

CMS: 100-04,20,130.6

E0433 Portable liquid oxygen system, rental; home liquefier used to fill portable liquid oxygen containers, includes portable containers, regulator, flowmeter, humidifier, cannula or mask and tubing, with or without supply reservoir and contents gauge Y ♿ (RR)

CMS: 100-04,20,130.6

E0434 Portable liquid oxygen system, rental; includes portable container, supply reservoir, humidifier, flowmeter, refill adaptor, contents gauge, cannula or mask, and tubing Y ♿ (RR)

CMS: 100-04,20,130.6

E0435 Portable liquid oxygen system, purchase; includes portable container, supply reservoir, flowmeter, humidifier, contents gauge, cannula or mask, tubing and refill adaptor EI

E0439 Stationary liquid oxygen system, rental; includes container, contents, regulator, flowmeter, humidifier, nebulizer, cannula or mask, & tubing Y ♿ (RR)

CMS: 100-04,20,130.6

E0440 Stationary liquid oxygen system, purchase; includes use of reservoir, contents indicator, regulator, flowmeter, humidifier, nebulizer, cannula or mask, and tubing EI

E0441 Stationary oxygen contents, gaseous, 1 month's supply = 1 unit Y ☑ ♿

CMS: 100-04,20,30.6

E0442 Stationary oxygen contents, liquid, 1 month's supply = 1 unit Y ☑ ♿

E0443 Portable oxygen contents, gaseous, 1 month's supply = 1 unit Y ☑ ♿

CMS: 100-04,20,30.6

E0444 Portable oxygen contents, liquid, 1 month's supply = 1 unit Y ☑ ♿

E0445 Oximeter device for measuring blood oxygen levels noninvasively N

E0446 Topical oxygen delivery system, not otherwise specified, includes all supplies and accessories A

E0447 Portable oxygen contents, liquid, 1 month's supply = 1 unit, prescribed amount at rest or nighttime exceeds 4 liters per minute (LPM)

E0455 Oxygen tent, excluding croup or pediatric tents Y

E0457 Chest shell (cuirass) EI

E0459 Chest wrap EI

E0462 Rocking bed, with or without side rails Y ♿ (RR)

E0465 Home ventilator, any type, used with invasive interface, (e.g., tracheostomy tube) Y ♿ (RR)

E0466 Home ventilator, any type, used with noninvasive interface, (e.g., mask, chest shell) Y ♿ (RR)

E0467 Home ventilator, multi-function respiratory device, also performs any or all of the additional functions of oxygen concentration, drug nebulization, aspiration, and cough stimulation, includes all accessories, components and supplies for all functions (RR)

E0470 Respiratory assist device, bi-level pressure capability, without backup rate feature, used with noninvasive interface, e.g., nasal or facial mask (intermittent assist device with continuous positive airway pressure device) Y ♿ (RR)

CMS: 100-03,240.4

E0471 Respiratory assist device, bi-level pressure capability, with back-up rate feature, used with noninvasive interface, e.g., nasal or facial mask (intermittent assist device with continuous positive airway pressure device) Y ♿ (RR)

CMS: 100-03,240.4

E0472 Respiratory assist device, bi-level pressure capability, with backup rate feature, used with invasive interface, e.g., tracheostomy tube (intermittent assist device with continuous positive airway pressure device) Y ♿ (RR)

CMS: 100-03,240.4

E0480 Percussor, electric or pneumatic, home model Y ♿ (RR)

E0481 Intrapulmonary percussive ventilation system and related accessories EI

E0482 Cough stimulating device, alternating positive and negative airway pressure Y ♿ (RR)

▲ **E0483** High frequency chest wall oscillation system, with full anterior and/or posterior thoracic region receiving simultaneous external oscillation, includes all accessories and supplies, each Y ☑ ♿ (RR)

E0484 Oscillatory positive expiratory pressure device, nonelectric, any type, each Y ☑ ♿ (NU, RR, UE)

E0485 Oral device/appliance used to reduce upper airway collapsibility, adjustable or nonadjustable, prefabricated, includes fitting and adjustment Y ♿ (NU, RR, UE)

E0486 Oral device/appliance used to reduce upper airway collapsibility, adjustable or nonadjustable, custom fabricated, includes fitting and adjustment Y ♿ (NU, RR, UE)

E0487 Spirometer, electronic, includes all accessories N

IPPB Machines

E0500   IPPB machine, all types, with built-in nebulization; manual or automatic valves; internal or external power source   Y ♿ (RR)

Intermittent Positive Pressure Breathing (IPPB) devices

- Battery pack and controls
- Nebulizer
- Nebulizer reservoir
- Oxygen supply tube
- IPPB unit in use

Humidifiers/Compressors/Nebulizers

E0550   Humidifier, durable for extensive supplemental humidification during IPPB treatments or oxygen delivery   Y ♿ (RR)

E0555   Humidifier, durable, glass or autoclavable plastic bottle type, for use with regulator or flowmeter   Y

E0560   Humidifier, durable for supplemental humidification during IPPB treatment or oxygen delivery   Y ♿ (NU, RR, UE)

E0561   Humidifier, nonheated, used with positive airway pressure device   Y ♿ (NU, RR, UE)
CMS: 100-03,240.4; 100-04,36,50.14

E0562   Humidifier, heated, used with positive airway pressure device   Y ♿ (NU, RR, UE)
CMS: 100-03,240.4; 100-04,36,50.14

E0565   Compressor, air power source for equipment which is not self-contained or cylinder driven   Y ♿ (RR)

E0570   Nebulizer, with compressor   Y ♿ (RR)

E0572   Aerosol compressor, adjustable pressure, light duty for intermittent use   Y ♿ (RR)

E0574   Ultrasonic/electronic aerosol generator with small volume nebulizer   Y ♿ (RR)

E0575   Nebulizer, ultrasonic, large volume   Y ♿ (RR)

E0580   Nebulizer, durable, glass or autoclavable plastic, bottle type, for use with regulator or flowmeter   Y ♿ (NU, RR, UE)

E0585   Nebulizer, with compressor and heater   Y ♿ (RR)

Pumps and Vaporizers

E0600   Respiratory suction pump, home model, portable or stationary, electric   Y ♿ (RR)

E0601   Continuous positive airway pressure (CPAP) device   Y ♿ (RR)
CMS: 100-03,240.4

E0602   Breast pump, manual, any type   M ♀ Y ♿ (NU, RR, UE)

E0603   Breast pump, electric (AC and/or DC), any type   M ♀ N

E0604   Breast pump, hospital grade, electric (AC and/or DC), any type   M ♀ A

E0605   Vaporizer, room type   Y ♿ (NU, RR, UE)

E0606   Postural drainage board   Y ♿ (RR)

Monitoring Devices

E0607   Home blood glucose monitor   Y ♿ (NU, RR, UE)
Medicare covers home blood testing devices for diabetic patients when the devices are prescribed by the patients' physicians. Many commercial payers provide this coverage to noninsulin dependent diabetics as well.

E0610   Pacemaker monitor, self-contained, (checks battery depletion, includes audible and visible check systems)   Y ♿ (NU, RR, UE)

E0615   Pacemaker monitor, self-contained, checks battery depletion and other pacemaker components, includes digital/visible check systems   Y ♿ (NU, RR, UE)

E0616   Implantable cardiac event recorder with memory, activator, and programmer   N

E0617   External defibrillator with integrated electrocardiogram analysis   Y ♿ (RR)

E0618   Apnea monitor, without recording feature   Y ♿ (RR)

E0619   Apnea monitor, with recording feature   Y ♿ (RR)

E0620   Skin piercing device for collection of capillary blood, laser, each   Y ♿ (RR)

Patient Lifts

E0621   Sling or seat, patient lift, canvas or nylon   Y ♿ (NU, RR, UE)

E0625   Patient lift, bathroom or toilet, not otherwise classified   EI

E0627   Seat lift mechanism, electric, any type   Y ♿ (NU, RR, UE)
CMS: 100-04,20,100; 100-04,20,130.2; 100-04,20,130.3; 100-04,20,130.4; 100-04,20,130.5

E0629   Seat lift mechanism, nonelectric, any type   Y ♿ (NU, RR, UE)
CMS: 100-04,20,100; 100-04,20,130.2; 100-04,20,130.3; 100-04,20,130.4; 100-04,20,130.5

E0630   Patient lift, hydraulic or mechanical, includes any seat, sling, strap(s), or pad(s)   Y ♿ (RR)

E0635   Patient lift, electric, with seat or sling   Y ♿ (RR)

E0636   Multipositional patient support system, with integrated lift, patient accessible controls   Y ♿ (RR)

E0637   Combination sit-to-stand frame/table system, any size including pediatric, with seat lift feature, with or without wheels   EI

E0638   Standing frame/table system, one position (e.g., upright, supine or prone stander), any size including pediatric, with or without wheels   EI

E0639   Patient lift, moveable from room to room with disassembly and reassembly, includes all components/accessories   EI ♿ (RR)

E0640   Patient lift, fixed system, includes all components/accessories   EI ♿ (RR)

E0641   Standing frame/table system, multi-position (e.g., 3-way stander), any size including pediatric, with or without wheels   EI

Special Coverage Instructions   Noncovered by Medicare   Carrier Discretion   ☑ Quantity Alert   ● New Code   ○ Recycled/Reinstated   ▲ Revised Code

© 2022 Optum, Inc.   A2–Z3 ASC Pmt   CMS: IOM   AHA: Coding Clinic   ♿ DMEPOS Paid   ⊘ SNF Excluded   E Codes — 35

Compression Devices

Code	Description
E0642	Standing frame/table system, mobile (dynamic stander), any size including pediatric
E0650	Pneumatic compressor, nonsegmental home model (NU, RR, UE)
E0651	Pneumatic compressor, segmental home model without calibrated gradient pressure (NU, RR, UE)
E0652	Pneumatic compressor, segmental home model with calibrated gradient pressure (NU, RR, UE)
E0655	Nonsegmental pneumatic appliance for use with pneumatic compressor, half arm (NU, RR, UE)
E0656	Segmental pneumatic appliance for use with pneumatic compressor, trunk (RR)
E0657	Segmental pneumatic appliance for use with pneumatic compressor, chest (RR)
E0660	Nonsegmental pneumatic appliance for use with pneumatic compressor, full leg (NU, RR, UE)
E0665	Nonsegmental pneumatic appliance for use with pneumatic compressor, full arm (NU, RR, UE)
E0666	Nonsegmental pneumatic appliance for use with pneumatic compressor, half leg (NU, RR, UE)
E0667	Segmental pneumatic appliance for use with pneumatic compressor, full leg (NU, RR, UE)
E0668	Segmental pneumatic appliance for use with pneumatic compressor, full arm (NU, RR, UE)
E0669	Segmental pneumatic appliance for use with pneumatic compressor, half leg (NU, RR, UE)
E0670	Segmental pneumatic appliance for use with pneumatic compressor, integrated, two full legs and trunk (NU, RR, UE)
E0671	Segmental gradient pressure pneumatic appliance, full leg (NU, RR, UE)
E0672	Segmental gradient pressure pneumatic appliance, full arm (NU, RR, UE)
E0673	Segmental gradient pressure pneumatic appliance, half leg (NU, RR, UE)
E0675	Pneumatic compression device, high pressure, rapid inflation/deflation cycle, for arterial insufficiency (unilateral or bilateral system) (RR)
E0676	Intermittent limb compression device (includes all accessories), not otherwise specified

Ultraviolet Light

Code	Description
E0691	Ultraviolet light therapy system, includes bulbs/lamps, timer and eye protection; treatment area 2 sq ft or less (NU, RR, UE)
E0692	Ultraviolet light therapy system panel, includes bulbs/lamps, timer and eye protection, 4 ft panel (NU, RR, UE)
E0693	Ultraviolet light therapy system panel, includes bulbs/lamps, timer and eye protection, 6 ft panel (NU, RR, UE)
E0694	Ultraviolet multidirectional light therapy system in 6 ft cabinet, includes bulbs/lamps, timer, and eye protection (NU, RR, UE)

Safety Equipment

E0700 Safety equipment, device or accessory, any type

Restraints (E0710)
Fabric wrist restraint
Padded leather restraints may feature a locking device
Body restraint
Fabric gait belt for assistance in walking (E0700)

Code	Description
E0705	Transfer device, any type, each (NU, RR, UE)
E0710	Restraints, any type (body, chest, wrist, or ankle)

Nerve Stimulators and Devices

E0720 Transcutaneous electrical nerve stimulation (TENS) device, two-lead, localized stimulation (NU)
A Certificate of Medical Necessity is required for the purchase of a TENS. It is not required for rentals.
CMS: 100-03,10.2; 100-03,160.27; 100-03,160.7.1; 100-04,20,30.1.2

E0730 Transcutaneous electrical nerve stimulation (TENS) device, four or more leads, for multiple nerve stimulation (NU)
A Certificate of Medical Necessity is required for the purchase of a TENS. It is not required for rentals.
CMS: 100-03,10.2; 100-03,160.27; 100-03,160.7.1; 100-04,20,30.1.2

E0731 Form-fitting conductive garment for delivery of TENS or NMES (with conductive fibers separated from the patient's skin by layers of fabric) (NU)
CMS: 100-03,10.2; 100-03,160.13

E0740 Nonimplanted pelvic floor electrical stimulator, complete system (RR)

E0744 Neuromuscular stimulator for scoliosis (RR)

E0745 Neuromuscular stimulator, electronic shock unit (RR)

E0746 Electromyography (EMG), biofeedback device
Biofeedback therapy is covered by Medicare only for re-education of specific muscles or for treatment of incapacitating muscle spasm or weakness.

E0747 Osteogenesis stimulator, electrical, noninvasive, other than spinal applications (NU, RR, UE)
Medicare covers noninvasive osteogenic stimulation for nonunion of long bone fractures, failed fusion, or congenital pseudoarthroses.

2023 HCPCS Level II

Code	Description
E0748	Osteogenesis stimulator, electrical, noninvasive, spinal applications Y (NU, RR, UE)
	Medicare covers noninvasive osteogenic stimulation as an adjunct to spinal fusion surgery for patients at high risk of pseudoarthroses due to previously failed spinal fusion, or for those undergoing fusion of three or more vertebrae.
E0749	Osteogenesis stimulator, electrical, surgically implanted N (RR)
	Medicare covers invasive osteogenic stimulation for nonunion of long bone fractures or as an adjunct to spinal fusion surgery for patients at high risk of pseudoarthroses due to previously failed spinal fusion, or for those undergoing fusion of three or more vertebrae. **CMS:** 100-04,4,190
E0755	Electronic salivary reflex stimulator (intraoral/noninvasive) EI
E0760	Osteogenesis stimulator, low intensity ultrasound, noninvasive Y (NU, RR, UE) **CMS:** 100-04,32,110.5
E0761	Nonthermal pulsed high frequency radiowaves, high peak power electromagnetic energy treatment device EI
E0762	Transcutaneous electrical joint stimulation device system, includes all accessories B (RR)
E0764	Functional neuromuscular stimulation, transcutaneous stimulation of sequential muscle groups of ambulation with computer control, used for walking by spinal cord injured, entire system, after completion of training program Y (RR)
E0765	FDA approved nerve stimulator, with replaceable batteries, for treatment of nausea and vomiting Y (NU, RR, UE)
E0766	Electrical stimulation device used for cancer treatment, includes all accessories, any type Y (RR)
E0769	Electrical stimulation or electromagnetic wound treatment device, not otherwise classified B **CMS:** 100-04,32,11.1
E0770	Functional electrical stimulator, transcutaneous stimulation of nerve and/or muscle groups, any type, complete system, not otherwise specified Y

Infusion Supplies

Code	Description
E0776	IV pole Y (NU, RR, UE)
E0779	Ambulatory infusion pump, mechanical, reusable, for infusion 8 hours or greater Y (RR)
E0780	Ambulatory infusion pump, mechanical, reusable, for infusion less than 8 hours Y (NU)
E0781	Ambulatory infusion pump, single or multiple channels, electric or battery operated, with administrative equipment, worn by patient Y (RR)
E0782	Infusion pump, implantable, nonprogrammable (includes all components, e.g., pump, catheter, connectors, etc.) N (NU, RR, UE) **CMS:** 100-04,4,190
E0783	Infusion pump system, implantable, programmable (includes all components, e.g., pump, catheter, connectors, etc.) N (NU, RR, UE) **CMS:** 100-04,4,190
E0784	External ambulatory infusion pump, insulin Y (RR) Covered by some commercial payers with preauthorization.
E0785	Implantable intraspinal (epidural/intrathecal) catheter used with implantable infusion pump, replacement N (KF) **CMS:** 100-04,4,190
E0786	Implantable programmable infusion pump, replacement (excludes implantable intraspinal catheter) N (NU, RR, UE)
E0787	External ambulatory infusion pump, insulin, dosage rate adjustment using therapeutic continuous glucose sensing
E0791	Parenteral infusion pump, stationary, single, or multichannel Y (RR)

Traction Equipment

Code	Description
E0830	Ambulatory traction device, all types, each N
E0840	Traction frame, attached to headboard, cervical traction Y (NU, RR, UE)
E0849	Traction equipment, cervical, free-standing stand/frame, pneumatic, applying traction force to other than mandible Y (RR)
E0850	Traction stand, freestanding, cervical traction Y (NU, RR, UE)
E0855	Cervical traction equipment not requiring additional stand or frame Y (RR)
E0856	Cervical traction device, with inflatable air bladder(s) Y (RR)
E0860	Traction equipment, overdoor, cervical Y (NU, RR, UE)
E0870	Traction frame, attached to footboard, extremity traction (e.g., Buck's) Y (NU, RR, UE)
E0890	Traction frame, attached to footboard, pelvic traction Y (NU, RR, UE)
E0900	Traction stand, freestanding, pelvic traction (e.g., Buck's) Y (NU, RR, UE)

Orthopedic Devices

Code	Description
E0910	Trapeze bars, also known as Patient Helper, attached to bed, with grab bar Y (RR)
E0911	Trapeze bar, heavy-duty, for patient weight capacity greater than 250 pounds, attached to bed, with grab bar Y (RR)
E0912	Trapeze bar, heavy-duty, for patient weight capacity greater than 250 pounds, freestanding, complete with grab bar Y (RR)
E0920	Fracture frame, attached to bed, includes weights Y (RR)
E0930	Fracture frame, freestanding, includes weights Y (RR)
E0935	Continuous passive motion exercise device for use on knee only Y (RR)
E0936	Continuous passive motion exercise device for use other than knee EI
E0940	Trapeze bar, freestanding, complete with grab bar Y (RR)
E0941	Gravity assisted traction device, any type Y (RR)
E0942	Cervical head harness/halter Y (NU, RR, UE)
E0944	Pelvic belt/harness/boot Y (NU, RR, UE)
E0945	Extremity belt/harness Y (NU, RR, UE)
E0946	Fracture, frame, dual with cross bars, attached to bed, (e.g., Balken, four-poster) Y (RR)
E0947	Fracture frame, attachments for complex pelvic traction Y (NU, RR, UE)
E0948	Fracture frame, attachments for complex cervical traction Y (NU, RR, UE)

Wheelchair Accessories

Code	Description
E0950	Wheelchair accessory, tray, each Y ☑ (NU, RR, UE)
E0951	Heel loop/holder, any type, with or without ankle strap, each Y ☑ (NU, RR, UE)
E0952	Toe loop/holder, any type, each Y ☑ (NU, RR, UE)

Special Coverage Instructions | Noncovered by Medicare | Carrier Discretion | ☑ Quantity Alert | ● New Code | ○ Recycled/Reinstated | ▲ Revised Code

© 2022 Optum, Inc.   A2-Z3 ASC Pmt   **CMS:** IOM   **AHA:** Coding Clinic   DMEPOS Paid   SNF Excluded

Durable Medical Equipment

E0953 — E1039

Code	Description
E0953	Wheelchair accessory, lateral thigh or knee support, any type including fixed mounting hardware, each (NU, RR, UE)
E0954	Wheelchair accessory, foot box, any type, includes attachment and mounting hardware, each foot (NU, RR, UE)
E0955	Wheelchair accessory, headrest, cushioned, any type, including fixed mounting hardware, each (RR)
E0956	Wheelchair accessory, lateral trunk or hip support, any type, including fixed mounting hardware, each (NU, RR, UE)
E0957	Wheelchair accessory, medial thigh support, any type, including fixed mounting hardware, each (NU, RR, UE)
E0958	Manual wheelchair accessory, one-arm drive attachment, each (RR)
E0959	Manual wheelchair accessory, adapter for amputee, each (NU, RR, UE)
E0960	Wheelchair accessory, shoulder harness/straps or chest strap, including any type mounting hardware (NU, RR, UE)
E0961	Manual wheelchair accessory, wheel lock brake extension (handle), each (NU, RR, UE)
E0966	Manual wheelchair accessory, headrest extension, each (NU, RR, UE)
E0967	Manual wheelchair accessory, hand rim with projections, any type, replacement only, each (NU, RR, UE)
E0968	Commode seat, wheelchair (RR)
E0969	Narrowing device, wheelchair (NU, RR, UE)
E0970	No. 2 footplates, except for elevating legrest See code(s): K0037, K0042
E0971	Manual wheelchair accessory, antitipping device, each (NU, RR, UE)
E0973	Wheelchair accessory, adjustable height, detachable armrest, complete assembly, each (NU, RR, UE)
E0974	Manual wheelchair accessory, antirollback device, each (NU, RR, UE)
E0978	Wheelchair accessory, positioning belt/safety belt/pelvic strap, each (NU, RR, UE)
E0980	Safety vest, wheelchair (NU, RR, UE)
E0981	Wheelchair accessory, seat upholstery, replacement only, each (NU, RR, UE)
E0982	Wheelchair accessory, back upholstery, replacement only, each (NU, RR, UE)
E0983	Manual wheelchair accessory, power add-on to convert manual wheelchair to motorized wheelchair, joystick control (RR)
E0984	Manual wheelchair accessory, power add-on to convert manual wheelchair to motorized wheelchair, tiller control (RR)
E0985	Wheelchair accessory, seat lift mechanism (RR)
E0986	Manual wheelchair accessory, push-rim activated power assist system (RR)
E0988	Manual wheelchair accessory, lever-activated, wheel drive, pair (RR)
E0990	Wheelchair accessory, elevating legrest, complete assembly, each (NU, RR, UE)
E0992	Manual wheelchair accessory, solid seat insert (NU, RR, UE)
E0994	Armrest, each (NU, RR, UE)
E0995	Wheelchair accessory, calf rest/pad, replacement only, each (NU, RR, UE)
E1002	Wheelchair accessory, power seating system, tilt only (RR)
E1003	Wheelchair accessory, power seating system, recline only, without shear reduction (RR)
E1004	Wheelchair accessory, power seating system, recline only, with mechanical shear reduction (RR)
E1005	Wheelchair accessory, power seating system, recline only, with power shear reduction (RR)
E1006	Wheelchair accessory, power seating system, combination tilt and recline, without shear reduction (RR)
E1007	Wheelchair accessory, power seating system, combination tilt and recline, with mechanical shear reduction (RR)
E1008	Wheelchair accessory, power seating system, combination tilt and recline, with power shear reduction (RR)
E1009	Wheelchair accessory, addition to power seating system, mechanically linked leg elevation system, including pushrod and legrest, each (NU, RR, UE)
E1010	Wheelchair accessory, addition to power seating system, power leg elevation system, including legrest, pair (RR)
E1011	Modification to pediatric size wheelchair, width adjustment package (not to be dispensed with initial chair) (NU, RR, UE)
E1012	Wheelchair accessory, addition to power seating system, center mount power elevating leg rest/platform, complete system, any type, each (RR)
E1014	Reclining back, addition to pediatric size wheelchair (RR)
E1015	Shock absorber for manual wheelchair, each (NU, RR, UE)
E1016	Shock absorber for power wheelchair, each (NU, RR, UE)
E1017	Heavy-duty shock absorber for heavy-duty or extra heavy-duty manual wheelchair, each (NU, RR, UE)
E1018	Heavy-duty shock absorber for heavy-duty or extra heavy-duty power wheelchair, each (NU, RR, UE)
E1020	Residual limb support system for wheelchair, any type (RR)
E1028	Wheelchair accessory, manual swingaway, retractable or removable mounting hardware for joystick, other control interface or positioning accessory (RR)
E1029	Wheelchair accessory, ventilator tray, fixed (RR)
E1030	Wheelchair accessory, ventilator tray, gimbaled (RR)
E1031	Rollabout chair, any and all types with castors 5 in or greater (RR)
E1035	Multi-positional patient transfer system, with integrated seat, operated by care giver, patient weight capacity up to and including 300 lbs (RR) **CMS:** 100-02,15,110
E1036	Multi-positional patient transfer system, extra-wide, with integrated seat, operated by caregiver, patient weight capacity greater than 300 lbs (RR)
E1037	Transport chair, pediatric size (RR)
E1038	Transport chair, adult size, patient weight capacity up to and including 300 pounds (RR)
E1039	Transport chair, adult size, heavy-duty, patient weight capacity greater than 300 pounds (RR)

Wheelchairs

E1050 Fully-reclining wheelchair, fixed full-length arms, swing-away detachable elevating legrests ⓎⓋ (RR)

E1060 Fully-reclining wheelchair, detachable arms, desk or full-length, swing-away detachable elevating legrests ⓎⓋ (RR)

E1070 Fully-reclining wheelchair, detachable arms (desk or full-length) swing-away detachable footrest ⓎⓋ (RR)

E1083 Hemi-wheelchair, fixed full-length arms, swing-away detachable elevating legrest ⓎⓋ (RR)

E1084 Hemi-wheelchair, detachable arms desk or full-length arms, swing-away detachable elevating legrests ⓎⓋ (RR)

E1085 Hemi-wheelchair, fixed full-length arms, swing-away detachable footrests ⒺⒾ
See code(s): K0002

E1086 Hemi-wheelchair, detachable arms, desk or full-length, swing-away detachable footrests ⒺⒾ
See code(s): K0002

E1087 High strength lightweight wheelchair, fixed full-length arms, swing-away detachable elevating legrests ⓎⓋ (RR)

E1088 High strength lightweight wheelchair, detachable arms desk or full-length, swing-away detachable elevating legrests ⓎⓋ (RR)

E1089 High-strength lightweight wheelchair, fixed-length arms, swing-away detachable footrest ⒺⒾ
See code(s): K0004

E1090 High-strength lightweight wheelchair, detachable arms, desk or full-length, swing-away detachable footrests ⒺⒾ
See code(s): K0004

E1092 Wide heavy-duty wheel chair, detachable arms (desk or full-length), swing-away detachable elevating legrests ⓎⓋ (RR)

E1093 Wide heavy-duty wheelchair, detachable arms, desk or full-length arms, swing-away detachable footrests ⓎⓋ (RR)

E1100 Semi-reclining wheelchair, fixed full-length arms, swing-away detachable elevating legrests ⓎⓋ (RR)

E1110 Semi-reclining wheelchair, detachable arms (desk or full-length) elevating legrest ⓎⓋ (RR)

E1130 Standard wheelchair, fixed full-length arms, fixed or swing-away detachable footrests ⒺⒾ
See code(s): K0001

E1140 Wheelchair, detachable arms, desk or full-length, swing-away detachable footrests ⒺⒾ
See code(s): K0001

E1150 Wheelchair, detachable arms, desk or full-length swing-away detachable elevating legrests ⓎⓋ (RR)

E1160 Wheelchair, fixed full-length arms, swing-away detachable elevating legrests ⓎⓋ (RR)

E1161 Manual adult size wheelchair, includes tilt in space ⓎⓋ (RR)

E1170 Amputee wheelchair, fixed full-length arms, swing-away detachable elevating legrests ⓎⓋ (RR)

E1171 Amputee wheelchair, fixed full-length arms, without footrests or legrest ⓎⓋ (RR)

E1172 Amputee wheelchair, detachable arms (desk or full-length) without footrests or legrest ⓎⓋ (RR)

E1180 Amputee wheelchair, detachable arms (desk or full-length) swing-away detachable footrests ⓎⓋ (RR)

E1190 Amputee wheelchair, detachable arms (desk or full-length) swing-away detachable elevating legrests ⓎⓋ (RR)

E1195 Heavy-duty wheelchair, fixed full-length arms, swing-away detachable elevating legrests ⓎⓋ (RR)

E1200 Amputee wheelchair, fixed full-length arms, swing-away detachable footrest ⓎⓋ (RR)

E1220 Wheelchair; specially sized or constructed, (indicate brand name, model number, if any) and justification Ⓨ

E1221 Wheelchair with fixed arm, footrests ⓎⓋ (RR)

E1222 Wheelchair with fixed arm, elevating legrests ⓎⓋ (RR)

E1223 Wheelchair with detachable arms, footrests ⓎⓋ (RR)

E1224 Wheelchair with detachable arms, elevating legrests ⓎⓋ (RR)

E1225 Wheelchair accessory, manual semi-reclining back, (recline greater than 15 degrees, but less than 80 degrees), each Ⓨ☑Ⓥ (RR)

E1226 Wheelchair accessory, manual fully reclining back, (recline greater than 80 degrees), each Ⓑ☑Ⓥ (NU, RR, UE)
See also K0028

E1227 Special height arms for wheelchair ⓎⓋ (NU, RR, UE)

E1228 Special back height for wheelchair ⓎⓋ (RR)

E1229 Wheelchair, pediatric size, not otherwise specified Ⓨ

E1230 Power operated vehicle (three- or four-wheel nonhighway), specify brand name and model number ⓎⓋ (NU, RR, UE)
Prior authorization is required by Medicare for this item.

E1231 Wheelchair, pediatric size, tilt-in-space, rigid, adjustable, with seating system ⓎⓋ (NU, RR, UE)

E1232 Wheelchair, pediatric size, tilt-in-space, folding, adjustable, with seating system ⓎⓋ (RR)

E1233 Wheelchair, pediatric size, tilt-in-space, rigid, adjustable, without seating system ⓎⓋ (RR)

E1234 Wheelchair, pediatric size, tilt-in-space, folding, adjustable, without seating system ⓎⓋ (RR)

E1235 Wheelchair, pediatric size, rigid, adjustable, with seating system ⓎⓋ (RR)

E1236 Wheelchair, pediatric size, folding, adjustable, with seating system ⓎⓋ (RR)

E1237 Wheelchair, pediatric size, rigid, adjustable, without seating system ⓎⓋ (RR)

E1238 Wheelchair, pediatric size, folding, adjustable, without seating system ⓎⓋ (RR)

E1239 Power wheelchair, pediatric size, not otherwise specified Ⓨ

E1240 Lightweight wheelchair, detachable arms, (desk or full-length) swing-away detachable, elevating legrest ⓎⓋ (RR)

E1250 Lightweight wheelchair, fixed full-length arms, swing-away detachable footrest ⒺⒾ
See code(s): K0003

E1260 Lightweight wheelchair, detachable arms (desk or full-length) swing-away detachable footrest ⒺⒾ
See code(s): K0003

E1270 Lightweight wheelchair, fixed full-length arms, swing-away detachable elevating legrests ⓎⓋ (RR)

E1280 Heavy-duty wheelchair, detachable arms (desk or full-length) elevating legrests ⓎⓋ (RR)

Durable Medical Equipment

Code	Description	Indicators
E1285	Heavy-duty wheelchair, fixed full-length arms, swing-away detachable footrest	EI
	See code(s): K0006	
E1290	Heavy-duty wheelchair, detachable arms (desk or full-length) swing-away detachable footrest	EI
	See code(s): K0006	
E1295	Heavy-duty wheelchair, fixed full-length arms, elevating legrest	Y ♿ (RR)
E1296	Special wheelchair seat height from floor	Y ♿ (NU, RR, UE)
E1297	Special wheelchair seat depth, by upholstery	Y ♿ (NU, RR, UE)
E1298	Special wheelchair seat depth and/or width, by construction	Y ♿ (NU, RR, UE)

Whirlpool - Equipment

Code	Description	Indicators
E1300	Whirlpool, portable (overtub type)	EI
E1310	Whirlpool, nonportable (built-in type)	Y ♿ (NU, RR, UE)

Additional Oxygen Related Equipment

Code	Description	Indicators
E1352	Oxygen accessory, flow regulator capable of positive inspiratory pressure	Y
E1353	Regulator	Y ♿
E1354	Oxygen accessory, wheeled cart for portable cylinder or portable concentrator, any type, replacement only, each	Y ☑
E1355	Stand/rack	Y ♿
E1356	Oxygen accessory, battery pack/cartridge for portable concentrator, any type, replacement only, each	Y ☑
E1357	Oxygen accessory, battery charger for portable concentrator, any type, replacement only, each	Y ☑
E1358	Oxygen accessory, DC power adapter for portable concentrator, any type, replacement only, each	Y ☑
E1372	Immersion external heater for nebulizer	Y ♿ (NU, RR, UE)
E1390	Oxygen concentrator, single delivery port, capable of delivering 85 percent or greater oxygen concentration at the prescribed flow rate	Y ♿ (RR)
	CMS: 100-04,20,130.6	
E1391	Oxygen concentrator, dual delivery port, capable of delivering 85 percent or greater oxygen concentration at the prescribed flow rate, each	Y ☑ ♿ (RR)
	CMS: 100-04,20,130.6	
E1392	Portable oxygen concentrator, rental	Y ♿ (RR)
	CMS: 100-04,20,130.6	
E1399	Durable medical equipment, miscellaneous	Y
	CMS: 100-04,20,30.9; 100-04,32,110.5	
E1405	Oxygen and water vapor enriching system with heated delivery	Y ♿ (RR)
	CMS: 100-04,20,20; 100-04,20,20.4	
E1406	Oxygen and water vapor enriching system without heated delivery	Y ♿ (RR)
	CMS: 100-04,20,20; 100-04,20,20.4	

Artificial Kidney Machines and Accessories

Code	Description	Indicators
E1500	Centrifuge, for dialysis	A ⊘
E1510	Kidney, dialysate delivery system kidney machine, pump recirculating, air removal system, flowrate meter, power off, heater and temperature control with alarm, IV poles, pressure gauge, concentrate container	A ⊘
E1520	Heparin infusion pump for hemodialysis	A ⊘
E1530	Air bubble detector for hemodialysis, each, replacement	A ☑ ⊘
E1540	Pressure alarm for hemodialysis, each, replacement	A ☑ ⊘
E1550	Bath conductivity meter for hemodialysis, each	A ☑ ⊘
E1560	Blood leak detector for hemodialysis, each, replacement	A ☑ ⊘
E1570	Adjustable chair, for ESRD patients	A ⊘
E1575	Transducer protectors/fluid barriers, for hemodialysis, any size, per 10	A ☑ ⊘
E1580	Unipuncture control system for hemodialysis	A ⊘
E1590	Hemodialysis machine	A ⊘
E1592	Automatic intermittent peritoneal dialysis system	A ⊘
E1594	Cycler dialysis machine for peritoneal dialysis	A ⊘
E1600	Delivery and/or installation charges for hemodialysis equipment	A ⊘
E1610	Reverse osmosis water purification system, for hemodialysis	A ⊘
E1615	Deionizer water purification system, for hemodialysis	A ⊘
E1620	Blood pump for hemodialysis, replacement	A ⊘
E1625	Water softening system, for hemodialysis	A ⊘
E1629	Tablo hemodialysis system for the billable dialysis service	
E1630	Reciprocating peritoneal dialysis system	A ⊘
E1632	Wearable artificial kidney, each	A ☑ ⊘
E1634	Peritoneal dialysis clamps, each	B ☑
E1635	Compact (portable) travel hemodialyzer system	A ⊘
E1636	Sorbent cartridges, for hemodialysis, per 10	A ☑ ⊘
E1637	Hemostats, each	A ☑ ⊘
E1639	Scale, each	A ☑ ⊘
E1699	Dialysis equipment, not otherwise specified	A ⊘
	CMS: 100-04,8,20	

Jaw Motion Rehabilitation System and Accessories

Code	Description	Indicators
E1700	Jaw motion rehabilitation system	Y ♿ (RR)
	Medicare jurisdiction: local contractor.	
E1701	Replacement cushions for jaw motion rehabilitation system, package of 6	Y ♿
	Medicare jurisdiction: local contractor.	
E1702	Replacement measuring scales for jaw motion rehabilitation system, package of 200	Y ☑ ♿
	Medicare jurisdiction: local contractor.	

Flexion/Extension Device

Code	Description	Indicators
E1800	Dynamic adjustable elbow extension/flexion device, includes soft interface material	Y ♿ (RR)
E1801	Static progressive stretch elbow device, extension and/or flexion, with or without range of motion adjustment, includes all components and accessories	Y ♿ (RR)
E1802	Dynamic adjustable forearm pronation/supination device, includes soft interface material	Y ♿ (RR)
E1805	Dynamic adjustable wrist extension/flexion device, includes soft interface material	Y ♿ (RR)
E1806	Static progressive stretch wrist device, flexion and/or extension, with or without range of motion adjustment, includes all components and accessories	Y ♿ (RR)

Special Coverage Instructions | **Noncovered by Medicare** | **Carrier Discretion** | ☑ Quantity Alert | ● New Code | ○ Recycled/Reinstated | ▲ Revised Code

A Age Edit **M** Maternity Edit ♀ Female Only ♂ Male Only **A**–**Y** OPPS Status Indicators

2023 HCPCS Level II

Durable Medical Equipment

Code	Description
E1810	Dynamic adjustable knee extension/flexion device, includes soft interface material Y & (RR)
E1811	Static progressive stretch knee device, extension and/or flexion, with or without range of motion adjustment, includes all components and accessories Y & (RR)
E1812	Dynamic knee, extension/flexion device with active resistance control Y & (RR)
E1815	Dynamic adjustable ankle extension/flexion device, includes soft interface material Y & (RR)
E1816	Static progressive stretch ankle device, flexion and/or extension, with or without range of motion adjustment, includes all components and accessories Y & (RR)
E1818	Static progressive stretch forearm pronation/supination device, with or without range of motion adjustment, includes all components and accessories Y & (RR)
E1820	Replacement soft interface material, dynamic adjustable extension/flexion device Y & (NU, RR, UE)
E1821	Replacement soft interface material/cuffs for bi-directional static progressive stretch device Y & (NU, RR, UE)
E1825	Dynamic adjustable finger extension/flexion device, includes soft interface material Y & (RR)
E1830	Dynamic adjustable toe extension/flexion device, includes soft interface material Y & (RR)
E1831	Static progressive stretch toe device, extension and/or flexion, with or without range of motion adjustment, includes all components and accessories Y & (RR)
E1840	Dynamic adjustable shoulder flexion/abduction/rotation device, includes soft interface material Y & (RR)
E1841	Static progressive stretch shoulder device, with or without range of motion adjustment, includes all components and accessories Y & (RR)

Other Devices

Code	Description
E1902	Communication board, nonelectronic augmentative or alternative communication device Y
E2000	Gastric suction pump, home model, portable or stationary, electric Y & (RR)
E2100	Blood glucose monitor with integrated voice synthesizer Y & (NU, RR, UE)
E2101	Blood glucose monitor with integrated lancing/blood sample Y & (NU, RR, UE)
▲ E2102	Adjunctive, nonimplanted continuous glucose monitor (CGM) or receiver (NU, RR, UE)
● E2103	Nonadjunctive, nonimplanted continuous glucose monitor (CGM) or receiver
E2120	Pulse generator system for tympanic treatment of inner ear endolymphatic fluid Y & (RR)

DME Wheelchair Accessory

Code	Description
E2201	Manual wheelchair accessory, nonstandard seat frame, width greater than or equal to 20 in and less than 24 in Y ☑ & (NU, RR, UE)
E2202	Manual wheelchair accessory, nonstandard seat frame width, 24-27 in Y ☑ & (NU, RR, UE)
E2203	Manual wheelchair accessory, nonstandard seat frame depth, 20 to less than 22 in Y ☑ & (NU, RR, UE)
E2204	Manual wheelchair accessory, nonstandard seat frame depth, 22 to 25 in Y ☑ & (NU, RR, UE)
E2205	Manual wheelchair accessory, handrim without projections (includes ergonomic or contoured), any type, replacement only, each Y ☑ & (NU, RR, UE)
E2206	Manual wheelchair accessory, wheel lock assembly, complete, replacement only, each Y ☑ & (NU, RR, UE)
E2207	Wheelchair accessory, crutch and cane holder, each Y ☑ & (NU, RR, UE)
E2208	Wheelchair accessory, cylinder tank carrier, each Y ☑ & (NU, RR, UE)
E2209	Accessory, arm trough, with or without hand support, each Y ☑ & (NU, RR, UE)
E2210	Wheelchair accessory, bearings, any type, replacement only, each Y ☑ & (NU, RR, UE)
E2211	Manual wheelchair accessory, pneumatic propulsion tire, any size, each Y ☑ & (NU, RR, UE)
E2212	Manual wheelchair accessory, tube for pneumatic propulsion tire, any size, each Y ☑ & (NU, RR, UE)
E2213	Manual wheelchair accessory, insert for pneumatic propulsion tire (removable), any type, any size, each Y ☑ & (NU, RR, UE)
E2214	Manual wheelchair accessory, pneumatic caster tire, any size, each Y ☑ & (NU, RR, UE)
E2215	Manual wheelchair accessory, tube for pneumatic caster tire, any size, each Y ☑ & (NU, RR, UE)
E2216	Manual wheelchair accessory, foam filled propulsion tire, any size, each Y ☑ & (NU, RR, UE)
E2217	Manual wheelchair accessory, foam filled caster tire, any size, each Y ☑ & (NU, RR, UE)
E2218	Manual wheelchair accessory, foam propulsion tire, any size, each Y ☑ & (NU, RR, UE)
E2219	Manual wheelchair accessory, foam caster tire, any size, each Y ☑ & (NU, RR, UE)
E2220	Manual wheelchair accessory, solid (rubber/plastic) propulsion tire, any size, replacement only, each Y ☑ & (NU, RR, UE)
E2221	Manual wheelchair accessory, solid (rubber/plastic) caster tire (removable), any size, replacement only, each Y ☑ & (NU, RR, UE)
E2222	Manual wheelchair accessory, solid (rubber/plastic) caster tire with integrated wheel, any size, replacement only, each Y ☑ & (NU, RR, UE)
E2224	Manual wheelchair accessory, propulsion wheel excludes tire, any size, replacement only, each Y ☑ & (NU, RR, UE)
E2225	Manual wheelchair accessory, caster wheel excludes tire, any size, replacement only, each Y ☑ & (NU, RR, UE)
E2226	Manual wheelchair accessory, caster fork, any size, replacement only, each Y ☑ & (NU, RR, UE)
E2227	Manual wheelchair accessory, gear reduction drive wheel, each Y ☑ & (RR)
E2228	Manual wheelchair accessory, wheel braking system and lock, complete, each Y ☑ & (RR)
E2230	Manual wheelchair accessory, manual standing system Y
E2231	Manual wheelchair accessory, solid seat support base (replaces sling seat), includes any type mounting hardware Y & (NU, RR, UE)
E2291	Back, planar, for pediatric size wheelchair including fixed attaching hardware Y

Special Coverage Instructions | Noncovered by Medicare | Carrier Discretion | ☑ Quantity Alert | ● New Code | ○ Recycled/Reinstated | ▲ Revised Code

© 2022 Optum, Inc. | A2-Z3 ASC Pmt | CMS: IOM | AHA: Coding Clinic | & DMEPOS Paid | ⊘ SNF Excluded | E Codes — 41

Code	Description
E2292	Seat, planar, for pediatric size wheelchair including fixed attaching hardware Y
E2293	Back, contoured, for pediatric size wheelchair including fixed attaching hardware Y
E2294	Seat, contoured, for pediatric size wheelchair including fixed attaching hardware Y
E2295	Manual wheelchair accessory, for pediatric size wheelchair, dynamic seating frame, allows coordinated movement of multiple positioning features Y
E2300	Wheelchair accessory, power seat elevation system, any type Y CMS: 100-04,20,30.9
E2301	Wheelchair accessory, power standing system, any type Y
E2310	Power wheelchair accessory, electronic connection between wheelchair controller and one power seating system motor, including all related electronics, indicator feature, mechanical function selection switch, and fixed mounting hardware Y (RR)
E2311	Power wheelchair accessory, electronic connection between wheelchair controller and 2 or more power seating system motors, including all related electronics, indicator feature, mechanical function selection switch, and fixed mounting hardware Y (RR)
E2312	Power wheelchair accessory, hand or chin control interface, mini-proportional remote joystick, proportional, including fixed mounting hardware Y (RR)
E2313	Power wheelchair accessory, harness for upgrade to expandable controller, including all fasteners, connectors and mounting hardware, each Y ☑ (RR)
E2321	Power wheelchair accessory, hand control interface, remote joystick, nonproportional, including all related electronics, mechanical stop switch, and fixed mounting hardware Y (RR)
E2322	Power wheelchair accessory, hand control interface, multiple mechanical switches, nonproportional, including all related electronics, mechanical stop switch, and fixed mounting hardware Y (RR)
E2323	Power wheelchair accessory, specialty joystick handle for hand control interface, prefabricated Y (NU, RR, UE)
E2324	Power wheelchair accessory, chin cup for chin control interface Y (NU, RR, UE)
E2325	Power wheelchair accessory, sip and puff interface, nonproportional, including all related electronics, mechanical stop switch, and manual swingaway mounting hardware Y (RR)
E2326	Power wheelchair accessory, breath tube kit for sip and puff interface Y (RR)
E2327	Power wheelchair accessory, head control interface, mechanical, proportional, including all related electronics, mechanical direction change switch, and fixed mounting hardware Y (RR)
E2328	Power wheelchair accessory, head control or extremity control interface, electronic, proportional, including all related electronics and fixed mounting hardware Y (RR)
E2329	Power wheelchair accessory, head control interface, contact switch mechanism, nonproportional, including all related electronics, mechanical stop switch, mechanical direction change switch, head array, and fixed mounting hardware Y (RR)
E2330	Power wheelchair accessory, head control interface, proximity switch mechanism, nonproportional, including all related electronics, mechanical stop switch, mechanical direction change switch, head array, and fixed mounting hardware Y (RR)
E2331	Power wheelchair accessory, attendant control, proportional, including all related electronics and fixed mounting hardware Y
E2340	Power wheelchair accessory, nonstandard seat frame width, 20-23 in Y ☑ (NU, RR, UE)
E2341	Power wheelchair accessory, nonstandard seat frame width, 24-27 in Y ☑ (NU, RR, UE)
E2342	Power wheelchair accessory, nonstandard seat frame depth, 20 or 21 in Y ☑ (NU, RR, UE)
E2343	Power wheelchair accessory, nonstandard seat frame depth, 22-25 in Y ☑ (NU, RR, UE)
E2351	Power wheelchair accessory, electronic interface to operate speech generating device using power wheelchair control interface Y (NU, RR, UE)
E2358	Power wheelchair accessory, group 34 nonsealed lead acid battery, each Y ☑
E2359	Power wheelchair accessory, group 34 sealed lead acid battery, each (e.g., gel cell, absorbed glass mat) Y ☑ (NU, RR, UE)
E2360	Power wheelchair accessory, 22 NF nonsealed lead acid battery, each Y ☑ (NU, RR, UE)
E2361	Power wheelchair accessory, 22 NF sealed lead acid battery, each (e.g., gel cell, absorbed glassmat) Y ☑ (NU, RR, UE)
E2362	Power wheelchair accessory, group 24 nonsealed lead acid battery, each Y ☑ (NU, RR, UE)
E2363	Power wheelchair accessory, group 24 sealed lead acid battery, each (e.g., gel cell, absorbed glassmat) Y ☑ (NU, RR, UE)
E2364	Power wheelchair accessory, U-1 nonsealed lead acid battery, each Y ☑ (NU, RR, UE)
E2365	Power wheelchair accessory, U-1 sealed lead acid battery, each (e.g., gel cell, absorbed glassmat) Y ☑ (NU, RR, UE)
E2366	Power wheelchair accessory, battery charger, single mode, for use with only one battery type, sealed or nonsealed, each Y ☑ (NU, RR, UE)
E2367	Power wheelchair accessory, battery charger, dual mode, for use with either battery type, sealed or nonsealed, each Y ☑ (NU, RR, UE)
E2368	Power wheelchair component, drive wheel motor, replacement only Y (RR)
E2369	Power wheelchair component, drive wheel gear box, replacement only Y (RR)
E2370	Power wheelchair component, integrated drive wheel motor and gear box combination, replacement only Y (RR)
E2371	Power wheelchair accessory, group 27 sealed lead acid battery, (e.g., gel cell, absorbed glassmat), each Y ☑ (NU, RR, UE)
E2372	Power wheelchair accessory, group 27 nonsealed lead acid battery, each Y ☑ (NU, RR, UE)
E2373	Power wheelchair accessory, hand or chin control interface, compact remote joystick, proportional, including fixed mounting hardware Y (RR)
E2374	Power wheelchair accessory, hand or chin control interface, standard remote joystick (not including controller), proportional, including all related electronics and fixed mounting hardware, replacement only Y (RR)

Code	Description
E2375	Power wheelchair accessory, nonexpandable controller, including all related electronics and mounting hardware, replacement only (RR)
E2376	Power wheelchair accessory, expandable controller, including all related electronics and mounting hardware, replacement only (RR)
E2377	Power wheelchair accessory, expandable controller, including all related electronics and mounting hardware, upgrade provided at initial issue (RR)
E2378	Power wheelchair component, actuator, replacement only (RR)
E2381	Power wheelchair accessory, pneumatic drive wheel tire, any size, replacement only, each (NU, RR, UE)
E2382	Power wheelchair accessory, tube for pneumatic drive wheel tire, any size, replacement only, each (NU, RR, UE)
E2383	Power wheelchair accessory, insert for pneumatic drive wheel tire (removable), any type, any size, replacement only, each (NU, RR, UE)
E2384	Power wheelchair accessory, pneumatic caster tire, any size, replacement only, each (NU, RR, UE)
E2385	Power wheelchair accessory, tube for pneumatic caster tire, any size, replacement only, each (NU, RR, UE)
E2386	Power wheelchair accessory, foam filled drive wheel tire, any size, replacement only, each (NU, RR, UE)
E2387	Power wheelchair accessory, foam filled caster tire, any size, replacement only, each (NU, RR, UE)
E2388	Power wheelchair accessory, foam drive wheel tire, any size, replacement only, each (NU, RR, UE)
E2389	Power wheelchair accessory, foam caster tire, any size, replacement only, each (NU, RR, UE)
E2390	Power wheelchair accessory, solid (rubber/plastic) drive wheel tire, any size, replacement only, each (NU, RR, UE)
E2391	Power wheelchair accessory, solid (rubber/plastic) caster tire (removable), any size, replacement only, each (NU, RR, UE)
E2392	Power wheelchair accessory, solid (rubber/plastic) caster tire with integrated wheel, any size, replacement only, each (NU, RR, UE)
E2394	Power wheelchair accessory, drive wheel excludes tire, any size, replacement only, each (NU, RR, UE)
E2395	Power wheelchair accessory, caster wheel excludes tire, any size, replacement only, each (NU, RR, UE)
E2396	Power wheelchair accessory, caster fork, any size, replacement only, each (NU, RR, UE)
E2397	Power wheelchair accessory, lithium-based battery, each (NU, RR, UE)
E2398	Wheelchair accessory, dynamic positioning hardware for back

Wound Therapy

Code	Description
E2402	Negative pressure wound therapy electrical pump, stationary or portable (RR)
	CMS: 100-02,7,40.1.2.8

Speech Generating Device

Code	Description
E2500	Speech generating device, digitized speech, using prerecorded messages, less than or equal to eight minutes recording time (NU, RR, UE)
E2502	Speech generating device, digitized speech, using prerecorded messages, greater than eight minutes but less than or equal to 20 minutes recording time (NU, RR, UE)
E2504	Speech generating device, digitized speech, using prerecorded messages, greater than 20 minutes but less than or equal to 40 minutes recording time (NU, RR, UE)
E2506	Speech generating device, digitized speech, using prerecorded messages, greater than 40 minutes recording time (NU, RR, UE)
E2508	Speech generating device, synthesized speech, requiring message formulation by spelling and access by physical contact with the device (NU, RR, UE)
E2510	Speech generating device, synthesized speech, permitting multiple methods of message formulation and multiple methods of device access (NU, RR, UE)
E2511	Speech generating software program, for personal computer or personal digital assistant (NU, RR, UE)
E2512	Accessory for speech generating device, mounting system (NU, RR, UE)
E2599	Accessory for speech generating device, not otherwise classified

Wheelchair Cushion

Code	Description
E2601	General use wheelchair seat cushion, width less than 22 in, any depth (NU, RR, UE)
E2602	General use wheelchair seat cushion, width 22 in or greater, any depth (NU, RR, UE)
E2603	Skin protection wheelchair seat cushion, width less than 22 in, any depth (NU, RR, UE)
E2604	Skin protection wheelchair seat cushion, width 22 in or greater, any depth (NU, RR, UE)
E2605	Positioning wheelchair seat cushion, width less than 22 in, any depth (NU, RR, UE)
E2606	Positioning wheelchair seat cushion, width 22 in or greater, any depth (NU, RR, UE)
E2607	Skin protection and positioning wheelchair seat cushion, width less than 22 in, any depth (NU, RR, UE)
E2608	Skin protection and positioning wheelchair seat cushion, width 22 in or greater, any depth (NU, RR, UE)
E2609	Custom fabricated wheelchair seat cushion, any size
E2610	Wheelchair seat cushion, powered
E2611	General use wheelchair back cushion, width less than 22 in, any height, including any type mounting hardware (NU, RR, UE)
E2612	General use wheelchair back cushion, width 22 in or greater, any height, including any type mounting hardware (NU, RR, UE)
E2613	Positioning wheelchair back cushion, posterior, width less than 22 in, any height, including any type mounting hardware (NU, RR, UE)
E2614	Positioning wheelchair back cushion, posterior, width 22 in or greater, any height, including any type mounting hardware (NU, RR, UE)
E2615	Positioning wheelchair back cushion, posterior-lateral, width less than 22 in, any height, including any type mounting hardware (NU, RR, UE)
E2616	Positioning wheelchair back cushion, posterior-lateral, width 22 in or greater, any height, including any type mounting hardware (NU, RR, UE)

Code	Description
E2617	Custom fabricated wheelchair back cushion, any size, including any type mounting hardware ⓨ
E2619	Replacement cover for wheelchair seat cushion or back cushion, each ⓨ ☑ ♿ (NU, RR, UE)
E2620	Positioning wheelchair back cushion, planar back with lateral supports, width less than 22 in, any height, including any type mounting hardware ⓨ ♿ (NU, RR, UE)
E2621	Positioning wheelchair back cushion, planar back with lateral supports, width 22 in or greater, any height, including any type mounting hardware ⓨ ♿ (NU, RR, UE)
E2622	Skin protection wheelchair seat cushion, adjustable, width less than 22 in, any depth ⓨ ♿ (NU, RR, UE)
E2623	Skin protection wheelchair seat cushion, adjustable, width 22 in or greater, any depth ⓨ ♿ (NU, RR, UE)
E2624	Skin protection and positioning wheelchair seat cushion, adjustable, width less than 22 in, any depth ⓨ ♿ (NU, RR, UE)
E2625	Skin protection and positioning wheelchair seat cushion, adjustable, width 22 in or greater, any depth ⓨ ♿ (NU, RR, UE)

Wheelchair Arm Support

Code	Description
E2626	Wheelchair accessory, shoulder elbow, mobile arm support attached to wheelchair, balanced, adjustable ⓨ ♿ (NU, RR, UE)
E2627	Wheelchair accessory, shoulder elbow, mobile arm support attached to wheelchair, balanced, adjustable Rancho type ⓨ ♿ (NU, RR, UE)
E2628	Wheelchair accessory, shoulder elbow, mobile arm support attached to wheelchair, balanced, reclining ⓨ ♿ (NU, RR, UE)
E2629	Wheelchair accessory, shoulder elbow, mobile arm support attached to wheelchair, balanced, friction arm support (friction dampening to proximal and distal joints) ⓨ ♿ (NU, RR, UE)
E2630	Wheelchair accessory, shoulder elbow, mobile arm support, monosuspension arm and hand support, overhead elbow forearm hand sling support, yoke type suspension support ⓨ ♿ (NU, RR, UE)
E2631	Wheelchair accessory, addition to mobile arm support, elevating proximal arm ⓨ ♿ (NU, RR, UE)
E2632	Wheelchair accessory, addition to mobile arm support, offset or lateral rocker arm with elastic balance control ⓨ ♿ (NU, RR, UE)
E2633	Wheelchair accessory, addition to mobile arm support, supinator ⓨ ♿ (NU, RR, UE)

Gait Trainer

Code	Description
E8000	Gait trainer, pediatric size, posterior support, includes all accessories and components EI
E8001	Gait trainer, pediatric size, upright support, includes all accessories and components EI
E8002	Gait trainer, pediatric size, anterior support, includes all accessories and components EI

Procedures/Professional Services (Temporary) G0008-G9999

The G codes are used to identify professional health care procedures and services that would otherwise be coded in CPT but for which there are no CPT codes. Please refer to your CPT book for possible alternate code(s).

Immunization Administration

G0008 Administration of influenza virus vaccine [S]
CMS: 100-02,12,40.11; 100-02,13,220; 100-02,13,220.1; 100-02,13,220.3; 100-02,15,50.4.4.2; 100-04,18,10.1.2; 100-04,18,10.2; 100-04,18,10.2.1; 100-04,18,10.2.2.1; 100-04,18,10.2.5.2; 100-04,18,10.3.1.1; 100-04,18,10.4; 100-04,18,10.4.1; 100-04,18,10.4.2; 100-04,18,10.4.3; 100-04,18,140.8; 1004-04,13,220.1
AHA: 3Q,18; 4Q,16

G0009 Administration of pneumococcal vaccine [S]
CMS: 100-02,12,40.11; 100-02,13,220; 100-02,13,220.1; 100-02,13,220.3; 100-02,15,50.4.4.2; 100-04,18,10.1.2; 100-04,18,10.2.1; 100-04,18,10.2.2.1; 100-04,18,10.2.5.2; 100-04,18,10.3.1.1; 100-04,18,10.4; 100-04,18,10.4.1; 100-04,18,10.4.2; 100-04,18,10.4.3; 100-04,18,140.8; 1004-04,13,220.1
AHA: 3Q,18; 4Q,16

G0010 Administration of hepatitis B vaccine [S]
CMS: 100-02,12,40.11; 100-02,13,220; 100-02,13,220.1; 100-02,13,220.3; 100-02,15,50.4.4.2; 100-04,18,10.1.2; 100-04,18,10.2.1; 100-04,18,10.2.2.1; 100-04,18,10.2.5.2; 100-04,18,10.3.1.1; 100-04,18,140.8; 1004-04,13,220.1
AHA: 3Q,18; 4Q,16

Semen Analysis

G0027 Semen analysis; presence and/or motility of sperm excluding Huhner ♂ Q

Quality Measures

G0028 ~~Documentation of medical reason(s) for not screening for tobacco use (e.g., limited life expectancy, other medical reason)~~

▲ **G0029** Tobacco screening not performed or tobacco cessation intervention not provided during the measurement period or in the 6 months prior to the measurement period

▲ **G0030** Patient screened for tobacco use and received tobacco cessation intervention during the measurement period or in the 6 months prior to the measurement period (counseling, pharmacotherapy, or both), if identified as a tobacco user

G0031 Palliative care services given to patient any time during the measurement period

G0032 Two or more antipsychotic prescriptions ordered for patients who had a diagnosis of schizophrenia, schizoaffective disorder, or bipolar disorder on or between January 1 of the year prior to the measurement period and the index prescription start date (IPSD) for antipsychotics

G0033 Two or more benzodiazepine prescriptions ordered for patients who had a diagnosis of seizure disorders, rapid eye movement sleep behavior disorder, benzodiazepine withdrawal, ethanol withdrawal, or severe generalized anxiety disorder on or between January 1 of the year prior to the measurement period and the IPSD for benzodiazepines

G0034 Patients receiving palliative care during the measurement period

G0035 Patient has any emergency department encounter during the performance period with place of service indicator 23

G0036 Patient or care partner decline assessment

G0037 On date of encounter, patient is not able to participate in assessment or screening, including nonverbal patients, delirious, severely aphasic, severely developmentally delayed, severe visual or hearing impairment and for those patients, no knowledgeable informant available

G0038 Clinician determines patient does not require referral

G0039 Patient not referred, reason not otherwise specified

G0040 Patient already receiving physical/occupational/speech/recreational therapy during the measurement period

G0041 Patient and/or care partner decline referral

G0042 Referral to physical, occupational, speech, or recreational therapy

G0043 Patients with mechanical prosthetic heart valve

G0044 Patients with moderate or severe mitral stenosis

G0045 Clinical follow-up and MRS score assessed at 90 days following endovascular stroke intervention

G0046 Clinical follow-up and MRS score not assessed at 90 days following endovascular stroke intervention

G0047 Pediatric patient with minor blunt head trauma and PECARN prediction criteria are not assessed

G0048 Patients who receive palliative care services any time during the intake period through the end of the measurement year

G0049 With maintenance hemodialysis (in-center and home HD) for the complete reporting month

G0050 Patients with a catheter that have limited life expectancy

G0051 Patients under hospice care in the current reporting month

G0052 Patients on peritoneal dialysis for any portion of the reporting month

G0053 Advancing rheumatology patient care MIPS value pathways

G0054 Coordinating stroke care to promote prevention and cultivate positive outcomes MIPS value pathways

G0055 Advancing care for heart disease MIPS value pathways

G0056 Optimizing chronic disease management MIPS value pathways

G0057 Proposed adopting best practices and promoting patient safety within emergency medicine MIPS value pathways

G0058 Improving care for lower extremity joint repair MIPS value pathways

G0059 Patient safety and support of positive experiences with anesthesia MIPS value pathways

G0060 Allergy/Immunology MIPS specialty set

G0061 Anesthesiology MIPS specialty set

G0062 Audiology MIPS specialty set

G0063 Cardiology MIPS specialty set

G0064 Certified Nurse Midwife MIPS specialty set

G0065 Chiropractic Medicine MIPS specialty set

G0066 Clinical Social Work MIPS specialty set

G0067 Dentistry MIPS specialty set

Professional Services

G0068 Professional services for the administration of anti-infective, pain management, chelation, pulmonary hypertension, inotropic, or other intravenous infusion drug or biological (excluding chemotherapy or other highly complex drug or biological) for each infusion drug administration calendar day in the individual's home, each 15 min
CMS: 100-04,20,180; 100-04,32,411.3; 100-04,32,411.4; 100-04,32,411.5; 100-04,32,411.6

G0069 Professional services for the administration of subcutaneous immunotherapy or other subcutaneous infusion drug or biological for each infusion drug administration calendar day in the individual's home, each 15 min
CMS: 100-04,20,180; 100-04,32,411.3; 100-04,32,411.4; 100-04,32,411.5; 100-04,32,411.6

Procedures/Professional Services (Temporary)

G0070 — G0109

G0070 Professional services for the administration of intravenous chemotherapy or other intravenous highly complex drug or biological infusion for each infusion drug administration calendar day in the individual's home, each 15 min
CMS: 100-04,20,180; 100-04,32,411.3; 100-04,32,411.4; 100-04,32,411.5; 100-04,32,411.6

G0071 Payment for communication technology-based services for 5 minutes or more of a virtual (nonface-to-face) communication between a rural health clinic (RHC) or federally qualified health center (FQHC) practitioner and RHC or FQHC patient, or 5 minutes or more of remote evaluation of recorded video and/or images by an RHC or FQHC practitioner, occurring in lieu of an office visit; RHC or FQHC only
CMS: 100-04,9,70.7

G0076 Brief (20 minutes) care management home visit for a new patient. For use only in a Medicare-approved CMMI model (services must be furnished within a beneficiary's home, domiciliary, rest home, assisted living and/or nursing facility)

G0077 Limited (30 minutes) care management home visit for a new patient. For use only in a Medicare-approved CMMI model (services must be furnished within a beneficiary's home, domiciliary, rest home, assisted living and/or nursing facility)

G0078 Moderate (45 minutes) care management home visit for a new patient. For use only in a Medicare-approved CMMI model (services must be furnished within a beneficiary's home, domiciliary, rest home, assisted living and/or nursing facility)

G0079 Comprehensive (60 minutes) care management home visit for a new patient. For use only in a Medicare-approved CMMI model (services must be furnished within a beneficiary's home, domiciliary, rest home, assisted living and/or nursing facility)

G0080 Extensive (75 minutes) care management home visit for a new patient. For use only in a Medicare-approved CMMI model (services must be furnished within a beneficiary's home, domiciliary, rest home, assisted living and/or nursing facility)

G0081 Brief (20 minutes) care management home visit for an existing patient. For use only in a Medicare-approved CMMI model (services must be furnished within a beneficiary's home, domiciliary, rest home, assisted living and/or nursing facility)

G0082 Limited (30 minutes) care management home visit for an existing patient. For use only in a Medicare-approved CMMI model (services must be furnished within a beneficiary's home, domiciliary, rest home, assisted living and/or nursing facility)

G0083 Moderate (45 minutes) care management home visit for an existing patient. For use only in a Medicare-approved CMMI model (services must be furnished within a beneficiary's home, domiciliary, rest home, assisted living and/or nursing facility)

G0084 Comprehensive (60 minutes) care management home visit for an existing patient. For use only in a Medicare-approved CMMI model (services must be furnished within a beneficiary's home, domiciliary, rest home, assisted living and/or nursing facility)

G0085 Extensive (75 minutes) care management home visit for an existing patient. For use only in a Medicare-approved CMMI model (services must be furnished within a beneficiary's home, domiciliary, rest home, assisted living and/or nursing facility)

G0086 Limited (30 minutes) care management home care plan oversight. For use only in a Medicare-approved CMMI model (services must be furnished within a beneficiary's home, domiciliary, rest home, assisted living and/or nursing facility)

G0087 Comprehensive (60 minutes) care management home care plan oversight. For use only in a Medicare-approved CMMI model (services must be furnished within a beneficiary's home, domiciliary, rest home, assisted living and/or nursing facility)

G0088 Professional services, initial visit, for the administration of anti-infective, pain management, chelation, pulmonary hypertension, inotropic, or other intravenous infusion drug or biological (excluding chemotherapy or other highly complex drug or biological) for each infusion drug administration calendar day in the individual's home, each 15 min
CMS: 100-04,32,411.3; 100-04,32,411.4; 100-04,32,411.5; 100-04,32,411.6

G0089 Professional services, initial visit, for the administration of subcutaneous immunotherapy or other subcutaneous infusion drug or biological for each infusion drug administration calendar day in the individual's home, each 15 min
CMS: 100-04,32,411.3; 100-04,32,411.4; 100-04,32,411.5; 100-04,32,411.6

G0090 Professional services, initial visit, for the administration of intravenous chemotherapy or other highly complex infusion drug or biological for each infusion drug administration calendar day in the individual's home, each 15 min
CMS: 100-04,32,411.3; 100-04,32,411.4; 100-04,32,411.5; 100-04,32,411.6

Screening Services

G0101 Cervical or vaginal cancer screening; pelvic and clinical breast examination
G0101 can be reported with an E/M code when a separately identifiable E/M service was provided.
CMS: 100-02,13,220; 100-02,13,220.1; 100-03,210.2; 100-04,18,10.1.2; 1004-04,13,220.1

G0102 Prostate cancer screening; digital rectal examination
CMS: 100-02,13,220; 100-02,13,220.1; 100-02,13,220.3; 100-04,18,10.1.2

G0103 Prostate cancer screening; prostate specific antigen test (PSA)
CMS: 100-04,18,10.1.2

G0104 Colorectal cancer screening; flexible sigmoidoscopy
Medicare covers colorectal screening for cancer via flexible sigmoidoscopy once every four years for patients 50 years or older.
CMS: 100-02,15,280.2.2; 100-04,18,10.1.2; 100-04,18,60; 100-04,18,60.1; 100-04,18,60.1.1; 100-04,18,60.2; 100-04,18,60.2.1; 100-04,18,60.6; 100-04,18,60.7

G0105 Colorectal cancer screening; colonoscopy on individual at high risk
An individual with ulcerative enteritis or a history of a malignant neoplasm of the lower gastrointestinal tract is considered at high-risk for colorectal cancer, as defined by CMS.
CMS: 100-02,15,280.2.2; 100-04,12,30.1; 100-04,18,10.1.2; 100-04,18,60; 100-04,18,60.1; 100-04,18,60.1.1; 100-04,18,60.2; 100-04,18,60.2.1; 100-04,18,60.2.2; 100-04,18,60.6; 100-04,18,60.7; 100-04,18,60.8; 100-04,23,30.2; 100-04,4,250.18
AHA: 2Q,18

G0106 Colorectal cancer screening; alternative to G0104, screening sigmoidoscopy, barium enema
CMS: 100-02,15,280.2.2; 100-04,18,10.1.2; 100-04,18,60; 100-04,18,60.1; 100-04,18,60.1.1; 100-04,18,60.2; 100-04,18,60.2.1; 100-04,18,60.6; 100-04,18,60.7

G0108 Diabetes outpatient self-management training services, individual, per 30 minutes
CMS: 100-02,13,220.3; 100-02,15,300; 100-02,15,300.2; 100-02,15,300.3; 100-02,15,300.4; 100-04,12,190.3; 100-04,12,190.3.6; 100-04,12,190.6; 100-04,12,190.6.1; 100-04,12,190.7; 100-04,18,10.1.2; 100-04,18,120.1; 100-04,4,300.6
AHA: 3Q,19

G0109 Diabetes outpatient self-management training services, group session (two or more), per 30 minutes
CMS: 100-02,15,300.2; 100-02,15,300.3; 100-04,12,190.3; 100-04,12,190.3.6; 100-04,12,190.6; 100-04,12,190.6.1; 100-04,12,190.7; 100-04,18,10.1.2; 100-04,4,300.6
AHA: 3Q,19

Procedures/Professional Services (Temporary)

G0117 Glaucoma screening for high risk patients furnished by an optometrist or ophthalmologist ⓢ ⊘
CMS: 100-02,13,220; 100-02,13,220.1; 100-02,13,220.3; 100-02,15,280.1; 100-04,18,10.1.2; 100-04,18,70.1.1; 1004-04,13,220.1

G0118 Glaucoma screening for high risk patient furnished under the direct supervision of an optometrist or ophthalmologist ⓢ ⊘
CMS: 100-02,13,220; 100-02,13,220.1; 100-02,13,220.3; 100-02,15,280.1; 100-04,18,10.1.2; 100-04,18,70.1.1; 1004-04,13,220.1

G0120 Colorectal cancer screening; alternative to G0105, screening colonoscopy, barium enema ⓢ
CMS: 100-02,15,280.2.2; 100-04,18,10.1.2; 100-04,18,60; 100-04,18,60.1; 100-04,18,60.1.1; 100-04,18,60.2; 100-04,18,60.2.1; 100-04,18,60.6; 100-04,18,60.7; 100-04,18,60.8

G0121 Colorectal cancer screening; colonoscopy on individual not meeting criteria for high risk Ⓣ A2
CMS: 100-02,15,280.2.2; 100-04,12,30.1; 100-04,18,10.1.2; 100-04,18,60; 100-04,18,60.1; 100-04,18,60.1.1; 100-04,18,60.2; 100-04,18,60.2.1; 100-04,18,60.2.2; 100-04,18,60.5; 100-04,18,60.6; 100-04,23,30.2; 100-04,4,250.18
AHA: 2Q,18

G0122 Colorectal cancer screening; barium enema E1
CMS: 100-04,18,60; 100-04,18,60.2; 100-04,18,60.2.1; 100-04,18,60.5; 100-04,18,60.6; 100-04,18,60.7; 100-04,18,60.8

G0123 Screening cytopathology, cervical or vaginal (any reporting system), collected in preservative fluid, automated thin layer preparation, screening by cytotechnologist under physician supervision A ♀ A
See also P3000-P3001.
CMS: 100-03,210.2.1; 100-04,18,10.1.2; 100-04,18,30.2.1; 100-04,18,30.5; 100-04,18,30.6

G0124 Screening cytopathology, cervical or vaginal (any reporting system), collected in preservative fluid, automated thin layer preparation, requiring interpretation by physician A ♀ B ⊘
See also P3000-P3001.
CMS: 100-03,210.2.1; 100-04,18,10.1.2; 100-04,18,30.2.1; 100-04,18,30.5; 100-04,18,30.6

Miscellaneous Services

G0127 Trimming of dystrophic nails, any number 01 ⊘
CMS: 100-02,15,290

G0128 Direct (face-to-face with patient) skilled nursing services of a registered nurse provided in a comprehensive outpatient rehabilitation facility, each 10 minutes beyond the first 5 minutes B ☑ ⊘
CMS: 100-02,12,30.1; 100-02,12,40.8; 100-02,17,40.1.2; 100-04,39,30.6; 100-04,39,30.8; 100-04,5,100.3; 100-04,5,20.4

G0129 Occupational therapy services requiring the skills of a qualified occupational therapist, furnished as a component of a partial hospitalization treatment program, per session (45 minutes or more) P ☑
CMS: 100-04,4,260.1; 100-04,4,260.1.1

G0130 Single energy x-ray absorptiometry (SEXA) bone density study, one or more sites; appendicular skeleton (peripheral) (e.g., radius, wrist, heel) ⓢ Z3
CMS: 100-04,18,10.1.2

G0141 Screening cytopathology smears, cervical or vaginal, performed by automated system, with manual rescreening, requiring interpretation by physician A ♀ B ⊘
CMS: 100-03,210.2.1; 100-04,18,10.1.2; 100-04,18,30.2.1; 100-04,18,30.5; 100-04,18,30.6

G0143 Screening cytopathology, cervical or vaginal (any reporting system), collected in preservative fluid, automated thin layer preparation, with manual screening and rescreening by cytotechnologist under physician supervision A ♀ A
CMS: 100-03,210.2.1; 100-04,18,10.1.2; 100-04,18,30.2.1; 100-04,18,30.5; 100-04,18,30.6

G0144 Screening cytopathology, cervical or vaginal (any reporting system), collected in preservative fluid, automated thin layer preparation, with screening by automated system, under physician supervision A ♀ A
CMS: 100-03,210.2.1; 100-04,18,30.2.1; 100-04,18,30.5; 100-04,18,30.6

G0145 Screening cytopathology, cervical or vaginal (any reporting system), collected in preservative fluid, automated thin layer preparation, with screening by automated system and manual rescreening under physician supervision A ♀ A
CMS: 100-03,210.2.1; 100-04,18,10.1.2; 100-04,18,30.2.1; 100-04,18,30.5; 100-04,18,30.6

G0147 Screening cytopathology smears, cervical or vaginal, performed by automated system under physician supervision A ♀ A
CMS: 100-03,210.2.1; 100-04,18,10.1.2; 100-04,18,30.2.1; 100-04,18,30.5; 100-04,18,30.6

G0148 Screening cytopathology smears, cervical or vaginal, performed by automated system with manual rescreening A ♀ A
CMS: 100-03,210.2.1; 100-04,18,10.1.2; 100-04,18,30.2.1; 100-04,18,30.5; 100-04,18,30.6

G0151 Services performed by a qualified physical therapist in the home health or hospice setting, each 15 minutes B ☑
CMS: 100-01,3,30.3; 100-04,10,40.2; 100-04,11,10; 100-04,11,130.1; 100-04,11,30.3

G0152 Services performed by a qualified occupational therapist in the home health or hospice setting, each 15 minutes B ☑
CMS: 100-01,3,30.3; 100-04,10,40.2; 100-04,11,10; 100-04,11,130.1; 100-04,11,30.3

G0153 Services performed by a qualified speech-language pathologist in the home health or hospice setting, each 15 minutes B ☑
CMS: 100-01,3,30.3; 100-04,10,40.2; 100-04,11,10; 100-04,11,130.1; 100-04,11,30.3

G0155 Services of clinical social worker in home health or hospice settings, each 15 minutes B ☑
CMS: 100-01,3,30.3; 100-04,10,40.2; 100-04,11,10; 100-04,11,130.1; 100-04,11,30.3

G0156 Services of home health/hospice aide in home health or hospice settings, each 15 minutes B ☑
CMS: 100-01,3,30.3; 100-04,10,40.2; 100-04,11,10; 100-04,11,130.1; 100-04,11,30.3

G0157 Services performed by a qualified physical therapist assistant in the home health or hospice setting, each 15 minutes B ☑
CMS: 100-04,10,40.2; 100-04,11,10

G0158 Services performed by a qualified occupational therapist assistant in the home health or hospice setting, each 15 minutes B ☑
CMS: 100-04,10,40.2; 100-04,11,10

G0159 Services performed by a qualified physical therapist, in the home health setting, in the establishment or delivery of a safe and effective physical therapy maintenance program, each 15 minutes B ☑
CMS: 100-04,10,40.2

G0160 Services performed by a qualified occupational therapist, in the home health setting, in the establishment or delivery of a safe and effective occupational therapy maintenance program, each 15 minutes B ☑
CMS: 100-04,10,40.2

Procedures/Professional Services (Temporary)

G0161 — Services performed by a qualified speech-language pathologist, in the home health setting, in the establishment or delivery of a safe and effective speech-language pathology maintenance program, each 15 minutes
CMS: 100-04,10,40.2

G0162 — Skilled services by a registered nurse (RN) for management and evaluation of the plan of care; each 15 minutes (the patient's underlying condition or complication requires an RN to ensure that essential nonskilled care achieves its purpose in the home health or hospice setting)
CMS: 100-04,10,40.2; 100-04,11,10

G0166 — External counterpulsation, per treatment session
CMS: 100-04,32,130; 100-04,32,130.1

G0168 — Wound closure utilizing tissue adhesive(s) only
CMS: 100-04,10,40.2

G0175 — Scheduled interdisciplinary team conference (minimum of three exclusive of patient care nursing staff) with patient present
CMS: 100-04,4,160

G0176 — Activity therapy, such as music, dance, art or play therapies not for recreation, related to the care and treatment of patient's disabling mental health problems, per session (45 minutes or more)
CMS: 100-04,4,260.1; 100-04,4,260.1.1; 100-04,4,260.5

G0177 — Training and educational services related to the care and treatment of patient's disabling mental health problems per session (45 minutes or more)
CMS: 100-04,4,260.1; 100-04,4,260.1.1

G0179 — Physician or allowed practitioner re-certification for Medicare-covered home health services under a home health plan of care (patient not present), including contacts with home health agency and review of reports of patient status required by physicians and allowed practitioners to affirm the initial implementation of the plan of care
CMS: 100-02,7,30.5.4; 100-04,10,20.1.2; 100-04,12,180; 100-04,12,180.1

G0180 — Physician or allowed practitioner certification for Medicare-covered home health services under a home health plan of care (patient not present), including contacts with home health agency and review of reports of patient status required by physicians or allowed practitioners to affirm the initial implementation of the plan of care
CMS: 100-02,7,30.5.4; 100-04,10,20.1.2; 100-04,12,180; 100-04,12,180.1

G0181 — Physician or allowed practitioner supervision of a patient receiving Medicare-covered services provided by a participating home health agency (patient not present) requiring complex and multidisciplinary care modalities involving regular physician or allowed practitioner development and/or revision of care plans
CMS: 100-04,12,100.1.4; 100-04,12,180; 100-04,12,180.1

G0182 — Physician supervision of a patient under a Medicare-approved hospice (patient not present) requiring complex and multidisciplinary care modalities involving regular physician development and/or revision of care plans, review of subsequent reports of patient status, review of laboratory and other studies, communication (including telephone calls) with other health care professionals involved in the patient's care, integration of new information into the medical treatment plan and/or adjustment of medical therapy, within a calendar month, 30 minutes or more
CMS: 100-04,11,40.1.3.1; 100-04,12,100.1.4; 100-04,12,180; 100-04,12,180.1

G0186 — Destruction of localized lesion of choroid (for example, choroidal neovascularization); photocoagulation, feeder vessel technique (one or more sessions)

G0219 — PET imaging whole body; melanoma for noncovered indications
CMS: 100-03,220.6.10; 100-03,220.6.12; 100-03,220.6.17; 100-03,220.6.3; 100-03,220.6.4; 100-03,220.6.6; 100-03,220.6.7; 100-04,13,60; 100-04,13,60.16

G0235 — PET imaging, any site, not otherwise specified
CMS: 100-03,220.6.10; 100-03,220.6.12; 100-03,220.6.13; 100-03,220.6.17; 100-03,220.6.2; 100-03,220.6.3; 100-03,220.6.4; 100-03,220.6.5; 100-03,220.6.6; 100-03,220.6.7; 100-03,220.6.9; 100-04,13,60; 100-04,13,60.13; 100-04,13,60.14; 100-04,13,60.16; 100-04,13,60.17

G0237 — Therapeutic procedures to increase strength or endurance of respiratory muscles, face-to-face, one-on-one, each 15 minutes (includes monitoring)
CMS: 100-02,12,30.1; 100-02,12,40.5

G0238 — Therapeutic procedures to improve respiratory function, other than described by G0237, one-on-one, face-to-face, per 15 minutes (includes monitoring)
CMS: 100-02,12,30.1; 100-02,12,40.5

G0239 — Therapeutic procedures to improve respiratory function or increase strength or endurance of respiratory muscles, two or more individuals (includes monitoring)
CMS: 100-02,12,30.1; 100-02,12,40.5

G0245 — Initial physician evaluation and management of a diabetic patient with diabetic sensory neuropathy resulting in a loss of protective sensation (LOPS) which must include: (1) the diagnosis of LOPS, (2) a patient history, (3) a physical examination that consists of at least the following elements: (a) visual inspection of the forefoot, hindfoot, and toe web spaces, (b) evaluation of a protective sensation, (c) evaluation of foot structure and biomechanics, (d) evaluation of vascular status and skin integrity, and (e) evaluation and recommendation of footwear, and (4) patient education
CMS: 100-04,32,80.2; 100-04,32,80.3; 100-04,32,80.6; 100-04,32,80.8

G0246 — Follow-up physician evaluation and management of a diabetic patient with diabetic sensory neuropathy resulting in a loss of protective sensation (LOPS) to include at least the following: (1) a patient history, (2) a physical examination that includes: (a) visual inspection of the forefoot, hindfoot, and toe web spaces, (b) evaluation of protective sensation, (c) evaluation of foot structure and biomechanics, (d) evaluation of vascular status and skin integrity, and (e) evaluation and recommendation of footwear, and (3) patient education
CMS: 100-03,70.2.1; 100-04,32,80; 100-04,32,80.2; 100-04,32,80.3; 100-04,32,80.6; 100-04,32,80.8

G0247 — Routine foot care by a physician of a diabetic patient with diabetic sensory neuropathy resulting in a loss of protective sensation (LOPS) to include the local care of superficial wounds (i.e., superficial to muscle and fascia) and at least the following, if present: (1) local care of superficial wounds, (2) debridement of corns and calluses, and (3) trimming and debridement of nails
CMS: 100-03,70.2.1; 100-04,32,80; 100-04,32,80.2; 100-04,32,80.3; 100-04,32,80.6; 100-04,32,80.8

G0248 — Demonstration, prior to initiation of home INR monitoring, for patient with either mechanical heart valve(s), chronic atrial fibrillation, or venous thromboembolism who meets Medicare coverage criteria, under the direction of a physician; includes: face-to-face demonstration of use and care of the INR monitor, obtaining at least one blood sample, provision of instructions for reporting home INR test results, and documentation of patient's ability to perform testing and report results
CMS: 100-03,190.11; 100-04,32,80

2023 HCPCS Level II

G0249 Provision of test materials and equipment for home INR monitoring of patient with either mechanical heart valve(s), chronic atrial fibrillation, or venous thromboembolism who meets Medicare coverage criteria; includes: provision of materials for use in the home and reporting of test results to physician; testing not occurring more frequently than once a week; testing materials, billing units of service include four tests
CMS: 100-03,190.11

G0250 Physician review, interpretation, and patient management of home INR testing for patient with either mechanical heart valve(s), chronic atrial fibrillation, or venous thromboembolism who meets Medicare coverage criteria; testing not occurring more frequently than once a week; billing units of service include four tests
CMS: 100-03,190.11

G0252 PET imaging, full and partial-ring PET scanners only, for initial diagnosis of breast cancer and/or surgical planning for breast cancer (e.g., initial staging of axillary lymph nodes)
CMS: 100-03,220.6.10; 100-03,220.6.3; 100-04,13,60; 100-04,13,60.16

G0255 Current perception threshold/sensory nerve conduction test, (SNCT) per limb, any nerve

G0257 Unscheduled or emergency dialysis treatment for an ESRD patient in a hospital outpatient department that is not certified as an ESRD facility
CMS: 100-04,4,200.2; 100-04,8,60.4.7

G0259 Injection procedure for sacroiliac joint; arthrography

G0260 Injection procedure for sacroiliac joint; provision of anesthetic, steroid and/or other therapeutic agent, with or without arthrography
AHA: 4Q,21

G0268 Removal of impacted cerumen (one or both ears) by physician on same date of service as audiologic function testing

G0269 Placement of occlusive device into either a venous or arterial access site, postsurgical or interventional procedure (e.g., angioseal plug, vascular plug)
AHA: 3Q,22

G0270 Medical nutrition therapy; reassessment and subsequent intervention(s) following second referral in same year for change in diagnosis, medical condition or treatment regimen (including additional hours needed for renal disease), individual, face-to-face with the patient, each 15 minutes
CMS: 100-04,12,190.3; 100-04,12,190.6; 100-04,12,190.6.1; 100-04,12,190.7; 100-04,18,10.1.2
AHA: 3Q,19

G0271 Medical nutrition therapy, reassessment and subsequent intervention(s) following second referral in same year for change in diagnosis, medical condition, or treatment regimen (including additional hours needed for renal disease), group (two or more individuals), each 30 minutes
CMS: 100-04,18,10.1.2

G0276 Blinded procedure for lumbar stenosis, percutaneous image-guided lumbar decompression (PILD) or placebo-control, performed in an approved coverage with evidence development (CED) clinical trial
CMS: 100-03,150.13; 100-04,32,330.1; 100-04,32,330.2

G0277 Hyperbaric oxygen under pressure, full body chamber, per 30 minute interval
CMS: 100-04,32,30.1

G0278 Iliac and/or femoral artery angiography, nonselective, bilateral or ipsilateral to catheter insertion, performed at the same time as cardiac catheterization and/or coronary angiography, includes positioning or placement of the catheter in the distal aorta or ipsilateral femoral or iliac artery, injection of dye, production of permanent images, and radiologic supervision and interpretation (List separately in addition to primary procedure)
AHA: 3Q,22

G0279 Diagnostic digital breast tomosynthesis, unilateral or bilateral (list separately in addition to 77065 or 77066)
CMS: 100-04,18,20.2; 100-04,18,20.2.1; 100-04,18,20.2.2; 100-04,18,20.6

G0281 Electrical stimulation, (unattended), to one or more areas, for chronic Stage III and Stage IV pressure ulcers, arterial ulcers, diabetic ulcers, and venous stasis ulcers not demonstrating measurable signs of healing after 30 days of conventional care, as part of a therapy plan of care
CMS: 100-02,15,220.4; 100-04,32,11.1; 100-04,5,10.3.2; 100-04,5,10.3.3

G0282 Electrical stimulation, (unattended), to one or more areas, for wound care other than described in G0281
CMS: 100-04,32,11.1

G0283 Electrical stimulation (unattended), to one or more areas for indication(s) other than wound care, as part of a therapy plan of care
CMS: 100-02,15,220.4; 100-04,5,10.3.2; 100-04,5,10.3.3

G0288 Reconstruction, computed tomographic angiography of aorta for surgical planning for vascular surgery

G0289 Arthroscopy, knee, surgical, for removal of loose body, foreign body, debridement/shaving of articular cartilage (chondroplasty) at the time of other surgical knee arthroscopy in a different compartment of the same knee
AHA: 4Q,20

G0293 Noncovered surgical procedure(s) using conscious sedation, regional, general, or spinal anesthesia in a Medicare qualifying clinical trial, per day

G0294 Noncovered procedure(s) using either no anesthesia or local anesthesia only, in a Medicare qualifying clinical trial, per day

G0295 Electromagnetic therapy, to one or more areas, for wound care other than described in G0329 or for other uses

G0296 Counseling visit to discuss need for lung cancer screening using low dose CT scan (LDCT) (service is for eligibility determination and shared decision making)
CMS: 100-02,13,220; 100-02,13,220.1; 100-02,13,220.3; 100-04,18,10.1.2; 100-04,18,220; 100-04,18,220.1; 100-04,18,220.2; 100-04,18,220.3; 100-04,18,220.4; 100-04,18,220.5; 1004-04,13,220.1
AHA: 3Q,19

G0299 Direct skilled nursing services of a registered nurse (RN) in the home health or hospice setting, each 15 minutes
CMS: 100-01,3,30.3; 100-04,10,40.2; 100-04,11,130.1; 100-04,11,30.3

G0300 Direct skilled nursing services of a licensed practical nurse (LPN) in the home health or hospice setting, each 15 minutes
CMS: 100-01,3,30.3; 100-04,10,40.2; 100-04,11,130.1; 100-04,11,30.3

G0302 Preoperative pulmonary surgery services for preparation for LVRS, complete course of services, to include a minimum of 16 days of services

G0303 Preoperative pulmonary surgery services for preparation for LVRS, 10 to 15 days of services

G0304 Preoperative pulmonary surgery services for preparation for LVRS, 1 to 9 days of services

Procedures/Professional Services (Temporary)

Code	Description
G0305	Postdischarge pulmonary surgery services after LVRS, minimum of 6 days of services
G0306	Complete CBC, automated (HgB, HCT, RBC, WBC, without platelet count) and automated WBC differential count CMS: 100-02,11,20.2
G0307	Complete CBC, automated (HgB, HCT, RBC, WBC; without platelet count) CMS: 100-02,11,20.2
G0308	~~Creation of subcutaneous pocket with insertion of 180 day implantable interstitial glucose sensor, including system activation and patient training~~
G0309	~~Removal of implantable interstitial glucose sensor with creation of subcutaneous pocket at different anatomic site and insertion of new 180 day implantable sensor, including system activation~~
G0310	Immunization counseling by a physician or other qualified health care professional when the vaccine(s) is not administered on the same date of service, 5-15 minutes time (This code is used for Medicaid billing purposes)
G0311	Immunization counseling by a physician or other qualified health care professional when the vaccine(s) is not administered on the same date of service, 16-30 minutes time (This code is used for Medicaid billing purposes)
G0312	Immunization counseling by a physician or other qualified health care professional when the vaccine(s) is not administered on the same date of service for ages under 21, 5-15 minutes time (This code is used for Medicaid billing purposes)
G0313	Immunization counseling by a physician or other qualified health care professional when the vaccine(s) is not administered on the same date of service for ages under 21, 16-30 minutes time (This code is used for Medicaid billing purposes)
G0314	Immunization counseling by a physician or other qualified health care professional for COVID-19, ages under 21, 16-30 minutes time (This code is used for the Medicaid Early and Periodic Screening, Diagnostic, and Treatment Benefit [EPSDT])
G0315	Immunization counseling by a physician or other qualified health care professional for COVID-19, ages under 21, 5-15 minutes time (This code is used for the Medicaid Early and Periodic Screening, Diagnostic, and Treatment Benefit [EPSDT])
G0316	Prolonged hospital inpatient or observation care evaluation and management service(s) beyond the total time for the primary service (when the primary service has been selected using time on the date of the primary service); each additional 15 minutes by the physician or qualified healthcare professional, with or without direct patient contact (list separately in addition to CPT codes 99223, 99233, and 99236 for hospital inpatient or observation care evaluation and management services). (Do not report G0316 on the same date of service as other prolonged services for evaluation and management codes 99358, 99359, 99418, 99415, 99416). (Do not report G0316 for any time unit less than 15 minutes)
G0317	Prolonged nursing facility evaluation and management service(s) beyond the total time for the primary service (when the primary service has been selected using time on the date of the primary service); each additional 15 minutes by the physician or qualified healthcare professional, with or without direct patient contact (list separately in addition to CPT codes 99306, 99310 for nursing facility evaluation and management services). (Do not report G0317 on the same date of service as other prolonged services for evaluation and management codes 99358, 99359, 99418). (Do not report G0317 for any time unit less than 15 minutes)
G0318	Prolonged home or residence evaluation and management service(s) beyond the total time for the primary service (when the primary service has been selected using time on the date of the primary service); each additional 15 minutes by the physician or qualified healthcare professional, with or without direct patient contact (list separately in addition to CPT codes 99345, 99350 for home or residence evaluation and management services). (Do not report G0318 on the same date of service as other prolonged services for evaluation and management codes 99358, 99359, 99417). (Do not report G0318 for any time unit less than 15 minutes)
G0320	Home health services furnished using synchronous telemedicine rendered via a real-time two-way audio and video telecommunications system
G0321	Home health services furnished using synchronous telemedicine rendered via telephone or other real-time interactive audio-only telecommunications system
G0322	The collection of physiologic data digitally stored and/or transmitted by the patient to the home health agency (i.e., remote patient monitoring)
G0323	Care management services for behavioral health conditions, at least 20 minutes of clinical psychologist or clinical social worker time, per calendar month. (These services include the following required elements: initial assessment or follow-up monitoring, including the use of applicable validated rating scales; behavioral health care planning in relation to behavioral/psychiatric health problems, including revision for patients who are not progressing or whose status changes; facilitating and coordinating treatment such as psychotherapy, coordination with and/or referral to physicians and practitioners who are authorized by Medicare to prescribe medications and furnish E/M services, counseling and/or psychiatric consultation; and continuity of care with a designated member of the care team)
G0327	Colorectal cancer screening; blood-based biomarker CMS: 100-04,18,10.1.2; 100-04,18,60; 100-04,18,60.1; 100-04,18,60.1.1; 100-04,18,60.2; 100-04,18,60.2.1; 100-04,18,60.6; 100-04,18,60.7; 100-04,18,60.8 AHA: 3Q,21
G0328	Colorectal cancer screening; fecal occult blood test, immunoassay, one to three simultaneous determinations CMS: 100-02,15,280.2.2; 100-04,16,70.8; 100-04,18,10.1.2; 100-04,18,60; 100-04,18,60.1; 100-04,18,60.1.1; 100-04,18,60.2; 100-04,18,60.2.1; 100-04,18,60.6; 100-04,18,60.7
G0329	Electromagnetic therapy, to one or more areas for chronic Stage III and Stage IV pressure ulcers, arterial ulcers, diabetic ulcers and venous stasis ulcers not demonstrating measurable signs of healing after 30 days of conventional care as part of a therapy plan of care CMS: 100-02,15,220.4; 100-04,32,11.2; 100-04,5,10.3.2; 100-04,5,10.3.3
G0330	Facility services for dental rehabilitation procedure(s) performed on a patient who requires monitored anesthesia (e.g., general, intravenous sedation (monitored anesthesia care) and use of an operating room
G0333	Pharmacy dispensing fee for inhalation drug(s); initial 30-day supply as a beneficiary
G0337	Hospice evaluation and counseling services, preelection CMS: 100-04,11,10
G0339	Image guided robotic linear accelerator-based stereotactic radiosurgery, complete course of therapy in one session or first session of fractionated treatment

2023 HCPCS Level II

Code	Description
G0340	Image guided robotic linear accelerator-based stereotactic radiosurgery, delivery including collimator changes and custom plugging, fractionated treatment, all lesions, per session, second through fifth sessions, maximum five sessions per course of treatment [B]
G0341	Percutaneous islet cell transplant, includes portal vein catheterization and infusion [C] **CMS:** 100-04,32,70
G0342	Laparoscopy for islet cell transplant, includes portal vein catheterization and infusion [C] **CMS:** 100-04,32,70
G0343	Laparotomy for islet cell transplant, includes portal vein catheterization and infusion [C] **CMS:** 100-04,32,70
G0372	Physician service required to establish and document the need for a power mobility device [M] **CMS:** 100-04,12,30.6.15; 100-04,12,30.6.15.4

Observation/Emergency Department Services

Code	Description
G0378	Hospital observation service, per hour [N] **CMS:** 100-02,6,20.6; 100-04,01,50.3.2; 100-04,4,290.1; 100-04,4,290.2.2; 100-04,4,290.4.1; 100-04,4,290.4.2; 100-04,4,290.4.3; 100-04,4,290.5.1; 100-04,4,290.5.2; 100-04,4,290.5.3
G0379	Direct admission of patient for hospital observation care [J] **CMS:** 100-02,6,20.6; 100-04,4,290.4.1; 100-04,4,290.4.2; 100-04,4,290.4.3; 100-04,4,290.5.1; 100-04,4,290.5.2; 100-04,4,290.5.3
G0380	Level 1 hospital emergency department visit provided in a type B emergency department; (the ED must meet at least one of the following requirements: (1) it is licensed by the state in which it is located under applicable state law as an emergency room or emergency department; (2) it is held out to the public (by name, posted signs, advertising, or other means) as a place that provides care for emergency medical conditions on an urgent basis without requiring a previously scheduled appointment; or (3) during the calendar year immediately preceding the calendar year in which a determination under 42 CFR 489.24 is being made, based on a representative sample of patient visits that occurred during that calendar year, it provides at least one-third of all of its outpatient visits for the treatment of emergency medical conditions on an urgent basis without requiring a previously scheduled appointment) [J] **CMS:** 100-04,4,160
G0381	Level 2 hospital emergency department visit provided in a type B emergency department; (the ED must meet at least one of the following requirements: (1) it is licensed by the state in which it is located under applicable state law as an emergency room or emergency department; (2) it is held out to the public (by name, posted signs, advertising, or other means) as a place that provides care for emergency medical conditions on an urgent basis without requiring a previously scheduled appointment; or (3) during the calendar year immediately preceding the calendar year in which a determination under 42 CFR 489.24 is being made, based on a representative sample of patient visits that occurred during that calendar year, it provides at least one-third of all of its outpatient visits for the treatment of emergency medical conditions on an urgent basis without requiring a previously scheduled appointment) [J] **CMS:** 100-04,4,160
G0382	Level 3 hospital emergency department visit provided in a type B emergency department; (the ED must meet at least one of the following requirements: (1) it is licensed by the state in which it is located under applicable state law as an emergency room or emergency department; (2) it is held out to the public (by name, posted signs, advertising, or other means) as a place that provides care for emergency medical conditions on an urgent basis without requiring a previously scheduled appointment; or (3) during the calendar year immediately preceding the calendar year in which a determination under 42 CFR 489.24 is being made, based on a representative sample of patient visits that occurred during that calendar year, it provides at least one-third of all of its outpatient visits for the treatment of emergency medical conditions on an urgent basis without requiring a previously scheduled appointment) [J] **CMS:** 100-04,4,160
G0383	Level 4 hospital emergency department visit provided in a type B emergency department; (the ED must meet at least one of the following requirements: (1) it is licensed by the state in which it is located under applicable state law as an emergency room or emergency department; (2) it is held out to the public (by name, posted signs, advertising, or other means) as a place that provides care for emergency medical conditions on an urgent basis without requiring a previously scheduled appointment; or (3) during the calendar year immediately preceding the calendar year in which a determination under 42 CFR 489.24 is being made, based on a representative sample of patient visits that occurred during that calendar year, it provides at least one-third of all of its outpatient visits for the treatment of emergency medical conditions on an urgent basis without requiring a previously scheduled appointment) [J] **CMS:** 100-04,4,160
G0384	Level 5 hospital emergency department visit provided in a type B emergency department; (the ED must meet at least one of the following requirements: (1) it is licensed by the state in which it is located under applicable state law as an emergency room or emergency department; (2) it is held out to the public (by name, posted signs, advertising, or other means) as a place that provides care for emergency medical conditions on an urgent basis without requiring a previously scheduled appointment; or (3) during the calendar year immediately preceding the calendar year in which a determination under 42 CFR 489.24 is being made, based on a representative sample of patient visits that occurred during that calendar year, it provides at least one-third of all of its outpatient visits for the treatment of emergency medical conditions on an urgent basis without requiring a previously scheduled appointment) [J] **CMS:** 100-04,4,160; 100-04,4,290.5.1

Other Services

Code	Description
G0390	Trauma response team associated with hospital critical care service [S] **CMS:** 100-04,4,160.1

Alcohol or Substance Abuse

Code	Description
G0396	Alcohol and/or substance (other than tobacco) misuse structured assessment (e.g., audit, dast), and brief intervention 15 to 30 minutes [S] **CMS:** 100-04,12,190.3; 100-04,12,190.6; 100-04,12,190.6.1; 100-04,12,190.7; 100-04,4,200.6 **AHA:** 3Q,19
G0397	Alcohol and/or substance (other than tobacco) misuse structured assessment (e.g., audit, dast), and intervention, greater than 30 minutes [S] **CMS:** 100-04,12,190.3; 100-04,12,190.6; 100-04,12,190.6.1; 100-04,12,190.7; 100-04,4,200.6 **AHA:** 3Q,19

Home Sleep Study

G0398 Home sleep study test (HST) with type II portable monitor, unattended; minimum of 7 channels: EEG, EOG, EMG, ECG/heart rate, airflow, respiratory effort and oxygen saturation
CMS: 100-03,240.4

G0399 Home sleep test (HST) with type III portable monitor, unattended; minimum of 4 channels: 2 respiratory movement/airflow, 1 ECG/heart rate and 1 oxygen saturation
CMS: 100-03,240.4

G0400 Home sleep test (HST) with type IV portable monitor, unattended; minimum of 3 channels
CMS: 100-03,240.4

Initial Physical Exam

G0402 Initial preventive physical examination; face-to-face visit, services limited to new beneficiary during the first 12 months of Medicare enrollment
CMS: 100-02,13,220; 100-02,13,220.1; 100-02,13,220.3; 100-04,12,100.1.1; 100-04,18,10.1.2; 100-04,18,140.6; 100-04,18,80; 100-04,18,80.1; 100-04,18,80.2; 100-04,18,80.3.3; 100-04,18,80.4; 1004-04,13,220.1

G0403 Electrocardiogram, routine ECG with 12 leads; performed as a screening for the initial preventive physical examination with interpretation and report
CMS: 100-04,18,10.1.2; 100-04,18,80; 100-04,18,80.1; 100-04,18,80.2

G0404 Electrocardiogram, routine ECG with 12 leads; tracing only, without interpretation and report, performed as a screening for the initial preventive physical examination
CMS: 100-04,18,10.1.2; 100-04,18,80; 100-04,18,80.1; 100-04,18,80.2; 100-04,18,80.3.3

G0405 Electrocardiogram, routine ECG with 12 leads; interpretation and report only, performed as a screening for the initial preventive physical examination
CMS: 100-04,18,10.1.2; 100-04,18,80; 100-04,18,80.1; 100-04,18,80.2

Follow-up Telehealth

G0406 Follow-up inpatient consultation, limited, physicians typically spend 15 minutes communicating with the patient via telehealth
CMS: 100-04,12,190.3; 100-04,12,190.3.1; 100-04,12,190.3.3; 100-04,12,190.3.5; 100-04,12,190.6; 100-04,12,190.6.1; 100-04,12,190.7
AHA: 3Q,19

G0407 Follow-up inpatient consultation, intermediate, physicians typically spend 25 minutes communicating with the patient via telehealth
CMS: 100-04,12,190.3; 100-04,12,190.3.1; 100-04,12,190.3.3; 100-04,12,190.3.5; 100-04,12,190.6; 100-04,12,190.6.1; 100-04,12,190.7
AHA: 3Q,19

G0408 Follow-up inpatient consultation, complex, physicians typically spend 35 minutes communicating with the patient via telehealth
CMS: 100-04,12,190.3; 100-04,12,190.3.1; 100-04,12,190.3.3; 100-04,12,190.3.5; 100-04,12,190.6; 100-04,12,190.6.1; 100-04,12,190.7
AHA: 3Q,19

Psychological Services

G0409 Social work and psychological services, directly relating to and/or furthering the patient's rehabilitation goals, each 15 minutes, face-to-face; individual (services provided by a CORF qualified social worker or psychologist in a CORF)
CMS: 100-02,12,30.1; 100-04,5,100.11; 100-04,5,100.4

G0410 Group psychotherapy other than of a multiple-family group, in a partial hospitalization setting, approximately 45 to 50 minutes
CMS: 100-04,4,260.1; 100-04,4,260.1.1

G0411 Interactive group psychotherapy, in a partial hospitalization setting, approximately 45 to 50 minutes
CMS: 100-04,4,260.1; 100-04,4,260.1.1

Fracture Care

G0412 Open treatment of iliac spine(s), tuberosity avulsion, or iliac wing fracture(s), unilateral or bilateral for pelvic bone fracture patterns which do not disrupt the pelvic ring, includes internal fixation, when performed

G0413 Percutaneous skeletal fixation of posterior pelvic bone fracture and/or dislocation, for fracture patterns which disrupt the pelvic ring, unilateral or bilateral, (includes ilium, sacroiliac joint and/or sacrum)

G0414 Open treatment of anterior pelvic bone fracture and/or dislocation for fracture patterns which disrupt the pelvic ring, unilateral or bilateral, includes internal fixation when performed (includes pubic symphysis and/or superior/inferior rami)

G0415 Open treatment of posterior pelvic bone fracture and/or dislocation, for fracture patterns which disrupt the pelvic ring, unilateral or bilateral, includes internal fixation, when performed (includes ilium, sacroiliac joint and/or sacrum)

Surgical Pathology

G0416 Surgical pathology, gross and microscopic examinations, for prostate needle biopsy, any method
AHA: 2Q,22

Educational Services

G0420 Face-to-face educational services related to the care of chronic kidney disease; individual, per session, per 1 hour
CMS: 100-02,15,200; 100-02,15,310; 100-02,15,310.1; 100-02,15,310.2; 100-02,15,310.4; 100-02,15,310.5; 100-04,12,190.3; 100-04,12,190.6; 100-04,12,190.6.1; 100-04,12,190.7
AHA: 3Q,19

G0421 Face-to-face educational services related to the care of chronic kidney disease; group, per session, per 1 hour
CMS: 100-02,15,200; 100-02,15,310; 100-02,15,310.1; 100-02,15,310.2; 100-02,15,310.4; 100-02,15,310.5; 100-04,12,190.3; 100-04,12,190.6; 100-04,12,190.6.1; 100-04,12,190.7
AHA: 3Q,19

Cardiac and Pulmonary Rehabilitation

G0422 Intensive cardiac rehabilitation; with or without continuous ECG monitoring with exercise, per session
CMS: 100-02,15,232; 100-04,32,140.2.2.1; 100-04,32,140.2.2.2; 100-04,32,140.3; 100-04,32,140.3.1; 100-08,15,4.2.8

G0423 Intensive cardiac rehabilitation; with or without continuous ECG monitoring; without exercise, per session
CMS: 100-02,15,232; 100-04,32,140.2.2.1; 100-04,32,140.2.2.2; 100-04,32,140.3; 100-04,32,140.3.1; 100-08,15,4.2.8

Inpatient Telehealth

G0425 Telehealth consultation, emergency department or initial inpatient, typically 30 minutes communicating with the patient via telehealth
CMS: 100-04,12,190.3; 100-04,12,190.3.1; 100-04,12,190.3.2; 100-04,12,190.6; 100-04,12,190.6.1; 100-04,12,190.7
AHA: 3Q,19

G0426 Telehealth consultation, emergency department or initial inpatient, typically 50 minutes communicating with the patient via telehealth
CMS: 100-04,12,190.3; 100-04,12,190.3.1; 100-04,12,190.3.2; 100-04,12,190.6; 100-04,12,190.6.1; 100-04,12,190.7
AHA: 3Q,19

2023 HCPCS Level II

G0427 Telehealth consultation, emergency department or initial inpatient, typically 70 minutes or more communicating with the patient via telehealth
CMS: 100-04,12,190.3; 100-04,12,190.3.1; 100-04,12,190.3.2; 100-04,12,190.6; 100-04,12,190.6.1; 100-04,12,190.7
AHA: 3Q,19

Defect Fillers

G0428 Collagen meniscus implant procedure for filling meniscal defects (e.g., CMI, collagen scaffold, Menaflex)
CMS: 100-03,150.12

G0429 Dermal filler injection(s) for the treatment of facial lipodystrophy syndrome (LDS) (e.g., as a result of highly active antiretroviral therapy)
CMS: 100-03,250.5; 100-04,32,260.1; 100-04,32,260.2.1; 100-04,32,260.2.2

Laboratory Services

G0432 Infectious agent antibody detection by enzyme immunoassay (EIA) technique, HIV-1 and/or HIV-2, screening
CMS: 100-03,190.14; 100-03,190.9; 100-03,210.7; 100-04,18,10.1.2; 100-04,18,130.1; 100-04,18,130.2; 100-04,18,130.3; 100-04,18,130.4; 100-04,18,130.5

G0433 Infectious agent antibody detection by enzyme-linked immunosorbent assay (ELISA) technique, HIV-1 and/or HIV-2, screening
CMS: 100-03,190.14; 100-03,190.9; 100-03,210.7; 100-04,16,70.8; 100-04,18,10.1.2; 100-04,18,130.1; 100-04,18,130.2; 100-04,18,130.3; 100-04,18,130.4; 100-04,18,130.5

G0435 Infectious agent antibody detection by rapid antibody test, HIV-1 and/or HIV-2, screening
CMS: 100-03,190.14; 100-03,190.9; 100-03,210.7; 100-04,18,10.1.2; 100-04,18,130.1; 100-04,18,130.2; 100-04,18,130.3; 100-04,18,130.4; 100-04,18,130.5

Counseling and Wellness Visit

G0438 Annual wellness visit; includes a personalized prevention plan of service (PPS), initial visit
CMS: 100-02,13,220; 100-02,13,220.1; 100-02,13,220.3; 100-02,15,280.5; 100-02,15,280.5.1; 100-04,12,100.1.1; 100-04,18,10.1.2; 100-04,18,140; 100-04,18,140.1; 100-04,18,140.5; 100-04,18,140.6; 100-04,18,140.8; 100-04,4,200.11; 1004-04,13,220.1
AHA: 3Q,19

G0439 Annual wellness visit, includes a personalized prevention plan of service (PPS), subsequent visit
CMS: 100-02,13,220; 100-02,13,220.1; 100-02,13,220.3; 100-02,15,280.5; 100-02,15,280.5.1; 100-04,12,100.1.1; 100-04,18,10.1.2; 100-04,18,140; 100-04,18,140.1; 100-04,18,140.5; 100-04,18,140.6; 100-04,18,140.8; 100-04,4,200.11; 1004-04,13,220.1
AHA: 3Q,19

Other Services

▲ **G0442** Annual alcohol misuse screening, 5 to 15 minutes
CMS: 100-03,210.8; 100-04,12,190.3; 100-04,12,190.6; 100-04,12,190.6.1; 100-04,12,190.7; 100-04,18,180; 100-04,18,180.1; 100-04,18,180.2; 100-04,18,180.3; 100-04,18,180.4; 100-04,18,180.5; 100-04,32,180.4; 100-04,32,180.5
AHA: 3Q,19

G0443 Brief face-to-face behavioral counseling for alcohol misuse, 15 minutes
CMS: 100-03,210.8; 100-04,12,190.3; 100-04,12,190.6; 100-04,12,190.6.1; 100-04,12,190.7; 100-04,18,180; 100-04,18,180.1; 100-04,18,180.2; 100-04,18,180.3; 100-04,18,180.4; 100-04,18,180.5; 100-04,32,180.4; 100-04,32,180.5
AHA: 3Q,19

▲ **G0444** Annual depression screening, 5 to 15 minutes
CMS: 100-04,12,190.3; 100-04,12,190.6; 100-04,12,190.6.1; 100-04,12,190.7; 100-04,18,190; 100-04,18,190.1; 100-04,18,190.2; 100-04,18,190.3
AHA: 3Q,19

G0445 Semiannual high intensity behavioral counseling to prevent STIs, individual, face-to-face, includes education skills training & guidance on how to change sexual behavior
CMS: 100-03,210.10; 100-04,12,190.3; 100-04,12,190.6; 100-04,12,190.6.1; 100-04,12,190.7; 100-04,18,170.1; 100-04,18,170.2; 100-04,18,170.3; 100-04,18,170.4; 100-04,18,170.4.1; 100-04,18,170.5
AHA: 3Q,19

G0446 Annual, face-to-face intensive behavioral therapy for cardiovascular disease, individual, 15 minutes
CMS: 100-03,210.11; 100-04,12,190.3; 100-04,12,190.6; 100-04,12,190.6.1; 100-04,12,190.7; 100-04,18,160; 100-04,18,160.1; 100-04,18,160.2.1; 100-04,18,160.2.2; 100-04,18,160.3; 100-04,18,160.4; 100-04,18,160.5
AHA: 3Q,19

G0447 Face-to-face behavioral counseling for obesity, 15 minutes
CMS: 100-03,210.12; 100-04,12,190.3; 100-04,12,190.6; 100-04,12,190.6.1; 100-04,12,190.7; 100-04,18,10.1.2; 100-04,18,200; 100-04,18,200.1; 100-04,18,200.2; 100-04,18,200.3; 100-04,18,200.4; 100-04,18,200.5
AHA: 3Q,19

G0448 Insertion or replacement of a permanent pacing cardioverter-defibrillator system with transvenous lead(s), single or dual chamber with insertion of pacing electrode, cardiac venous system, for left ventricular pacing
CMS: 100-04,32,270; 100-04,32,270.1; 100-04,32,270.2; 100-04,32,270.3

G0451 Development testing, with interpretation and report, per standardized instrument form
CMS: 100-02,15,220.4; 100-04,5,10.3.2; 100-04,5,10.3.3

Molecular Pathology

G0452 Molecular pathology procedure; physician interpretation and report

Neurophysiology Monitoring

G0453 Continuous intraoperative neurophysiology monitoring, from outside the operating room (remote or nearby), per patient, (attention directed exclusively to one patient) each 15 minutes (list in addition to primary procedure)

Documentation and Preparation

G0454 Physician documentation of face-to-face visit for durable medical equipment determination performed by nurse practitioner, physician assistant or clinical nurse specialist

G0455 Preparation with instillation of fecal microbiota by any method, including assessment of donor specimen

Prostate Brachytherapy

G0458 Low dose rate (LDR) prostate brachytherapy services, composite rate

Inpatient Telehealth Pharmacologic Management

G0459 Inpatient telehealth pharmacologic management, including prescription, use, and review of medication with no more than minimal medical psychotherapy
CMS: 100-04,12,190.3; 100-04,12,190.6; 100-04,12,190.6.1; 100-04,12,190.7
AHA: 3Q,19

Other Wound/Ulcer Care

G0460 Autologous platelet rich plasma for nondiabetic chronic wounds/ulcers, including phlebotomy, centrifugation, and all other preparatory procedures, administration and dressings, per treatment T
CMS: 100-03,270.3; 100-04,32,11.3.1; 100-04,32,11.3.2; 100-04,32,11.3.3; 100-04,32,11.3.4; 100-04,32,11.3.5; 100-04,32,11.3.6
AHA: 3Q,22

Hospital Outpatient Visit

G0463 Hospital outpatient clinic visit for assessment and management of a patient J
CMS: 100-04,4,160.2; 100-04,4,260.1; 100-04,4,260.1.1; 100-04,4,290.5.1; 100-04,4,290.5.3; 100-04,6,20.1.1.2; 100-04,6,30.4.1
AHA: 4Q,20; 2Q,20

Platelet Rich Plasma

G0465 Autologous platelet rich plasma (PRP) for diabetic chronic wounds/ulcers, using an FDA-cleared device (includes administration, dressings, phlebotomy, centrifugation, and all other preparatory procedures, per treatment)
CMS: 100-04,32,11.3.1; 100-04,32,11.3.2; 100-04,32,11.3.3; 100-04,32,11.3.4; 100-04,32,11.3.5; 100-04,32,11.3.6
AHA: 3Q,22

Federally Qualified Health Center Visits

G0466 Federally qualified health center (FQHC) visit, new patient A
CMS: 100-04,9,60.6

G0467 Federally qualified health center (FQHC) visit, established patient A
CMS: 100-04,9,60.6

G0468 Federally qualified health center (FQHC) visit, initial preventive physical exam (IPPE) or annual wellness visit (AWV) A
CMS: 100-04,9,60.6

G0469 Federally qualified health center (FQHC) visit, mental health, new patient A
CMS: 100-04,9,60.6

G0470 Federally qualified health center (FQHC) visit, mental health, established patient A
CMS: 100-04,9,60.6

HHA and SNF Specimen Collection

G0471 Collection of venous blood by venipuncture or urine sample by catheterization from an individual in a skilled nursing facility (SNF) or by a laboratory on behalf of a home health agency (HHA) A
CMS: 100-04,16,60.1.4

Hepatitis C Screening

G0472 Hepatitis C antibody screening for individual at high risk and other covered indication(s) A
CMS: 100-02,13,220; 100-02,13,220.1; 100-02,13,220.3; 100-03,210.13; 100-04,18,10.1.2; 100-04,18,210; 100-04,18,210.2; 100-04,18,210.3; 100-04,18,210.4; 1004-04,13,220.1

Behavioral Counseling

G0473 Face-to-face behavioral counseling for obesity, group (2-10), 30 minutes S
CMS: 100-04,18,10.1.2; 100-04,18,200.1; 100-04,18,200.2; 100-04,18,200.3; 100-04,18,200.4; 100-04,18,200.5

Screening Measures

G0475 HIV antigen/antibody, combination assay, screening A
CMS: 100-03,210.7; 100-04,18,130.1; 100-04,18,130.2; 100-04,18,130.3; 100-04,18,130.5

G0476 Infectious agent detection by nucleic acid (DNA or RNA); human papillomavirus HPV), high-risk types (e.g., 16, 18, 31, 33, 35, 39, 45, 51, 52, 56, 58, 59, 68) for cervical cancer screening, must be performed in addition to pap test ♀ A
CMS: 100-03,210.2.1; 100-04,18,30.2.1; 100-04,18,30.5; 100-04,18,30.6; 100-04,18,30.8; 100-04,18,30.9

Drug Testing

G0480 Drug test(s), definitive, utilizing (1) drug identification methods able to identify individual drugs and distinguish between structural isomers (but not necessarily stereoisomers), including, but not limited to, GC/MS (any type, single or tandem) and LC/MS (any type, single or tandem and excluding immunoassays (e.g., IA, EIA, ELISA, EMIT, FPIA) and enzymatic methods (e.g., alcohol dehydrogenase)), (2) stable isotope or other universally recognized internal standards in all samples (e.g., to control for matrix effects, interferences and variations in signal strength), and (3) method or drug-specific calibration and matrix-matched quality control material (e.g., to control for instrument variations and mass spectral drift); qualitative or quantitative, all sources, includes specimen validity testing, per day; 1-7 drug class(es), including metabolite(s) if performed Q
AHA: 2Q,22; 1Q,18

G0481 Drug test(s), definitive, utilizing (1) drug identification methods able to identify individual drugs and distinguish between structural isomers (but not necessarily stereoisomers), including, but not limited to, GC/MS (any type, single or tandem) and LC/MS (any type, single or tandem and excluding immunoassays (e.g., IA, EIA, ELISA, EMIT, FPIA) and enzymatic methods (e.g., alcohol dehydrogenase)), (2) stable isotope or other universally recognized internal standards in all samples (e.g., to control for matrix effects, interferences and variations in signal strength), and (3) method or drug-specific calibration and matrix-matched quality control material (e.g., to control for instrument variations and mass spectral drift); qualitative or quantitative, all sources, includes specimen validity testing, per day; 8-14 drug class(es), including metabolite(s) if performed Q
AHA: 2Q,22; 1Q,18

G0482 Drug test(s), definitive, utilizing (1) drug identification methods able to identify individual drugs and distinguish between structural isomers (but not necessarily stereoisomers), including, but not limited to, GC/MS (any type, single or tandem) and LC/MS (any type, single or tandem and excluding immunoassays (e.g., IA, EIA, ELISA, EMIT, FPIA) and enzymatic methods (e.g., alcohol dehydrogenase)), (2) stable isotope or other universally recognized internal standards in all samples (e.g., to control for matrix effects, interferences and variations in signal strength), and (3) method or drug-specific calibration and matrix-matched quality control material (e.g., to control for instrument variations and mass spectral drift); qualitative or quantitative, all sources, includes specimen validity testing, per day; 15-21 drug class(es), including metabolite(s) if performed Q
AHA: 2Q,22; 1Q,18

G0483 Drug test(s), definitive, utilizing (1) drug identification methods able to identify individual drugs and distinguish between structural isomers (but not necessarily stereoisomers), including, but not limited to, GC/MS (any type, single or tandem) and LC/MS (any type, single or tandem and excluding immunoassays (e.g., IA, EIA, ELISA, EMIT, FPIA) and enzymatic methods (e.g., alcohol dehydrogenase)), (2) stable isotope or other universally recognized internal standards in all samples (e.g., to control for matrix effects, interferences and variations in signal strength), and (3) method or drug-specific calibration and matrix-matched quality control material (e.g., to control for instrument variations and mass spectral drift); qualitative or quantitative, all sources, includes specimen validity testing, per day; 22 or more drug class(es), including metabolite(s) if performed Q
AHA: 2Q,22; 1Q,18

Home Health Nursing Visit

G0490 Face-to-face home health nursing visit by a rural health clinic (RHC) or federally qualified health center (FQHC) in an area with a shortage of home health agencies; (services limited to RN or LPN only) [A]

Dialysis Procedures

G0491 Dialysis procedure at a Medicare certified ESRD facility for acute kidney injury without ESRD [B]
CMS: 100-04,8,40; 100-04,8,50.2

G0492 Dialysis procedure with single evaluation by a physician or other qualified health care professional for acute kidney injury without ESRD [B]

Skilled Nursing Services

G0493 Skilled services of a registered nurse (RN) for the observation and assessment of the patient's condition, each 15 minutes (the change in the patient's condition requires skilled nursing personnel to identify and evaluate the patient's need for possible modification of treatment in the home health or hospice setting) [B]
CMS: 100-04,10,40.2

G0494 Skilled services of a licensed practical nurse (LPN) for the observation and assessment of the patient's condition, each 15 minutes (the change in the patient's condition requires skilled nursing personnel to identify and evaluate the patient's need for possible modification of treatment in the home health or hospice setting) [B]
CMS: 100-04,10,40.2

G0495 Skilled services of a registered nurse (RN), in the training and/or education of a patient or family member, in the home health or hospice setting, each 15 minutes [B]
CMS: 100-04,10,40.2

G0496 Skilled services of a licensed practical nurse (LPN), in the training and/or education of a patient or family member, in the home health or hospice setting, each 15 minutes [B]
CMS: 100-04,10,40.2

Chemotherapy Infusion

G0498 Chemotherapy administration, intravenous infusion technique; initiation of infusion in the office/clinic setting using office/clinic pump/supplies, with continuation of the infusion in the community setting (e.g., home, domiciliary, rest home or assisted living) using a portable pump provided by the office/clinic, includes follow up office/clinic visit at the conclusion of the infusion [S]
AHA: 2Q,17

Hepatitis B Screening

G0499 Hepatitis B screening in nonpregnant, high-risk individual includes hepatitis B surface antigen (HBSAG), antibodies to HBSAG (anti-HBS) and antibodies to hepatitis B core antigen (anti-HBC), and is followed by a neutralizing confirmatory test, when performed, only for an initially reactive HBSAG result [A]
CMS: 100-03,1,210.6; 100-04,18,230; 100-04,18,230.1; 100-04,18,230.2; 100-04,18,230.3; 100-04,18,230.4

Moderate Sedation

G0500 Moderate sedation services provided by the same physician or other qualified health care professional performing a gastrointestinal endoscopic service that sedation supports, requiring the presence of an independent trained observer to assist in the monitoring of the patient's level of consciousness and physiological status; initial 15 minutes of intra-service time; patient age 5 years or older (additional time may be reported with 99153, as appropriate) [N]
CMS: 100-04,18,60.1.1

Mobility-Assistive Technology

G0501 Resource-intensive services for patients for whom the use of specialized mobility-assistive technology (such as adjustable height chairs or tables, patient lift, and adjustable padded leg supports) is medically necessary and used during the provision of an office/outpatient, evaluation and management visit (list separately in addition to primary service) [N]

Care Management Services

G0506 Comprehensive assessment of and care planning for patients requiring chronic care management services (list separately in addition to primary monthly care management service) [N]
AHA: 3Q,19

Telehealth Consultation

G0508 Telehealth consultation, critical care, initial, physicians typically spend 60 minutes communicating with the patient and providers via telehealth [B]
AHA: 3Q,19

G0509 Telehealth consultation, critical care, subsequent, physicians typically spend 50 minutes communicating with the patient and providers via telehealth [B]
AHA: 3Q,19

RHC or FQHC General Care Management

G0511 Rural health clinic or federally qualified health center (RHC or FQHC) only, general care management, 20 minutes or more of clinical staff time for chronic care management services or behavioral health integration services directed by an RHC or FQHC practitioner (physician, NP, PA, or CNM), per calendar month [A]
CMS: 100-02,13,230.2; 100-04,9,70.8

G0512 Rural health clinic or federally qualified health center (RHC/FQHC) only, psychiatric collaborative care model (psychiatric COCM), 60 minutes or more of clinical staff time for psychiatric COCM services directed by an RHC or FQHC practitioner (physician, NP, PA, or CNM) and including services furnished by a behavioral health care manager and consultation with a psychiatric consultant, per calendar month [A]
CMS: 100-02,13,230.2; 100-02,13,230.3; 100-04,9,70.8

Prolonged Services

G0513 Prolonged preventive service(s) (beyond the typical service time of the primary procedure), in the office or other outpatient setting requiring direct patient contact beyond the usual service; first 30 minutes (list separately in addition to code for preventive service) [N]
AHA: 3Q,19

G0514 Prolonged preventive service(s) (beyond the typical service time of the primary procedure), in the office or other outpatient setting requiring direct patient contact beyond the usual service; each additional 30 minutes (list separately in addition to code G0513 for additional 30 minutes of preventive service) [N]
AHA: 3Q,19

Drug Delivery Implants

G0516 Insertion of nonbiodegradable drug delivery implants, four or more (services for subdermal rod implant) [01] [N]

G0517 Removal of nonbiodegradable drug delivery implants, four or more (services for subdermal implants) [01] [N]

G0518 Removal with reinsertion, nonbiodegradable drug delivery implants, four or more (services for subdermal implants) [01] [N]

Procedures/Professional Services (Temporary)

Drug Test(s)

G0659 Drug test(s), definitive, utilizing drug identification methods able to identify individual drugs and distinguish between structural isomers (but not necessarily stereoisomers), including but not limited to GC/MS (any type, single or tandem) and LC/MS (any type, single or tandem), excluding immunoassays (e.g., IA, EIA, ELISA, EMIT, FPIA) and enzymatic methods (e.g., alcohol dehydrogenase), performed without method or drug-specific calibration, without matrix-matched quality control material, or without use of stable isotope or other universally recognized internal standard(s) for each drug, drug metabolite or drug class per specimen; qualitative or quantitative, all sources, includes specimen validity testing, per day, any number of drug classes
AHA: 2Q,22

Quality Measures

G0913 Improvement in visual function achieved within 90 days following cataract surgery

G0914 Patient care survey was not completed by patient

G0915 Improvement in visual function not achieved within 90 days following cataract surgery

G0916 Satisfaction with care achieved within 90 days following cataract surgery

▲ **G0917** Patient care survey was not completed by patient

G0918 Satisfaction with care not achieved within 90 days following cataract surgery

Clinical Decision Support Mechanism

G1001 Clinical Decision Support Mechanism eviCore, as defined by the Medicare Appropriate Use Criteria Program

G1002 Clinical Decision Support Mechanism MedCurrent, as defined by the Medicare Appropriate Use Criteria Program

G1003 Clinical Decision Support Mechanism Medicalis, as defined by the Medicare Appropriate Use Criteria Program

G1004 Clinical Decision Support Mechanism National Decision Support Company, as defined by the Medicare Appropriate Use Criteria Program

G1007 Clinical Decision Support Mechanism AIM Specialty Health, as defined by the Medicare Appropriate Use Criteria Program

G1008 Clinical Decision Support Mechanism Cranberry Peak, as defined by the Medicare Appropriate Use Criteria Program

~~**G1009** Clinical Decision Support Mechanism Sage Health Management Solutions, as defined by the Medicare Appropriate Use Criteria Program~~

G1010 Clinical Decision Support Mechanism Stanson, as defined by the Medicare Appropriate Use Criteria Program

G1011 Clinical Decision Support Mechanism, qualified tool not otherwise specified, as defined by the Medicare Appropriate Use Criteria Program

G1012 Clinical Decision Support Mechanism AgileMD, as defined by the Medicare Appropriate Use Criteria Program

G1013 Clinical Decision Support Mechanism EvidenceCare ImagingCare, as defined by the Medicare Appropriate Use Criteria Program

G1014 Clinical Decision Support Mechanism InveniQA Semantic Answers in Medicine, as defined by the Medicare Appropriate Use Criteria Program

G1015 Clinical Decision Support Mechanism Reliant Medical Group, as defined by the Medicare Appropriate Use Criteria Program

G1016 Clinical Decision Support Mechanism Speed of Care, as defined by the Medicare Appropriate Use Criteria Program

G1017 Clinical Decision Support Mechanism HealthHelp, as defined by the Medicare Appropriate Use Criteria Program

G1018 Clinical Decision Support Mechanism INFINX, as defined by the Medicare Appropriate Use Criteria Program

G1019 Clinical Decision Support Mechanism LogicNets, as defined by the Medicare Appropriate Use Criteria Program

G1020 Clinical Decision Support Mechanism Curbside Clinical Augmented Workflow, as defined by the Medicare Appropriate Use Criteria Program

G1021 Clinical Decision Support Mechanism EHealthLine Clinical Decision Support Mechanism, as defined by the Medicare Appropriate Use Criteria Program

G1022 Clinical Decision Support Mechanism Intermountain Clinical Decision Support Mechanism, as defined by the Medicare Appropriate Use Criteria Program

G1023 Clinical Decision Support Mechanism Persivia Clinical Decision Support, as defined by the Medicare Appropriate Use Criteria Program

G1024 Clinical decision support mechanism Radrite, as defined by the Medicare Appropriate Use Criteria Program

Patient-Month Quality Measures

G1025 Patient-months where there are more than one Medicare capitated payment (MCP) provider listed for the month

G1026 The number of adult patient-months in the denominator who were on maintenance hemodialysis using a catheter continuously for 3 months or longer under the care of the same practitioner or group partner as of the last hemodialysis session of the reporting month

G1027 The number of adult patient-months in the denominator who were on maintenance hemodialysis under the care of the same practitioner or group partner as of the last hemodialysis session of the reporting month using a catheter continuously for less than 3 months

Nasal Naloxone

G1028 Take-home supply of nasal naloxone; 2-pack of 8 mg per 0.1 ml nasal spray (provision of the services by a Medicare-enrolled Opioid Treatment Program); list separately in addition to code for primary procedure
CMS: 100-02,17,20; 100-02,17,40.1.1; 100-04,39,30.6.1

Convulsive Therapy Procedure

G2000 Blinded administration of convulsive therapy procedure, either electroconvulsive therapy (ECT, current covered gold standard) or magnetic seizure therapy (MST, noncovered experimental therapy), performed in an approved IDE-based clinical trial, per treatment session

Assessments, Evaluations, and CMMI Home Visits

G2001 Brief (20 minutes) in-home visit for a new patient postdischarge. For use only in a Medicare-approved CMMI model. (Services must be furnished within a beneficiary's home, domiciliary, rest home, assisted living and/or nursing facility within 90 days following discharge from an inpatient facility and no more than nine times.)

G2002 Limited (30 minutes) in-home visit for a new patient postdischarge. For use only in a Medicare-approved CMMI model. (Services must be furnished within a beneficiary's home, domiciliary, rest home, assisted living and/or nursing facility within 90 days following discharge from an inpatient facility and no more than nine times.)

G2003 Moderate (45 minutes) in-home visit for a new patient postdischarge. For use only in a Medicare-approved CMMI model. (Services must be furnished within a beneficiary's home, domiciliary, rest home, assisted living and/or nursing facility within 90 days following discharge from an inpatient facility and no more than nine times.)

G2004 Comprehensive (60 minutes) in-home visit for a new patient postdischarge. For use only in a Medicare-approved CMMI model. (Services must be furnished within a beneficiary's home, domiciliary, rest home, assisted living and/or nursing facility within 90 days following discharge from an inpatient facility and no more than nine times.)

G2005 Extensive (75 minutes) in-home visit for a new patient postdischarge. For use only in a Medicare-approved CMMI model. (Services must be furnished within a beneficiary's home, domiciliary, rest home, assisted living and/or nursing facility within 90 days following discharge from an inpatient facility and no more than nine times.)

G2006 Brief (20 minutes) in-home visit for an existing patient postdischarge. For use only in a Medicare-approved CMMI model. (Services must be furnished within a beneficiary's home, domiciliary, rest home, assisted living and/or nursing facility within 90 days following discharge from an inpatient facility and no more than nine times.)

G2007 Limited (30 minutes) in-home visit for an existing patient postdischarge. For use only in a Medicare-approved CMMI model. (Services must be furnished within a beneficiary's home, domiciliary, rest home, assisted living and/or nursing facility within 90 days following discharge from an inpatient facility and no more than nine times.)

G2008 Moderate (45 minutes) in-home visit for an existing patient postdischarge. For use only in a Medicare-approved CMMI model. (Services must be furnished within a beneficiary's home, domiciliary, rest home, assisted living and/or nursing facility within 90 days following discharge from an inpatient facility and no more than nine times.)

G2009 Comprehensive (60 minutes) in-home visit for an existing patient postdischarge. For use only in a Medicare-approved CMMI model. (Services must be furnished within a beneficiary's home, domiciliary, rest home, assisted living and/or nursing facility within 90 days following discharge from an inpatient facility and no more than nine times.)

G2010 Remote evaluation of recorded video and/or images submitted by an established patient (e.g., store and forward), including interpretation with follow-up with the patient within 24 business hours, not originating from a related E/M service provided within the previous 7 days nor leading to an E/M service or procedure within the next 24 hours or soonest available appointment

G2011 Alcohol and/or substance (other than tobacco) misuse structured assessment (e.g., audit, dast), and brief intervention, 5-14 minutes

G2012 Brief communication technology-based service, e.g., virtual check-in, by a physician or other qualified health care professional who can report evaluation and management services, provided to an established patient, not originating from a related E/M service provided within the previous 7 days nor leading to an E/M service or procedure within the next 24 hours or soonest available appointment; 5-10 minutes of medical discussion

G2013 Extensive (75 minutes) in-home visit for an existing patient postdischarge. For use only in a Medicare-approved CMMI model. (Services must be furnished within a beneficiary's home, domiciliary, rest home, assisted living and/or nursing facility within 90 days following discharge from an inpatient facility and no more than nine times.)

G2014 Limited (30 minutes) care plan oversight. For use only in a Medicare-approved CMMI model. (Services must be furnished within a beneficiary's home, domiciliary, rest home, assisted living and/or nursing facility within 90 days following discharge from an inpatient facility and no more than nine times.)

G2015 Comprehensive (60 minutes) home care plan oversight. For use only in a Medicare-approved CMMI model. (Services must be furnished within a beneficiary's home, domiciliary, rest home, assisted living and/or nursing facility within 90 days following discharge from an inpatient facility.)

Treatment in Place

G2020 Services for high intensity clinical services associated with the initial engagement and outreach of beneficiaries assigned to the SIP component of the PCF model (do not bill with chronic care management codes)
AHA: 2Q,21

G2021 Health care practitioners rendering treatment in place (TIP)

G2022 A model participant (ambulance supplier/provider), the beneficiary refuses services covered under the model (transport to an alternate destination/treatment in place)

COVID-19 Specimen Collection
May be reported by clinical diagnostic laboratories.

G2023 Specimen collection for Severe Acute Respiratory Syndrome Coronavirus 2 (SARS-CoV-2) (Coronavirus disease [COVID-19]), any specimen source
AHA: 2Q,20

G2024 Specimen collection for severe acute respiratory syndrome coronavirus 2 (SARS-CoV-2) (coronavirus disease [COVID-19]) from an individual in a SNF or by a laboratory on behalf of a HHA, any specimen source
AHA: 2Q,20

G2025 Payment for a telehealth distant site service furnished by a Rural Health Clinic (RHC) or Federally Qualified Health Center (FQHC) only
AHA: 2Q,20

Device Evaluation/Interrogation

G2066 Interrogation device evaluation(s), (remote) up to 30 days; implantable cardiovascular physiologic monitor system, implantable loop recorder system, or subcutaneous cardiac rhythm monitor system, remote data acquisition(s), receipt of transmissions and technician review, technical support and distribution of results

Medication Assisted Treatment and Other Services

G2067 Medication assisted treatment, methadone; weekly bundle including dispensing and/or administration, substance use counseling, individual and group therapy, and toxicology testing, if performed (provision of the services by a Medicare-enrolled opioid treatment program)
CMS: 100-02,17,20; 100-02,17,40.1.1; 100-02,17,40.1.2; 100-04,26,10.5; 100-04,39,30.6; 100-04,39,30.6.1; 100-04,39,30.7; 100-04,39,30.8; 100-04,39,30.9; 100-04,39,40; 100-04,39,40.2; 100-04,39,50; 100-04,39,50.1

G2068 Medication assisted treatment, buprenorphine (oral); weekly bundle including dispensing and/or administration, substance use counseling, individual and group therapy, and toxicology testing if performed (provision of the services by a Medicare-enrolled opioid treatment program)
CMS: 100-02,17,20; 100-02,17,40.1.1; 100-02,17,40.1.2; 100-04,26,10.5; 100-04,39,30.6; 100-04,39,30.6.1; 100-04,39,30.7; 100-04,39,30.8; 100-04,39,30.9; 100-04,39,40; 100-04,39,40.2; 100-04,39,50; 100-04,39,50.1

G2069 Medication assisted treatment, buprenorphine (injectable); weekly bundle including dispensing and/or administration, substance use counseling, individual and group therapy, and toxicology testing if performed (provision of the services by a Medicare-enrolled opioid treatment program)

CMS: 100-02,17,20; 100-02,17,40.1.1; 100-02,17,40.1.2; 100-04,26,10.5; 100-04,39,30.6; 100-04,39,30.6.1; 100-04,39,30.7; 100-04,39,30.8; 100-04,39,30.9; 100-04,39,40; 100-04,39,40.2; 100-04,39,50; 100-04,39,50.1

G2070 Medication assisted treatment, buprenorphine (implant insertion); weekly bundle including dispensing and/or administration, substance use counseling, individual and group therapy, and toxicology testing if performed (provision of the services by a Medicare-enrolled opioid treatment program)

CMS: 100-02,17,20; 100-02,17,40.1.1; 100-02,17,40.1.2; 100-04,26,10.5; 100-04,39,30.6; 100-04,39,30.6.1; 100-04,39,30.7; 100-04,39,30.8; 100-04,39,30.9; 100-04,39,40; 100-04,39,40.2; 100-04,39,50; 100-04,39,50.1

G2071 Medication assisted treatment, buprenorphine (implant removal); weekly bundle including dispensing and/or administration, substance use counseling, individual and group therapy, and toxicology testing if performed (provision of the services by a Medicare-enrolled opioid treatment program)

CMS: 100-02,17,20; 100-02,17,40.1.1; 100-02,17,40.1.2; 100-04,26,10.5; 100-04,39,30.6; 100-04,39,30.6.1; 100-04,39,30.7; 100-04,39,30.8; 100-04,39,30.9; 100-04,39,40; 100-04,39,40.2; 100-04,39,50; 100-04,39,50.1

G2072 Medication assisted treatment, buprenorphine (implant insertion and removal); weekly bundle including dispensing and/or administration, substance use counseling, individual and group therapy, and toxicology testing if performed (provision of the services by a Medicare-enrolled opioid treatment program)

CMS: 100-02,17,20; 100-02,17,40.1.1; 100-02,17,40.1.2; 100-04,26,10.5; 100-04,39,30.6; 100-04,39,30.6.1; 100-04,39,30.7; 100-04,39,30.8; 100-04,39,30.9; 100-04,39,40; 100-04,39,40.2; 100-04,39,50; 100-04,39,50.1

G2073 Medication assisted treatment, naltrexone; weekly bundle including dispensing and/or administration, substance use counseling, individual and group therapy, and toxicology testing if performed (provision of the services by a Medicare-enrolled opioid treatment program)

CMS: 100-02,17,20; 100-02,17,40.1.1; 100-02,17,40.1.2; 100-04,26,10.5; 100-04,39,30.6; 100-04,39,30.6.1; 100-04,39,30.7; 100-04,39,30.8; 100-04,39,30.9; 100-04,39,40; 100-04,39,40.2; 100-04,39,50; 100-04,39,50.1

G2074 Medication assisted treatment, weekly bundle not including the drug, including substance use counseling, individual and group therapy, and toxicology testing if performed (provision of the services by a Medicare-enrolled opioid treatment program)

CMS: 100-02,17,20; 100-02,17,40.1.1; 100-02,17,40.1.2; 100-04,26,10.5; 100-04,39,30.2; 100-04,39,30.3; 100-04,39,30.6; 100-04,39,30.6.1; 100-04,39,30.7; 100-04,39,30.8; 100-04,39,30.9; 100-04,39,40; 100-04,39,40.2; 100-04,39,50; 100-04,39,50.1

G2075 Medication assisted treatment, medication not otherwise specified; weekly bundle including dispensing and/or administration, substance use counseling, individual and group therapy, and toxicology testing, if performed (provision of the services by a Medicare-enrolled opioid treatment program)

CMS: 100-02,17,20; 100-02,17,40.1.1; 100-02,17,40.1.2; 100-04,26,10.5; 100-04,39,30.4; 100-04,39,30.6; 100-04,39,30.6.1; 100-04,39,30.7; 100-04,39,30.8; 100-04,39,30.9; 100-04,39,40; 100-04,39,40.2; 100-04,39,50; 100-04,39,50.1

G2076 Intake activities, including initial medical examination that is a complete, fully documented physical evaluation and initial assessment by a program physician or a primary care physician, or an authorized health care professional under the supervision of a program physician qualified personnel that includes preparation of a treatment plan that includes the patient's short-term goals and the tasks the patient must perform to complete the short-term goals; the patient's requirements for education, vocational rehabilitation, and employment; and the medical, psycho-social, economic, legal, or other supportive services that a patient needs, conducted by qualified personnel (provision of the services by a Medicare-enrolled opioid treatment program); list separately in addition to code for primary procedure

CMS: 100-02,17,20; 100-02,17,40.1.1; 100-02,17,40.1.2; 100-04,26,10.5; 100-04,39,30.6; 100-04,39,30.6.1; 100-04,39,30.7; 100-04,39,30.8; 100-04,39,30.9; 100-04,39,40; 100-04,39,40.2; 100-04,39,50; 100-04,39,50.1

G2077 Periodic assessment; assessing periodically by qualified personnel to determine the most appropriate combination of services and treatment (provision of the services by a Medicare-enrolled opioid treatment program); list separately in addition to code for primary procedure

CMS: 100-02,17,20; 100-02,17,40.1.1; 100-02,17,40.1.2; 100-04,26,10.5; 100-04,39,30.6; 100-04,39,30.6.1; 100-04,39,30.7; 100-04,39,30.8; 100-04,39,30.9; 100-04,39,40; 100-04,39,40.2; 100-04,39,50; 100-04,39,50.1

G2078 Take home supply of methadone; up to 7 additional day supply (provision of the services by a Medicare-enrolled opioid treatment program); list separately in addition to code for primary procedure

CMS: 100-02,17,20; 100-02,17,40.1.1; 100-02,17,40.1.2; 100-04,26,10.5; 100-04,39,30.6; 100-04,39,30.6.1; 100-04,39,30.7; 100-04,39,30.8; 100-04,39,30.9; 100-04,39,40; 100-04,39,40.2; 100-04,39,50; 100-04,39,50.1

G2079 Take home supply of buprenorphine (oral); up to 7 additional day supply (provision of the services by a Medicare-enrolled opioid treatment program); list separately in addition to code for primary procedure

CMS: 100-02,17,20; 100-02,17,40.1.1; 100-02,17,40.1.2; 100-04,26,10.5; 100-04,39,30.6; 100-04,39,30.6.1; 100-04,39,30.7; 100-04,39,30.8; 100-04,39,30.9; 100-04,39,40; 100-04,39,40.2; 100-04,39,50; 100-04,39,50.1

G2080 Each additional 30 minutes of counseling in a week of medication assisted treatment, (provision of the services by a Medicare-enrolled opioid treatment program); list separately in addition to code for primary procedure

CMS: 100-02,17,20; 100-02,17,40.1.1; 100-02,17,40.1.2; 100-04,26,10.5; 100-04,39,30.5; 100-04,39,30.6; 100-04,39,30.6.1; 100-04,39,30.7; 100-04,39,30.8; 100-04,39,30.9; 100-04,39,40; 100-04,39,40.2; 100-04,39,50; 100-04,39,50.1

G2081 Patients age 66 and older in institutional special needs plans (SNP) or residing in long-term care with a POS code 32, 33, 34, 54 or 56 for more than 90 consecutive days during the measurement period   **A**

G2082 Office or other outpatient visit for the evaluation and management of an established patient that requires the supervision of a physician or other qualified health care professional and provision of up to 56 mg of esketamine nasal self administration, includes 2 hours post administration observation

G2083 Office or other outpatient visit for the evaluation and management of an established patient that requires the supervision of a physician or other qualified health care professional and provision of greater than 56 mg esketamine nasal self administration, includes 2 hours post administration observation

Code	Description
G2086	Office-based treatment for opioid use disorder, including development of the treatment plan, care coordination, individual therapy and group therapy and counseling; at least 70 minutes in the first calendar month AHA: 1Q,20
G2087	Office-based treatment for opioid use disorder, including care coordination, individual therapy and group therapy and counseling; at least 60 minutes in a subsequent calendar month AHA: 1Q,20
G2088	Office-based treatment for opioid use disorder, including care coordination, individual therapy and group therapy and counseling; each additional 30 minutes beyond the first 120 minutes (list separately in addition to code for primary procedure) AHA: 1Q,20
G2090	Patients 66 years of age and older with at least one claim/encounter for frailty during the measurement period and a dispensed medication for dementia during the measurement period or the year prior to the measurement period A
G2091	Patients 66 years of age and older with at least one claim/encounter for frailty during the measurement period and either one acute inpatient encounter with a diagnosis of advanced illness or two outpatient, observation, ED or nonacute inpatient encounters on different dates of service with an advanced illness diagnosis during the measurement period or the year prior to the measurement period A
G2092	Angiotensin converting enzyme (ACE) inhibitor or angiotensin receptor blocker (ARB) or angiotensin receptor-neprilysin inhibitor (ARNI) therapy prescribed or currently being taken
G2093	Documentation of medical reason(s) for not prescribing ACE inhibitor or ARB or ARNI therapy (e.g., hypotensive patients who are at immediate risk of cardiogenic shock, hospitalized patients who have experienced marked azotemia, allergy, intolerance, other medical reasons)
G2094	Documentation of patient reason(s) for not prescribing ACE inhibitor or ARB or ARNI therapy (e.g., patient declined, other patient reasons)
~~G2095~~	~~Documentation of system reason(s) for not prescribing ACE inhibitor or ARB or ARNI therapy (e.g., other system reasons)~~
G2096	Angiotensin converting enzyme (ACE) inhibitor or angiotensin receptor blocker (ARB) or angiotensin receptor-neprilysin inhibitor (ARNI) therapy was not prescribed, reason not given
G2097	Episodes where the patient had a competing diagnosis on or within 3 days after the episode date (e.g., intestinal infection, pertussis, bacterial infection, Lyme disease, otitis media, acute sinusitis, chronic sinusitis, infection of the adenoids, prostatitis, cellulitis, mastoiditis, or bone infections, acute lymphadenitis, impetigo, skin staph infections, pneumonia/gonococcal infections, venereal disease (syphilis, chlamydia, inflammatory diseases [female reproductive organs]), infections of the kidney, cystitis or UTI)
G2098	Patients 66 years of age and older with at least one claim/encounter for frailty during the measurement period and a dispensed medication for dementia during the measurement period or the year prior to the measurement period A
G2099	Patients 66 years of age and older with at least one claim/encounter for frailty during the measurement period and either one acute inpatient encounter with a diagnosis of advanced illness or two outpatient, observation, ED or nonacute inpatient encounters on different dates of service with an advanced illness diagnosis during the measurement period or the year prior to the measurement period A
G2100	Patients 66 years of age and older with at least one claim/encounter for frailty during the measurement period and a dispensed medication for dementia during the measurement period or the year prior to the measurement period A
G2101	Patients 66 years of age and older with at least one claim/encounter for frailty during the measurement period and either one acute inpatient encounter with a diagnosis of advanced illness or two outpatient, observation, ED or nonacute inpatient encounters on different dates of service with an advanced illness diagnosis during the measurement period or the year prior to the measurement period A
G2105	Patient age 66 or older in institutional special needs plans (SNP) or residing in long-term care with POS code 32, 33, 34, 54 or 56 for more than 90 consecutive days during the measurement period A
G2106	Patients 66 years of age and older with at least one claim/encounter for frailty during the measurement period and a dispensed medication for dementia during the measurement period or the year prior to the measurement period A
G2107	Patients 66 years of age and older with at least one claim/encounter for frailty during the measurement period and either one acute inpatient encounter with a diagnosis of advanced illness or two outpatient, observation, ED or nonacute inpatient encounters on different dates of service with an advanced illness diagnosis during the measurement period or the year prior to the measurement period A
G2108	Patient age 66 or older in institutional special needs plans (SNP) or residing in long-term care with POS code 32, 33, 34, 54 or 56 for more than 90 consecutive days during the measurement period A
G2109	Patients 66 years of age and older with at least one claim/encounter for frailty during the measurement period and a dispensed medication for dementia during the measurement period or the year prior to the measurement period A
G2110	Patients 66 years of age and older with at least one claim/encounter for frailty during the measurement period and either one acute inpatient encounter with a diagnosis of advanced illness or two outpatient, observation, ED or nonacute inpatient encounters on different dates of service with an advanced illness diagnosis during the measurement period or the year prior to the measurement period A
G2112	Patient receiving <=5 mg daily prednisone (or equivalent), or RA activity is worsening, or glucocorticoid use is for less than 6 months
G2113	Patient receiving >5 mg daily prednisone (or equivalent) for longer than 6 months, and improvement or no change in disease activity
G2115	Patients 66 - 80 years of age with at least one claim/encounter for frailty during the measurement period and a dispensed medication for dementia during the measurement period or the year prior to the measurement period A
G2116	Patients 66 - 80 years of age with at least one claim/encounter for frailty during the measurement period and either one acute inpatient encounter with a diagnosis of advanced illness or two outpatient, observation, ED or nonacute inpatient encounters on different dates of service with an advanced illness diagnosis during the measurement period or the year prior to the measurement period A
G2118	Patients 81 years of age and older with at least one claim/encounter for frailty during the measurement period A
G2121	Depression, anxiety, apathy, and psychosis assessed
G2122	Depression, anxiety, apathy, and psychosis not assessed

Procedures/Professional Services (Temporary)

Code	Description
G2125	Patients 81 years of age and older with at least one claim/encounter for frailty during the six months prior to the measurement period through December 31 of the measurement period **A**
G2126	Patients 66 - 80 years of age with at least one claim/encounter for frailty during the measurement period and either one acute inpatient encounter with a diagnosis of advanced illness or two outpatient, observation, ED or nonacute inpatient encounters on different dates of service with an advanced illness diagnosis during the measurement period or the year prior to the measurement period **A**
G2127	Patients 66 - 80 years of age with at least one claim/encounter for frailty during the measurement period and a dispensed medication for dementia during the measurement period or the year prior to the measurement period **A**
G2128	Documentation of medical reason(s) for not on a daily aspirin or other antiplatelet (e.g., history of gastrointestinal bleed, intracranial bleed, blood disorders, idiopathic thrombocytopenic purpura (ITP), gastric bypass or documentation of active anticoagulant use during the measurement period)
G2129	Procedure related BP's not taken during an outpatient visit. Examples include same day surgery, ambulatory service center, GI, lab, dialysis, infusion center, chemotherapy
▲ G2136	Back pain measured by the visual analog scale (VAS) or numeric pain scale at 3 months (6 to 20 weeks) postoperatively was less than or equal to 3.0 or back pain measured by the visual analog scale (VAS) or numeric pain scale within 3 months preoperatively and at 3 months (6 to 20 weeks) postoperatively demonstrated an improvement of 5.0 points or greater
▲ G2137	Back pain measured by the visual analog scale (VAS) or numeric pain scale at 3 months (6 to 20 weeks) postoperatively was greater than 3.0 and back pain measured by the visual analog scale (VAS) or numeric pain scale within 3 months preoperatively and at 3 months (6 to 20 weeks) postoperatively demonstrated less than an improvement of 5.0 points
▲ G2138	Back pain as measured by the visual analog scale (VAS) or numeric pain scale at 1 year (9 to 15 months) postoperatively was less than or equal to 3.0 or back pain measured by the visual analog scale (VAS) or numeric pain scale within 3 months preoperatively and at 1 year (9 to 15 months) postoperatively demonstrated an improvement of 5.0 points or greater
▲ G2139	Back pain measured by the visual analog scale (VAS) or numeric pain scale at 1 year (9 to 15 months) postoperatively was greater than 3.0 and back pain measured by the visual analog scale (VAS) or numeric pain scale within 3 months preoperatively and at 1 year (9 to 15 months) postoperatively demonstrated less than an improvement of 5.0 points
▲ G2140	Leg pain measured by the visual analog scale (VAS) or numeric pain scale at 3 months (6 to 20 weeks) postoperatively was less than or equal to 3.0 or leg pain measured by the visual analog scale (VAS) or numeric pain scale within 3 months preoperatively and at 3 months (6 to 20 weeks) postoperatively demonstrated an improvement of 5.0 points or greater **AHA:** 2Q,21
▲ G2141	Leg pain measured by the visual analog scale (VAS) or numeric pain scale at 3 months (6 to 20 weeks) postoperatively was greater than 3.0 and leg pain measured by the visual analog scale (VAS) or numeric pain scale within 3 months preoperatively and at 3 months (6 to 20 weeks) postoperatively demonstrated less than an improvement of 5.0 points
G2142	Functional status measured by the Oswestry Disability Index (ODI version 2.1a) at 1 year (9 to 15 months) postoperatively was less than or equal to 22 or functional status measured by the ODI version 2.1a within 3 months preoperatively and at 1 year (9 to 15 months) postoperatively demonstrated an improvement of 30 points or greater
G2143	Functional status measured by the Oswestry Disability Index (ODI version 2.1a) at 1 year (9 to 15 months) postoperatively was greater than 22 and functional status measured by the ODI version 2.1a within 3 months preoperatively and at 1 year (9 to 15 months) postoperatively demonstrated an improvement of less than 30 points
G2144	Functional status measured by the Oswestry Disability Index (ODI version 2.1a) at 3 months (6 to 20 weeks) postoperatively was less than or equal to 22 or functional status measured by the ODI version 2.1a within 3 months preoperatively and at 3 months (6 to 20 weeks) postoperatively demonstrated an improvement of 30 points or greater
G2145	Functional status measured by the Oswestry Disability Index (ODI version 2.1a) at 3 months (6 to 20 weeks) postoperatively was greater than 22 and functional status measured by the ODI version 2.1a within 3 months preoperatively and at 3 months (6 to 20 weeks) postoperatively demonstrated an improvement of less than 30 points
▲ G2146	Leg pain as measured by the visual analog scale (VAS) or numeric pain scale at 1 year (9 to 15 months) postoperatively was less than or equal to 3.0 or leg pain measured by the visual analog scale (VAS) or numeric pain scale within 3 months preoperatively and at 1 year (9 to 15 months) postoperatively demonstrated an improvement of 5.0 points or greater
▲ G2147	Leg pain measured by the visual analog scale (VAS) or numeric pain scale at 1 year (9 to 15 months) postoperatively was greater than 3.0 and leg pain measured by the visual analog scale (VAS) or numeric pain scale within 3 months preoperatively and at 1 year (9 to 15 months) postoperatively demonstrated less than an improvement of 5.0 points
G2148	Multimodal pain management was used
G2149	Documentation of medical reason(s) for not using multimodal pain management (e.g., allergy to multiple classes of analgesics, intubated patient, hepatic failure, patient reports no pain during PACU stay, other medical reason(s))
G2150	Multimodal pain management was not used
G2151	Documentation stating patient has a diagnosis of a degenerative neurological condition such as ALS, MS, or Parkinson's diagnosed at any time before or during the episode of care
▲ G2152	Residual score for the neck impairment successfully calculated and the score was equal to zero (0) or greater than zero (> 0)
▲ G2167	Residual score for the neck impairment successfully calculated and the score was less than zero (< 0)

Home Health

Code	Description
G2168	Services performed by a physical therapist assistant in the home health setting in the delivery of a safe and effective physical therapy maintenance program, each 15 minutes
G2169	Services performed by an occupational therapist assistant in the home health setting in the delivery of a safe and effective occupational therapy maintenance program, each 15 minutes

Arteriovenous Fistual Creation

Code	Description
G2170	~~Percutaneous arteriovenous fistula creation (AVF), direct, any site, by tissue approximation using thermal resistance energy, and secondary procedures to redirect blood flow (e.g., transluminal balloon angioplasty, coil embolization) when performed, and includes all imaging and radiologic guidance, supervision and interpretation, when performed~~ To report, see ~36836

Code	Description
G2171	Percutaneous arteriovenous fistula creation (AVF), direct, any site, using magnetic-guided arterial and venous catheters and radiofrequency energy, including flow-directing procedures (e.g., vascular coil embolization with radiologic supervision and interpretation, when performed) and fistulogram(s); angiography, venography, and/or ultrasound, with radiologic supervision and interpretation, when performed To report, see ~36837

Quality Measures

Code	Description
G2172	All inclusive payment for services related to highly coordinated and integrated opioid use disorder (OUD) treatment services furnished for the demonstration project AHA: 2Q,21
G2173	URI episodes where the patient had a comorbid condition during the 12 months prior to or on the episode date (e.g., tuberculosis, neutropenia, cystic fibrosis, chronic bronchitis, pulmonary edema, respiratory failure, rheumatoid lung disease)
▲ G2174	URI episodes when the patient had an active prescription of antibiotics in the 30 days prior to the episode date or is still active the same day of the encounter
G2175	Episodes where the patient had a comorbid condition during the 12 months prior to or on the episode date (e.g., tuberculosis, neutropenia, cystic fibrosis, chronic bronchitis, pulmonary edema, respiratory failure, rheumatoid lung disease)
G2176	Outpatient, ED, or observation visits that result in an inpatient admission
G2177	Acute bronchitis/bronchiolitis episodes when the patient had a new or refill prescription of antibiotics (table 1) in the 30 days prior to the episode date
G2178	Clinician documented that patient was not an eligible candidate for lower extremity neurological exam measure, for example patient bilateral amputee; patient has condition that would not allow them to accurately respond to a neurological exam (dementia, Alzheimer's, etc.); patient has previously documented diabetic peripheral neuropathy with loss of protective sensation
G2179	Clinician documented that patient had medical reason for not performing lower extremity neurological exam
G2180	Clinician documented that patient was not an eligible candidate for evaluation of footwear as patient is bilateral lower extremity amputee
G2181	BMI not documented due to medical reason or patient refusal of height or weight measurement
▲ G2182	Patient receiving first-time biologic and/or immune response modifier therapy
G2183	Documentation patient unable to communicate and informant not available
G2184	Patient does not have a caregiver
G2185	Documentation caregiver is trained and certified in dementia care
G2186	Patient /caregiver dyad has been referred to appropriate resources and connection to those resources is confirmed
G2187	Patients with clinical indications for imaging of the head: head trauma
G2188	Patients with clinical indications for imaging of the head: new or change in headache above 50 years of age
G2189	Patients with clinical indications for imaging of the head: abnormal neurologic exam
G2190	Patients with clinical indications for imaging of the head: headache radiating to the neck
G2191	Patients with clinical indications for imaging of the head: positional headaches
G2192	Patients with clinical indications for imaging of the head: temporal headaches in patients over 55 years of age
G2193	Patients with clinical indications for imaging of the head: new onset headache in preschool children or younger (<6 years of age)
G2194	Patients with clinical indications for imaging of the head: new onset headache in pediatric patients with disabilities for which headache is a concern as inferred from behavior
G2195	Patients with clinical indications for imaging of the head: occipital headache in children
G2196	Patient identified as an unhealthy alcohol user when screened for unhealthy alcohol use using a systematic screening method
G2197	Patient screened for unhealthy alcohol use using a systematic screening method and not identified as an unhealthy alcohol user
G2198	~~Documentation of medical reason(s) for not screening for unhealthy alcohol use using a systematic screening method (e.g., limited life expectancy, other medical reasons)~~
▲ G2199	Patient not screened for unhealthy alcohol use using a systematic screening method
G2200	Patient identified as an unhealthy alcohol user received brief counseling
G2201	~~Documentation of medical reason(s) for not providing brief counseling (e.g., limited life expectancy, other medical reasons)~~
▲ G2202	Patient did not receive brief counseling if identified as an unhealthy alcohol user
G2203	~~Documentation of medical reason(s) for not providing brief counseling if identified as an unhealthy alcohol user (e.g., limited life expectancy, other medical reasons)~~
▲ G2204	Patients between 45 and 85 years of age who received a screening colonoscopy during the performance period
G2205	Patients with pregnancy during adjuvant treatment course
G2206	Patient received adjuvant treatment course including both chemotherapy and HER2-targeted therapy
▲ G2207	Reason for not administering adjuvant treatment course including both chemotherapy and HER2-targeted therapy (e.g., poor performance status (ECOG 3-4; Karnofsky <=50), cardiac contraindications, insufficient renal function, insufficient hepatic function, other active or secondary cancer diagnoses, other medical contraindications, patients who died during initial treatment course or transferred during or after initial treatment course)
G2208	Patient did not receive adjuvant treatment course including both chemotherapy and HER2-targeted therapy
G2209	Patient refused to participate
▲ G2210	Residual score for the neck impairment not measured because the patient did not complete the neck FS PROM at initial evaluation and/or near discharge, reason not given
G2211	Visit complexity inherent to evaluation and management associated with medical care services that serve as the continuing focal point for all needed health care services and/or with medical care services that are part of ongoing care related to a patient's single, serious condition or a complex condition. (add-on code, list separately in addition to office/outpatient evaluation and management visit, new or established)

Procedures/Professional Services (Temporary)

▲ **G2212** Prolonged office or other outpatient evaluation and management service(s) beyond the maximum required time of the primary procedure which has been selected using total time on the date of the primary service; each additional 15 minutes by the physician or qualified healthcare professional, with or without direct patient contact (list separately in addition to CPT codes 99205, 99215, 99483 for office or other outpatient evaluation and management services.) (Do not report G2212 on the same date of service as codes 99358, 99359, 99415, 99416). (Do not report G2212 for any time unit less than 15 minutes)
CMS: 100-04,12,30.6.18

G2213 Initiation of medication for the treatment of opioid use disorder in the emergency department setting, including assessment, referral to ongoing care, and arranging access to supportive services (list separately in addition to code for primary procedure)

G2214 Initial or subsequent psychiatric collaborative care management, first 30 minutes in a month of behavioral health care manager activities, in consultation with a psychiatric consultant, and directed by the treating physician or other qualified health care professional

G2215 Take home supply of nasal naloxone; 2-pack of 4 mg per 0.1 ml nasal spray (provision of the services by a Medicare-enrolled Opioid Treatment Program); list separately in addition to code for primary procedure
CMS: 100-02,17,20; 100-02,17,40.1.1; 100-02,17,40.1.2; 100-04,39,30.6; 100-04,39,30.6.1; 100-04,39,30.7; 100-04,39,30.8; 100-04,39,40

G2216 Take home supply of injectable naloxone (provision of the services by a Medicare-enrolled opioid treatment program); list separately in addition to code for primary procedure
CMS: 100-02,17,20; 100-02,17,40.1.1; 100-02,17,40.1.2; 100-04,39,30.6; 100-04,39,30.6.1; 100-04,39,30.7; 100-04,39,30.8; 100-04,39,40

G2250 Remote assessment of recorded video and/or images submitted by an established patient (e.g., store and forward), including interpretation with follow-up with the patient within 24 business hours, not originating from a related service provided within the previous 7 days nor leading to a service or procedure within the next 24 hours or soonest available appointment

G2251 Brief communication technology-based service, e.g. virtual check-in, by a qualified health care professional who cannot report evaluation and management services, provided to an established patient, not originating from a related service provided within the previous 7 days nor leading to a service or procedure within the next 24 hours or soonest available appointment; 5-10 minutes of clinical discussion

G2252 Brief communication technology-based service, e.g. virtual check-in, by a physician or other qualified health care professional who can report evaluation and management services, provided to an established patient, not originating from a related EM service provided within the previous 7 days nor leading to an EM service or procedure within the next 24 hours or soonest available appointment; 11-20 minutes of medical discussion

Chronic Pain Management

● **G3002** Chronic pain management and treatment, monthly bundle including, diagnosis; assessment and monitoring; administration of a validated pain rating scale or tool; the development, implementation, revision, and/or maintenance of a person-centered care plan that includes strengths, goals, clinical needs, and desired outcomes; overall treatment management; facilitation and coordination of any necessary behavioral health treatment; medication management; pain and health literacy counseling; any necessary chronic pain related crisis care; and ongoing communication and care coordination between relevant practitioners furnishing care e.g., physical therapy and occupational therapy, complementary and integrative approaches, and community-based care, as appropriate. Requires initial face-to-face visit at least 30 minutes provided by a physician or other qualified health professional; first 30 minutes personally provided by physician or other qualified health care professional, per calendar month. (When using G3002, 30 minutes must be met or exceeded)

● **G3003** Each additional 15 minutes of chronic pain management and treatment by a physician or other qualified health care professional, per calendar month. (List separately in addition to code for G3002. When using G3003, 15 minutes must be met or exceeded)

MIPS Specialty Sets

Code	Description
G4000	Dermatology MIPS specialty set
G4001	Diagnostic Radiology MIPS specialty set
G4002	Electrophysiology Cardiac Specialist MIPS specialty set
G4003	Emergency Medicine MIPS specialty set
G4004	Endocrinology MIPS specialty set
G4005	Family Medicine MIPS specialty set
G4006	Gastroenterology MIPS specialty set
G4007	General Surgery MIPSspecialty set
G4008	Geriatrics MIPS specialty set
G4009	Hospitalists MIPS specialty set
G4010	Infectious Disease MIPS specialty set
G4011	Internal Medicine MIPS specialty set
G4012	Interventional Radiology MIPS specialty set
▲ G4013	Mental/behavioral and Psychiatry MIPS specialty set
G4014	Nephrology MIPS specialty set
G4015	Neurology MIPS specialty set
G4016	Neurosurgical MIPS specialty set
G4017	Nutrition/Dietician MIPS specialty set
G4018	Obstetrics/Gynecology MIPS specialty set
G4019	Oncology/Hematology MIPS specialty set
▲ G4020	Ophthalmology/Optometry MIPS specialty set
G4021	Orthopedic surgery MIPS specialty set
G4022	Otolaryngology MIPS specialty set
G4023	Pathology MIPS specialty set
G4024	Pediatrics MIPS specialty set
G4025	Physical Medicine MIPS specialty set
G4026	Physical Therapy/Occupational Therapy MIPS specialty set
G4027	Plastic Surgery MIPS specialty set
G4028	Podiatry MIPS specialty set
G4029	Preventive Medicine MIPS specialty set

2023 HCPCS Level II · G8465

Code	Description
G4030	Pulmonology MIPS specialty set
G4031	Radiation Oncology MIPS specialty set
G4032	Rheumatology MIPS specialty set
G4033	Skilled Nursing Facility MIPS specialty set
G4034	Speech Language Pathology MIPS specialty set
G4035	Thoracic Surgery MIPS specialty set
G4036	Urgent Care MIPS specialty set
G4037	Urology MIPS specialty set
G4038	Vascular Surgery MIPS specialty set

Radiation Therapy

Code	Description	
G6001	Ultrasonic guidance for placement of radiation therapy fields	B
G6002	Stereoscopic x-ray guidance for localization of target volume for the delivery of radiation therapy	B
G6003	Radiation treatment delivery, single treatment area, single port or parallel opposed ports, simple blocks or no blocks: up to 5 mev	B
G6004	Radiation treatment delivery, single treatment area, single port or parallel opposed ports, simple blocks or no blocks: 6-10 mev	B
G6005	Radiation treatment delivery, single treatment area, single port or parallel opposed ports, simple blocks or no blocks: 11-19 mev	B
G6006	Radiation treatment delivery, single treatment area, single port or parallel opposed ports, simple blocks or no blocks: 20 mev or greater	B
G6007	Radiation treatment delivery, two separate treatment areas, three or more ports on a single treatment area, use of multiple blocks: up to 5 mev	B
G6008	Radiation treatment delivery, two separate treatment areas, three or more ports on a single treatment area, use of multiple blocks: 6-10 mev	B
G6009	Radiation treatment delivery, two separate treatment areas, three or more ports on a single treatment area, use of multiple blocks: 11-19 mev	B
G6010	Radiation treatment delivery, two separate treatment areas, three or more ports on a single treatment area, use of multiple blocks: 20 mev or greater	B
G6011	Radiation treatment delivery, three or more separate treatment areas, custom blocking, tangential ports, wedges, rotational beam, compensators, electron beam; up to 5 mev	B
G6012	Radiation treatment delivery, three or more separate treatment areas, custom blocking, tangential ports, wedges, rotational beam, compensators, electron beam; 6-10 mev	B
G6013	Radiation treatment delivery, three or more separate treatment areas, custom blocking, tangential ports, wedges, rotational beam, compensators, electron beam; 11-19 mev	B
G6014	Radiation treatment delivery, three or more separate treatment areas, custom blocking, tangential ports, wedges, rotational beam, compensators, electron beam; 20 mev or greater	B
G6015	Intensity modulated treatment delivery, single or multiple fields/arcs, via narrow spatially and temporally modulated beams, binary, dynamic MLC, per treatment session	B
G6016	Compensator-based beam modulation treatment delivery of inverse planned treatment using three or more high resolution (milled or cast) compensator, convergent beam modulated fields, per treatment session	B
G6017	Intra-fraction localization and tracking of target or patient motion during delivery of radiation therapy (e.g., 3D positional tracking, gating, 3D surface tracking), each fraction of treatment	B

Quality Measures

Code	Description	
G8395	Left ventricular ejection fraction (LVEF) ≥ 40% or documentation as normal or mildly depressed left ventricular systolic function	M
G8396	Left ventricular ejection fraction (LVEF) not performed or documented	M
G8397	Dilated macular or fundus exam performed, including documentation of the presence or absence of macular edema and level of severity of retinopathy	M
G8399	Patient with documented results of a central dual-energy x-ray absorptiometry (DXA) ever being performed	M
G8400	Patient with central dual-energy x-ray absorptiometry (DXA) results not documented, reason not given	M
G8404	Lower extremity neurological exam performed and documented	M
G8405	Lower extremity neurological exam not performed	M
G8410	Footwear evaluation performed and documented	M
G8415	Footwear evaluation was not performed	M
G8416	Clinician documented that patient was not an eligible candidate for footwear evaluation measure	M
G8417	BMI is documented above normal parameters and a follow-up plan is documented	M
G8418	BMI is documented below normal parameters and a follow-up plan is documented	M
G8419	BMI documented outside normal parameters, no follow-up plan documented, no reason given	M
G8420	BMI is documented within normal parameters and no follow-up plan is required	M
G8421	BMI not documented and no reason is given	M
G8427	Eligible clinician attests to documenting in the medical record they obtained, updated, or reviewed the patient's current medications	M
G8428	Current list of medications not documented as obtained, updated, or reviewed by the eligible clinician, reason not given	M
G8430	Documentation of a medical reason(s) for not documenting, updating, or reviewing the patient's current medications list (e.g., patient is in an urgent or emergent medical situation)	M
G8431	Screening for depression is documented as being positive and a follow-up plan is documented	M
G8432	Depression screening not documented, reason not given	M
G8433	Screening for depression not completed, documented patient or medical reason	M
G8450	Beta-blocker therapy prescribed	M
▲ G8451	Beta-blocker therapy for LVEF <=40% not prescribed for reasons documented by the clinician (e.g., low blood pressure, fluid overload, asthma, patients recently treated with an intravenous positive inotropic agent, allergy, intolerance, other medical reasons, patient declined, other patient reasons)	M
G8452	Beta-blocker therapy not prescribed	M
G8465	High or very high risk of recurrence of prostate cancer	M

Special Coverage Instructions · Noncovered by Medicare · Carrier Discretion · ☑ Quantity Alert · ● New Code · ○ Recycled/Reinstated · ▲ Revised Code

© 2022 Optum, Inc. · A2–Z3 ASC Pmt · CMS: IOM · AHA: Coding Clinic · DMEPOS Paid · SNF Excluded · G Codes — 63

Procedures/Professional Services (Temporary)

G8473 — G8654

Code	Description
G8473	Angiotensin converting enzyme (ACE) inhibitor or angiotensin receptor blocker (ARB) therapy prescribed M
G8474	Angiotensin converting enzyme (ACE) inhibitor or angiotensin receptor blocker (ARB) therapy not prescribed for reasons documented by the clinician (e.g., allergy, intolerance, pregnancy, renal failure due to ACE inhibitor, diseases of the aortic or mitral valve, other medical reasons) or (e.g., patient declined, other patient reasons) or (e.g., lack of drug availability, other reasons attributable to the health care system) M
G8475	Angiotensin converting enzyme (ACE) inhibitor or angiotensin receptor blocker (ARB) therapy not prescribed, reason not given M
G8476	Most recent blood pressure has a systolic measurement of < 140 mm Hg and a diastolic measurement of < 90 mm Hg M
G8477	Most recent blood pressure has a systolic measurement of >=140 mm Hg and/or a diastolic measurement of >=90 mm Hg M
G8478	Blood pressure measurement not performed or documented, reason not given M
G8482	Influenza immunization administered or previously received M
G8483	Influenza immunization was not administered for reasons documented by clinician (e.g., patient allergy or other medical reasons, patient declined or other patient reasons, vaccine not available or other system reasons) M
G8484	Influenza immunization was not administered, reason not given M
G8506	Patient receiving angiotensin converting enzyme (ACE) inhibitor or angiotensin receptor blocker (ARB) therapy M
G8510	Screening for depression is documented as negative, a follow-up plan is not required M
G8511	Screening for depression documented as positive, follow-up plan not documented, reason not given M
G8535	Elder maltreatment screen not documented; documentation that patient is not eligible for the elder maltreatment screen at the time of the encounter M
G8536	No documentation of an elder maltreatment screen, reason not given M
▲ G8539	Functional outcome assessment documented as positive using a standardized tool and a care plan based on identified deficiencies is documented within 2 days of the functional outcome assessment M
G8540	Functional outcome assessment not documented as being performed, documentation the patient is not eligible for a functional outcome assessment using a standardized tool at the time of the encounter M
G8541	Functional outcome assessment using a standardized tool, not documented, reason not given M
G8542	Functional outcome assessment using a standardized tool is documented; no functional deficiencies identified, care plan not required M
▲ G8543	Documentation of a positive functional outcome assessment using a standardized tool; care plan not documented within 2 days of assessment, reason not given M
G8559	Patient referred to a physician (preferably a physician with training in disorders of the ear) for an otologic evaluation
G8560	Patient has a history of active drainage from the ear within the previous 90 days M
G8561	Patient is not eligible for the referral for otologic evaluation for patients with a history of active drainage measure M
G8562	Patient does not have a history of active drainage from the ear within the previous 90 days M
G8563	Patient not referred to a physician (preferably a physician with training in disorders of the ear) for an otologic evaluation, reason not given M
G8564	Patient was referred to a physician (preferably a physician with training in disorders of the ear) for an otologic evaluation, reason not specified M
G8565	Verification and documentation of sudden or rapidly progressive hearing loss M
G8566	Patient is not eligible for the "referral for otologic evaluation for sudden or rapidly progressive hearing loss" measure
G8567	Patient does not have verification and documentation of sudden or rapidly progressive hearing loss M
G8568	Patient was not referred to a physician (preferably a physician with training in disorders of the ear) for an otologic evaluation, reason not given M
G8569	Prolonged postoperative intubation (> 24 hrs) required M
G8570	Prolonged postoperative intubation (> 24 hrs) not required M
G8575	Developed postoperative renal failure or required dialysis M
G8576	No postoperative renal failure/dialysis not required M
G8577	Re-exploration required due to mediastinal bleeding with or without tamponade, graft occlusion, valve dysfunction or other cardiac reason M
G8578	Re-exploration not required due to mediastinal bleeding with or without tamponade, graft occlusion, valve dysfunction or other cardiac reason M
G8598	Aspirin or another antiplatelet therapy used M
G8599	Aspirin or another antiplatelet therapy not used, reason not given M
▲ G8600	IV thrombolytic therapy initiated within 4.5 hours (≤ 270 minutes) of time last known well M
▲ G8601	IV thrombolytic therapy not initiated within 4.5 hours (= 270 minutes) of time last known well for reasons documented by clinician (e.g., patient enrolled in clinical trial for stroke, patient admitted for elective carotid intervention, patient received tenecteplase (TNK)) M
▲ G8602	IV thrombolytic therapy not initiated within 4.5 hours (≤ 270 minutes) of time last known well, reason not given M
G8633	Pharmacologic therapy (other than minerals/vitamins) for osteoporosis prescribed M
G8635	Pharmacologic therapy for osteoporosis was not prescribed, reason not given M
▲ G8647	Residual score for the knee impairment successfully calculated and the score was equal to zero (0) or greater than zero (> 0) M ☑
▲ G8648	Residual score for the knee impairment successfully calculated and the score was less than zero (< 0) M ☑
▲ G8650	Residual score for the knee impairment not measured because the patient did not complete the LEPF PROM at initial evaluation and/or near discharge, reason not given M
▲ G8651	Residual score for the hip impairment successfully calculated and the score was equal to zero (0) or greater than zero (> 0) M ☑
▲ G8652	Residual score for the hip impairment successfully calculated and the score was less than zero (< 0) M ☑
▲ G8654	Residual score for the hip impairment not measured because the patient did not complete the LEPF PROM at initial evaluation and/or near discharge, reason not given M

Special Coverage Instructions | Noncovered by Medicare | Carrier Discretion | ☑ Quantity Alert | ● New Code | ○ Recycled/Reinstated | ▲ Revised Code

A Age Edit | M Maternity Edit | ♀ Female Only | ♂ Male Only | A-Y OPPS Status Indicators

Code	Description
▲ G8655	Residual score for the lower leg, foot or ankle impairment successfully calculated and the score was equal to zero (0) or greater than zero (> 0)
▲ G8656	Residual score for the lower leg, foot or ankle impairment successfully calculated and the score was less than zero (< 0)
▲ G8658	Residual score for the lower leg, foot or ankle impairment not measured because the patient did not complete the LEPF PROM at initial evaluation and/or near discharge, reason not given
▲ G8659	Residual score for the low back impairment successfully calculated and the score was equal to zero (0) or greater than zero (> 0)
▲ G8660	Residual score for the low back impairment successfully calculated and the score was less than zero (< 0)
G8661	Risk-adjusted functional status change residual score for the low back impairment not measured because the patient did not complete the FS status survey near discharge, patient not appropriate
▲ G8662	Residual score for the low back impairment not measured because the patient did not complete the low back FS PROM at initial evaluation and/or near discharge, reason not given
▲ G8663	Residual score for the shoulder impairment successfully calculated and the score was equal to zero (0) or greater than zero (> 0)
▲ G8664	Residual score for the shoulder impairment successfully calculated and the score was less than zero (< 0)
▲ G8666	Residual score for the shoulder impairment not measured because the patient did not complete the shoulder FS PROM at initial evaluation and/or near discharge, reason not given
▲ G8667	Residual score for the elbow, wrist or hand impairment successfully calculated and the score was equal to zero (0) or greater than zero (> 0)
▲ G8668	Residual score for the elbow, wrist or hand impairment successfully calculated and the score was less than zero (< 0)
▲ G8670	Residual score for the elbow, wrist or hand impairment not measured because the patient did not complete the elbow/wrist/hand FS PROM at initial evaluation and/or near discharge, reason not given
▲ G8694	Left ventricular ejection fraction (LVEF) < = 40% or documentation of moderate or severe LVSD
▲ G8708	Patient not prescribed antibiotic
G8709	URI episodes when the patient had competing diagnoses on or three days after the episode date (e.g., intestinal infection, pertussis, bacterial infection, Lyme disease, otitis media, acute sinusitis, acute pharyngitis, acute tonsillitis, chronic sinusitis, infection of the pharynx/larynx/tonsils/adenoids, prostatitis, cellulitis, mastoiditis, or bone infections, acute lymphadenitis, impetigo, skin staph infections, pneumonia/gonococcal infections, venereal disease (syphilis, chlamydia, inflammatory diseases [female reproductive organs]), infections of the kidney, cystitis or UTI, and acne)
▲ G8710	Patient prescribed antibiotic
▲ G8711	Prescribed antibiotic on or within 3 days after the episode date
G8712	Antibiotic not prescribed or dispensed
G8721	PT category (primary tumor), PN category (regional lymph nodes), and histologic grade were documented in pathology report
G8722	Documentation of medical reason(s) for not including the PT category, the PN category or the histologic grade in the pathology report (e.g., re-excision without residual tumor; noncarcinomasanal canal)
G8723	Specimen site is other than anatomic location of primary tumor
G8724	PT category, PN category and histologic grade were not documented in the pathology report, reason not given
G8733	Elder maltreatment screen documented as positive and a follow-up plan is documented
▲ G8734	Elder maltreatment screen documented as negative, follow-up is not required
G8735	Elder maltreatment screen documented as positive, follow-up plan not documented, reason not given
G8749	Absence of signs of melanoma (tenderness, jaundice, localized neurologic signs such as weakness, or any other sign suggesting systemic spread) or absence of symptoms of melanoma (cough, dyspnea, pain, paresthesia, or any other symptom suggesting the possibility of systemic spread of melanoma)
G8752	Most recent systolic blood pressure < 140 mm Hg
G8753	Most recent systolic blood pressure ≥ 140 mm Hg
G8754	Most recent diastolic blood pressure < 90 mm Hg
G8755	Most recent diastolic blood pressure ≥ 90 mm Hg
G8756	No documentation of blood pressure measurement, reason not given
G8783	Normal blood pressure reading documented, follow-up not required
G8785	Blood pressure reading not documented, reason not given
G8797	Specimen site other than anatomic location of esophagus
G8798	Specimen site other than anatomic location of prostate
G8806	Performance of trans-abdominal or trans-vaginal ultrasound and pregnancy location documented
G8807	Transabdominal or transvaginal ultrasound not performed for reasons documented by clinician (e.g., patient has visited the ED multiple times within 72 hours, patient has a documented intrauterine pregnancy (IUP))
G8808	Transabdominal or transvaginal ultrasound not performed, reason not given
G8815	Documented reason in the medical records for why the statin therapy was not prescribed (i.e., lower extremity bypass was for a patient with nonartherosclerotic disease)
G8816	Statin medication prescribed at discharge
G8817	Statin therapy not prescribed at discharge, reason not given
G8818	Patient discharge to home no later than postoperative day #7
G8825	Patient not discharged to home by postoperative day #7
G8826	Patient discharged to home no later than postoperative day #2 following EVAR
G8833	Patient not discharged to home by postoperative day #2 following EVAR
G8834	Patient discharged to home no later than postoperative day #2 following CEA
G8838	Patient not discharged to home by postoperative day #2 following CEA

Code	Description
G8839	Sleep apnea symptoms assessed, including presence or absence of snoring and daytime sleepiness
G8840	Documentation of reason(s) for not documenting an assessment of sleep symptoms (e.g., patient didn't have initial daytime sleepiness, patient visited between initial testing and initiation of therapy)
G8841	Sleep apnea symptoms not assessed, reason not given
▲ G8842	Apnea hypopnea index (AHI), respiratory disturbance index (RDI) or respiratory event index (REI) documented or measured within 2 months of initial evaluation for suspected obstructive sleep apnea
▲ G8843	Documentation of reason(s) for not measuring an apnea hypopnea index (AHI), a respiratory disturbance index (RDI), or a respiratory event index (REI) within 2 months of initial evaluation for suspected obstructive sleep apnea (e.g., medical, neurological, or psychiatric disease that prohibits successful completion of a sleep study, patients for whom a sleep study would present a bigger risk than benefit or would pose an undue burden, dementia, patients who decline AHI/RDI/REI measurement, patients who had a financial reason for not completing testing, test was ordered but not completed, patients decline because their insurance (payer) does not cover the expense))
▲ G8844	Apnea hypopnea index (AHI), respiratory disturbance index (RDI), or respiratory event index (REI) not documented or measured within 2 months of initial evaluation for suspected obstructive sleep apnea, reason not given
G8845	Positive airway pressure therapy prescribed
G8846	Moderate or severe obstructive sleep apnea (apnea hypopnea index (AHI) or respiratory disturbance index (RDI) of 15 or greater)
G8849	Documentation of reason(s) for not prescribing positive airway pressure therapy (e.g., patient unable to tolerate, alternative therapies use, patient declined, financial, insurance coverage)
G8850	Positive airway pressure therapy not prescribed, reason not given
G8851	Objective measurement of adherence to positive airway pressure therapy, documented
▲ G8852	Positive airway pressure therapy was prescribed
▲ G8854	Documentation of reason(s) for not objectively measuring adherence to positive airway pressure therapy (e.g., patient didn't bring data from continuous positive airway pressure [CPAP], therapy not yet initiated, not available on machine)
G8855	Objective measurement of adherence to positive airway pressure therapy not performed, reason not given
G8856	Referral to a physician for an otologic evaluation performed
G8857	Patient is not eligible for the referral for otologic evaluation measure (e.g., patients who are already under the care of a physician for acute or chronic dizziness)
G8858	Referral to a physician for an otologic evaluation not performed, reason not given
G8863	Patients not assessed for risk of bone loss, reason not given
G8864	Pneumococcal vaccine administered or previously received
G8865	Documentation of medical reason(s) for not administering or previously receiving pneumococcal vaccine (e.g., patient allergic reaction, potential adverse drug reaction)
G8866	Documentation of patient reason(s) for not administering or previously receiving pneumococcal vaccine (e.g., patient refusal)
G8867	Pneumococcal vaccine not administered or previously received, reason not given
G8869	Patient has documented immunity to hepatitis B and initiating anti-TNF therapy
G8875	Clinician diagnosed breast cancer preoperatively by a minimally invasive biopsy method
G8876	Documentation of reason(s) for not performing minimally invasive biopsy to diagnose breast cancer preoperatively (e.g., lesion too close to skin, implant, chest wall, etc., lesion could not be adequately visualized for needle biopsy, patient condition prevents needle biopsy [weight, breast thickness, etc.], duct excision without imaging abnormality, prophylactic mastectomy, reduction mammoplasty, excisional biopsy performed by another physician)
G8877	Clinician did not attempt to achieve the diagnosis of breast cancer preoperatively by a minimally invasive biopsy method, reason not given
G8878	Sentinel lymph node biopsy procedure performed
G8880	Documentation of reason(s) sentinel lymph node biopsy not performed (e.g., reasons could include but not limited to: noninvasive cancer, incidental discovery of breast cancer on prophylactic mastectomy, incidental discovery of breast cancer on reduction mammoplasty, preoperative biopsy proven lymph node (LN) metastases, inflammatory carcinoma, Stage III locally advanced cancer, recurrent invasive breast cancer, clinically node positive after neoadjuvant systemic therapy, patient refusal after informed consent, patient with significant age, comorbidities, or limited life expectancy and favorable tumor; adjuvant systemic therapy unlikely to change)
G8881	Stage of breast cancer is greater than T1N0M0 or T2N0M0
G8882	Sentinel lymph node biopsy procedure not performed, reason not given
G8883	Biopsy results reviewed, communicated, tracked and documented
G8884	Clinician documented reason that patient's biopsy results were not reviewed
G8885	Biopsy results not reviewed, communicated, tracked or documented
G8907	Patient documented not to have experienced any of the following events: a burn prior to discharge; a fall within the facility; wrong site/side/patient/procedure/implant event; or a hospital transfer or hospital admission upon discharge from the facility
G8908	Patient documented to have received a burn prior to discharge
G8909	Patient documented not to have received a burn prior to discharge
G8910	Patient documented to have experienced a fall within ASC
G8911	Patient documented not to have experienced a fall within ASC
G8912	Patient documented to have experienced a wrong site, wrong side, wrong patient, wrong procedure or wrong implant event
G8913	Patient documented not to have experienced a wrong site, wrong side, wrong patient, wrong procedure or wrong implant event

Code	Description
G8914	Patient documented to have experienced a hospital transfer or hospital admission upon discharge from ASC
G8915	Patient documented not to have experienced a hospital transfer or hospital admission upon discharge from ASC
G8916	Patient with preoperative order for IV antibiotic surgical site infection (SSI) prophylaxis, antibiotic initiated on time
G8917	Patient with preoperative order for IV antibiotic surgical site infection (SSI) prophylaxis, antibiotic not initiated on time
G8918	Patient without preoperative order for IV antibiotic surgical site infection (SSI) prophylaxis
▲ G8923	Left ventricular ejection fraction (LVEF) <= 40% or documentation of moderately or severely depressed left ventricular systolic function
G8924	Spirometry test results demonstrate FEV1/FVC < 70%, FEV1 < 60% predicted and patient has COPD symptoms (e.g., dyspnea, cough/sputum, wheezing)
▲ G8934	Left ventricular ejection fraction (LVEF) <=40% or documentation of moderately or severely depressed left ventricular systolic function
G8935	Clinician prescribed angiotensin converting enzyme (ACE) inhibitor or angiotensin receptor blocker (ARB) therapy
G8936	Clinician documented that patient was not an eligible candidate for angiotensin converting enzyme (ACE) inhibitor or angiotensin receptor blocker (ARB) therapy (e.g., allergy, intolerance, pregnancy, renal failure due to ACE inhibitor, diseases of the aortic or mitral valve, other medical reasons) or (e.g., patient declined, other patient reasons) or (e.g., lack of drug availability, other reasons attributable to the health care system)
G8937	Clinician did not prescribe angiotensin converting enzyme (ACE) inhibitor or angiotensin receptor blocker (ARB) therapy, reason not given
G8941	Elder maltreatment screen documented as positive, follow-up plan not documented, documentation the patient is not eligible for follow-up plan at the time of the encounter
▲ G8942	Functional outcomes assessment using a standardized tool is documented within the previous 30 days and care plan, based on identified deficiencies is documented within two days of the functional outcome assessment
G8944	AJCC melanoma cancer stage 0 through IIC melanoma
G8946	Minimally invasive biopsy method attempted but not diagnostic of breast cancer (e.g., high risk lesion of breast such as atypical ductal hyperplasia, lobular neoplasia, atypical lobular hyperplasia, lobular carcinoma in situ, atypical columnar hyperplasia, flat epithelial atypia, radial scar, complex sclerosing lesion, papillary lesion, or any lesion with spindle cells)
G8950	Elevated or hypertensive blood pressure reading documented, and the indicated follow-up is documented
G8952	Elevated or hypertensive blood pressure reading documented, indicated follow-up not documented, reason not given
G8955	Most recent assessment of adequacy of volume management documented
G8956	Patient receiving maintenance hemodialysis in an outpatient dialysis facility
G8958	Assessment of adequacy of volume management not documented, reason not given
G8961	Cardiac stress imaging test primarily performed on low-risk surgery patient for preoperative evaluation within 30 days preceding this surgery
G8962	Cardiac stress imaging test performed on patient for any reason including those who did not have low risk surgery or test that was performed more than 30 days preceding low risk surgery
G8963	Cardiac stress imaging performed primarily for monitoring of asymptomatic patient who had PCI wihin 2 years
G8964	Cardiac stress imaging test performed primarily for any other reason than monitoring of asymptomatic patient who had PCI wthin 2 years (e.g., symptomatic patient, patient greater than 2 years since PCI, initial evaluation, etc.)
G8965	Cardiac stress imaging test primarily performed on low CHD risk patient for initial detection and risk assessment
G8966	Cardiac stress imaging test performed on symptomatic or higher than low CHD risk patient or for any reason other than initial detection and risk assessment
G8967	FDA-approved oral anticoagulant is prescribed
▲ G8968	Documentation of medical reason(s) for not prescribing an FDA-approved anticoagulant (e.g., present or planned atrial appendage occlusion or ligation)
G8969	Documentation of patient reason(s) for not prescribing an oral anticoagulant that is FDA-approved for the prevention of thromboembolism (e.g., patient preference for not receiving anticoagulation)
G8970	No risk factors or one moderate risk factor for thromboembolism

Coordinated Care

Code	Description
G9001	Coordinated care fee, initial rate
G9002	Coordinated care fee
G9003	Coordinated care fee, risk adjusted high, initial
G9004	Coordinated care fee, risk adjusted low, initial
G9005	Coordinated care fee risk adjusted maintenance
G9006	Coordinated care fee, home monitoring
G9007	Coordinated care fee, scheduled team conference
G9008	Coordinated care fee, physician coordinated care oversight services
G9009	Coordinated care fee, risk adjusted maintenance, Level 3
G9010	Coordinated care fee, risk adjusted maintenance, Level 4
G9011	Coordinated care fee, risk adjusted maintenance, Level 5
G9012	Other specified case management service not elsewhere classified

Demonstration Project

Code	Description
G9013	ESRD demo basic bundle Level I
G9014	ESRD demo expanded bundle including venous access and related services
G9016	Smoking cessation counseling, individual, in the absence of or in addition to any other evaluation and management service, per session (6-10 minutes) [demo project code only] CMS: 100-03,210.4.1
G9050	Oncology; primary focus of visit; work-up, evaluation, or staging at the time of cancer diagnosis or recurrence (for use in a Medicare-approved demonstration project)
G9051	Oncology; primary focus of visit; treatment decision-making after disease is staged or restaged, discussion of treatment options, supervising/coordinating active cancer-directed therapy or managing consequences of cancer-directed therapy (for use in a Medicare-approved demonstration project)

Procedures/Professional Services (Temporary)

G9052 — Oncology; primary focus of visit; surveillance for disease recurrence for patient who has completed definitive cancer-directed therapy and currently lacks evidence of recurrent disease; cancer-directed therapy might be considered in the future (for use in a Medicare-approved demonstration project) [EI]

G9053 — Oncology; primary focus of visit; expectant management of patient with evidence of cancer for whom no cancer-directed therapy is being administered or arranged at present; cancer-directed therapy might be considered in the future (for use in a Medicare-approved demonstration project) [EI]

G9054 — Oncology; primary focus of visit; supervising, coordinating or managing care of patient with terminal cancer or for whom other medical illness prevents further cancer treatment; includes symptom management, end-of-life care planning, management of palliative therapies (for use in a Medicare-approved demonstration project) [EI]

G9055 — Oncology; primary focus of visit; other, unspecified service not otherwise listed (for use in a Medicare-approved demonstration project) [EI]

G9056 — Oncology; practice guidelines; management adheres to guidelines (for use in a Medicare-approved demonstration project) [EI]

G9057 — Oncology; practice guidelines; management differs from guidelines as a result of patient enrollment in an institutional review board-approved clinical trial (for use in a Medicare-approved demonstration project) [EI]

G9058 — Oncology; practice guidelines; management differs from guidelines because the treating physician disagrees with guideline recommendations (for use in a Medicare-approved demonstration project) [EI]

G9059 — Oncology; practice guidelines; management differs from guidelines because the patient, after being offered treatment consistent with guidelines, has opted for alternative treatment or management, including no treatment (for use in a Medicare-approved demonstration project) [EI]

G9060 — Oncology; practice guidelines; management differs from guidelines for reason(s) associated with patient comorbid illness or performance status not factored into guidelines (for use in a Medicare-approved demonstration project) [EI]

G9061 — Oncology; practice guidelines; patient's condition not addressed by available guidelines (for use in a Medicare-approved demonstration project) [EI]

G9062 — Oncology; practice guidelines; management differs from guidelines for other reason(s) not listed (for use in a Medicare-approved demonstration project) [EI]

G9063 — Oncology; disease status; limited to nonsmall cell lung cancer; extent of disease initially established as Stage I (prior to neoadjuvant therapy, if any) with no evidence of disease progression, recurrence, or metastases (for use in a Medicare-approved demonstration project) [M]

G9064 — Oncology; disease status; limited to nonsmall cell lung cancer; extent of disease initially established as Stage II (prior to neoadjuvant therapy, if any) with no evidence of disease progression, recurrence, or metastases (for use in a Medicare-approved demonstration project) [M]

G9065 — Oncology; disease status; limited to nonsmall cell lung cancer; extent of disease initially established as Stage III a (prior to neoadjuvant therapy, if any) with no evidence of disease progression, recurrence, or metastases (for use in a Medicare-approved demonstration project) [M]

G9066 — Oncology; disease status; limited to nonsmall cell lung cancer; Stage III B-IV at diagnosis, metastatic, locally recurrent, or progressive (for use in a Medicare-approved demonstration project) [M]

G9067 — Oncology; disease status; limited to nonsmall cell lung cancer; extent of disease unknown, staging in progress, or not listed (for use in a Medicare-approved demonstration project) [M]

G9068 — Oncology; disease status; limited to small cell and combined small cell/nonsmall cell; extent of disease initially established as limited with no evidence of disease progression, recurrence, or metastases (for use in a Medicare-approved demonstration project) [M]

G9069 — Oncology; disease status; small cell lung cancer, limited to small cell and combined small cell/nonsmall cell; extensive Stage at diagnosis, metastatic, locally recurrent, or progressive (for use in a Medicare-approved demonstration project) [M]

G9070 — Oncology; disease status; small cell lung cancer, limited to small cell and combined small cell/nonsmall; extent of disease unknown, staging in progress, or not listed (for use in a Medicare-approved demonstration project) [M]

G9071 — Oncology; disease status; invasive female breast cancer (does not include ductal carcinoma in situ); adenocarcinoma as predominant cell type; Stage I or Stage IIA-IIB; or T3, N1, M0; and ER and/or PR positive; with no evidence of disease progression, recurrence, or metastases (for use in a Medicare-approved demonstration project) [♀][M]

G9072 — Oncology; disease status; invasive female breast cancer (does not include ductal carcinoma in situ); adenocarcinoma as predominant cell type; Stage I, or Stage IIA-IIB; or T3, N1, M0; and ER and PR negative; with no evidence of disease progression, recurrence, or metastases (for use in a Medicare-approved demonstration project) [♀][M]

G9073 — Oncology; disease status; invasive female breast cancer (does not include ductal carcinoma in situ); adenocarcinoma as predominant cell type; Stage IIIA-IIIB; and not T3, N1, M0; and ER and/or PR positive; with no evidence of disease progression, recurrence, or metastases (for use in a Medicare-approved demonstration project) [♀][M]

G9074 — Oncology; disease status; invasive female breast cancer (does not include ductal carcinoma in situ); adenocarcinoma as predominant cell type; Stage IIIA-IIIB; and not T3, N1, M0; and ER and PR negative; with no evidence of disease progression, recurrence, or metastases (for use in a Medicare-approved demonstration project) [♀][M]

G9075 — Oncology; disease status; invasive female breast cancer (does not include ductal carcinoma in situ); adenocarcinoma as predominant cell type; M1 at diagnosis, metastatic, locally recurrent, or progressive (for use in a Medicare-approved demonstration project) [♀][M]

G9077 — Oncology; disease status; prostate cancer, limited to adenocarcinoma as predominant cell type; T1-T2c and Gleason 2-7 and PSA < or equal to 20 at diagnosis with no evidence of disease progression, recurrence, or metastases (for use in a Medicare-approved demonstration project) [♂]

G9078 — Oncology; disease status; prostate cancer, limited to adenocarcinoma as predominant cell type; T2 or T3a Gleason 8-10 or PSA > 20 at diagnosis with no evidence of disease progression, recurrence, or metastases (for use in a Medicare-approved demonstration project) [♂]

G9079 — Oncology; disease status; prostate cancer, limited to adenocarcinoma as predominant cell type; T3b-T4, any N; any T, N1 at diagnosis with no evidence of disease progression, recurrence, or metastases (for use in a Medicare-approved demonstration project) [♂]

G9080 Oncology; disease status; prostate cancer, limited to adenocarcinoma; after initial treatment with rising PSA or failure of PSA decline (for use in a Medicare-approved demonstration project) ♂ M

G9083 Oncology; disease status; prostate cancer, limited to adenocarcinoma; extent of disease unknown, staging in progress, or not listed (for use in a Medicare-approved demonstration project) ♂ M

G9084 Oncology; disease status; colon cancer, limited to invasive cancer, adenocarcinoma as predominant cell type; extent of disease initially established as T1-3, N0, M0 with no evidence of disease progression, recurrence or metastases (for use in a Medicare-approved demonstration project) M

G9085 Oncology; disease status; colon cancer, limited to invasive cancer, adenocarcinoma as predominant cell type; extent of disease initially established as T4, N0, M0 with no evidence of disease progression, recurrence, or metastases (for use in a Medicare-approved demonstration project) M

G9086 Oncology; disease status; colon cancer, limited to invasive cancer, adenocarcinoma as predominant cell type; extent of disease initially established as T1-4, N1-2, M0 with no evidence of disease progression, recurrence, or metastases (for use in a Medicare-approved demonstration project) M

G9087 Oncology; disease status; colon cancer, limited to invasive cancer, adenocarcinoma as predominant cell type; M1 at diagnosis, metastatic, locally recurrent, or progressive with current clinical, radiologic, or biochemical evidence of disease (for use in a Medicare-approved demonstration project) M

G9088 Oncology; disease status; colon cancer, limited to invasive cancer, adenocarcinoma as predominant cell type; M1 at diagnosis, metastatic, locally recurrent, or progressive without current clinical, radiologic, or biochemical evidence of disease (for use in a Medicare-approved demonstration project) M

G9089 Oncology; disease status; colon cancer, limited to invasive cancer, adenocarcinoma as predominant cell type; extent of disease unknown, staging in progress or not listed (for use in a Medicare-approved demonstration project) M

G9090 Oncology; disease status; rectal cancer, limited to invasive cancer, adenocarcinoma as predominant cell type; extent of disease initially established as T1-2, N0, M0 (prior to neoadjuvant therapy, if any) with no evidence of disease progression, recurrence, or metastases (for use in a Medicare-approved demonstration project) M

G9091 Oncology; disease status; rectal cancer, limited to invasive cancer, adenocarcinoma as predominant cell type; extent of disease initially established as T3, N0, M0 (prior to neoadjuvant therapy, if any) with no evidence of disease progression, recurrence, or metastases (for use in a Medicare-approved demonstration project) M

G9092 Oncology; disease status; rectal cancer, limited to invasive cancer, adenocarcinoma as predominant cell type; extent of disease initially established as T1-3, N1-2, M0 (prior to neoadjuvant therapy, if any) with no evidence of disease progression, recurrence or metastases (for use in a Medicare-approved demonstration project) M

G9093 Oncology; disease status; rectal cancer, limited to invasive cancer, adenocarcinoma as predominant cell type; extent of disease initially established as T4, any N, M0 (prior to neoadjuvant therapy, if any) with no evidence of disease progression, recurrence, or metastases (for use in a Medicare-approved demonstration project) M

G9094 Oncology; disease status; rectal cancer, limited to invasive cancer, adenocarcinoma as predominant cell type; M1 at diagnosis, metastatic, locally recurrent, or progressive (for use in a Medicare-approved demonstration project) M

G9095 Oncology; disease status; rectal cancer, limited to invasive cancer, adenocarcinoma as predominant cell type; extent of disease unknown, staging in progress or not listed (for use in a Medicare-approved demonstration project) M

G9096 Oncology; disease status; esophageal cancer, limited to adenocarcinoma or squamous cell carcinoma as predominant cell type; extent of disease initially established as T1-T3, N0-N1 or NX (prior to neoadjuvant therapy, if any) with no evidence of disease progression, recurrence, or metastases (for use in a Medicare-approved demonstration project) M

G9097 Oncology; disease status; esophageal cancer, limited to adenocarcinoma or squamous cell carcinoma as predominant cell type; extent of disease initially established as T4, any N, M0 (prior to neoadjuvant therapy, if any) with no evidence of disease progression, recurrence, or metastases (for use in a Medicare-approved demonstration project) M

G9098 Oncology; disease status; esophageal cancer, limited to adenocarcinoma or squamous cell carcinoma as predominant cell type; M1 at diagnosis, metastatic, locally recurrent, or progressive (for use in a Medicare-approved demonstration project) M

G9099 Oncology; disease status; esophageal cancer, limited to adenocarcinoma or squamous cell carcinoma as predominant cell type; extent of disease unknown, staging in progress, or not listed (for use in a Medicare-approved demonstration project) M

G9100 Oncology; disease status; gastric cancer, limited to adenocarcinoma as predominant cell type; post R0 resection (with or without neoadjuvant therapy) with no evidence of disease recurrence, progression, or metastases (for use in a Medicare-approved demonstration project) M

G9101 Oncology; disease status; gastric cancer, limited to adenocarcinoma as predominant cell type; post R1 or R2 resection (with or without neoadjuvant therapy) with no evidence of disease progression, or metastases (for use in a Medicare-approved demonstration project) M

G9102 Oncology; disease status; gastric cancer, limited to adenocarcinoma as predominant cell type; clinical or pathologic M0, unresectable with no evidence of disease progression, or metastases (for use in a Medicare-approved demonstration project) M

G9103 Oncology; disease status; gastric cancer, limited to adenocarcinoma as predominant cell type; clinical or pathologic M1 at diagnosis, metastatic, locally recurrent, or progressive (for use in a Medicare-approved demonstration project) M

G9104 Oncology; disease status; gastric cancer, limited to adenocarcinoma as predominant cell type; extent of disease unknown, staging in progress, or not listed (for use in a Medicare-approved demonstration project) M

G9105 Oncology; disease status; pancreatic cancer, limited to adenocarcinoma as predominant cell type; post R0 resection without evidence of disease progression, recurrence, or metastases (for use in a Medicare-approved demonstration project) M

G9106 Oncology; disease status; pancreatic cancer, limited to adenocarcinoma; post R1 or R2 resection with no evidence of disease progression, or metastases (for use in a Medicare-approved demonstration project) M

Procedures/Professional Services (Temporary)

G9107 — Oncology; disease status; pancreatic cancer, limited to adenocarcinoma; unresectable at diagnosis, M1 at diagnosis, metastatic, locally recurrent, or progressive (for use in a Medicare-approved demonstration project) Ⓜ

G9108 — Oncology; disease status; pancreatic cancer, limited to adenocarcinoma; extent of disease unknown, staging in progress, or not listed (for use in a Medicare-approved demonstration project) Ⓜ

G9109 — Oncology; disease status; head and neck cancer, limited to cancers of oral cavity, pharynx and larynx with squamous cell as predominant cell type; extent of disease initially established as T1-T2 and N0, M0 (prior to neoadjuvant therapy, if any) with no evidence of disease progression, recurrence, or metastases (for use in a Medicare-approved demonstration project) Ⓜ

G9110 — Oncology; disease status; head and neck cancer, limited to cancers of oral cavity, pharynx and larynx with squamous cell as predominant cell type; extent of disease initially established as T3-4 and/or N1-3, M0 (prior to neoadjuvant therapy, if any) with no evidence of disease progression, recurrence, or metastases (for use in a Medicare-approved demonstration project) Ⓜ

G9111 — Oncology; disease status; head and neck cancer, limited to cancers of oral cavity, pharynx and larynx with squamous cell as predominant cell type; M1 at diagnosis, metastatic, locally recurrent, or progressive (for use in a Medicare-approved demonstration project) Ⓜ

G9112 — Oncology; disease status; head and neck cancer, limited to cancers of oral cavity, pharynx and larynx with squamous cell as predominant cell type; extent of disease unknown, staging in progress, or not listed (for use in a Medicare-approved demonstration project) Ⓜ

G9113 — Oncology; disease status; ovarian cancer, limited to epithelial cancer; pathologic Stage IA-B (Grade 1) without evidence of disease progression, recurrence, or metastases (for use in a Medicare-approved demonstration project) ♀ Ⓜ

G9114 — Oncology; disease status; ovarian cancer, limited to epithelial cancer; pathologic Stage IA-B (Grade 2-3); or Stage IC (all grades); or Stage II; without evidence of disease progression, recurrence, or metastases (for use in a Medicare-approved demonstration project) ♀ Ⓜ

G9115 — Oncology; disease status; ovarian cancer, limited to epithelial cancer; pathologic Stage III-IV; without evidence of progression, recurrence, or metastases (for use in a Medicare-approved demonstration project) ♀ Ⓜ

G9116 — Oncology; disease status; ovarian cancer, limited to epithelial cancer; evidence of disease progression, or recurrence, and/or platinum resistance (for use in a Medicare-approved demonstration project) ♀ Ⓜ

G9117 — Oncology; disease status; ovarian cancer, limited to epithelial cancer; extent of disease unknown, staging in progress, or not listed (for use in a Medicare-approved demonstration project) ♀ Ⓜ

G9123 — Oncology; disease status; chronic myelogenous leukemia, limited to Philadelphia chromosome positive and/or BCR-ABL positive; chronic phase not in hematologic, cytogenetic, or molecular remission (for use in a Medicare-approved demonstration project) Ⓜ

G9124 — Oncology; disease status; chronic myelogenous leukemia, limited to Philadelphia chromosome positive and/or BCR-ABL positive; accelerated phase not in hematologic cytogenetic, or molecular remission (for use in a Medicare-approved demonstration project) Ⓜ

G9125 — Oncology; disease status; chronic myelogenous leukemia, limited to Philadelphia chromosome positive and/or BCR-ABL positive; blast phase not in hematologic, cytogenetic, or molecular remission (for use in a Medicare-approved demonstration project) Ⓜ

G9126 — Oncology; disease status; chronic myelogenous leukemia, limited to Philadelphia chromosome positive and/or BCR-ABL positive; in hematologic, cytogenetic, or molecular remission (for use in a Medicare-approved demonstration project) Ⓜ

G9128 — Oncology; disease status; limited to multiple myeloma, systemic disease; smoldering, Stage I (for use in a Medicare-approved demonstration project) Ⓜ

G9129 — Oncology; disease status; limited to multiple myeloma, systemic disease; Stage II or higher (for use in a Medicare-approved demonstration project) Ⓜ

G9130 — Oncology; disease status; limited to multiple myeloma, systemic disease; extent of disease unknown, staging in progress, or not listed (for use in a Medicare-approved demonstration project) Ⓜ

G9131 — Oncology; disease status; invasive female breast cancer (does not include ductal carcinoma in situ); adenocarcinoma as predominant cell type; extent of disease unknown, staging in progress, or not listed (for use in a Medicare-approved demonstration project) ♀ Ⓜ

G9132 — Oncology; disease status; prostate cancer, limited to adenocarcinoma; hormone-refractory/androgen-independent (e.g., rising PSA on antiandrogen therapy or postorchiectomy); clinical metastases (for use in a Medicare-approved demonstration project) ♂ Ⓜ

G9133 — Oncology; disease status; prostate cancer, limited to adenocarcinoma; hormone-responsive; clinical metastases or M1 at diagnosis (for use in a Medicare-approved demonstration project) ♂ Ⓜ

G9134 — Oncology; disease status; non-Hodgkin's lymphoma, any cellular classification; Stage I, II at diagnosis, not relapsed, not refractory (for use in a Medicare-approved demonstration project) Ⓜ

G9135 — Oncology; disease status; non-Hodgkin's lymphoma, any cellular classification; Stage III, IV, not relapsed, not refractory (for use in a Medicare-approved demonstration project) Ⓜ

G9136 — Oncology; disease status; non-Hodgkin's lymphoma, transformed from original cellular diagnosis to a second cellular classification (for use in a Medicare-approved demonstration project) Ⓜ

G9137 — Oncology; disease status; non-Hodgkin's lymphoma, any cellular classification; relapsed/refractory (for use in a Medicare-approved demonstration project) Ⓜ

G9138 — Oncology; disease status; non-Hodgkin's lymphoma, any cellular classification; diagnostic evaluation, stage not determined, evaluation of possible relapse or nonresponse to therapy, or not listed (for use in a Medicare-approved demonstration project) Ⓜ

G9139 — Oncology; disease status; chronic myelogenous leukemia, limited to Philadelphia chromosome positive and/or BCR-ABL positive; extent of disease unknown, staging in progress, not listed (for use in a Medicare-approved demonstration project) Ⓜ

2023 HCPCS Level II G9254

G9140 Frontier Extended Stay Clinic demonstration; for a patient stay in a clinic approved for the CMS demonstration project; the following measures should be present: the stay must be equal to or greater than 4 hours; weather or other conditions must prevent transfer or the case falls into a category of monitoring and observation cases that are permitted by the rules of the demonstration; there is a maximum Frontier Extended Stay Clinic (FESC) visit of 48 hours, except in the case when weather or other conditions prevent transfer; payment is made on each period up to 4 hours, after the first 4 hours

Warfarin Testing

G9143 Warfarin responsiveness testing by genetic technique using any method, any number of specimen(s)
CMS: 100-03,90.1; 100-04,32,250.1; 100-04,32,250.2; 100-04,32,250.3

Outpatient IV Insulin TX

G9147 Outpatient Intravenous Insulin Treatment (OIVIT) either pulsatile or continuous, by any means, guided by the results of measurements for: respiratory quotient; and/or, urine urea nitrogen (UUN); and/or, arterial, venous or capillary glucose; and/or potassium concentration
CMS: 100-03,40.7; 100-04,4,320.1; 100-04,4,320.2

Quality Assurance

G9148 National Committee for Quality Assurance-Level 1 Medical Home

G9149 National Committee for Quality Assurance-Level 2 Medical Home

G9150 National Committee for Quality Assurance-Level 3 Medical Home

G9151 MAPCP Demonstration-state provided services

G9152 MAPCP Demonstration-Community Health Teams

G9153 MAPCP Demonstration-Physician Incentive Pool

Wheelchair Evaluation

G9156 Evaluation for wheelchair requiring face-to-face visit with physician

Monitor

G9157 Transesophageal Doppler used for cardiac monitoring
CMS: 100-04,32,310; 100-04,32,310.2; 100-04,32,310.3

BPCI Services

G9187 Bundled payments for care improvement initiative home visit for patient assessment performed by a qualified health care professional for individuals not considered homebound including, but not limited to, assessment of safety, falls, clinical status, fluid status, medication reconciliation/management, patient compliance with orders/plan of care, performance of activities of daily living, appropriateness of care setting; (for use only in the Medicare-approved bundled payments for care improvement initiative); may not be billed for a 30-day period covered by a transitional care management code

Miscellaneous Quality Measures

G9188 Beta-blocker therapy not prescribed, reason not given

G9189 Beta-blocker therapy prescribed or currently being taken

G9190 Documentation of medical reason(s) for not prescribing beta-blocker therapy (e.g., allergy, intolerance, other medical reasons)

G9191 Documentation of patient reason(s) for not prescribing beta-blocker therapy (e.g., patient declined, other patient reasons)

G9192 Documentation of system reason(s) for not prescribing beta-blocker therapy (e.g., other reasons attributable to the health care system)

G9196 Documentation of medical reason(s) for not ordering a first or second generation cephalosporin for antimicrobial prophylaxis (e.g., patients enrolled in clinical trials, patients with documented infection prior to surgical procedure of interest, patients who were receiving antibiotics more than 24 hours prior to surgery [except colon surgery patients taking oral prophylactic antibiotics], patients who were receiving antibiotics within 24 hours prior to arrival [except colon surgery patients taking oral prophylactic antibiotics], other medical reason(s))

G9197 Documentation of order for first or second generation cephalosporin for antimicrobial prophylaxis

G9198 Order for first or second generation cephalosporin for antimicrobial prophylaxis was not documented, reason not given

G9212 DSM-IVTM criteria for major depressive disorder documented at the initial evaluation

G9213 DSM-IV-TR criteria for major depressive disorder not documented at the initial evaluation, reason not otherwise specified

G9223 Pneumocystis jiroveci pneumonia prophylaxis prescribed within 3 months of low CD4+ cell count below 500 cells/mm3 or a CD4 percentage below 15%

G9225 Foot exam was not performed, reason not given

G9226 Foot examination performed (includes examination through visual inspection, sensory exam with 10-g monofilament plus testing any one of the following: vibration using 128-Hz tuning fork, pinprick sensation, ankle reflexes, or vibration perception threshold, and pulse exam; report when all of the three components are completed)

G9227 Functional outcome assessment documented, care plan not documented, documentation the patient is not eligible for a care plan at the time of the encounter

G9228 Chlamydia, gonorrhea and syphilis screening results documented (report when results are present for all of the three screenings)

G9229 Chlamydia, gonorrhea, and syphilis screening results not documented (patient refusal is the only allowed exception)

G9230 Chlamydia, gonorrhea, and syphilis not screened, reason not given

G9231 Documentation of end stage renal disease (ESRD), dialysis, renal transplant before or during the measurement period or pregnancy during the measurement period

G9242 Documentation of viral load equal to or greater than 200 copies/ml or viral load not performed

G9243 Documentation of viral load less than 200 copies/ml

G9246 Patient did not have at least one medical visit in each 6 month period of the 24 month measurement period, with a minimum of 60 days between medical visits

G9247 Patient had at least one medical visit in each 6 month period of the 24 month measurement period, with a minimum of 60 days between medical visits

G9250 Documentation of patient pain brought to a comfortable level within 48 hours from initial assessment

G9251 Documentation of patient with pain not brought to a comfortable level within 48 hours from initial assessment

G9254 Documentation of patient discharged to home later than post-operative day 2 following CAS

Special Coverage Instructions | Noncovered by Medicare | Carrier Discretion | ☑ Quantity Alert | ● New Code | ○ Recycled/Reinstated | ▲ Revised Code

© 2022 Optum, Inc. | A2-Z3 ASC Pmt | CMS: IOM | AHA: Coding Clinic | DMEPOS Paid | SNF Excluded | G Codes — 71

Code	Description
G9255	Documentation of patient discharged to home no later than post operative day 2 following CAS
G9273	Blood pressure has a systolic value of < 140 and a diastolic value of < 90
G9274	Blood pressure has a systolic value of = 140 and a diastolic value of = 90 or systolic value < 140 and diastolic value = 90 or systolic value = 140 and diastolic value < 90
G9275	Documentation that patient is a current nontobacco user
G9276	Documentation that patient is a current tobacco user
G9277	Documentation that the patient is on daily aspirin or antiplatelet or has documentation of a valid contraindication or exception to aspirin/antiplatelet; contraindications/exceptions include anticoagulant use, allergy to aspirin or antiplatelets, history of gastrointestinal bleed and bleeding disorder. Additionally, the following exceptions documented by the physician as a reason for not taking daily aspirin or antiplatelet are acceptable (use of nonsteroidal anti-inflammatory agents, documented risk for drug interaction, uncontrolled hypertension defined as > 180 systolic or > 110 diastolic or gastroesophageal reflux)
G9278	Documentation that the patient is not on daily aspirin or antiplatelet regimen
G9279	Pneumococcal screening performed and documentation of vaccination received prior to discharge
G9280	Pneumococcal vaccination not administered prior to discharge, reason not specified
G9281	Screening performed and documentation that vaccination not indicated/patient refusal
G9282	Documentation of medical reason(s) for not reporting the histological type or NSCLC-NOS classification with an explanation (e.g., biopsy taken for other purposes in a patient with a history of nonsmall cell lung cancer or other documented medical reasons)
G9283	Nonsmall cell lung cancer biopsy and cytology specimen report documents classification into specific histologic type or classified as NSCLC-NOS with an explanation
G9284	Nonsmall cell lung cancer biopsy and cytology specimen report does not document classification into specific histologic type or classified as NSCLC-NOS with an explanation
G9285	Specimen site other than anatomic location of lung or is not classified as nonsmall cell lung cancer
G9286	Antibiotic regimen prescribed within 10 days after onset of symptoms
G9287	Antibiotic regimen not prescribed within 10 days after onset of symptoms
G9288	Documentation of medical reason(s) for not reporting the histological type or NSCLC-NOS classification with an explanation (e.g., a solitary fibrous tumor in a person with a history of nonsmall cell carcinoma or other documented medical reasons)
G9289	Nonsmall cell lung cancer biopsy and cytology specimen report documents classification into specific histologic type or classified as NSCLC-NOS with an explanation
G9290	Nonsmall cell lung cancer biopsy and cytology specimen report does not document classification into specific histologic type or classified as NSCLC-NOS with an explanation
G9291	Specimen site other than anatomic location of lung, is not classified as nonsmall cell lung cancer or classified as NSCLC-NOS
G9292	Documentation of medical reason(s) for not reporting PT category and a statement on thickness and ulceration and for PT1, mitotic rate (e.g., negative skin biopsies in a patient with a history of melanoma or other documented medical reasons)
G9293	Pathology report does not include the PT category and a statement on thickness and ulceration and for PT1, mitotic rate
G9294	Pathology report includes the PT category and a statement on thickness and ulceration and for PT1, mitotic rate
G9295	Specimen site other than anatomic cutaneous location
G9296	Patients with documented shared decision-making including discussion of conservative (nonsurgical) therapy (e.g., NSAIDs, analgesics, weight loss, exercise, injections) prior to the procedure
G9297	Shared decision-making including discussion of conservative (nonsurgical) therapy (e.g., NSAIDs, analgesics, weight loss, exercise, injections) prior to the procedure, not documented, reason not given
G9298	Patients who are evaluated for venous thromboembolic and cardiovascular risk factors within 30 days prior to the procedure (e.g., history of DVT, PE, MI, arrhythmia and stroke)
G9299	Patients who are not evaluated for venous thromboembolic and cardiovascular risk factors within 30 days prior to the procedure (e.g., history of DVT, PE, MI, arrhythmia and stroke, reason not given)
G9305	Intervention for presence of leak of endoluminal contents through an anastomosis not required
G9306	Intervention for presence of leak of endoluminal contents through an anastomosis required
G9307	No return to the operating room for a surgical procedure, for complications of the principal operative procedure, within 30 days of the principal operative procedure
G9308	Unplanned return to the operating room for a surgical procedure, for complications of the principal operative procedure, within 30 days of the principal operative procedure
G9309	No unplanned hospital readmission within 30 days of principal procedure
G9310	Unplanned hospital readmission within 30 days of principal procedure
G9311	No surgical site infection
G9312	Surgical site infection
G9313	Amoxicillin, with or without clavulanate, not prescribed as first line antibiotic at the time of diagnosis for documented reason
G9314	Amoxicillin, with or without clavulanate, not prescribed as first line antibiotic at the time of diagnosis, reason not given
▲ G9315	Amoxicillin, with or without clavulanate, prescribed as a first line antibiotic at the time of diagnosis
G9316	Documentation of patient-specific risk assessment with a risk calculator based on multi-institutional clinical data, the specific risk calculator used, and communication of risk assessment from risk calculator with the patient or family
G9317	Documentation of patient-specific risk assessment with a risk calculator based on multi-institutional clinical data, the specific risk calculator used, and communication of risk assessment from risk calculator with the patient or family not completed

Code	Description
G9318	Imaging study named according to standardized nomenclature
G9319	Imaging study not named according to standardized nomenclature, reason not given
G9321	Count of previous CT (any type of CT) and cardiac nuclear medicine (myocardial perfusion) studies documented in the 12-month period prior to the current study
G9322	Count of previous CT and cardiac nuclear medicine (myocardial perfusion) studies not documented in the 12-month period prior to the current study, reason not given
G9341	Search conducted for prior patient CT studies completed at nonaffiliated external health care facilities or entities within the past 12-months and are available through a secure, authorized, media-free, shared archive prior to an imaging study being performed
G9342	Search not conducted prior to an imaging study being performed for prior patient CT studies completed at nonaffiliated external health care facilities or entities within the past 12 months and are available through a secure, authorized, media-free, shared archive, reason not given
G9344	Due to system reasons search not conducted for DICOM format images for prior patient CT imaging studies completed at nonaffiliated external health care facilities or entities within the past 12 months that are available through a secure, authorized, media-free, shared archive (e.g., nonaffiliated external health care facilities or entities does not have archival abilities through a shared archival system)
G9345	Follow-up recommendations documented according to recommended guidelines for incidentally detected pulmonary nodules (e.g., follow-up CT imaging studies needed or that no follow-up is needed) based at a minimum on nodule size and patient risk factors
G9347	Follow-up recommendations not documented according to recommended guidelines for incidentally detected pulmonary nodules, reason not given
G9351	More than one CT scan of the paranasal sinuses ordered or received within 90 days after diagnosis
G9352	More than one CT scan of the paranasal sinuses ordered or received within 90 days after the date of diagnosis, reason not given
G9353	More than one CT scan of the paranasal sinuses ordered or received within 90 days after the date of diagnosis for documented reasons (e.g., patients with complications, second CT obtained prior to surgery, other medical reasons)
G9354	One CT scan or no CT scan of the paranasal sinuses ordered within 90 days after the date of diagnosis
G9355	Elective delivery (without medical indication) by Cesarean birth or induction of labor not performed (<39 weeks of gestation)
G9356	Elective delivery (without medical indication) by Cesarean birth or induction of labor performed (<39 weeks of gestation)
G9357	Post-partum screenings, evaluations and education performed
G9358	Post-partum screenings, evaluations and education not performed
G9359	~~Documentation of negative or managed positive TB screen with further evidence that TB is not active prior to treatment with a biologic immune response modifier~~
G9360	~~No documentation of negative or managed positive TB screen~~
G9361	Medical indication for delivery by Cesarean birth or induction of labor (<39 weeks of gestation) [documentation of reason(s) for elective delivery (e.g., hemorrhage and placental complications, hypertension, preeclampsia and eclampsia, rupture of membranes (premature or prolonged), maternal conditions complicating pregnancy/delivery, fetal conditions complicating pregnancy/delivery, late pregnancy, prior uterine surgery, or participation in clinical trial)]
G9364	Sinusitis caused by, or presumed to be caused by, bacterial infection
G9367	At least two orders for high risk medications from the same drug class
G9368	At least two orders for high risk medications from the same drug class not ordered
G9380	Patient offered assistance with end of life issues during the measurement period
G9382	Patient not offered assistance with end of life issues during the measurement period
G9383	Patient received screening for HCV infection within the 12 month reporting period
G9384	Documentation of medical reason(s) for not receiving annual screening for HCV infection (e.g., decompensated cirrhosis indicating advanced disease [i.e., ascites, esophageal variceal bleeding, hepatic encephalopathy], hepatocellular carcinoma, waitlist for organ transplant, limited life expectancy, other medical reasons)
G9385	Documentation of patient reason(s) for not receiving annual screening for HCV infection (e.g., patient declined, other patient reasons)
G9386	Screening for HCV infection not received within the twelve-month reporting period, reason not given
G9393	Patient with an initial PHQ-9 score greater than nine who achieves remission at twelve months as demonstrated by a twelve-month (+/- 30 days) PHQ-9 score of less than five
G9394	Patient who had a diagnosis of bipolar disorder or personality disorder, death, permanent nursing home resident or receiving hospice or palliative care any time during the measurement or assessment period
G9395	Patient with an initial PHQ-9 score greater than nine who did not achieve remission at twelve months as demonstrated by a twelve-month (+/- 30 days) PHQ-9 score greater than or equal to five
G9396	Patient with an initial PHQ-9 score greater than nine who was not assessed for remission at twelve months (+/- 30 days)
G9402	Patient received follow-up within 30 days after discharge
G9403	Clinician documented reason patient was not able to complete 30-day follow-up from acute inpatient setting discharge (e.g., patient death prior to follow-up visit, patient noncompliant for visit follow-up)
▲ G9404	Patient did not receive follow-up within 30 days after discharge
G9405	Patient received follow up within 7 days after discharge
G9406	Clinician documented reason patient was not able to complete 7-day follow-up from acute inpatient setting discharge (i.e., patient death prior to follow-up visit, patient noncompliance for visit follow-up)
▲ G9407	Patient did not receive follow-up within 7 days after discharge
G9408	Patients with cardiac tamponade and/or pericardiocentesis occurring within 30 days

Procedures/Professional Services (Temporary)

Code	Description
G9409	Patients without cardiac tamponade and/or pericardiocentesis occurring within 30 days Ⓜ
G9410	Patient admitted within 180 days, status post CIED implantation, replacement, or revision with an infection requiring device removal or surgical revision Ⓜ
G9411	Patient not admitted within 180 days, status post CIED implantation, replacement, or revision with an infection requiring device removal or surgical revision Ⓜ
G9412	Patient admitted within 180 days, status post CIED implantation, replacement, or revision with an infection requiring device removal or surgical revision Ⓜ
G9413	Patient not admitted within 180 days, status post CIED implantation, replacement, or revision with an infection requiring device removal or surgical revision Ⓜ
G9414	Patient had one dose of meningococcal vaccine (serogroups A, C, W, Y) on or between the patient's 11th and 13th birthdays Ⓜ
G9415	Patient did not have one dose of meningococcal vaccine (serogroups A, C, W, Y) on or between the patient's 11th and 13th birthdays Ⓜ
G9416	Patient had one tetanus, diphtheria toxoids and acellular pertussis vaccine (TDaP) on or between the patient's 10th and 13th birthdays Ⓜ
G9417	Patient did not have one tetanus, diphtheria toxoids and acellular pertussis vaccine (TDaP) on or between the patient's 10th and 13th birthdays Ⓜ
▲ G9418	Primary nonsmall cell lung cancer lung biopsy and cytology specimen report documents classification into specific histologic type following IASLC guidance or classified as NSCLC-NOS with an explanation Ⓜ
G9419	Documentation of medical reason(s) for not including the histological type or NSCLC-NOS classification with an explanation (e.g. specimen insufficient or non-diagnostic, specimen does not contain cancer, or other documented medical reasons) Ⓜ
G9420	Specimen site other than anatomic location of lung or is not classified as primary nonsmall cell lung cancer Ⓜ
G9421	Primary nonsmall cell lung cancer lung biopsy and cytology specimen report does not document classification into specific histologic type or histologic type does not follow IASLC guidance or is classified as NSCLC-NOS but without an explanation Ⓜ
G9422	Primary lung carcinoma resection report documents PT category, PN category and for nonsmall cell lung cancer, histologic type (e.g., squamous cell carcinoma, adenocarcinoma and not NSCLC-NOS) Ⓜ
G9423	Documentation of medical reason for not including PT category, PN category and histologic type (for patient with appropriate exclusion criteria [e.g., metastatic disease, benign tumors, malignant tumors other than carcinomas, inadequate surgical specimens]) Ⓜ
G9424	Specimen site other than anatomic location of lung, or classified as NSCLC-NOS Ⓜ
G9425	Primary lung carcinoma resection report does not document PT category, PN category and for nonsmall cell lung cancer, histologic type (e.g., squamous cell carcinoma, adenocarcinoma) Ⓜ
G9426	Improvement in median time from ED arrival to initial ED oral or parenteral pain medication administration performed for ED admitted patients Ⓜ
G9427	Improvement in median time from ED arrival to initial ED oral or parenteral pain medication administration not performed for ED admitted patients Ⓜ
G9428	Pathology report includes the PT category, thickness, ulceration and mitotic rate, peripheral and deep margin status and presence or absence of microsatellitosis for invasive tumors Ⓜ
G9429	Documentation of medical reason(s) for not including PT category, thickness, ulceration and mitotic rate, peripheral and deep margin status and presence or absence of microsatellitosis for invasive tumors (e.g., negative skin biopsies, insufficient tissue, or other documented medical reasons) Ⓜ
G9430	Specimen site other than anatomic cutaneous location Ⓜ
G9431	Pathology report does not include the PT category, thickness, ulceration and mitotic rate, peripheral and deep margin status and presence or absence of microsatellitosis for invasive tumors Ⓜ
G9432	Asthma well-controlled based on the ACT, C-ACT, ACQ, or ATAQ score and results documented Ⓜ
G9434	Asthma not well-controlled based on the ACT, C-ACT, ACQ, or ATAQ score, or specified asthma control tool not used, reason not given Ⓜ
G9451	Patient received one-time screening for HCV infection Ⓜ
G9452	Documentation of medical reason(s) for not receiving one-time screening for HCV infection (e.g., decompensated cirrhosis indicating advanced disease [i.e., ascites, esophageal variceal bleeding, hepatic encephalopathy], hepatocellular carcinoma, waitlist for organ transplant, limited life expectancy, other medical reasons) Ⓜ
G9453	Documentation of patient reason(s) for not receiving one-time screening for HCV infection (e.g., patient declined, other patient reasons) Ⓜ
G9454	One-time screening for HCV infection not received within 12-month reporting period and no documentation of prior screening for HCV infection, reason not given Ⓜ
G9455	Patient underwent abdominal imaging with ultrasound, contrast enhanced CT or contrast MRI for HCC Ⓜ
G9456	Documentation of medical or patient reason(s) for not ordering or performing screening for HCC. Medical reason: comorbid medical conditions with expected survival < 5 years, hepatic decompensation and not a candidate for liver transplantation, or other medical reasons; patient reasons: patient declined or other patient reasons (e.g., cost of tests, time related to accessing testing equipment) Ⓜ
G9457	Patient did not undergo abdominal imaging and did not have a documented reason for not undergoing abdominal imaging in the submission period Ⓜ
G9458	Patient documented as tobacco user and received tobacco cessation intervention (must include at least one of the following: advice given to quit smoking or tobacco use, counseling on the benefits of quitting smoking or tobacco use, assistance with or referral to external smoking or tobacco cessation support programs, or current enrollment in smoking or tobacco use cessation program) if identified as a tobacco user Ⓜ
G9459	Currently a tobacco nonuser Ⓜ
G9460	Tobacco assessment or tobacco cessation intervention not performed, reason not given Ⓜ
G9468	Patient not receiving corticosteroids greater than or equal to 10 mg/day of prednisone equivalents for 60 or greater consecutive days or a single prescription equating to 600 mg prednisone or greater for all fills Ⓜ

Special Coverage Instructions | Noncovered by Medicare | Carrier Discretion | ☑ Quantity Alert | ● New Code | ○ Recycled/Reinstated | ▲ Revised Code

74 — G Codes | Ⓐ Age Edit | Ⓜ Maternity Edit | ♀ Female Only | ♂ Male Only | Ⓐ-Ⓨ OPPS Status Indicators | © 2022 Optum, Inc.

G9470	Patients not receiving corticosteroids greater than or equal to 10 mg/day of prednisone equivalents for 60 or greater consecutive days or a single prescription equating to 600 mg prednisone or greater for all fills ⓜ
G9471	Within the past 2 years, central dual-energy x-ray absorptiometry (DXA) not ordered or documented ⓜ

Hospice Services

G9473	Services performed by chaplain in the hospice setting, each 15 minutes Ⓑ
G9474	Services performed by dietary counselor in the hospice setting, each 15 minutes Ⓑ
G9475	Services performed by other counselor in the hospice setting, each 15 minutes Ⓑ
G9476	Services performed by volunteer in the hospice setting, each 15 minutes Ⓑ
G9477	Services performed by care coordinator in the hospice setting, each 15 minutes Ⓑ
G9478	Services performed by other qualified therapist in the hospice setting, each 15 minutes Ⓑ
G9479	Services performed by qualified pharmacist in the hospice setting, each 15 minutes Ⓑ

Medicare Care Choice Model Program

G9480	Admission to Medicare Care Choice Model Program (MCCM) Ⓑ

CMS Innovation Center Demonstration Project

G9481	Remote in-home visit for the evaluation and management of a new patient for use only in a Medicare-approved CMS Innovation Center Demonstration Project, which requires these three key components: a problem focused history; a problem focused examination; straightforward medical decision making, furnished in real time using interactive audio and video technology. Counseling and coordination of care with other physicians, other qualified health care professionals or agencies are provided consistent with the nature of the problem(s) and the needs of the patient or the family or both. Usually, the presenting problem(s) are self limited or minor. Typically, 10 minutes are spent with the patient or family or both via real time, audio and video intercommunications technology Ⓑ
G9482	Remote in-home visit for the evaluation and management of a new patient for use only in a Medicare-approved CMS Innovation Center Demonstration Project, which requires these three key components: an expanded problem focused history; an expanded problem focused examination; straightforward medical decision making, furnished in real time using interactive audio and video technology. Counseling and coordination of care with other physicians, other qualified health care professionals or agencies are provided consistent with the nature of the problem(s) and the needs of the patient or the family or both. Usually, the presenting problem(s) are of low to moderate severity. Typically, 20 minutes are spent with the patient or family or both via real time, audio and video intercommunications technology Ⓑ
G9483	Remote in-home visit for the evaluation and management of a new patient for use only in a Medicare-approved CMS Innovation Center Demonstration Project, which requires these three key components: a detailed history; a detailed examination; medical decision making of low complexity, furnished in real time using interactive audio and video technology. Counseling and coordination of care with other physicians, other qualified health care professionals or agencies are provided consistent with the nature of the problem(s) and the needs of the patient or the family or both. Usually, the presenting problem(s) are of moderate severity. Typically, 30 minutes are spent with the patient or family or both via real time, audio and video intercommunications technology Ⓑ
G9484	Remote in-home visit for the evaluation and management of a new patient for use only in a Medicare-approved CMS Innovation Center Demonstration Project, which requires these three key components: a comprehensive history; a comprehensive examination; medical decision making of moderate complexity, furnished in real time using interactive audio and video technology. Counseling and coordination of care with other physicians, other qualified health care professionals or agencies are provided consistent with the nature of the problem(s) and the needs of the patient or the family or both. Usually, the presenting problem(s) are of moderate to high severity. Typically, 45 minutes are spent with the patient or family or both via real time, audio and video intercommunications technology Ⓑ
G9485	Remote in-home visit for the evaluation and management of a new patient for use only in a Medicare-approved CMS Innovation Center Demonstration Project, which requires these three key components: a comprehensive history; a comprehensive examination; medical decision making of high complexity, furnished in real time using interactive audio and video technology. Counseling and coordination of care with other physicians, other qualified health care professionals or agencies are provided consistent with the nature of the problem(s) and the needs of the patient or the family or both. Usually, the presenting problem(s) are of moderate to high severity. Typically, 60 minutes are spent with the patient or family or both via real time, audio and video intercommunications technology Ⓑ
G9486	Remote in-home visit for the evaluation and management of an established patient for use only in a Medicare-approved CMS Innovation Center Demonstration Project, which requires at least two of the following three key components: a problem focused history; a problem focused examination; straightforward medical decision making, furnished in real time using interactive audio and video technology. Counseling and coordination of care with other physicians, other qualified health care professionals or agencies are provided consistent with the nature of the problem(s) and the needs of the patient or the family or both. Usually, the presenting problem(s) are self limited or minor. Typically, 10 minutes are spent with the patient or family or both via real time, audio and video intercommunications technology Ⓑ

Procedures/Professional Services (Temporary)

Code	Description
G9487	Remote in-home visit for the evaluation and management of an established patient for use only in a Medicare-approved CMS Innovation Center Demonstration Project, which requires at least two of the following three key components: an expanded problem focused history; an expanded problem focused examination; medical decision making of low complexity, furnished in real time using interactive audio and video technology. Counseling and coordination of care with other physicians, other qualified health care professionals or agencies are provided consistent with the nature of the problem(s) and the needs of the patient or the family or both. Usually, the presenting problem(s) are of low to moderate severity. Typically, 15 minutes are spent with the patient or family or both via real time, audio and video intercommunications technology ⓑ
G9488	Remote in-home visit for the evaluation and management of an established patient for use only in a Medicare-approved CMS Innovation Center Demonstration Project, which requires at least two of the following three key components: a detailed history; a detailed examination; medical decision making of moderate complexity, furnished in real time using interactive audio and video technology. Counseling and coordination of care with other physicians, other qualified health care professionals or agencies are provided consistent with the nature of the problem(s) and the needs of the patient or the family or both. Usually, the presenting problem(s) are of moderate to high severity. Typically, 25 minutes are spent with the patient or family or both via real time, audio and video intercommunications technology ⓑ
G9489	Remote in-home visit for the evaluation and management of an established patient for use only in a Medicare-approved CMS Innovation Center Demonstration Project, which requires at least two of the following three key components: a comprehensive history; a comprehensive examination; medical decision making of high complexity, furnished in real time using interactive audio and video technology. Counseling and coordination of care with other physicians, other qualified health care professionals or agencies are provided consistent with the nature of the problem(s) and the needs of the patient or the family or both. Usually, the presenting problem(s) are of moderate to high severity. Typically, 40 minutes are spent with the patient or family or both via real time, audio and video intercommunications technology ⓑ
G9490	CMS Innovation Center Models, home visit for patient assessment performed by clinical staff for an individual not considered homebound, including, but not necessarily limited to patient assessment of clinical status, safety/fall prevention, functional status/ambulation, medication reconciliation/management, compliance with orders/plan of care, performance of activities of daily living, and ensuring beneficiary connections to community and other services. (For use only in Medicare-approved CMS Innovation Center Models); may not be billed for a 30 day period covered by a transitional care management code ⓑ

Quality Measures

Code	Description
G9497	Received instruction from the anesthesiologist or proxy prior to the day of surgery to abstain from smoking on the day of surgery Ⓜ
G9498	Antibiotic regimen prescribed Ⓜ
▲ G9500	Radiation exposure indices documented in final report for procedure using fluoroscopy Ⓜ
▲ G9501	Radiation exposure indices not documented in final report for procedure using fluoroscopy, reason not given Ⓜ
G9502	Documentation of medical reason for not performing foot exam (i.e., patients who have had either a bilateral amputation above or below the knee, or both a left and right amputation above or below the knee before or during the measurement period) Ⓜ
G9504	Documented reason for not assessing hepatitis B virus (HBV) status (e.g., patient not initiating anti-TNF therapy, patient declined) prior to initiating anti-TNF therapy Ⓜ
G9505	Antibiotic regimen prescribed within 10 days after onset of symptoms for documented medical reason Ⓜ
G9506	Biologic immune response modifier prescribed
G9507	Documentation that the patient is on a statin medication or has documentation of a valid contraindication or exception to statin medications; contraindications/exceptions that can be defined by diagnosis codes include pregnancy during the measurement period, active liver disease, rhabdomyolysis, end stage renal disease on dialysis and heart failure; provider documented contraindications/exceptions include breastfeeding during the measurement period, woman of child-bearing age not actively taking birth control, allergy to statin, drug interaction (HIV protease inhibitors, nefazodone, cyclosporine, gemfibrozil, and danazol) and intolerance (with supporting documentation of trying a statin at least once within the last 5 years or diagnosis codes for myositis or toxic myopathy related to drugs) Ⓜ
G9508	Documentation that the patient is not on a statin medication Ⓜ
G9509	Adult patients 18 years of age or older with major depression or dysthymia who reached remission at twelve months as demonstrated by a twelve-month (+/-60 days) PHQ-9 or PHQ-9M score of less than 5 Ⓜ
G9510	Adult patients 18 years of age or older with major depression or dysthymia who did not reach remission at 12 months as demonstrated by a 12 month (+/-60 days) PHQ-9 or PHQ-9M score of less than 5. Either PHQ-9 or PHQ-9M score was not assessed or is greater than or equal to 5 Ⓜ
G9511	Index PHQ-9 or PHQ-9M score greater than 9 documented during the twelve-month denominator identification period Ⓜ
G9512	Individual had a PDC of 0.8 or greater Ⓜ
G9513	Individual did not have a PDC of 0.8 or greater Ⓜ
G9514	Patient required a return to the operating room within 90 days of surgery Ⓜ
G9515	Patient did not require a return to the operating room within 90 days of surgery Ⓜ
G9516	Patient achieved an improvement in visual acuity, from their preoperative level, within 90 days of surgery Ⓜ
G9517	Patient did not achieve an improvement in visual acuity, from their preoperative level, within 90 days of surgery, reason not given Ⓜ
G9518	Documentation of active injection drug use Ⓜ
G9519	Patient achieves final refraction (spherical equivalent) +/- 1.0 diopters of their planned refraction within 90 days of surgery Ⓜ
G9520	Patient does not achieve final refraction (spherical equivalent) +/- 1.0 diopters of their planned refraction within 90 days of surgery Ⓜ
G9521	Total number of emergency department visits and inpatient hospitalizations less than two in the past 12 months Ⓜ
G9522	Total number of emergency department visits and inpatient hospitalizations equal to or greater than two in the past 12 months or patient not screened, reason not given Ⓜ

Blunt Head Trauma

G9529 Patient with minor blunt head trauma had an appropriate indication(s) for a head CT ⓜ

G9530 Patient presented with a minor blunt head trauma and had a head CT ordered for trauma by an emergency care provider ⓜ

G9531 Patient has documentation of ventricular shunt, brain tumor, multisystem trauma, or is currently taking an antiplatelet medication including: abciximab, anagrelide, cangrelor, cilostazol, clopidogrel, dipyridamole, eptifibatide, prasugrel, ticlopidine, ticagrelor, tirofiban, or vorapaxar ⓜ

G9533 Patient with minor blunt head trauma did not have an appropriate indication(s) for a head CT ⓜ

Miscellaneous Quality Measures

G9537 Imaging needed as part of a clinical trial; or other clinician ordered the study ⓜ

G9539 Intent for potential removal at time of placement ⓜ

G9540 Patient alive 3 months post procedure ⓜ

G9541 Filter removed within 3 months of placement ⓜ

G9542 Documented reassessment for the appropriateness of filter removal within 3 months of placement ⓜ

G9543 Documentation of at least two attempts to reach the patient to arrange a clinical reassessment for the appropriateness of filter removal within 3 months of placement ⓜ

G9544 Patients that do not have the filter removed, documented reassessment for the appropriateness of filter removal, or documentation of at least two attempts to reach the patient to arrange a clinical reassessment for the appropriateness of filter removal within 3 months of placement ⓜ

G9547 Cystic renal lesion that is simple appearing (Bosniak I or II), or adrenal lesion less than or equal to 1.0 cm or adrenal lesion greater than 1.0 cm but less than or equal to 4.0 cm classified as likely benign by unenhanced CT or washout protocol CT, or MRI with in- and opposed-phase sequences or other equivalent institutional imaging protocols ⓜ

G9548 Final reports for imaging studies stating no follow up imaging is recommended ⓜ

G9549 Documentation of medical reason(s) that follow up imaging is indicated (e.g., patient has lymphadenopathy, signs of metastasis or an active diagnosis or history of cancer, and other medical reason(s)) ⓜ

G9550 Final reports for imaging studies with follow-up imaging recommended, or final reports that do not include a specific recommendation of no follow-up ⓜ

G9551 Final reports for imaging studies without an incidentally found lesion noted ⓜ

G9552 Incidental thyroid nodule < 1.0 cm noted in report ⓜ

G9553 Prior thyroid disease diagnosis ⓜ

G9554 Final reports for CT, CTA, MRI or MRA of the chest or neck with follow-up imaging recommended ⓜ

G9555 Documentation of medical reason(s) for recommending follow up imaging (e.g., patient has multiple endocrine neoplasia, patient has cervical lymphadenopathy, other medical reason(s)) ⓜ

G9556 Final reports for CT, CTA, MRI or MRA of the chest or neck with follow-up imaging not recommended ⓜ

G9557 Final reports for CT, CTA, MRI or MRA studies of the chest or neck without an incidentally found thyroid nodule < 1.0 cm noted or no nodule found ⓜ

Stroke Therapy

G9580 Door to puncture time of 90 minutes or less ⓜ

G9582 Door to puncture time of greater than 90 minutes, no reason given ⓜ

Blunt Head Trauma

G9593 Pediatric patient with minor blunt head trauma classified as low risk according to the PECARN prediction rules ⓜ

G9594 Patient presented with a minor blunt head trauma and had a head CT ordered for trauma by an emergency care provider ⓜ

G9595 Patient has documentation of ventricular shunt, brain tumor, or coagulopathy ⓜ

G9596 Pediatric patient had a head CT for trauma ordered by someone other than an emergency care provider or was ordered for a reason other than trauma ⓜ

G9597 Pediatric patient with minor blunt head trauma not classified as low risk according to the PECARN prediction rules ⓜ

Aortic Aneurysm

G9598 Aortic aneurysm 5.5-5.9 cm maximum diameter on centerline formatted CT or minor diameter on axial formatted CT ⓜ

G9599 Aortic aneurysm 6.0 cm or greater maximum diameter on centerline formatted CT or minor diameter on axial formatted CT ⓜ

Patient Survey

G9603 Patient survey score improved from baseline following treatment ⓜ

G9604 Patient survey results not available ⓜ

G9605 Patient survey score did not improve from baseline following treatment ⓜ

Intraoperative Cystoscopy

G9606 Intraoperative cystoscopy performed to evaluate for lower tract injury ⓜ

G9607 Documented medical reasons for not performing intraoperative cystoscopy (e.g., urethral pathology precluding cystoscopy, any patient who has a congenital or acquired absence of the urethra) or in the case of patient death ⓜ

G9608 Intraoperative cystoscopy not performed to evaluate for lower tract injury ⓜ

Aspirin/Antiplatelet Therapy

G9609 Documentation of an order for antiplatelet agents ⓜ

G9610 Documentation of medical reason(s) in the patient's record for not ordering antiplatelet agents ⓜ

G9611 Order for antiplatelet agents was not documented in the patient's record, reason not given ⓜ

Colonoscopy Documentation

G9612 Photodocumentation of two or more cecal landmarks to establish a complete examination ⓜ

G9613 Documentation of postsurgical anatomy (e.g., right hemicolectomy, ileocecal resection, etc.) ⓜ

G9614 Photodocumentation of less than two cecal landmarks (i.e., no cecal landmarks or only one cecal landmark) to establish a complete examination ⓜ

Uterine Malignancy Screening

G9618 ~~Documentation of screening for uterine malignancy or those that had an ultrasound and/or endometrial sampling of any kind~~

Code	Description
G9620	~~Patient not screened for uterine malignancy, or those that have not had an ultrasound and/or endometrial sampling of any kind, reason not given~~

Alcohol Use

Code	Description
G9621	Patient identified as an unhealthy alcohol user when screened for unhealthy alcohol use using a systematic screening method and received brief counseling M
G9622	Patient not identified as an unhealthy alcohol user when screened for unhealthy alcohol use using a systematic screening method M
G9623	~~Documentation of medical reason(s) for not screening for unhealthy alcohol use (e.g., limited life expectancy, other medical reasons)~~
▲ G9624	Patient not screened for unhealthy alcohol use using a systematic screening method or patient did not receive brief counseling if identified as an unhealthy alcohol user M

Bladder/Ureter Injury

Code	Description
G9625	Patient sustained bladder injury at the time of surgery or discovered subsequently up to 30 days post-surgery M
G9626	Documented medical reason for not reporting bladder injury (e.g., gynecologic or other pelvic malignancy documented, concurrent surgery involving bladder pathology, injury that occurs during urinary incontinence procedure, patient death from nonmedical causes not related to surgery, patient died during procedure without evidence of bladder injury) M
G9627	Patient did not sustain bladder injury at the time of surgery nor discovered subsequently up to 30 days post-surgery M
G9628	Patient sustained bowel injury at the time of surgery or discovered subsequently up to 30 days post-surgery M
G9629	Documented medical reasons for not reporting bowel injury (e.g., gynecologic or other pelvic malignancy documented, planned (e.g., not due to an unexpected bowel injury) resection and/or re-anastomosis of bowel, or patient death from nonmedical causes not related to surgery, patient died during procedure without evidence of bowel injury) M
G9630	Patient did not sustain a bowel injury at the time of surgery nor discovered subsequently up to 30 days post-surgery M
G9631	~~Patient sustained ureter injury at the time of surgery or discovered subsequently up to 30 days postsurgery~~
G9632	~~Documented medical reasons for not reporting ureter injury (e.g., gynecologic or other pelvic malignancy documented, concurrent surgery involving bladder pathology, injury that occurs during a urinary incontinence procedure, patient death from nonmedical causes not related to surgery, patient died during procedure without evidence of ureter injury)~~
G9633	~~Patient did not sustain ureter injury at the time of surgery nor discovered subsequently up to 30 days postsurgery~~

Quality Measures

Code	Description
G9637	Final reports with documentation of one or more dose reduction techniques (e.g., automated exposure control, adjustment of the mA and/or kV according to patient size, use of iterative reconstruction technique) M
G9638	Final reports without documentation of one or more dose reduction techniques (e.g., automated exposure control, adjustment of the mA and/or kV according to patient size, use of iterative reconstruction technique) M
G9642	Current smoker (e.g., cigarette, cigar, pipe, e-cigarette or marijuana) M
G9643	Elective surgery M
G9644	Patients who abstained from smoking prior to anesthesia on the day of surgery or procedure M
G9645	Patients who did not abstain from smoking prior to anesthesia on the day of surgery or procedure M
G9646	Patients with 90 day MRS score of 0 to 2 M
G9648	Patients with 90 day MRS score greater than 2 M

Psoriasis Therapy

Code	Description
G9649	Psoriasis assessment tool documented meeting any one of the specified benchmarks (e.g., (PGA; 5-point or 6-point scale), body surface area (BSA), psoriasis area and severity index (PASI) and/or dermatology life quality index (DLQI)) M
G9651	Psoriasis assessment tool documented not meeting any one of the specified benchmarks (e.g., (PGA; 5-point or 6-point scale), body surface area (BSA), psoriasis area and severity index (PASI) and/or dermatology life quality index (DLQI)) or psoriasis assessment tool not documented M

Anesthesia Services

Code	Description
G9654	Monitored anesthesia care (MAC) M
G9655	A transfer of care protocol or handoff tool/checklist that includes the required key handoff elements is used M
G9656	Patient transferred directly from anesthetizing location to PACU or other non-ICU location M
G9658	A transfer of care protocol or handoff tool/checklist that includes the required key handoff elements is not used M

Reason for Colonoscopy

Code	Description
G9659	Patients greater than or equal to 86 years of age who underwent a screening colonoscopy and did not have a history of colorectal cancer or other valid medical reason for the colonoscopy, including: iron deficiency anemia, lower gastrointestinal bleeding, Crohn's disease (i.e., regional enteritis), familial adenomatous polyposis, Lynch syndrome (i.e., hereditary nonpolyposis colorectal cancer), inflammatory bowel disease, ulcerative colitis, abnormal finding of gastrointestinal tract, or changes in bowel habits M
G9660	Documentation of medical reason(s) for a colonoscopy performed on a patient greater than or equal to 86 years of age (e.g., iron deficiency anemia, lower gastrointestinal bleeding, Crohn's disease (i.e., regional enteritis), familial history of adenomatous polyposis, Lynch syndrome (i.e., hereditary nonpolyposis colorectal cancer), inflammatory bowel disease, ulcerative colitis, abnormal finding of gastrointestinal tract, or changes in bowel habits M
G9661	Patients greater than or equal to 86 years of age who received a colonoscopy for an assessment of signs/symptoms of GI tract illness, and/or because the patient meets high risk criteria, and/or to follow-up on previously diagnosed advanced lesions M

Statin Therapy

Code	Description
▲ G9662	Previously diagnosed or have a diagnosis of clinical ASCVD, including ASCVD procedure M
▲ G9663	Any LDL-C laboratory result >= 190 mg/dl M
G9664	Patients who are currently statin therapy users or received an order (prescription) for statin therapy M
G9665	Patients who are not currently statin therapy users or did not receive an order (prescription) for statin therapy M

Cardiovascular Measures

Code	Description
G9674	Patients with clinical ASCVD diagnosis M

2023 HCPCS Level II — G9719

Code	Description
G9675	Patients who have ever had a fasting or direct laboratory result of LDL-C = 190 mg/dl Ⓜ
G9676	Patients aged 40 to 75 years at the beginning of the measurement period with type 1 or type 2 diabetes and with an ldl-c result of 70-189 mg/dl recorded as the highest fasting or direct laboratory test result in the measurement year or during the two years prior to the beginning of the measurement period Ⓜ

Oncology Demonstration Project

Code	Description
~~G9678~~	~~Oncology Care Model (OCM) Monthly Enhanced Oncology Services (MEOS) payment for OCM-enhanced services. G9678 payments may only be made to OCM practitioners for OCM beneficiaries for the furnishment of enhanced services as defined in the OCM participation agreement~~

Nursing Facility Care

Code	Description
G9679	Onsite acute care treatment of a nursing facility resident with pneumonia. May only be billed once per day per beneficiary Ⓑ
G9680	Onsite acute care treatment of a nursing facility resident with CHF. May only be billed once per day per beneficiary Ⓑ
G9681	Onsite acute care treatment of a nursing facility resident with COPD or asthma. May only be billed once per day per beneficiary Ⓑ
G9682	Onsite acute care treatment of a nursing facility resident with a skin infection. May only be billed once per day per beneficiary Ⓑ
G9683	Facility service(s) for the onsite acute care treatment of a nursing facility resident with fluid or electrolyte disorder. (May only be billed once per day per beneficiary.) This service is for a demonstration project Ⓑ
G9684	Onsite acute care treatment of a nursing facility resident for a UTI. May only be billed once per day per beneficiary Ⓑ
G9685	Physician service or other qualified health care professional for the evaluation and management of a beneficiary's acute change in condition in a nursing facility. This service is for a demonstration project Ⓜ

Other Quality Measures

Code	Description
G9687	Hospice services provided to patient any time during the measurement period Ⓜ
G9688	Patients using hospice services any time during the measurement period Ⓜ
G9689	Patient admitted for performance of elective carotid intervention Ⓜ
G9690	Patient receiving hospice services any time during the measurement period Ⓜ
G9691	Patient had hospice services any time during the measurement period Ⓜ
G9692	Hospice services received by patient any time during the measurement period Ⓜ
G9693	Patient use of hospice services any time during the measurement period Ⓜ
G9694	Hospice services utilized by patient any time during the measurement period Ⓜ
G9695	Long-acting inhaled bronchodilator prescribed Ⓜ
G9696	Documentation of medical reason(s) for not prescribing a long-acting inhaled bronchodilator Ⓜ
G9697	Documentation of patient reason(s) for not prescribing a long-acting inhaled bronchodilator Ⓜ
G9698	Documentation of system reason(s) for not prescribing a long-acting inhaled bronchodilator Ⓜ
G9699	Long-acting inhaled bronchodilator not prescribed, reason not otherwise specified Ⓜ
G9700	Patients who use hospice services any time during the measurement period Ⓜ
G9702	Patients who use hospice services any time during the measurement period Ⓜ
G9703	Episodes where the patient is taking antibiotics (table 1) in the 30 days prior to the episode date, or had an active prescription on the episode date Ⓜ
G9704	AJCC breast cancer Stage I: T1 mic or T1a documented Ⓜ
G9705	AJCC breast cancer Stage I: T1b (tumor > 0.5 cm but <= 1 cm in greatest dimension) documented Ⓜ
G9706	Low (or very low) risk of recurrence, prostate cancer
G9707	Patient received hospice services any time during the measurement period Ⓜ
G9708	Women who had a bilateral mastectomy or who have a history of a bilateral mastectomy or for whom there is evidence of a right and a left unilateral mastectomy
G9709	Hospice services used by patient any time during the measurement period Ⓜ
G9710	Patient was provided hospice services any time during the measurement period Ⓜ
G9711	Patients with a diagnosis or past history of total colectomy or colorectal cancer Ⓜ
G9712	Documentation of medical reason(s) for prescribing or dispensing antibiotic (e.g., intestinal infection, pertussis, bacterial infection, lyme disease, otitis media, acute sinusitis, acute pharyngitis, acute tonsillitis, chronic sinusitis, infection of the pharynx/larynx/tonsils/adenoids, prostatitis, cellulitis/mastoiditis/bone infections, acute lymphadenitis, impetigo, skin staph infections, pneumonia, gonococcal infections/venereal disease (syphilis, chlamydia, inflammatory diseases [female reproductive organs]), infections of the kidney, cystitis/UTI, acne, HIV disease/asymptomatic HIV, cystic fibrosis, disorders of the immune system, malignancy neoplasms, chronic bronchitis, emphysema, bronchiectasis, extrinsic allergic alveolitis, chronic airway obstruction, chronic obstructive asthma, pneumoconiosis and other lung disease due to external agents, other diseases of the respiratory system, and tuberculosis Ⓜ
G9713	Patients who use hospice services any time during the measurement period Ⓜ
G9714	Patient is using hospice services any time during the measurement period Ⓜ
G9715	Patients who use hospice services any time during the measurement period Ⓜ
G9716	BMI is documented as being outside of normal parameters, follow-up plan is not completed for documented medical reason Ⓜ
G9717	Documentation stating the patient has had a diagnosis of depression or has had a diagnosis of bipolar disorder Ⓜ
~~G9718~~	~~Hospice services for patient provided any time during the measurement period~~
G9719	Patient is not ambulatory, bed ridden, immobile, confined to chair, wheelchair bound, dependent on helper pushing wheelchair, independent in wheelchair or minimal help in wheelchair Ⓜ

Procedures/Professional Services (Temporary)   G9675 — G9719

Procedures/Professional Services (Temporary)

G9720 — G9772

Code	Description
G9720	Hospice services for patient occurred any time during the measurement period [M]
G9721	Patient not ambulatory, bed ridden, immobile, confined to chair, wheelchair bound, dependent on helper pushing wheelchair, independent in wheelchair or minimal help in wheelchair [M]
G9722	Documented history of renal failure or baseline serum creatinine >= 4.0 mg/dl; renal transplant recipients are not considered to have preoperative renal failure, unless, since transplantation the CR has been or is 4.0 or higher [M]
G9723	Hospice services for patient received any time during the measurement period [M]
G9724	Patients who had documentation of use of anticoagulant medications overlapping the measurement year [M]
G9725	Patients who use hospice services any time during the measurement period [M]
G9726	Patient refused to participate [M]
G9727	Patient unable to complete the LEPF PROM at initial evaluation and/or discharge due to blindness, illiteracy, severe mental incapacity or language incompatibility and an adequate proxy is not available [M]
G9728	Patient refused to participate [M]
G9729	Patient unable to complete the LEPF PROM at initial evaluation and/or discharge due to blindness, illiteracy, severe mental incapacity or language incompatibility and an adequate proxy is not available [M]
G9730	Patient refused to participate [M]
G9731	Patient unable to complete the LEPF PROM at initial evaluation and/or discharge due to blindness, illiteracy, severe mental incapacity or language incompatibility and an adequate proxy is not available [M]
G9732	Patient refused to participate [M]
G9733	Patient unable to complete the low back FS PROM at initial evaluation and/or discharge due to blindness, illiteracy, severe mental incapacity or language incompatibility and an adequate proxy is not available [M]
G9734	Patient refused to participate [M]
G9735	Patient unable to complete the shoulder FS PROM at initial evaluation and/or discharge due to blindness, illiteracy, severe mental incapacity or language incompatibility and an adequate proxy is not available [M]
G9736	Patient refused to participate [M]
G9737	Patient unable to complete the elbow/wrist/hand FS PROM at initial evaluation and/or discharge due to blindness, illiteracy, severe mental incapacity or language incompatibility and an adequate proxy is not available [M]
G9740	Hospice services given to patient any time during the measurement period [M]
G9741	Patients who use hospice services any time during the measurement period [M]
G9744	Patient not eligible due to active diagnosis of hypertension [M]
G9745	Documented reason for not screening or recommending a follow-up for high blood pressure [M]
G9746	Patient has mitral stenosis or prosthetic heart valves or patient has transient or reversible cause of AF (e.g., pneumonia, hyperthyroidism, pregnancy, cardiac surgery) [M]
G9751	Patient died at any time during the 24-month measurement period [M]
G9752	Emergency surgery [M]
G9753	Documentation of medical reason for not conducting a search for DICOM format images for prior patient CT imaging studies completed at nonaffiliated external healthcare facilities or entities within the past 12 months that are available through a secure, authorized, media-free, shared archive (e.g., trauma, acute myocardial infarction, stroke, aortic aneurysm where time is of the essence) [M]
G9754	A finding of an incidental pulmonary nodule [M]
G9755	Documentation of medical reason(s) for not including a recommended interval and modality for follow-up or for no follow-up, and source of recommendations (e.g., patients with unexplained fever, immunocompromised patients who are at risk for infection) [M]
G9756	Surgical procedures that included the use of silicone oil [M]
G9757	Surgical procedures that included the use of silicone oil [M]
G9758	Patient in hospice at any time during the measurement period [M]
G9760	Patients who use hospice services any time during the measurement period [M]
G9761	Patients who use hospice services any time during the measurement period [M]
G9762	Patient had at least two HPV vaccines (with at least 146 days between the two) or three HPV vaccines on or between the patient's 9th and 13th birthdays [M]
G9763	Patient did not have at least two HPV vaccines (with at least 146 days between the two) or three HPV vaccines on or between the patient's 9th and 13th birthdays [M]
G9764	Patient has been treated with a systemic medication for psoriasis vulgaris [M]
G9765	Documentation that the patient declined change in medication or alternative therapies were unavailable, has documented contraindications, or has not been treated with a systemic medication for at least six consecutive months (e.g., experienced adverse effects or lack of efficacy with all other therapy options) in order to achieve better disease control as measured by PGA, BSA, PASI, or DLQI [M]
G9766	Patients who are transferred from one institution to another with a known diagnosis of CVA for endovascular stroke treatment [M]
G9767	Hospitalized patients with newly diagnosed CVA considered for endovascular stroke treatment [M]
G9768	Patients who utilize hospice services any time during the measurement period [M]
G9769	Patient had a bone mineral density test in the past two years or received osteoporosis medication or therapy in the past 12 months [M]
G9770	Peripheral nerve block (PNB) [M]
G9771	At least one body temperature measurement equal to or greater than 35.5 degrees celsius (or 95.9 degrees fahrenheit) achieved within the 30 minutes immediately before or the 15 minutes immediately after anesthesia end time [M]
G9772	Documentation of medical reason(s) for not achieving at least one body temperature measurement equal to or greater than 35.5 degrees Celsius (or 95.9 degrees Fahrenheit) within the 30 minutes immediately before or the 15 minutes immediately after anesthesia end time (e.g., emergency cases, intentional hypothermia, etc.) [M]

2023 HCPCS Level II

Code	Description
G9773	At least one body temperature measurement equal to or greater than 35.5 degrees celsius (or 95.9 degrees fahrenheit) not achieved within the 30 minutes immediately before or the 15 minutes immediately after anesthesia end time, reason not given M
G9774	Patients who have had a hysterectomy
G9775	Patient received at least two prophylactic pharmacologic antiemetic agents of different classes preoperatively and/or intraoperatively M
G9776	Documentation of medical reason for not receiving at least two prophylactic pharmacologic antiemetic agents of different classes preoperatively and/or intraoperatively (e.g., intolerance or other medical reason) M
G9777	Patient did not receive at least two prophylactic pharmacologic antiemetic agents of different classes preoperatively and/or intraoperatively M
G9778	Patients who have a diagnosis of pregnancy at any time during the measurement period
G9779	Patients who are breastfeeding at any time during the measurement period M
G9780	Patients who have a diagnosis of rhabdomyolysis at any time during the measurement period M
▲ G9781	Documentation of medical reason(s) for not currently being a statin therapy user or receiving an order (prescription) for statin therapy (e.g., patients with statin-associated muscle symptoms or an allergy to statin medication therapy, patients who are receiving palliative or hospice care, patients with active liver disease or hepatic disease or insufficiency, patients with end stage renal disease [ESRD], or other medical reasons) M
G9782	History of or active diagnosis of familial hypercholesterolemia M
G9784	Pathologists/dermatopathologists providing a second opinion on a biopsy M
G9785	Pathology report diagnosing cutaneous basal cell carcinoma, squamous cell carcinoma, or melanoma (to include in situ disease) sent from the pathologist/dermatopathologist to the biopsying clinician for review within 7 days from the time when the tissue specimen was received by the pathologist M
G9786	Pathology report diagnosing cutaneous basal cell carcinoma, squamous cell carcinoma, or melanoma (to include in situ disease) was not sent from the pathologist/dermatopathologist to the biopsying clinician for review within 7 days from the time when the tissue specimen was received by the pathologist M
G9787	Patient alive as of the last day of the measurement year M
G9788	Most recent BP is less than or equal to 140/90 mm Hg M
▲ G9789	Blood pressure recorded during inpatient stays, emergency room visits, or urgent care visits M
G9790	Most recent BP is greater than 140/90 mm Hg, or blood pressure not documented M
G9791	Most recent tobacco status is tobacco free M
G9792	Most recent tobacco status is not tobacco free M
G9793	Patient is currently on a daily aspirin or other antiplatelet M
G9794	Documentation of medical reason(s) for not on a daily aspirin or other antiplatelet (e.g., history of gastrointestinal bleed, intracranial bleed, idiopathic thrombocytopenic purpura (ITP), gastric bypass or documentation of active anticoagulant use during the measurement period) M
G9795	Patient is not currently on a daily aspirin or other antiplatelet M
G9796	Patient is currently on a statin therapy M
G9797	Patient is not on a statin therapy M
G9805	Patients who use hospice services any time during the measurement period M
G9806	Patients who received cervical cytology or an HPV test M
G9807	Patients who did not receive cervical cytology or an HPV test M
G9808	~~Any patients who had no asthma controller medications dispensed during the measurement year~~
G9809	~~Patients who use hospice services any time during the measurement period~~
G9810	~~Patient achieved a PDC of at least 75% for their asthma controller medication~~
G9811	~~Patient did not achieve a PDC of at least 75% for their asthma controller medication~~
G9812	Patient died including all deaths occurring during the hospitalization in which the operation was performed, even if after 30 days, and those deaths occurring after discharge from the hospital, but within 30 days of the procedure M
G9813	Patient did not die within 30 days of the procedure or during the index hospitalization M
G9818	Documentation of sexual activity M
G9819	Patients who use hospice services any time during the measurement period M
G9820	Documentation of a chlamydia screening test with proper follow-up M
G9821	No documentation of a chlamydia screening test with proper follow-up M
G9822	Patients who had an endometrial ablation procedure during the 12 months prior to the index date (exclusive of the index date) M
G9823	Endometrial sampling or hysteroscopy with biopsy and results documented during the 12 months prior to the index date (exclusive of the index date) of the endometrial ablation M
G9824	Endometrial sampling or hysteroscopy with biopsy and results not documented during the 12 months prior to the index date (exclusive of the index date) of the endometrial ablation M
G9830	HER2/neu positive M
G9831	AJCC Stage at breast cancer diagnosis = II or III M
G9832	AJCC Stage at breast cancer diagnosis = I (Ia or Ib) and T-Stage at breast cancer diagnosis does not equal = T1, T1a, T1b M
G9838	Patient has metastatic disease at diagnosis M
G9839	Anti-EGFR monoclonal antibody therapy M
G9840	RAS (KRAS and NRAS) gene mutation testing performed before initiation of anti-EGFR MoAb M
G9841	RAS (KRAS and NRAS) gene mutation testing not performed before initiation of anti-EGFR MoAb M
G9842	Patient has metastatic disease at diagnosis M
G9843	RAS (KRAS or NRAS) gene mutation M
G9844	Patient did not receive anti-EGFR monoclonal antibody therapy M
G9845	Patient received anti-EGFR monoclonal antibody therapy M
G9846	Patients who died from cancer M
▲ G9847	Patient received systemic cancer-directed therapy in the last 14 days of life M

Special Coverage Instructions | Noncovered by Medicare | Carrier Discretion | ☑ Quantity Alert | ● New Code | ○ Recycled/Reinstated | ▲ Revised Code

© 2022 Optum, Inc. | A2-Z3 ASC Pmt | CMS: IOM | AHA: Coding Clinic | DMEPOS Paid | ⊘ SNF Excluded | G Codes — 81

Code	Description
▲ G9848	Patient did not receive systemic cancer-directed therapy in the last 14 days of life [M]
G9852	Patients who died from cancer [M]
G9853	Patient admitted to the ICU in the last 30 days of life [M]
G9854	Patient was not admitted to the ICU in the last 30 days of life [M]
G9858	Patient enrolled in hospice [M]
G9859	Patients who died from cancer [M]
G9860	Patient spent less than three days in hospice care [M]
G9861	Patient spent greater than or equal to three days in hospice care [M]
G9862	Documentation of medical reason(s) for not recommending at least a 10 year follow-up interval (e.g., inadequate prep, familial or personal history of colonic polyps, patient had no adenoma and age is = 66 years old, or life expectancy < 10 years old, other medical reasons) [M]
G9868	Receipt and analysis of remote, asynchronous images for dermatologic and/or ophthalmologic evaluation, for use only in a Medicare-approved CMMI model, less than 10 minutes [B] AHA: 2Q,21
G9869	Receipt and analysis of remote, asynchronous images for dermatologic and/or ophthalmologic evaluation, for use only in a Medicare-approved CMMI model, 10 to 20 minutes [B] AHA: 2Q,21
G9870	Receipt and analysis of remote, asynchronous images for dermatologic and/or ophthalmologic evaluation, for use only in a Medicare-approved CMMI model, more than 20 minutes [B] AHA: 2Q,21
G9873	First Medicare Diabetes Prevention Program (MDPP) core session was attended by an MDPP beneficiary under the MDPP Expanded Model (EM). A core session is an MDPP service that: (1) is furnished by an MDPP supplier during months 1 through 6 of the MDPP services period; (2) is approximately 1 hour in length; and (3) adheres to a CDC-approved DPP curriculum for core sessions [M]
G9874	Four total Medicare Diabetes Prevention Program (MDPP) core sessions were attended by an MDPP beneficiary under the MDPP Expanded Model (EM). A core session is an MDPP service that: (1) is furnished by an MDPP supplier during months 1 through 6 of the MDPP services period; (2) is approximately 1 hour in length; and (3) adheres to a CDC-approved DPP curriculum for core sessions [M]
G9875	Nine total Medicare Diabetes Prevention Program (MDPP) core sessions were attended by an MDPP beneficiary under the MDPP Expanded Model (EM). A core session is an MDPP service that: (1) is furnished by an MDPP supplier during months 1 through 6 of the MDPP services period; (2) is approximately 1 hour in length; and (3) adheres to a CDC-approved DPP curriculum for core sessions [M]
G9876	Two Medicare Diabetes Prevention Program (MDPP) core maintenance sessions (MS) were attended by an MDPP beneficiary in months (mo) 7-9 under the MDPP Expanded Model (EM). A core maintenance session is an MDPP service that: (1) is furnished by an MDPP supplier during months 7 through 12 of the MDPP services period; (2) is approximately 1 hour in length; and (3) adheres to a CDC-approved DPP curriculum for maintenance sessions. The beneficiary did not achieve at least 5% weight loss (WL) from his/her baseline weight, as measured by at least one in-person weight measurement at a core maintenance session in months 7-9 [M]
G9877	Two Medicare Diabetes Prevention Program (MDPP) core maintenance sessions (MS) were attended by an MDPP beneficiary in months (mo) 10-12 under the MDPP Expanded Model (EM). A core maintenance session is an MDPP service that: (1) is furnished by an MDPP supplier during months 7 through 12 of the MDPP services period; (2) is approximately 1 hour in length; and (3) adheres to a CDC-approved DPP curriculum for maintenance sessions. The beneficiary did not achieve at least 5% weight loss (WL) from his/her baseline weight, as measured by at least one in-person weight measurement at a core maintenance session in months 10-12 [M]
G9878	Two Medicare Diabetes Prevention Program (MDPP) core maintenance sessions (MS) were attended by an MDPP beneficiary in months (mo) 7-9 under the MDPP Expanded Model (EM). A core maintenance session is an MDPP service that: (1) is furnished by an MDPP supplier during months 7 through 12 of the MDPP services period; (2) is approximately 1 hour in length; and (3) adheres to a CDC-approved DPP curriculum for maintenance sessions. The beneficiary achieved at least 5% weight loss (WL) from his/her baseline weight, as measured by at least one in-person weight measurement at a core maintenance session in months 7-9 [M]
G9879	Two Medicare Diabetes Prevention Program (MDPP) core maintenance sessions (MS) were attended by an MDPP beneficiary in months (mo) 10-12 under the MDPP Expanded Model (EM). A core maintenance session is an MDPP service that: (1) is furnished by an MDPP supplier during months 7 through 12 of the MDPP services period; (2) is approximately 1 hour in length; and (3) adheres to a CDC-approved DPP curriculum for maintenance sessions. The beneficiary achieved at least 5% weight loss (WL) from his/her baseline weight, as measured by at least one in-person weight measurement at a core maintenance session in months 10-12 [M]
G9880	The MDPP beneficiary achieved at least 5% weight loss (WL) from his/her baseline weight in months 1-12 of the MDPP services period under the MDPP Expanded Model (EM). This is a one-time payment available when a beneficiary first achieves at least 5% weight loss from baseline as measured by an in-person weight measurement at a core session or core maintenance session [M]
G9881	The MDPP beneficiary achieved at least 9% weight loss (WL) from his/her baseline weight in months 1-24 under the MDPP Expanded Model (EM). This is a one-time payment available when a beneficiary first achieves at least 9% weight loss from baseline as measured by an in-person weight measurement at a core session, core maintenance session, or ongoing maintenance session [M]
G9882	Two Medicare Diabetes Prevention Program (MDPP) ongoing maintenance sessions (MS) were attended by an MDPP beneficiary in months (mo) 13-15 under the MDPP Expanded Model (EM). An ongoing maintenance session is an MDPP service that: (1) is furnished by an MDPP supplier during months 13 through 24 of the MDPP services period; (2) is approximately 1 hour in length; and (3) adheres to a CDC-approved DPP curriculum for maintenance sessions. The beneficiary maintained at least 5% weight loss (WL) from his/her baseline weight, as measured by at least one in-person weight measurement at an ongoing maintenance session in months 13-15 [M]

2023 HCPCS Level II — G9920

Code	Description
G9883	Two Medicare Diabetes Prevention Program (MDPP) ongoing maintenance sessions (MS) were attended by an MDPP beneficiary in months (mo) 16-18 under the MDPP Expanded Model (EM). An ongoing maintenance session is an MDPP service that: (1) is furnished by an MDPP supplier during months 13 through 24 of the MDPP services period; (2) is approximately 1 hour in length; and (3) adheres to a CDC-approved DPP curriculum for maintenance sessions. The beneficiary maintained at least 5% weight loss (WL) from his/her baseline weight, as measured by at least one in-person weight measurement at an ongoing maintenance session in months 16-18 Ⓜ
G9884	Two Medicare Diabetes Prevention Program (MDPP) ongoing maintenance sessions (MS) were attended by an MDPP beneficiary in months (mo) 19-21 under the MDPP Expanded Model (EM). An ongoing maintenance session is an MDPP service that: (1) is furnished by an MDPP supplier during months 13 through 24 of the MDPP services period; (2) is approximately 1 hour in length; and (3) adheres to a CDC-approved DPP curriculum for maintenance sessions. The beneficiary maintained at least 5% weight loss (WL) from his/her baseline weight, as measured by at least one in-person weight measurement at an ongoing maintenance session in months 19-21 Ⓜ
G9885	Two Medicare Diabetes Prevention Program (MDPP) ongoing maintenance sessions (MS) were attended by an MDPP beneficiary in months (mo) 22-24 under the MDPP Expanded Model (EM). An ongoing maintenance session is an MDPP service that: (1) is furnished by an MDPP supplier during months 13 through 24 of the MDPP services period; (2) is approximately 1 hour in length; and (3) adheres to a CDC-approved DPP curriculum for maintenance sessions. The beneficiary maintained at least 5% weight loss (WL) from his/her baseline weight, as measured by at least one in-person weight measurement at an ongoing maintenance session in months 22-24 Ⓜ
G9890	Bridge Payment: A one-time payment for the first Medicare Diabetes Prevention Program (MDPP) core session, core maintenance session, or ongoing maintenance session furnished by an MDPP supplier to an MDPP beneficiary during months 1-24 of the MDPP Expanded Model (EM) who has previously received MDPP services from a different MDPP supplier under the MDPP Expanded Model. A supplier may only receive one bridge payment per MDPP beneficiary Ⓜ
G9891	MDPP session reported as a line-item on a claim for a payable MDPP Expanded Model (EM) HCPCS code for a session furnished by the billing supplier under the MDPP Expanded Model and counting toward achievement of the attendance performance goal for the payable MDPP Expanded Model HCPCS code. (This code is for reporting purposes only) Ⓜ
G9892	Documentation of patient reason(s) for not performing a dilated macular examination Ⓜ
G9893	Dilated macular exam was not performed, reason not otherwise specified Ⓜ
G9894	Androgen deprivation therapy prescribed/administered in combination with external beam radiotherapy to the prostate Ⓜ
G9895	Documentation of medical reason(s) for not prescribing/administering androgen deprivation therapy in combination with external beam radiotherapy to the prostate (e.g., salvage therapy) Ⓜ
G9896	Documentation of patient reason(s) for not prescribing/administering androgen deprivation therapy in combination with external beam radiotherapy to the prostate Ⓜ
G9897	Patients who were not prescribed/administered androgen deprivation therapy in combination with external beam radiotherapy to the prostate, reason not given Ⓜ
G9898	Patients age 66 or older in institutional special needs plans (SNP) or residing in long-term care with POS code 32, 33, 34, 54, or 56 for more than 90 consecutive days during the measurement period Ⓜ
G9899	Screening, diagnostic, film, digital or digital breast tomosynthesis (3D) mammography results documented and reviewed Ⓜ
G9900	Screening, diagnostic, film, digital or digital breast tomosynthesis (3D) mammography results were not documented and reviewed, reason not otherwise specified Ⓜ
G9901	Patient age 66 or older in institutional special needs plans (SNP) or residing in long-term care with POS code 32, 33, 34, 54, or 56 for more than 90 consecutive days during the measurement period Ⓜ
G9902	Patient screened for tobacco use and identified as a tobacco user Ⓜ
G9903	Patient screened for tobacco use and identified as a tobacco nonuser Ⓜ
G9904	~~Documentation of medical reason(s) for not screening for tobacco use (e.g., limited life expectancy, other medical reason)~~
▲ G9905	Patient not screened for tobacco use Ⓜ
▲ G9906	Patient identified as a tobacco user received tobacco cessation intervention during the measurement period or in the 6 months prior to the measurement period (counseling and/or pharmacotherapy) Ⓜ
G9907	~~Documentation of medical reason(s) for not providing tobacco cessation intervention on the date of the encounter or within the previous 12 months (e.g., limited life expectancy, other medical reason)~~
▲ G9908	Patient identified as tobacco user did not receive tobacco cessation intervention during the measurement period or in the 6 months prior to the measurement period (counseling and/or pharmacotherapy) Ⓜ
G9909	~~Documentation of medical reason(s) for not providing tobacco cessation intervention on the date of the encounter or within the previous 12 months if identified as a tobacco user (e.g., limited life expectancy, other medical reason)~~
G9910	Patients age 66 or older in institutional special needs plans (SNP) or residing in long-term care with POS code 32, 33, 34, 54 or 56 for more than 90 consecutive days during the measurement period Ⓜ
G9911	Clinically node negative (T1N0M0 or T2N0M0) invasive breast cancer before or after neoadjuvant systemic therapy Ⓜ
G9912	Hepatitis B virus (HBV) status assessed and results interpreted prior to initiating anti-TNF (tumor necrosis factor) therapy Ⓜ
▲ G9913	Hepatitis B virus (HBV) status not assessed and results interpreted prior to initiating anti-TNF (tumor necrosis factor) therapy, reason not otherwise specified Ⓜ
G9914	Patient receiving an anti-TNF agent Ⓜ
G9915	No record of HBV results documented Ⓜ
G9916	Functional status performed once in the last 12 months Ⓜ
G9917	Documentation of advanced stage dementia and caregiver knowledge is limited Ⓜ
G9918	Functional status not performed, reason not otherwise specified Ⓜ
G9919	Screening performed and positive and provision of recommendations Ⓜ
G9920	Screening performed and negative Ⓜ

Procedures/Professional Services (Temporary) — G9921–G9978

Code	Description
G9921	No screening performed, partial screening performed or positive screen without recommendations and reason is not given or otherwise specified
G9922	Safety concerns screen provided and if positive then documented mitigation recommendations
G9923	Safety concerns screen provided and negative
G9925	Safety concerns screening not provided, reason not otherwise specified
G9926	Safety concerns screening positive screen is without provision of mitigation recommendations, including but not limited to referral to other resources
G9927	Documentation of system reason(s) for not prescribing an FDA-approved anticoagulation due to patient being currently enrolled in a clinical trial related to AF/atrial flutter treatment
G9928	FDA-approved anticoagulant not prescribed, reason not given
G9929	Patient with transient or reversible cause of AF (e.g., pneumonia, hyperthyroidism, pregnancy, cardiac surgery)
G9930	Patients who are receiving comfort care only
G9931	Documentation of CHA2DS2-VASc risk score of 0 or 1 for men; or 0, 1, or 2 for women
G9932	~~Documentation of patient reason(s) for not having records of negative or managed positive TB screen (e.g., patient does not return for Mantoux (PPD) skin test evaluation)~~
G9938	Patients age 66 or older in institutional special needs plans (SNP) or residing in long-term care with POS code 32, 33, 34, 54, or 56 for more than 90 consecutive days during the six months prior to the measurement period through December 31 of the measurement period
G9939	Pathologist(s)/dermatopathologist(s) is the same clinician who performed the biopsy
G9940	Documentation of medical reason(s) for not on a statin (e.g., pregnancy, in vitro fertilization, clomiphene Rx, ESRD, cirrhosis, muscular pain and disease during the measurement period or prior year)
G9942	~~Patient had any additional spine procedures performed on the same date as the lumbar discectomy/laminectomy~~
▲ G9943	Back pain was not measured by the visual analog scale (VAS) or numeric pain scale at three months (6 to 20 weeks) postoperatively
G9945	Patient had cancer, acute fracture or infection related to the lumbar spine or patient had neuromuscular, idiopathic or congenital lumbar scoliosis
▲ G9946	Back pain was not measured by the visual analog scale (VAS) or numeric pain scale at one year (9 to 15 months) postoperatively
G9948	~~Patient had any additional spine procedures performed on the same date as the lumbar discectomy/laminectomy~~
▲ G9949	Leg pain was not measured by the visual analog scale (VAS) or numeric pain scale at three months (6 to 20 weeks) postoperatively
G9954	Patient exhibits 2 or more risk factors for postoperative vomiting
G9955	Cases in which an inhalational anesthetic is used only for induction
G9956	Patient received combination therapy consisting of at least two prophylactic pharmacologic antiemetic agents of different classes preoperatively and/or intraoperatively
G9957	Documentation of medical reason for not receiving combination therapy consisting of at least two prophylactic pharmacologic antiemetic agents of different classes preoperatively and/or intraoperatively (e.g., intolerance or other medical reason)
G9958	Patient did not receive combination therapy consisting of at least two prophylactic pharmacologic antiemetic agents of different classes preoperatively and/or intraoperatively
G9959	Systemic antimicrobials not prescribed
G9960	Documentation of medical reason(s) for prescribing systemic antimicrobials
G9961	Systemic antimicrobials prescribed
G9962	Embolization endpoints are documented separately for each embolized vessel and ovarian artery angiography or embolization performed in the presence of variant uterine artery anatomy
G9963	Embolization endpoints are not documented separately for each embolized vessel or ovarian artery angiography or embolization not performed in the presence of variant uterine artery anatomy
G9964	Patient received at least one well-child visit with a PCP during the performance period
G9965	Patient did not receive at least one well-child visit with PCP during the performance period
▲ G9968	Patient was referred to another clinician or specialist during the measurement period
▲ G9969	Clinician who referred the patient to another clinician received a report from the clinician to whom the patient was referred
▲ G9970	Clinician who referred the patient to another clinician did not receive a report from the clinician to whom the patient was referred
G9974	Dilated macular exam performed, including documentation of the presence or absence of macular thickening or geographic atrophy or hemorrhage and the level of macular degeneration severity
G9975	Documentation of medical reason(s) for not performing a dilated macular examination
G9976	Documentation of patient reason(s) for not performing a dilated macular examination
G9977	Dilated macular exam was not performed, reason not otherwise specified
G9978	Remote in-home visit for the evaluation and management of a new patient for use only in a Medicare-approved Bundled Payments for Care Improvement Advanced (BPCI Advanced) model episode of care, which requires these three key components: a problem focused history; a problem focused examination; straightforward medical decision making, furnished in real time using interactive audio and video technology. Counseling and coordination of care with other physicians, other qualified health care professionals or agencies are provided consistent with the nature of the problem(s) and the needs of the patient or the family or both. Usually, the presenting problem(s) are self limited or minor. Typically, 10 minutes are spent with the patient or family or both via real time, audio and video intercommunications technology

2023 HCPCS Level II

G9979 Remote in-home visit for the evaluation and management of a new patient for use only in a Medicare-approved Bundled Payments for Care Improvement Advanced (BPCI Advanced) model episode of care, which requires these three key components: an expanded problem focused history; an expanded problem focused examination; straightforward medical decision making, furnished in real time using interactive audio and video technology. Counseling and coordination of care with other physicians, other qualified health care professionals or agencies are provided consistent with the nature of the problem(s) and the needs of the patient or the family or both. Usually, the presenting problem(s) are of low to moderate severity. Typically, 20 minutes are spent with the patient or family or both via real time, audio and video intercommunications technology

G9980 Remote in-home visit for the evaluation and management of a new patient for use only in a Medicare-approved Bundled Payments for Care Improvement Advanced (BPCI Advanced) model episode of care, which requires these three key components: a detailed history; a detailed examination; medical decision making of low complexity, furnished in real time using interactive audio and video technology. Counseling and coordination of care with other physicians, other qualified health care professionals or agencies are provided consistent with the nature of the problem(s) and the needs of the patient or the family or both. Usually, the presenting problem(s) are of moderate severity. Typically, 30 minutes are spent with the patient or family or both via real time, audio and video intercommunications technology

G9981 Remote in-home visit for the evaluation and management of a new patient for use only in a Medicare-approved Bundled Payments for Care Improvement Advanced (BPCI Advanced) model episode of care, which requires these three key components: a comprehensive history; a comprehensive examination; medical decision making of moderate complexity, furnished in real time using interactive audio and video technology. Counseling and coordination of care with other physicians, other qualified health care professionals or agencies are provided consistent with the nature of the problem(s) and the needs of the patient or the family or both. Usually, the presenting problem(s) are of moderate to high severity. Typically, 45 minutes are spent with the patient or family or both via real time, audio and video intercommunications technology

G9982 Remote in-home visit for the evaluation and management of a new patient for use only in a Medicare-approved Bundled Payments for Care Improvement Advanced (BPCI Advanced) model episode of care, which requires these three key components: a comprehensive history; a comprehensive examination; medical decision making of high complexity, furnished in real time using interactive audio and video technology. Counseling and coordination of care with other physicians, other qualified health care professionals or agencies are provided consistent with the nature of the problem(s) and the needs of the patient or the family or both. Usually, the presenting problem(s) are of moderate to high severity. Typically, 60 minutes are spent with the patient or family or both via real time, audio and video intercommunications technology

G9983 Remote in-home visit for the evaluation and management of an established patient for use only in a Medicare-approved Bundled Payments for Care Improvement Advanced (BPCI Advanced) model episode of care, which requires at least two of the following three key components: a problem focused history; a problem focused examination; straightforward medical decision making, furnished in real time using interactive audio and video technology. Counseling and coordination of care with other physicians, other qualified health care professionals or agencies are provided consistent with the nature of the problem(s) and the needs of the patient or the family or both. Usually, the presenting problem(s) are self limited or minor. Typically, 10 minutes are spent with the patient or family or both via real time, audio and video intercommunications technology

G9984 Remote in-home visit for the evaluation and management of an established patient for use only in a Medicare-approved Bundled Payments for Care Improvement Advanced (BPCI Advanced) model episode of care, which requires at least two of the following three key components: an expanded problem focused history; an expanded problem focused examination; medical decision making of low complexity, furnished in real time using interactive audio and video technology. Counseling and coordination of care with other physicians, other qualified health care professionals or agencies are provided consistent with the nature of the problem(s) and the needs of the patient or the family or both. Usually, the presenting problem(s) are of low to moderate severity. Typically, 15 minutes are spent with the patient or family or both via real time, audio and video intercommunications technology

G9985 Remote in-home visit for the evaluation and management of an established patient for use only in a Medicare-approved Bundled Payments for Care Improvement Advanced (BPCI Advanced) model episode of care, which requires at least two of the following three key components: a detailed history; a detailed examination; medical decision making of moderate complexity, furnished in real time using interactive audio and video technology. Counseling and coordination of care with other physicians, other qualified health care professionals or agencies are provided consistent with the nature of the problem(s) and the needs of the patient or the family or both. Usually, the presenting problem(s) are of moderate to high severity. Typically, 25 minutes are spent with the patient or family or both via real time, audio and video intercommunications technology

G9986 Remote in-home visit for the evaluation and management of an established patient for use only in a Medicare-approved Bundled Payments for Care Improvement Advanced (BPCI Advanced) model episode of care, which requires at least two of the following three key components: a comprehensive history; a comprehensive examination; medical decision making of high complexity, furnished in real time using interactive audio and video technology. Counseling and coordination of care with other physicians, other qualified health care professionals or agencies are provided consistent with the nature of the problem(s) and the needs of the patient or the family or both. Usually, the presenting problem(s) are of moderate to high severity. Typically, 40 minutes are spent with the patient or family or both via real time, audio and video intercommunications technology

Procedures/Professional Services (Temporary)

G9987 — G9999

Code	Description
G9987	Bundled Payments for Care Improvement Advanced (BPCI Advanced) model home visit for patient assessment performed by clinical staff for an individual not considered homebound, including, but not necessarily limited to patient assessment of clinical status, safety/fall prevention, functional status/ambulation, medication reconciliation/management, compliance with orders/plan of care, performance of activities of daily living, and ensuring beneficiary connections to community and other services; for use only for a BPCI Advanced model episode of care; may not be billed for a 30-day period covered by a transitional care management code
G9988	Palliative care services provided to patient any time during the measurement period
G9989	~~Documentation of medical reason(s) for not administering pneumococcal vaccine (e.g., adverse reaction to vaccine)~~
▲ G9990	Patient did not receive any pneumococcal conjugate or polysaccharide vaccine on or after their 60th birthday and before the end of the measurement period
▲ G9991	Patient received any pneumococcal conjugate or polysaccharide vaccine on or after their 60th birthday and before the end of the measurement period
G9992	Palliative care services used by patient any time during the measurement period
▲ G9993	Patient was provided palliative care services any time during the measurement period
G9994	Patient is using palliative care services any time during the measurement period
G9995	Patients who use palliative care services any time during the measurement period
G9996	Documentation stating the patient has received or is currently receiving palliative or hospice care
G9997	Documentation of patient pregnancy anytime during the measurement period prior to and including the current encounter
G9998	Documentation of medical reason(s) for an interval of less than 3 years since the last colonoscopy (e.g., last colonoscopy incomplete, last colonoscopy had inadequate prep, piecemeal removal of adenomas, last colonoscopy found greater than 10 adenomas, or patient at high risk for colon cancer [Crohn's disease, ulcerative colitis, lower gastrointestinal bleeding, personal or family history of colon cancer, hereditary colorectal cancer syndromes])
G9999	Documentation of system reason(s) for an interval of less than 3 years since the last colonoscopy (e.g., unable to locate previous colonoscopy report, previous colonoscopy report was incomplete)

Alcohol and Drug Abuse Treatment Services H0001-H2037

The H codes are used by those state Medicaid agencies that are mandated by state law to establish separate codes for identifying mental health services that include alcohol and drug treatment services.

Code	Description
H0001	Alcohol and/or drug assessment
H0002	Behavioral health screening to determine eligibility for admission to treatment program
H0003	Alcohol and/or drug screening; laboratory analysis of specimens for presence of alcohol and/or drugs
H0004	Behavioral health counseling and therapy, per 15 minutes ☑
H0005	Alcohol and/or drug services; group counseling by a clinician
H0006	Alcohol and/or drug services; case management
H0007	Alcohol and/or drug services; crisis intervention (outpatient)
H0008	Alcohol and/or drug services; subacute detoxification (hospital inpatient)
H0009	Alcohol and/or drug services; acute detoxification (hospital inpatient)
H0010	Alcohol and/or drug services; subacute detoxification (residential addiction program inpatient)
H0011	Alcohol and/or drug services; acute detoxification (residential addiction program inpatient)
H0012	Alcohol and/or drug services; subacute detoxification (residential addiction program outpatient)
H0013	Alcohol and/or drug services; acute detoxification (residential addiction program outpatient)
H0014	Alcohol and/or drug services; ambulatory detoxification
H0015	Alcohol and/or drug services; intensive outpatient (treatment program that operates at least 3 hours/day and at least 3 days/week and is based on an individualized treatment plan), including assessment, counseling; crisis intervention, and activity therapies or education
H0016	Alcohol and/or drug services; medical/somatic (medical intervention in ambulatory setting)
H0017	Behavioral health; residential (hospital residential treatment program), without room and board, per diem ☑
H0018	Behavioral health; short-term residential (nonhospital residential treatment program), without room and board, per diem ☑
H0019	Behavioral health; long-term residential (nonmedical, nonacute care in a residential treatment program where stay is typically longer than 30 days), without room and board, per diem ☑
H0020	Alcohol and/or drug services; methadone administration and/or service (provision of the drug by a licensed program)
H0021	Alcohol and/or drug training service (for staff and personnel not employed by providers)
H0022	Alcohol and/or drug intervention service (planned facilitation)
H0023	Behavioral health outreach service (planned approach to reach a targeted population)
H0024	Behavioral health prevention information dissemination service (one-way direct or nondirect contact with service audiences to affect knowledge and attitude)
H0025	Behavioral health prevention education service (delivery of services with target population to affect knowledge, attitude and/or behavior)
H0026	Alcohol and/or drug prevention process service, community-based (delivery of services to develop skills of impactors)
H0027	Alcohol and/or drug prevention environmental service (broad range of external activities geared toward modifying systems in order to mainstream prevention through policy and law)
H0028	Alcohol and/or drug prevention problem identification and referral service (e.g., student assistance and employee assistance programs), does not include assessment
H0029	Alcohol and/or drug prevention alternatives service (services for populations that exclude alcohol and other drug use e.g., alcohol free social events)
H0030	Behavioral health hotline service
H0031	Mental health assessment, by nonphysician
H0032	Mental health service plan development by nonphysician
H0033	Oral medication administration, direct observation
H0034	Medication training and support, per 15 minutes ☑
H0035	Mental health partial hospitalization, treatment, less than 24 hours ☑
H0036	Community psychiatric supportive treatment, face-to-face, per 15 minutes ☑
H0037	Community psychiatric supportive treatment program, per diem ☑
H0038	Self-help/peer services, per 15 minutes ☑
H0039	Assertive community treatment, face-to-face, per 15 minutes ☑
H0040	Assertive community treatment program, per diem ☑
H0041	Foster care, child, nontherapeutic, per diem A ☑
H0042	Foster care, child, nontherapeutic, per month A ☑
H0043	Supported housing, per diem ☑
H0044	Supported housing, per month ☑
H0045	Respite care services, not in the home, per diem ☑
H0046	Mental health services, not otherwise specified
H0047	Alcohol and/or other drug abuse services, not otherwise specified
H0048	Alcohol and/or other drug testing: collection and handling only, specimens other than blood
H0049	Alcohol and/or drug screening
H0050	Alcohol and/or drug services, brief intervention, per 15 minutes ☑
H1000	Prenatal care, at-risk assessment M ♀
H1001	Prenatal care, at-risk enhanced service; antepartum management M ♀
H1002	Prenatal care, at risk enhanced service; care coordination M ♀
H1003	Prenatal care, at-risk enhanced service; education M ♀
H1004	Prenatal care, at-risk enhanced service; follow-up home visit M ♀
H1005	Prenatal care, at-risk enhanced service package (includes H1001-H1004) M ♀
H1010	Nonmedical family planning education, per session ☑
H1011	Family assessment by licensed behavioral health professional for state defined purposes
H2000	Comprehensive multidisciplinary evaluation
H2001	Rehabilitation program, per 1/2 day ☑
H2010	Comprehensive medication services, per 15 minutes ☑

Alcohol and Drug Abuse Treatment Services

Code	Description
H2011	Crisis intervention service, per 15 minutes ☑
H2012	Behavioral health day treatment, per hour ☑
H2013	Psychiatric health facility service, per diem ☑
H2014	Skills training and development, per 15 minutes ☑
H2015	Comprehensive community support services, per 15 minutes ☑
H2016	Comprehensive community support services, per diem ☑
H2017	Psychosocial rehabilitation services, per 15 minutes ☑
H2018	Psychosocial rehabilitation services, per diem ☑
H2019	Therapeutic behavioral services, per 15 minutes ☑
H2020	Therapeutic behavioral services, per diem ☑
H2021	Community-based wrap-around services, per 15 minutes ☑
H2022	Community-based wrap-around services, per diem ☑
H2023	Supported employment, per 15 minutes ☑
H2024	Supported employment, per diem ☑
H2025	Ongoing support to maintain employment, per 15 minutes ☑
H2026	Ongoing support to maintain employment, per diem ☑
H2027	Psychoeducational service, per 15 minutes ☑
H2028	Sexual offender treatment service, per 15 minutes ☑
H2029	Sexual offender treatment service, per diem ☑
H2030	Mental health clubhouse services, per 15 minutes ☑
H2031	Mental health clubhouse services, per diem ☑
H2032	Activity therapy, per 15 minutes ☑
H2033	Multisystemic therapy for juveniles, per 15 minutes ☑
H2034	Alcohol and/or drug abuse halfway house services, per diem ☑
H2035	Alcohol and/or other drug treatment program, per hour ☑
H2036	Alcohol and/or other drug treatment program, per diem ☑
H2037	Developmental delay prevention activities, dependent child of client, per 15 minutes Ⓐ ☑
● H2038	Skills training and development, per diem

Special Coverage Instructions | **Noncovered by Medicare** | **Carrier Discretion** | ☑ Quantity Alert ● New Code ○ Recycled/Reinstated ▲ Revised Code

Ⓐ Age Edit   Ⓜ Maternity Edit   ♀ Female Only   ♂ Male Only   Ⓐ-Ⓨ OPPS Status Indicators

2023 HCPCS Level II J0270

J Codes Drugs J0120-J8499

J codes include drugs that ordinarily cannot be self-administered, chemotherapy drugs, immunosuppressive drugs, inhalation solutions, and other miscellaneous drugs and solutions.

Miscellaneous Drugs

J0120 Injection, tetracycline, up to 250 mg [N] [N1] ☑
AHA: 4Q,18

J0121 Injection, omadacycline, 1 mg [K2]
Use this code for Nuzyra.
AHA: 4Q,19

J0122 Injection, eravacycline, 1 mg [N1]
Use this code for Xerava.
AHA: 4Q,19

J0129 Injection, abatacept, 10 mg (code may be used for Medicare when drug administered under the direct supervision of a physician, not for use when drug is self-administered) [K] [K2] ☑
Use this code for Orencia.
CMS: 100-02,15,50.5
AHA: 4Q,18

J0130 Injection abciximab, 10 mg [N] [N1] ☑
Use this code for ReoPro.
AHA: 4Q,18

▲ **J0131** Injection, acetaminophen, not otherwise specified, 10 mg [N] [N1] ☑
AHA: 4Q,18

J0132 Injection, acetylcysteine, 100 mg [N] [N1] ☑
Use this code for Acetadote.
AHA: 4Q,18

J0133 Injection, acyclovir, 5 mg [N] [N1] ☑
Use this code for Zovirax.
CMS: 100-04,20,180; 100-04,32,411.3
AHA: 4Q,18

● **J0134** Injection, acetaminophen (Fresenius Kabi) not therapeutically equivalent to J0131, 10 mg
Use this code for acetaminophen manufactured by Fresenius Kabi.

J0135 Injection, adalimumab, 20 mg [K] [K2] ☑
Use this code for Humira.
CMS: 100-02,15,50.5
AHA: 4Q,18

● **J0136** Injection, acetaminophen (B. Braun) not therapeutically equivalent to J0131, 10 mg
Use this code for acetaminophen manufactured by B. Braun.

J0153 Injection, adenosine, 1 mg (not to be used to report any adenosine phosphate compounds) [N] [N1] ☑
Use this code for Adenocard, Adenoscan.
AHA: 4Q,18

J0171 Injection, adrenalin, epinephrine, 0.1 mg [N] [N1] ☑
AHA: 4Q,18

J0172 Injection, aducanumab-avwa, 2 mg [K2]
Use this code for Aduhelm.
AHA: 1Q,22

● **J0173** Injection, epinephrine (Belcher) not therapeutically equivalent to J0171, 0.1 mg
Use this code for epinephrine manufactured by Belcher.

J0178 Injection, aflibercept, 1 mg [K] [K2] ☑
Use this code for Eylea.
AHA: 4Q,18

J0179 Injection, brolucizumab-dbll, 1 mg [K2]
Use this code for Beovu.
AHA: 1Q,20

J0180 Injection, agalsidase beta, 1 mg [K] [K2] ☑
Use this code for Fabrazyme.
AHA: 4Q,18

J0185 Injection, aprepitant, 1 mg [K2]
Use this code for Cinvanti.
AHA: 1Q,19; 4Q,18

J0190 Injection, biperiden lactate, per 5 mg [EI] ☑
AHA: 4Q,18

J0200 Injection, alatrofloxacin mesylate, 100 mg [EI] ☑
AHA: 4Q,18

J0202 Injection, alemtuzumab, 1 mg [K] [K2] ☑
Use this code for Lemtrada.
AHA: 4Q,18; 1Q,16

J0205 Injection, alglucerase, per 10 units [EI] ☑
Use this code for Ceredase.
AHA: 4Q,18

J0207 Injection, amifostine, 500 mg [K] [K2] ☑
Use this code for Ethyol.
AHA: 4Q,18

J0210 Injection, methyldopate HCl, up to 250 mg [N] ☑
Use this code for Aldomet.
AHA: 4Q,18

J0215 Injection, alefacept, 0.5 mg [EI] ☑
Use this for Amevive.
AHA: 4Q,18

● **J0219** Injection, avalglucosidase alfa-ngpt, 4 mg [K2]
Use this code for Nexviazyme.
AHA: 2Q,22

J0220 Injection, alglucosidase alfa, 10 mg, not otherwise specified [K] [K2] ☑
Use this code for Myozyme.
AHA: 4Q,18

J0221 Injection, alglucosidase alfa, (Lumizyme), 10 mg [K] [K2] ☑
AHA: 4Q,18

J0222 Injection, patisiran, 0.1 mg [K2]
Use this code for Onpattro.
AHA: 4Q,19

J0223 Injection, givosiran, 0.5 mg [K2]
Use this code for Givlaari.
AHA: 2Q,20

J0224 Injection, lumasiran, 0.5 mg [K2]
AHA: 3Q,21

● **J0225** Injection, vutrisiran, 1 mg

J0248 Injection, remdesivir, 1 mg
AHA: 1Q,22

J0256 Injection, alpha 1-proteinase inhibitor (human), not otherwise specified, 10 mg [K] [K2] ☑
Use this code for Aralast, Aralast NP, Prolastin C, Zemira.
AHA: 4Q,18

J0257 Injection, alpha 1 proteinase inhibitor (human), (GLASSIA), 10 mg [K] [K2] ☑
AHA: 4Q,18

J0270 Injection, alprostadil, 1.25 mcg (code may be used for Medicare when drug administered under the direct supervision of a physician, not for use when drug is self-administered) [B] ☑
Use this code for Alprostadil, Caverject, Edex, Prostin VR Pediatric.
AHA: 4Q,18

Drugs Administered Other Than Oral Method — J0120 — J0270

Special Coverage Instructions | Noncovered by Medicare | Carrier Discretion | ☑ Quantity Alert ● New Code ○ Recycled/Reinstated ▲ Revised Code

© 2022 Optum, Inc. [A2]-[Z3] ASC Pmt CMS: IOM AHA: Coding Clinic DMEPOS Paid SNF Excluded J Codes — 89

Drugs Administered Other Than Oral Method

J0275 — J0520

Code	Description
J0275	Alprostadil urethral suppository (code may be used for Medicare when drug administered under the direct supervision of a physician, not for use when drug is self-administered) [B] ☑ Use this code for Muse. **AHA:** 4Q,18
J0278	Injection, amikacin sulfate, 100 mg [N] [N1] ☑ Use this code for Amikin. **AHA:** 4Q,18
J0280	Injection, aminophyllin, up to 250 mg [N] [N1] ☑ **AHA:** 4Q,18
J0282	Injection, amiodarone HCl, 30 mg [N] [N1] ☑ Use this code for Cordarone IV. **AHA:** 4Q,18
● J0283	Injection, amiodarone HCl (Nexterone), 30 mg
J0285	Injection, amphotericin B, 50 mg [N] [N1] ☑ Use this for Amphocin, Fungizone. **CMS:** 100-04,20,180; 100-04,32,411.3 **AHA:** 4Q,18
J0287	Injection, amphotericin B lipid complex, 10 mg [K] [K2] ☑ Use this code for Abelcet. **CMS:** 100-04,20,180; 100-04,32,411.3 **AHA:** 4Q,18
J0288	Injection, amphotericin B cholesteryl sulfate complex, 10 mg [EI] ☑ Use this code for Amphotec. **CMS:** 100-04,20,180; 100-04,32,411.3 **AHA:** 4Q,18
J0289	Injection, amphotericin B liposome, 10 mg [K] [K2] ☑ Use this code for Ambisome. **CMS:** 100-04,20,180; 100-04,32,411.3 **AHA:** 4Q,18
J0290	Injection, ampicillin sodium, 500 mg [N] [N1] ☑ **AHA:** 4Q,18
J0291	Injection, plazomicin, 5 mg [K2] Use this code for Zemdri. **AHA:** 4Q,19
J0295	Injection, ampicillin sodium/sulbactam sodium, per 1.5 g [N] [N1] ☑ Use this code for Unasyn. **AHA:** 4Q,18
J0300	Injection, amobarbital, up to 125 mg [K] [K2] ☑ Use this code for Amytal. **AHA:** 4Q,18
J0330	Injection, succinylcholine chloride, up to 20 mg [N] [N1] ☑ Use this code for Anectine, Quelicin. **AHA:** 4Q,18
J0348	Injection, anidulafungin, 1 mg [N] [N1] ☑ Use this code for Eraxis. **AHA:** 4Q,18
J0350	Injection, anistreplase, per 30 units [EI] ☑ Use this code for Eminase. **AHA:** 4Q,18
J0360	Injection, hydralazine HCl, up to 20 mg [N] [N1] ☑ **AHA:** 4Q,18
J0364	Injection, apomorphine HCl, 1 mg [EI] ☑ Use this code for Apokyn. **CMS:** 100-02,15,50.5 **AHA:** 4Q,18
J0365	Injection, aprotinin, 10,000 kiu [EI] ☑ Use this code for Trasylol. **AHA:** 4Q,18
J0380	Injection, metaraminol bitartrate, per 10 mg [N] ☑ Use this code for Aramine. **AHA:** 4Q,18
J0390	Injection, chloroquine HCl, up to 250 mg [N] [K2] ☑ Use this code for Aralen. **AHA:** 4Q,18
J0395	Injection, arbutamine HCl, 1 mg [EI] ☑ **AHA:** 4Q,18
J0400	Injection, aripiprazole, intramuscular, 0.25 mg [K] [N1] ☑ Use this code for Abilify. **AHA:** 4Q,18
J0401	Injection, aripiprazole, extended release, 1 mg [K] [K2] ☑ Use this code for the Abilify Maintena kit. **AHA:** 4Q,18
J0456	Injection, azithromycin, 500 mg [N] [N1] ☑ Use this code for Zithromax. **AHA:** 4Q,18
J0461	Injection, atropine sulfate, 0.01 mg [N] [N1] ☑ Use this code for AtroPen. **AHA:** 4Q,18
J0470	Injection, dimercaprol, per 100 mg [K] [N1] ☑ Use this code for BAL. **AHA:** 4Q,18
J0475	Injection, baclofen, 10 mg [K] [K2] ☑ Use this code for Lioresal, Gablofen. **AHA:** 4Q,18
J0476	Injection, baclofen, 50 mcg for intrathecal trial [K] [N1] ☑ Use this code for Lioresal, Gablofen. **AHA:** 4Q,18
J0480	Injection, basiliximab, 20 mg [K] [K2] ☑ Use this code for Simulect. **AHA:** 4Q,18
J0485	Injection, belatacept, 1 mg [K] [K2] ☑ Use this code for Nulojix. **AHA:** 4Q,18
J0490	Injection, belimumab, 10 mg [K] [K2] ☑ Use this code for BENLYSTA. **AHA:** 4Q,18
● J0491	Injection, anifrolumab-fnia, 1 mg [K2] Use this code for Saphnello. **AHA:** 2Q,22
J0500	Injection, dicyclomine HCl, up to 20 mg [N] [N1] ☑ Use this code for Bentyl. **AHA:** 4Q,18
J0515	Injection, benztropine mesylate, per 1 mg [N] [N1] ☑ Use this code for Cogentin. **AHA:** 4Q,18
J0517	Injection, benralizumab, 1 mg [K2] Use this code for Fasenra. **AHA:** 1Q,19; 4Q,18
J0520	Injection, bethanechol chloride, Myotonachol or Urecholine, up to 5 mg [EI] ☑ **AHA:** 4Q,18

2023 HCPCS Level II

Drugs Administered Other Than Oral Method

J0558 — Injection, penicillin G benzathine and penicillin G procaine, 100,000 units N K2 ☑
Use this code for Bicillin CR, Bicillin CR 900/300, Bicillin CR Tubex.
AHA: 4Q,18

J0561 — Injection, penicillin G benzathine, 100,000 units K K2 ☑
AHA: 4Q,18

J0565 — Injection, bezlotoxumab, 10 mg G K2
Use this code for Zinplava.
AHA: 4Q,18; 1Q,18

J0567 — Injection, cerliponase alfa, 1 mg
Use this code for Brineura.
AHA: 1Q,19; 4Q,18

J0570 — Buprenorphine implant, 74.2 mg G K2 ☑
Use this code for Probuphine.
AHA: 1Q,17

J0571 — Buprenorphine, oral, 1 mg EI ☑
Use this code for Subutex.

J0572 — Buprenorphine/naloxone, oral, less than or equal to 3 mg buprenorphine EI ☑
Use this code for Bunavail, Suboxone, Zubsolv.

J0573 — Buprenorphine/naloxone, oral, greater than 3 mg, but less than or equal to 6 mg buprenorphine EI ☑
Use this code for Bunavail, Suboxone, Zubsolv.

J0574 — Buprenorphine/naloxone, oral, greater than 6 mg, but less than or equal to 10 mg buprenorphine EI ☑
Use this code for Bunavail, Suboxone.

J0575 — Buprenorphine/naloxone, oral, greater than 10 mg buprenorphine EI ☑
Use this code for Suboxone.

J0583 — Injection, bivalirudin, 1 mg N N1 ☑
Use this code for Angiomax.
AHA: 4Q,18

J0584 — Injection, burosumab-twza, 1 mg K2
Use this code for Crysvita.
CMS: 100-04,4,260.1; 100-04,4,260.1.1
AHA: 1Q,19; 4Q,18

J0585 — Injection, onabotulinumtoxinA, 1 unit K K2 ☑
Use this code for Botox, Botox Cosmetic.
AHA: 2Q,21; 4Q,18

J0586 — Injection, abobotulinumtoxinA, 5 units K K2 ☑
Use this code for Dysport.
AHA: 4Q,18

J0587 — Injection, rimabotulinumtoxinB, 100 units K K2 ☑
Use this code for Myobloc.
AHA: 4Q,18

J0588 — Injection, incobotulinumtoxinA, 1 unit K K2 ☑
Use this code for XEOMIN.
AHA: 4Q,18

J0591 — Injection, deoxycholic acid, 1 mg
Use this code for Kybella.
AHA: 2Q,20

J0592 — Injection, buprenorphine HCl, 0.1 mg N N1 ☑
Use this code for Buprenex.
AHA: 4Q,18

J0593 — Injection, lanadelumab-flyo, 1 mg (code may be used for Medicare when drug administered under direct supervision of a physician, not for use when drug is self-administered)
Use this code for Takhzyro.
AHA: 4Q,19

J0594 — Injection, busulfan, 1 mg K K2 ☑
Use this code for Busulfex.
AHA: 4Q,18

J0595 — Injection, butorphanol tartrate, 1 mg N N1 ☑
Use this code for Stadol.
AHA: 4Q,18

J0596 — Injection, C1 esterase inhibitor (recombinant), Ruconest, 10 units K K2 ☑
CMS: 100-02,15,50.5
AHA: 4Q,18; 1Q,16

J0597 — Injection, C1 esterase inhibitor (human), Berinert, 10 units K K2 ☑
AHA: 4Q,18

J0598 — Injection, C1 esterase inhibitor (human), Cinryze, 10 units K K2 ☑
AHA: 4Q,18

J0599 — Injection, C1 esterase inhibitor (human), (Haegarda), 10 units N1
AHA: 1Q,19; 4Q,18

J0600 — Injection, edetate calcium disodium, up to 1,000 mg K K2 ☑
Use this code for Calcium Disodium Versenate, Calcium EDTA.
AHA: 4Q,18

J0604 — Cinacalcet, oral, 1 mg, (for ESRD on dialysis) B
Use this code for Sensipar.
AHA: 4Q,18; 1Q,18

J0606 — Injection, etelcalcetide, 0.1 mg K N1
Use this code for Parsabiv.
AHA: 4Q,18; 2Q,18; 1Q,18

▲ **J0610** — Injection, calcium gluconate (Fresenius Kabi), per 10 ml N N1 ☑
Use this code for calcium gluconate manufactured by Fresenius Kabi.
AHA: 4Q,18

● **J0611** — Injection, calcium gluconate (WG Critical Care), per 10 ml
Use this code for calcium gluconate manufactured by WG Critical Care.

J0620 — Injection, calcium glycerophosphate and calcium lactate, per 10 ml N N1 ☑
AHA: 4Q,18

J0630 — Injection, calcitonin salmon, up to 400 units K K2 ☑
Use this code for Calcimar, Miacalcin.
CMS: 100-04,10,90.1
AHA: 4Q,18

J0636 — Injection, calcitriol, 0.1 mcg N N1 ☑
Use this code for Calcijex.
AHA: 4Q,18

J0637 — Injection, caspofungin acetate, 5 mg K N1 ☑
Use this code for Cancidas.
AHA: 4Q,18

J0638 — Injection, canakinumab, 1 mg K K2 ☑
Use this code for ILARIS.
AHA: 4Q,18

J0640 — Injection, leucovorin calcium, per 50 mg N N1 ☑
AHA: 4Q,18

J0641 — Injection, levoleucovorin, not otherwise specified, 0.5 mg K N1 ☑
AHA: 4Q,19; 4Q,18

J0642 — Injection, levoleucovorin (Khapzory), 0.5 mg K2
AHA: 1Q,20; 4Q,19

Special Coverage Instructions | Noncovered by Medicare | Carrier Discretion | ☑ Quantity Alert ● New Code ○ Recycled/Reinstated ▲ Revised Code

© 2022 Optum, Inc. | A2-Z3 ASC Pmt | CMS: IOM | AHA: Coding Clinic | DMEPOS Paid | ⊘ SNF Excluded

J Codes — 91

Drugs Administered Other Than Oral Method

J0670 — J0875

Code	Description
J0670	Injection, mepivacaine HCl, per 10 ml
	Use this code for Carbocaine, Polocaine, Isocaine HCl, Scandonest
	AHA: 4Q,18
● J0689	Injection, cefazolin sodium (Baxter), not therapeutically equivalent to J0690, 500 mg
	Use this code for cefazolin sodium manufactured by Baxter.
J0690	Injection, cefazolin sodium, 500 mg
	AHA: 4Q,18
J0691	Injection, lefamulin, 1 mg
	Use this code for Xenleta.
	AHA: 2Q,20
J0692	Injection, cefepime HCl, 500 mg
	AHA: 4Q,18
J0694	Injection, cefoxitin sodium, 1 g
	AHA: 4Q,18
J0695	Injection, ceftolozane 50 mg and tazobactam 25 mg
	Use this code for Zerbaxa.
	AHA: 4Q,18; 1Q,16
J0696	Injection, ceftriaxone sodium, per 250 mg
	AHA: 4Q,18
J0697	Injection, sterile cefuroxime sodium, per 750 mg
	AHA: 4Q,18
J0698	Injection, cefotaxime sodium, per g
	AHA: 4Q,18
J0699	Injection, cefiderocol, 10 mg
	Use this code for Fetroja.
	AHA: 4Q,21
● J0701	Injection, cefepime HCl (Baxter), not therapeutically equivalent to Maxipime, 500 mg
	Use this code for cefepime HCl manufactured by Baxter.
J0702	Injection, betamethasone acetate 3 mg and betamethasone sodium phosphate 3 mg
	AHA: 4Q,18
● J0703	Injection, cefepime HCl (B. Braun), not therapeutically equivalent to Maxipime, 500 mg
	Use this code for cefepime HCl manufactured by B. Braun.
J0706	Injection, caffeine citrate, 5 mg
	AHA: 4Q,18
J0710	Injection, cephapirin sodium, up to 1 g
	AHA: 4Q,18
J0712	Injection, ceftaroline fosamil, 10 mg
	AHA: 4Q,18
J0713	Injection, ceftazidime, per 500 mg
	AHA: 4Q,18
J0714	Injection, ceftazidime and avibactam, 0.5 g/0.125 g
	Use this code for Avycaz.
	AHA: 4Q,18; 1Q,16
J0715	Injection, ceftizoxime sodium, per 500 mg
	AHA: 4Q,18
J0716	Injection, Centruroides immune f(ab)2, up to 120 mg
	Use this code for Anascorp.
	AHA: 4Q,18
J0717	Injection, certolizumab pegol, 1 mg (code may be used for Medicare when drug administered under the direct supervision of a physician, not for use when drug is self-administered)
	CMS: 100-02,15,50.5
	AHA: 4Q,18
J0720	Injection, chloramphenicol sodium succinate, up to 1 g
	AHA: 4Q,18
J0725	Injection, chorionic gonadotropin, per 1,000 USP units
	CMS: 100-02,15,50.5
	AHA: 4Q,18
J0735	Injection, clonidine HCl, 1 mg
	AHA: 4Q,18
● J0739	Injection, cabotegravir, 1 mg
	Use this code for Cabenuva.
	AHA: 3Q,22
J0740	Injection, cidofovir, 375 mg
	AHA: 4Q,18
J0741	Injection, cabotegravir and rilpivirine, 2 mg/3 mg
	Use this code for Cabenuva.
	AHA: 4Q,21
J0742	Injection, imipenem 4 mg, cilastatin 4 mg and relebactam 2 mg
	Use this code for Recarbrio.
	AHA: 2Q,20
J0743	Injection, cilastatin sodium; imipenem, per 250 mg
	AHA: 4Q,18
J0744	Injection, ciprofloxacin for intravenous infusion, 200 mg
	AHA: 4Q,18
J0745	Injection, codeine phosphate, per 30 mg
J0770	Injection, colistimethate sodium, up to 150 mg
	AHA: 4Q,18
J0775	Injection, collagenase, clostridium histolyticum, 0.01 mg
	AHA: 4Q,18
J0780	Injection, prochlorperazine, up to 10 mg
	AHA: 4Q,18
J0791	Injection, crizanlizumab-tmca, 5 mg
	Use this code for ADAKVEO.
	AHA: 2Q,20
J0795	Injection, corticorelin ovine triflutate, 1 mcg
	AHA: 4Q,18
J0800	Injection, corticotropin, up to 40 units
	CMS: 100-02,15,50.5
	AHA: 4Q,18
J0834	Injection, cosyntropin, 0.25 mg
	Use this code for Cortrosyn.
	AHA: 4Q,18
J0840	Injection, crotalidae polyvalent immune fab (ovine), up to 1 g
	AHA: 4Q,18
J0841	Injection, crotalidae immune F(ab')2 (equine), 120 mg
	Use this code for Anavip.
	CMS: 100-04,4,260.1; 100-04,4,260.1.1
	AHA: 1Q,19; 4Q,18
J0850	Injection, cytomegalovirus immune globulin intravenous (human), per vial
	AHA: 4Q,18
J0875	Injection, dalbavancin, 5 mg
	Use this code for Dalvance.
	AHA: 4Q,18; 1Q,16

Legend: Special Coverage Instructions · Noncovered by Medicare · Carrier Discretion · ☑ Quantity Alert · ● New Code · ○ Recycled/Reinstated · ▲ Revised Code

92 — J Codes · A Age Edit · M Maternity Edit · ♀ Female Only · ♂ Male Only · A-Y OPPS Status Indicators · © 2022 Optum, Inc.

Drugs Administered Other Than Oral Method

Code	Description
● J0877	Injection, daptomycin (Hospira), not therapeutically equivalent to J0878, 1 mg Use this code for daptomycin manufactured by Hospira.
J0878	Injection, daptomycin, 1 mg [K] [N1] ☑ Use this code for Cubicin. **AHA:** 4Q,18
● J0879	Injection, difelikefalin, 0.1 mcg, (for ESRD on dialysis) Use this code for Korsuva. **AHA:** 2Q,22
J0881	Injection, darbepoetin alfa, 1 mcg (non-ESRD use) [K] [K2] ☑ Use this code for Aranesp. **CMS:** 100-03,110.21; 100-04,17,80.12 **AHA:** 4Q,18
J0882	Injection, darbepoetin alfa, 1 mcg (for ESRD on dialysis) [K] [K2] ☑ ⊘ Use this code for Aranesp. **CMS:** 100-04,8,60.4; 100-04,8,60.4.1; 100-04,8,60.4.2; 100-04,8,60.4.5.1; 100-04,8,60.4.6.3; 100-04,8,60.4.6.4; 100-04,8,60.4.6.5 **AHA:** 4Q,18
J0883	Injection, argatroban, 1 mg (for non-ESRD use) [K] [K2] ☑ **AHA:** 4Q,18
J0884	Injection, argatroban, 1 mg (for ESRD on dialysis) [K] [K2] ☑ **AHA:** 4Q,18
J0885	Injection, epoetin alfa, (for non-ESRD use), 1000 units [K] [K2] ☑ Use this code for Epogen/Procrit. **CMS:** 100-03,110.21; 100-04,17,80.12 **AHA:** 4Q,18
J0887	Injection, epoetin beta, 1 mcg, (for ESRD on dialysis) [N] [N1] ☑ Use this code for Mircera. **AHA:** 4Q,18
J0888	Injection, epoetin beta, 1 mcg (for non-ESRD use) [K] [K2] ☑ Use this code for Mircera. **AHA:** 4Q,18
J0890	Injection, peginesatide, 0.1 mg (for ESRD on dialysis) [E1] ☑ Use this code for Omontys. **CMS:** 100-04,8,60.4; 100-04,8,60.4.1; 100-04,8,60.4.2; 100-04,8,60.4.5.1; 100-04,8,60.4.7 **AHA:** 4Q,18
● J0891	Injection, argatroban (Accord), not therapeutically equivalent to J0883, 1 mg (for non-ESRD use) Use this code for argatroban manufactured by Accord; for non-ESRD use.
● J0892	Injection, argatroban (Accord), not therapeutically equivalent to J0884, 1 mg (for ESRD on dialysis) Use this code for argatroban manufactured by Accord; for patients on ESRD dialysis.
● J0893	Injection, decitabine (Sun Pharma) not therapeutically equivalent to J0894, 1 mg Use this code for decitabine manufactured by Sun Pharma.
J0894	Injection, decitabine, 1 mg [K] [K2] ☑ ⊘ Use this code for Dacogen. **AHA:** 4Q,18
J0895	Injection, deferoxamine mesylate, 500 mg [N] [N1] ☑ Use this code for Desferal. **CMS:** 100-04,20,180; 100-04,32,411.3 **AHA:** 4Q,18
J0896	Injection, luspatercept-aamt, 0.25 mg [K2] Use this code for REBLOZYL. **AHA:** 2Q,20
J0897	Injection, denosumab, 1 mg [K] [K2] ☑ Use this code for XGEVA, Prolia. **CMS:** 100-04,10,90.1 **AHA:** 4Q,18; 1Q,16
● J0898	Injection, argatroban (AuroMedics), not therapeutically equivalent to J0883, 1 mg (for non-ESRD use) Use this code for argatroban manufactured by AuroMedics; for non-ESRD use.
● J0899	Injection, argatroban (AuroMedics), not therapeutically equivalent to J0884, 1 mg (for ESRD on dialysis) Use this code for argatroban manufactured by AuroMedics; for patients on ESRD dialysis.
J0945	Injection, brompheniramine maleate, per 10 mg [N] [N1] ☑ **AHA:** 4Q,18
J1000	Injection, depo-estradiol cypionate, up to 5 mg [N] [N1] ☑ Use this code for depGynogen, Depogen, Estradiol Cypionate. **AHA:** 4Q,18
J1020	Injection, methylprednisolone acetate, 20 mg [N] [N1] ☑ Use this code for Depo-Medrol. **AHA:** 3Q,19; 4Q,18
J1030	Injection, methylprednisolone acetate, 40 mg [N] [N1] ☑ Use this code for DepoMedalone40, Depo-Medrol, Sano-Drol. **AHA:** 3Q,19; 4Q,18
J1040	Injection, methylprednisolone acetate, 80 mg [N] [N1] ☑ Use this code for Cortimed, DepMedalone, DepoMedalone 80, Depo-Medrol, Duro Cort, Methylcotolone, Pri-Methylate, Sano-Drol. **AHA:** 4Q,18
J1050	Injection, medroxyprogesterone acetate, 1 mg [N] [N1] ☑ **AHA:** 4Q,18
J1071	Injection, testosterone cypionate, 1 mg [N] [N1] ☑ Use this code for Depo-testostrone. **AHA:** 4Q,18
J1094	Injection, dexamethasone acetate, 1 mg [N] [N1] ☑ Use this code for Cortastat LA, Dalalone L.A., Dexamethasone Acetate Anhydrous, Dexone LA. **AHA:** 4Q,18
J1095	Injection, dexamethasone 9%, intraocular, 1 mcg [K2] **AHA:** 1Q,19; 4Q,18
J1096	Dexamethasone, lacrimal ophthalmic insert, 0.1 mg [K2] Use this code for Dextenza. **AHA:** 4Q,19
J1097	Phenylephrine 10.16 mg/ml and ketorolac 2.88 mg/ml ophthalmic irrigation solution, 1 ml [K2] Use this code for Omidria. **AHA:** 4Q,19
J1100	Injection, dexamethasone sodium phosphate, 1 mg [N] [N1] ☑ Use this code for Cortastat, Dalalone, Decaject, Dexone, Solurex, Adrenocort, Primethasone, Dexasone, Dexim, Medidex, Spectro-Dex. **AHA:** 4Q,18
J1110	Injection, dihydroergotamine mesylate, per 1 mg [K] [N1] ☑ Use this code for D.H.E. 45. **AHA:** 4Q,18
J1120	Injection, acetazolamide sodium, up to 500 mg [N] [N1] ☑ Use this code for Diamox. **AHA:** 4Q,18
J1130	Injection, diclofenac sodium, 0.5 mg [K] [N1] ☑ Use this code for Dyloject. **AHA:** 4Q,18; 1Q,17

Special Coverage Instructions | Noncovered by Medicare | Carrier Discretion | ☑ Quantity Alert ● New Code ○ Recycled/Reinstated ▲ Revised Code

© 2022 Optum, Inc. | [A2]-[Z3] ASC Pmt | **CMS:** IOM | **AHA:** Coding Clinic | ⚕ DMEPOS Paid | ⊘ SNF Excluded | J Codes — 93

Drugs Administered Other Than Oral Method

J1160 — Injection, digoxin, up to 0.5 mg [N][N1][✓]
Use this code for Lanoxin.
AHA: 4Q,18

J1162 — Injection, digoxin immune fab (ovine), per vial [K][K2][✓]
Use this code for Digibind, Digifab.
AHA: 4Q,18

J1165 — Injection, phenytoin sodium, per 50 mg [N][N1][✓]
Use this code for Dilantin.
AHA: 4Q,18

J1170 — Injection, hydromorphone, up to 4 mg [N][N1][✓]
Use this code for Dilaudid, Dilaudid-HP.
CMS: 100-04,20,180; 100-04,32,411.3
AHA: 4Q,18

J1180 — Injection, dyphylline, up to 500 mg [EI][✓]
AHA: 4Q,18

J1190 — Injection, dexrazoxane HCl, per 250 mg [K][K2][✓]
Use this code for Zinecard.
AHA: 4Q,18

J1200 — Injection, diphenhydramine HCl, up to 50 mg [N][N1][✓]
Use this code for Benadryl, Benahist 10, Benahist 50, Benoject-10, Benoject-50, Bena-D 10, Bena-D 50, Nordryl, Dihydrex, Dimine, Diphenacen-50, Hyrexin-50, Truxadryl, Wehdryl.
AHA: 4Q,18

J1201 — Injection, cetirizine HCl, 0.5 mg [K2]
Use this code for Quzytiir.
AHA: 2Q,20

J1205 — Injection, chlorothiazide sodium, per 500 mg [N][N1][✓]
Use this code for Diuril Sodium.
AHA: 4Q,18

J1212 — Injection, DMSO, dimethyl sulfoxide, 50%, 50 ml [K][K2][✓]
Use this code for Rimso 50. DMSO is covered only as a treatment of interstitial cystitis.
AHA: 4Q,18

J1230 — Injection, methadone HCl, up to 10 mg [N][N1][✓]
Use this code for Dolophine HCl.
AHA: 4Q,18

J1240 — Injection, dimenhydrinate, up to 50 mg [N][N1][✓]
Use this code for Dramamine, Dinate, Dommanate, Dramanate, Dramilin, Dramocen, Dramoject, Dymenate, Hydrate, Marmine, Wehamine.
AHA: 4Q,18

J1245 — Injection, dipyridamole, per 10 mg [N][N1][✓]
Use this code for Persantine IV.
AHA: 4Q,18

J1250 — Injection, dobutamine HCl, per 250 mg [N][N1][✓]
CMS: 100-04,20,180; 100-04,32,411.3
AHA: 4Q,18

J1260 — Injection, dolasetron mesylate, 10 mg [N][N1][✓]
Use this code for Anzemet.
AHA: 4Q,18

J1265 — Injection, dopamine HCl, 40 mg [N][N1][✓]
CMS: 100-04,20,180; 100-04,32,411.3
AHA: 4Q,18

J1267 — Injection, doripenem, 10 mg [N][N1][✓]
Use this code for Doribax.
AHA: 4Q,18

J1270 — Injection, doxercalciferol, 1 mcg [N][N1][✓]
Use this code for Hectorol.
AHA: 4Q,18

J1290 — Injection, ecallantide, 1 mg [K][K2][✓]
Use this code for KALBITOR.
AHA: 4Q,18

J1300 — Injection, eculizumab, 10 mg [K][K2][✓]
Use this code for Soliris.
AHA: 4Q,18

J1301 — Injection, edaravone, 1 mg [K2]
Use this code for Radicava.
AHA: 1Q,19; 4Q,18

● **J1302** — Injection, sutimlimab-jome, 10 mg [K2]
Use this code for Enjaymo.

J1303 — Injection, ravulizumab-cwvz, 10 mg [K2]
Use this code for Ultomiris.
AHA: 4Q,19

J1305 — Injection, evinacumab-dgnb, 5 mg [K2]
Use this code for Evkeeza.
AHA: 4Q,21

● **J1306** — Injection, inclisiran, 1 mg [K2]
Use this code for Leqvio.
AHA: 3Q,22

J1320 — Injection, amitriptyline HCl, up to 20 mg [N][N1][✓]
Use this code for Elavil.
AHA: 4Q,18

J1322 — Injection, elosulfase alfa, 1 mg [K][K2][✓]
Use this code for Vimizim.
AHA: 4Q,18

J1324 — Injection, enfuvirtide, 1 mg [EI][✓]
Use this code for Fuzeon.
CMS: 100-02,15,50.5
AHA: 4Q,18

J1325 — Injection, epoprostenol, 0.5 mg [N][N1][✓]
Use this code for Flolan and Veletri. See K0455 for infusion pump for epoprosterol.
CMS: 100-04,20,180; 100-04,32,411.3
AHA: 4Q,18

J1327 — Injection, eptifibatide, 5 mg [K][K2][✓]
Use this code for Integrilin.
AHA: 4Q,18

J1330 — Injection, ergonovine maleate, up to 0.2 mg [N][✓]
Medicare jurisdiction: local contractor. Use this code for Ergotrate Maleate.
AHA: 4Q,18

J1335 — Injection, ertapenem sodium, 500 mg [N][N1][✓]
Use this code for Invanz.
AHA: 4Q,18

J1364 — Injection, erythromycin lactobionate, per 500 mg [K][N1][✓]
AHA: 4Q,18

J1380 — Injection, estradiol valerate, up to 10 mg [N][N1][✓]
Use this code for Delestrogen, Dioval, Dioval XX, Dioval 40, Duragen-10, Duragen-20, Duragen-40, Estradiol L.A., Estradiol L.A. 20, Estradiol L.A. 40, Gynogen L.A. 10, Gynogen L.A. 20, Gynogen L.A. 40, Valergen 10, Valergen 20, Valergen 40, Estra-L 20, Estra-L 40, L.A.E. 20.
AHA: 4Q,18

J1410 — Injection, estrogen conjugated, per 25 mg [K][K2][✓]
Use this code for Natural Estrogenic Substance, Premarin Intravenous, Primestrin Aqueous.
AHA: 4Q,18

J1426 — Injection, casimersen, 10 mg [K2]
Use this code for Amondys 45.
AHA: 4Q,21

Special Coverage Instructions | Noncovered by Medicare | Carrier Discretion | ☑ Quantity Alert ● New Code ○ Recycled/Reinstated ▲ Revised Code

94 — J Codes | Ⓐ Age Edit Ⓜ Maternity Edit ♀ Female Only ♂ Male Only | A-Y OPPS Status Indicators | © 2022 Optum, Inc.

J1427 Injection, viltolarsen, 10 mg
Use this code for Viltepso.
AHA: 1Q,21

J1428 Injection, eteplirsen, 10 mg
Use this code for Exondys 51.
AHA: 4Q,18; 1Q,18

J1429 Injection, golodirsen, 10 mg
Use this code for Vyondys 53.
AHA: 2Q,20

J1430 Injection, ethanolamine oleate, 100 mg
Use this code for Ethamolin.
AHA: 4Q,18

J1435 Injection, estrone, per 1 mg
Use this code for Estone Aqueous, Estragyn, Estro-A, Estrone, Estronol, Theelin Aqueous, Estone 5, Kestrone 5.
AHA: 4Q,18

J1436 Injection, etidronate disodium, per 300 mg
Use this code for Didronel.
AHA: 4Q,18

J1437 Injection, ferric derisomaltose, 10 mg
Use this code for Monoferric.
AHA: 4Q,20

J1438 Injection, etanercept, 25 mg (code may be used for Medicare when drug administered under the direct supervision of a physician, not for use when drug is self-administered)
Use this code for Enbrel.
CMS: 100-02,15,50.5
AHA: 4Q,18

J1439 Injection, ferric carboxymaltose, 1 mg
Use this code for Injectafer.
AHA: 4Q,18

J1442 Injection, filgrastim (G-CSF), excludes biosimilars, 1 mcg
Use this code for Neupogen.
AHA: 4Q,18

J1443 Injection, ferric pyrophosphate citrate solution (Triferic), 0.1 mg of iron
Use this code for Triferic solution.
AHA: 4Q,18; 1Q,16

J1444 Injection, ferric pyrophosphate citrate powder, 0.1 mg of iron
Use this code for Triferic powder.
AHA: 3Q,19

J1445 Injection, ferric pyrophosphate citrate solution (Triferic AVNU), 0.1 mg of iron
AHA: 4Q,21

J1447 Injection, tbo-filgrastim, 1 mcg
Use this code for Granix.
AHA: 4Q,18; 1Q,16

J1448 Injection, trilaciclib, 1 mg
Use this code for Cosela.
AHA: 4Q,21

J1450 Injection, fluconazole, 200 mg
Use this code for Diflucan.
CMS: 100-02,15,50.6
AHA: 4Q,18

J1451 Injection, fomepizole, 15 mg
Use this code for Antizol.
CMS: 100-02,15,50.6
AHA: 4Q,18

J1452 Injection, fomivirsen sodium, intraocular, 1.65 mg
Use this code for Vitravene.
CMS: 100-02,15,50.4.2; 100-02,15,50.6
AHA: 4Q,18

J1453 Injection, fosaprepitant, 1 mg
Use this code for Emend.
CMS: 100-02,15,50.6
AHA: 4Q,18

J1454 Injection, fosnetupitant 235 mg and palonosetron 0.25 mg
Use this code for Akynzeo.
CMS: 100-02,15,50.6
AHA: 1Q,19; 4Q,18

J1455 Injection, foscarnet sodium, per 1,000 mg
Use this code for Foscavir.
CMS: 100-02,15,50.6; 100-04,20,180; 100-04,32,411.3
AHA: 4Q,18

● **J1456** Injection, fosaprepitant (Teva), not therapeutically equivalent to J1453, 1 mg
Use this code for fosaprepitant manufactured by Teva.
CMS: 100-02,15,50.6

J1457 Injection, gallium nitrate, 1 mg
Use this code for Ganite.
CMS: 100-02,15,50.6; 100-04,20,180; 100-04,32,411.3
AHA: 4Q,18

J1458 Injection, galsulfase, 1 mg
Use this code for Naglazyme.
CMS: 100-02,15,50.6
AHA: 4Q,18

J1459 Injection, immune globulin (Privigen), intravenous, nonlyophilized (e.g., liquid), 500 mg
CMS: 100-02,15,50.6
AHA: 4Q,18

J1460 Injection, gamma globulin, intramuscular, 1 cc
Use this code for GamaSTAN SD.
CMS: 100-02,15,50.6; 100-04,17,80.6
AHA: 4Q,18

● **J1551** Injection, immune globulin (Cutaquig), 100 mg
CMS: 100-02,15,50.6; 100-04,32,411.3
AHA: 3Q,22

J1554 Injection, immune globulin (Asceniv), 500 mg
CMS: 100-02,15,50.6
AHA: 1Q,21

J1555 Injection, immune globulin (Cuvitru), 100 mg
CMS: 100-02,15,50.6; 100-04,20,180; 100-04,32,411.3
AHA: 4Q,18; 1Q,18

J1556 Injection, immune globulin (Bivigam), 500 mg
CMS: 100-02,15,50.6
AHA: 4Q,18

J1557 Injection, immune globulin, (Gammaplex), intravenous, nonlyophilized (e.g., liquid), 500 mg
CMS: 100-02,15,50.6
AHA: 4Q,18

J1558 Injection, immune globulin (xembify), 100 mg
CMS: 100-02,15,50.6; 100-04,32,411.3
AHA: 2Q,20

J1559 Injection, immune globulin (Hizentra), 100 mg
CMS: 100-02,15,50.6; 100-04,20,180; 100-04,32,411.3
AHA: 4Q,18

Drugs Administered Other Than Oral Method

J1560 — Injection, gamma globulin, intramuscular, over 10 cc [K] [K2] [✓]
Use this code for GamaSTAN SD.
CMS: 100-02,15,50.6; 100-04,17,80.6
AHA: 4Q,18

J1561 — Injection, immune globulin, (Gamunex/Gamunex-C/Gammaked), nonlyophilized (e.g., liquid), 500 mg [K] [K2] [✓]
CMS: 100-02,15,50.6; 100-04,20,180; 100-04,32,411.3
AHA: 4Q,18

J1562 — Injection, immune globulin (Vivaglobin), 100 mg [EI] [✓]
CMS: 100-02,15,50.6; 100-04,20,180; 100-04,32,411.3
AHA: 4Q,18

J1566 — Injection, immune globulin, intravenous, lyophilized (e.g., powder), not otherwise specified, 500 mg [K] [K2] [✓]
Use this code for Carimune, Gammagard S/D, Iveegam, Polygam, Polygam S/D.
CMS: 100-02,15,50.6
AHA: 4Q,18

J1568 — Injection, immune globulin, (Octagam), intravenous, nonlyophilized (e.g., liquid), 500 mg [K] [K2] [✓]
CMS: 100-02,15,50.6
AHA: 4Q,18

J1569 — Injection, immune globulin, (Gammagard liquid), nonlyophilized, (e.g., liquid), 500 mg [K] [K2] [✓]
CMS: 100-02,15,50.6; 100-04,20,180; 100-04,32,411.3
AHA: 4Q,18

J1570 — Injection, ganciclovir sodium, 500 mg [N] [N1] [✓]
Use this code for Cytovene.
CMS: 100-04,20,180; 100-04,32,411.3
AHA: 4Q,18

J1571 — Injection, hepatitis B immune globulin (Hepagam B), intramuscular, 0.5 ml [K] [K2] [✓]
AHA: 4Q,18

J1572 — Injection, immune globulin, (Flebogamma/Flebogamma Dif), intravenous, nonlyophilized (e.g., liquid), 500 mg [K] [K2] [✓]
AHA: 4Q,18

J1573 — Injection, hepatitis B immune globulin (Hepagam B), intravenous, 0.5 ml [K] [K2] [✓]
AHA: 4Q,18

● **J1574** — Injection, ganciclovir sodium (Exela) not therapeutically equivalent to J1570, 500 mg
Use this code for ganciclovir manufactured by Exela.

J1575 — Injection, immune globulin/hyaluronidase, 100 mg immuneglobulin [K] [K2] [✓]
Use this code for HyQvia.
CMS: 100-04,20,180; 100-04,32,411.3
AHA: 4Q,18; 1Q,16

J1580 — Injection, garamycin, gentamicin, up to 80 mg [N] [N1] [✓]
Use this code for Gentamicin Sulfate, Jenamicin.
AHA: 4Q,18

J1595 — Injection, glatiramer acetate, 20 mg [K] [K2] [✓]
Use this code for Copaxone.
CMS: 100-02,15,50.5
AHA: 4Q,18

J1599 — Injection, immune globulin, intravenous, nonlyophilized (e.g., liquid), not otherwise specified, 500 mg [N] [N1] [✓]
AHA: 4Q,18

J1600 — Injection, gold sodium thiomalate, up to 50 mg [EI] [✓]
Use this code for Myochrysine.
CMS: 100-04,4,20.6.4
AHA: 4Q,18

J1602 — Injection, golimumab, 1 mg, for intravenous use [K] [K2] [✓]
Use this code for Simponi.
AHA: 4Q,18

J1610 — Injection, glucagon HCl, per 1 mg [K] [K2] [✓]
Use this code for Glucagen.
AHA: 4Q,18

● **J1611** — Injection, glucagon HCl (Fresenius Kabi), not therapeutically equivalent to J1610, per 1 mg
Use this code for glucagon HCl manufactured by Fresenius Kabi.

J1620 — Injection, gonadorelin HCl, per 100 mcg [EI] [✓]
Use this code for Factrel, Lutrepulse.
AHA: 4Q,18

J1626 — Injection, granisetron HCl, 100 mcg [N] [N1] [✓]
Use this code for Kytril.
CMS: 100-04,4,20.6.4
AHA: 4Q,18

J1627 — Injection, granisetron, extended-release, 0.1 mg [G] [K2]
Use this code for Sustol.
AHA: 4Q,18; 1Q,18

J1628 — Injection, guselkumab, 1 mg [K2]
Use this code for Tremfya.
AHA: 1Q,19; 4Q,18

J1630 — Injection, haloperidol, up to 5 mg [N] [N1] [✓]
Use this code for Haldol.
CMS: 100-04,4,20.6.4
AHA: 4Q,18

J1631 — Injection, haloperidol decanoate, per 50 mg [N] [N1] [✓]
Use this code for Haldol Decanoate-50.
CMS: 100-04,4,20.6.4
AHA: 4Q,18

J1632 — Injection, brexanolone, 1 mg [K2]
Use this code for Zulresso.
AHA: 4Q,20

J1640 — Injection, hemin, 1 mg [K] [K2] [✓]
Use this code for Panhematin.
AHA: 4Q,18

J1642 — Injection, heparin sodium, (heparin lock flush), per 10 units [N] [N1] [✓]
Use this code for Hep-Lock, Hep-Lock U/P, Hep-Pak, Lok-Pak.
CMS: 100-04,4,20.6.4
AHA: 4Q,18

● **J1643** — Injection, heparin sodium (Pfizer), not therapeutically equivalent to J1644, per 1000 units
Use this code for heparin sodium manufactured by Pfizer.

J1644 — Injection, Heparin sodium, per 1000 units [N] [N1] [✓]
Use this code for Heparin Sodium, Liquaemin Sodium.
CMS: 100-04,4,20.6.4
AHA: 4Q,18

J1645 — Injection, dalteparin sodium, per 2500 IU [N] [N1] [✓]
Use this code for Fragmin.
CMS: 100-02,15,50.5; 100-04,4,20.6.4
AHA: 4Q,18

J1650 — Injection, enoxaparin sodium, 10 mg [N] [N1] [✓]
Use this code for Lovenox.
CMS: 100-02,15,50.5; 100-04,4,20.6.4
AHA: 4Q,18

J1652 — Injection, fondaparinux sodium, 0.5 mg [N] [N1] [✓]
Use this code for Atrixtra.
CMS: 100-02,15,50.5
AHA: 4Q,18

2023 HCPCS Level II

J1655 Injection, tinzaparin sodium, 1000 IU
Use this code for Innohep.
CMS: 100-02,15,50.5; 100-04,4,20.6.4
AHA: 4Q,18

J1670 Injection, tetanus immune globulin, human, up to 250 units
Use this code for HyperTET SD.
AHA: 4Q,18

J1675 Injection, histrelin acetate, 10 mcg
Use this code for Supprelin LA.
AHA: 4Q,18

J1700 Injection, hydrocortisone acetate, up to 25 mg
Use this code for Hydrocortone Acetate.
CMS: 100-04,4,20.6.4
AHA: 4Q,18

J1710 Injection, hydrocortisone sodium phosphate, up to 50 mg
Use this code for Hydrocortone Phosphate.
CMS: 100-04,4,20.6.4
AHA: 4Q,18

J1720 Injection, hydrocortisone sodium succinate, up to 100 mg
Use this code for Solu-Cortef, A-Hydrocort.
CMS: 100-04,4,20.6.4
AHA: 4Q,18

J1726 Injection, hydroxyprogesterone caproate, (Makena), 10 mg
AHA: 4Q,18; 1Q,18

J1729 Injection, hydroxyprogesterone caproate, not otherwise specified, 10 mg
AHA: 4Q,18; 1Q,18

J1730 Injection, diazoxide, up to 300 mg
AHA: 4Q,18

J1738 Injection, meloxicam, 1 mg
Use this code for Anjeso.
AHA: 4Q,20

J1740 Injection, ibandronate sodium, 1 mg
Use this code for Boniva.
AHA: 4Q,18

J1741 Injection, ibuprofen, 100 mg
Use this code for Caldolor.
AHA: 4Q,18

J1742 Injection, ibutilide fumarate, 1 mg
Use this code for Corvert.
AHA: 4Q,18

J1743 Injection, idursulfase, 1 mg
Use this code for Elaprase.
AHA: 4Q,18

J1744 Injection, icatibant, 1 mg
Use this code for Firazyr.
CMS: 100-02,15,50.5
AHA: 4Q,18

J1745 Injection, infliximab, excludes biosimilar, 10 mg
Use this code for Remicade.
AHA: 4Q,18

J1746 Injection, ibalizumab-uiyk, 10 mg
Use this code for Trogarzo.
CMS: 100-04,4,260.1; 100-04,4,260.1.1
AHA: 1Q,19; 4Q,18

J1750 Injection, iron dextran, 50 mg
Use this code for INFeD.
AHA: 4Q,18

J1756 Injection, iron sucrose, 1 mg
Use this code for Venofer.
CMS: 100-04,8,60.2.4; 100-04,8,60.2.4.2
AHA: 4Q,18

J1786 Injection, imiglucerase, 10 units
Use this code for Cerezyme.
AHA: 4Q,18

J1790 Injection, droperidol, up to 5 mg
Use this code for Inapsine.
CMS: 100-04,4,20.6.4
AHA: 4Q,18

J1800 Injection, propranolol HCl, up to 1 mg
Use this code for Inderal.
CMS: 100-04,4,20.6.4
AHA: 4Q,18

J1810 Injection, droperidol and fentanyl citrate, up to 2 ml ampule
AHA: 4Q,18

J1815 Injection, insulin, per 5 units
Use this code for Humalog, Humulin, Iletin, Insulin Lispo, Lantus, Levemir, NPH, Pork insulin, Regular insulin, Ultralente, Velosulin, Humulin R, Iletin II Regular Pork, Insulin Purified Pork, Relion, Lente Iletin I, Novolin R, Humulin R U-500.
CMS: 100-04,4,20.6.4
AHA: 4Q,18

J1817 Insulin for administration through DME (i.e., insulin pump) per 50 units
Use this code for Humalog, Humulin, Vesolin BR, Iletin II NPH Pork, Lispro-PFC, Novolin, Novolog, Novolog Flexpen, Novolog Mix, Relion Novolin.
AHA: 4Q,18

J1823 Injection, inebilizumab-cdon, 1 mg
Use this code for Uplinza.
AHA: 1Q,21

J1826 Injection, interferon beta-1a, 30 mcg
Use this code for AVONEX, Rebif.
AHA: 4Q,18

J1830 Injection interferon beta-1b, 0.25 mg (code may be used for Medicare when drug administered under the direct supervision of a physician, not for use when drug is self-administered)
Use this code for Betaseron.
CMS: 100-02,15,50.5
AHA: 4Q,18

J1833 Injection, isavuconazonium, 1 mg
Use this code for Cresemba.
AHA: 4Q,18; 1Q,16

J1835 Injection, itraconazole, 50 mg
Use this code for Sporonox IV.
CMS: 100-04,4,20.6.4
AHA: 4Q,18

J1840 Injection, kanamycin sulfate, up to 500 mg
Use this code for Kantrex.
CMS: 100-04,4,20.6.4
AHA: 4Q,18

J1850 Injection, kanamycin sulfate, up to 75 mg
Use this code for Kantrex.
CMS: 100-04,4,20.6.4
AHA: 4Q,18

Drugs Administered Other Than Oral Method

J1885 Injection, ketorolac tromethamine, per 15 mg N N1 ☑
Use this code for Toradol.
CMS: 100-04,4,20.6.4
AHA: 4Q,18

J1890 Injection, cephalothin sodium, up to 1 g N N1 ☑
CMS: 100-04,4,20.6.4
AHA: 4Q,18

J1930 Injection, lanreotide, 1 mg K K2 ☑
Use this code for Somatuline.
AHA: 4Q,18

J1931 Injection, laronidase, 0.1 mg K K2 ☑
Use this code for Aldurazyme.
AHA: 4Q,18

● **J1932** Injection, lanreotide, (Cipla), 1 mg K2

J1940 Injection, furosemide, up to 20 mg N N1 ☑
Use this code for Lasix.
CMS: 100-04,4,20.6.4
AHA: 4Q,18

J1943 Injection, aripiprazole lauroxil, (Aristada Initio), 1 mg K2
AHA: 4Q,19

J1944 Injection, aripiprazole lauroxil, (Aristada), 1 mg K2
AHA: 4Q,19

J1945 Injection, lepirudin, 50 mg EI ☑
Use this code for Refludan.
This drug is used for patients with heparin-induced thrombocytopenia.
AHA: 4Q,18

J1950 Injection, leuprolide acetate (for depot suspension), per 3.75 mg K K2 ☑
Use this code for Lupron Depot-Pedi.
AHA: 2Q,19; 4Q,18

J1951 Injection, leuprolide acetate for depot suspension (Fensolvi), 0.25 mg K2
AHA: 3Q,21

J1952 Leuprolide injectable, camcevi, 1 mg K2
Use this code for Camcevi.
AHA: 1Q,22

J1953 Injection, levetiracetam, 10 mg N N1 ☑
Use this code for Keppra.
AHA: 4Q,18

J1955 Injection, levocarnitine, per 1 g B ☑
Use this code for Carnitor.
AHA: 4Q,18

J1956 Injection, levofloxacin, 250 mg N N1 ☑
Use this code for Levaquin.
CMS: 100-04,4,20.6.4
AHA: 4Q,18

J1960 Injection, levorphanol tartrate, up to 2 mg N N1 ☑
Use this code for Levo-Dromoran.
CMS: 100-04,4,20.6.4
AHA: 4Q,18

J1980 Injection, hyoscyamine sulfate, up to 0.25 mg N N1 ☑
Use this code for Levsin.
CMS: 100-04,4,20.6.4
AHA: 4Q,18

J1990 Injection, chlordiazepoxide HCl, up to 100 mg N N1 ☑
Use this code for Librium.
CMS: 100-04,4,20.6.4
AHA: 4Q,18

J2001 Injection, lidocaine HCl for intravenous infusion, 10 mg N N1 ☑
Use this code for Xylocaine.
CMS: 100-04,4,20.6.4
AHA: 4Q,18

J2010 Injection, lincomycin HCl, up to 300 mg N N1 ☑
Use this code for Lincocin.
CMS: 100-04,4,20.6.4
AHA: 4Q,18

J2020 Injection, linezolid, 200 mg N N1 ☑
Use this code for Zyvok.
AHA: 4Q,18

● **J2021** Injection, linezolid (Hospira) not therapeutically equivalent to J2020, 200 mg
Use this code for linezolid manufactured by Hospira.

J2060 Injection, lorazepam, 2 mg N N1 ☑
Use this code for Ativan.
CMS: 100-04,4,20.6.4
AHA: 4Q,18

J2062 Loxapine for inhalation, 1 mg
Use this code for Adasuve.
AHA: 1Q,19

J2150 Injection, mannitol, 25% in 50 ml N N1 ☑
Use this code for Osmitrol.
CMS: 100-04,4,20.6.4
AHA: 4Q,18

J2170 Injection, mecasermin, 1 mg N N1 ☑
Use this code for Iplex, Increlex.
CMS: 100-02,15,50.5; 100-04,4,20.6.4
AHA: 4Q,18

J2175 Injection, meperidine HCl, per 100 mg N N1 ☑
Use this code for Demerol.
CMS: 100-04,20,180; 100-04,32,411.3; 100-04,4,20.6.4
AHA: 4Q,18

J2180 Injection, meperidine and promethazine HCl, up to 50 mg N N1 ☑
Use this code for Mepergan Injection.
CMS: 100-04,4,20.6.4
AHA: 4Q,18

J2182 Injection, mepolizumab, 1 mg G K2 ☑
Use this code for Nucala.
AHA: 4Q,18

● **J2184** Injection, meropenem (B. Braun) not therapeutically equivalent to J2185, 100 mg
Use this code for meropenem manufactured by B. Braun.

J2185 Injection, meropenem, 100 mg N N1 ☑
Use this code for Merrem.
CMS: 100-04,4,20.6.4
AHA: 4Q,18

J2186 Injection, meropenem, vaborbactam, 10 mg/10 mg, (20 mg) K2
Use this code for Vabomere.
CMS: 100-04,4,260.1; 100-04,4,260.1.1
AHA: 1Q,19; 4Q,18

J2210 Injection, methylergonovine maleate, up to 0.2 mg N N1 ☑
Use this code for Methergine.
CMS: 100-04,4,20.6.4
AHA: 4Q,18

Special Coverage Instructions | Noncovered by Medicare | Carrier Discretion | ☑ Quantity Alert | ● New Code | ○ Recycled/Reinstated | ▲ Revised Code

98 — J Codes | **A** Age Edit | **M** Maternity Edit | ♀ Female Only | ♂ Male Only | **A-Y** OPPS Status Indicators | © 2022 Optum, Inc.

J2212 Injection, methylnaltrexone, 0.1 mg
Use this code for Relistor.
CMS: 100-02,15,50.5
AHA: 4Q,18

● **J2247** Injection, micafungin sodium (Par Pharm) not therapeutically equivalent to J2248, 1 mg
Use this code for micafungin sodium manufactured by Par Pharm.

J2248 Injection, micafungin sodium, 1 mg
Use this code for Mycamine.
AHA: 4Q,18

J2250 Injection, midazolam HCl, per 1 mg
Use this code for Versed.
CMS: 100-04,4,20.6.4
AHA: 4Q,18

● **J2251** Injection, midazolam HCl (WG Critical Care) not therapeutically equivalent to J2250, per 1 mg
Use this code for midazolam HCl manufactured by WG Critical Care.

J2260 Injection, milrinone lactate, 5 mg
Use this code for Primacor.
CMS: 100-04,20,180; 100-04,32,411.3; 100-04,4,20.6.4
AHA: 4Q,18

J2265 Injection, minocycline HCl, 1 mg
Use this code for MINOCIN.
AHA: 4Q,18

J2270 Injection, morphine sulfate, up to 10 mg
Use this code for Depodur, Infumorph.
CMS: 100-04,20,180; 100-04,4,20.6.4
AHA: 4Q,18

● **J2272** Injection, morphine sulfate (Fresenius Kabi) not therapeutically equivalent to J2270, up to 10 mg
Use this code for morphine sulfate manufactured by Fresenius Kabi.

J2274 Injection, morphine sulfate, preservative free for epidural or intrathecal use, 10 mg
Use this code for DepoDur, Astromorph PF, Durarmorph PF.
CMS: 100-04,20,180
AHA: 4Q,18

J2278 Injection, ziconotide, 1 mcg
Use this code for Prialt.
CMS: 100-04,20,180
AHA: 4Q,18

J2280 Injection, moxifloxacin, 100 mg
Use this code for Avelox.
CMS: 100-04,4,20.6.4
AHA: 4Q,18

● **J2281** Injection, moxifloxacin (Fresenius Kabi) not therapeutically equivalent to J2280, 100 mg
Use this code for moxifloxacin manufactured by Fresenius Kabi.

J2300 Injection, nalbuphine HCl, per 10 mg
Use this code for Nubain.
CMS: 100-04,4,20.6.4
AHA: 4Q,18

J2310 Injection, naloxone HCl, per 1 mg
Use this code for Narcan.
AHA: 4Q,18

● **J2311** Injection, naloxone HCl (Zimhi), 1 mg
Use this code for naloxone HCl (Zimhi) manufactured by Adamis.

J2315 Injection, naltrexone, depot form, 1 mg
Use this code for Vivitrol.
AHA: 4Q,18

J2320 Injection, nandrolone decanoate, up to 50 mg
AHA: 4Q,18

J2323 Injection, natalizumab, 1 mg
Use this code for Tysabri.
AHA: 4Q,18

J2325 Injection, nesiritide, 0.1 mg
Use this code for Natrecor.
CMS: 100-03,200.1
AHA: 4Q,18

J2326 Injection, nusinersen, 0.1 mg
Use this code for Spinraza.
AHA: 1Q,21; 1Q,20; 4Q,18; 1Q,18

● **J2327** Injection, risankizumab-rzaa, intravenous, 1 mg

J2350 Injection, ocrelizumab, 1 mg
Use this code for Ocrevus.
AHA: 4Q,18; 1Q,18

J2353 Injection, octreotide, depot form for intramuscular injection, 1 mg
Use this code for Sandostatin LAR.
AHA: 4Q,18

J2354 Injection, octreotide, nondepot form for subcutaneous or intravenous injection, 25 mcg
Use this code for Sandostatin.
CMS: 100-02,15,50.5
AHA: 4Q,18

J2355 Injection, oprelvekin, 5 mg
Use this code for Neumega.
AHA: 4Q,18

● **J2356** Injection, tezepelumab-ekko, 1 mg
Use this code for Tezspire.
AHA: 3Q,22

J2357 Injection, omalizumab, 5 mg
Use this code for Xolair.
AHA: 4Q,18

J2358 Injection, olanzapine, long-acting, 1 mg
Use this code for ZYPREXA RELPREVV.
AHA: 4Q,18

J2360 Injection, orphenadrine citrate, up to 60 mg
Use this code for Norflex.
AHA: 4Q,18

J2370 Injection, phenylephrine HCl, up to 1 ml
AHA: 4Q,18

J2400 ~~Injection, chloroprocaine HCl, per 30 ml~~
To report, see ~J2401, J2402

● **J2401** Injection, chloroprocaine HCl, per 1 mg

● **J2402** Injection, chloroprocaine HCl (Clorotekal), per 1 mg
Use this code for chloroprocaine HCl (Clorotekal) manufactured by B. Braun.

J2405 Injection, ondansetron HCl, per 1 mg
Use this code for Zofran.
AHA: 4Q,18

J2406 Injection, oritavancin (Kimyrsa), 10 mg
AHA: 4Q,21

J2407 Injection, oritavancin (Orbactiv), 10 mg
Use this code for Orbactiv.
AHA: 4Q,18; 1Q,16

J2410 Injection, oxymorphone HCl, up to 1 mg
Use this code for Numorphan, Oxymorphone HCl.
AHA: 4Q,18

Drugs Administered Other Than Oral Method

J2425 — J2777

J2425 Injection, palifermin, 50 mcg
Use this code for Kepivance.
AHA: 4Q,18

J2426 Injection, paliperidone palmitate extended release, 1 mg
Use this code for INVEGA SUSTENNA.
AHA: 4Q,18

J2430 Injection, pamidronate disodium, per 30 mg
Use this code for Aredia.
AHA: 4Q,18

J2440 Injection, papaverine HCl, up to 60 mg
AHA: 4Q,18

J2460 Injection, oxytetracycline HCl, up to 50 mg
Use this code for Terramycin IM.
AHA: 4Q,18

J2469 Injection, palonosetron HCl, 25 mcg
Use this code for Aloxi.
AHA: 4Q,18

J2501 Injection, paricalcitol, 1 mcg
Use this code For Zemplar.
AHA: 4Q,18

J2502 Injection, pasireotide long acting, 1 mg
Use this code for Signifor LAR.
AHA: 4Q,18; 1Q,16

J2503 Injection, pegaptanib sodium, 0.3 mg
Use this code for Macugen.
AHA: 4Q,18

J2504 Injection, pegademase bovine, 25 IU
Use this code for Adagen.
AHA: 4Q,18

J2506 Injection, pegfilgrastim, excludes biosimilar, 0.5 mg
Use this code for Neulasta.
AHA: 1Q,22

J2507 Injection, pegloticase, 1 mg
Use this code for KRYSTEXXA.
AHA: 4Q,18

J2510 Injection, penicillin G procaine, aqueous, up to 600,000 units
Use this code for Wycillin, Duracillin A.S., Pfizerpen A.S., Crysticillin 300 A.S., Crysticillin 600 A.S.
AHA: 4Q,18

J2513 Injection, pentastarch, 10% solution, 100 ml
AHA: 4Q,18

J2515 Injection, pentobarbital sodium, per 50 mg
Use this code for Nembutal Sodium Solution.
AHA: 4Q,18

J2540 Injection, penicillin G potassium, up to 600,000 units
Use this code for Pfizerpen.
AHA: 4Q,18

J2543 Injection, piperacillin sodium/tazobactam sodium, 1 g/0.125 g (1.125 g)
Use this code for Zosyn.
AHA: 4Q,18

J2545 Pentamidine isethionate, inhalation solution, FDA-approved final product, noncompounded, administered through DME, unit dose form, per 300 mg
Use this code for Nebupent, Pentam 300.

J2547 Injection, peramivir, 1 mg
Use this code for Rapivab.
AHA: 4Q,18; 1Q,16

J2550 Injection, promethazine HCl, up to 50 mg
Use this code for Phenergan.
AHA: 4Q,18

J2560 Injection, phenobarbital sodium, up to 120 mg
AHA: 4Q,18

J2562 Injection, plerixafor, 1 mg
Use this code for Mozobil.
AHA: 4Q,18

J2590 Injection, oxytocin, up to 10 units
Use this code for Pitocin, Syntocinon.
AHA: 4Q,18

J2597 Injection, desmopressin acetate, per 1 mcg
Use this code for DDAVP.
AHA: 4Q,18

J2650 Injection, prednisolone acetate, up to 1 ml
AHA: 4Q,18

J2670 Injection, tolazoline HCl, up to 25 mg
AHA: 4Q,18

J2675 Injection, progesterone, per 50 mg
Use this code for Gesterone, Gestrin.
AHA: 4Q,18

J2680 Injection, fluphenazine decanoate, up to 25 mg
AHA: 4Q,18

J2690 Injection, procainamide HCl, up to 1 g
Use this code for Pronestyl.
AHA: 4Q,18

J2700 Injection, oxacillin sodium, up to 250 mg
Use this code for Bactocill
AHA: 4Q,18

J2704 Injection, propofol, 10 mg
Use this code for Diprivan.
AHA: 4Q,18

J2710 Injection, neostigmine methylsulfate, up to 0.5 mg
Use this code for Prostigmin.
AHA: 4Q,18

J2720 Injection, protamine sulfate, per 10 mg
AHA: 4Q,18

J2724 Injection, protein C concentrate, intravenous, human, 10 IU
AHA: 4Q,18

J2725 Injection, protirelin, per 250 mcg
Use this code for Thyrel TRH.
AHA: 4Q,18

J2730 Injection, pralidoxime chloride, up to 1 g
Use this code for Protopam Chloride.
AHA: 4Q,18

J2760 Injection, phentolamine mesylate, up to 5 mg
Use this code for Regitine.
AHA: 4Q,18

J2765 Injection, metoclopramide HCl, up to 10 mg
Use this code for Reglan.
AHA: 4Q,18

J2770 Injection, quinupristin/dalfopristin, 500 mg (150/350)
Use this code for Synercid.
AHA: 4Q,18

● **J2777** Injection, faricimab-svoa, 0.1 mg
Use this code for Vabysmo.

2023 HCPCS Level II — J3000

Drugs Administered Other Than Oral Method — J2778–J3000

J2778 Injection, ranibizumab, 0.1 mg
Use this code for Lucentis.
AHA: 4Q,18

● **J2779** Injection, ranibizumab, via intravitreal implant (Susvimo), 0.1 mg
AHA: 3Q,22

J2780 Injection, ranitidine HCl, 25 mg
Use this code for Zantac.
AHA: 4Q,18

J2783 Injection, rasburicase, 0.5 mg
Use this code for Elitek.
AHA: 4Q,18

J2785 Injection, regadenoson, 0.1 mg
Use this code for Lexiscan.
AHA: 4Q,18

J2786 Injection, reslizumab, 1 mg
Use this code for Cinqair.
AHA: 4Q,18; 4Q,16

J2787 Riboflavin 5'-phosphate, ophthalmic solution, up to 3 ml
Use this code for Photrexa Viscous.
CMS: 100-04,4,260.1; 100-04,4,260.1.1
AHA: 1Q,19

J2788 Injection, Rho D immune globulin, human, minidose, 50 mcg (250 IU)
Use this code for RhoGam, MiCRhoGAM.
AHA: 4Q,18

J2790 Injection, Rho D immune globulin, human, full dose, 300 mcg (1500 IU)
Use this code for RhoGam, HypRho SD.
AHA: 4Q,18

J2791 Injection, Rho D immune globulin (human), (Rhophylac), intramuscular or intravenous, 100 IU
Use this for Rhophylac.
AHA: 4Q,18

J2792 Injection, Rho D immune globulin, intravenous, human, solvent detergent, 100 IU
Use this code for WINRho SDF.
AHA: 4Q,18

J2793 Injection, rilonacept, 1 mg
Use this code for Arcalyst.
CMS: 100-02,15,50.5
AHA: 4Q,18

J2794 Injection, risperidone (RISPERDAL CONSTA), 0.5 mg
AHA: 4Q,18

J2795 Injection, ropivacaine HCl, 1 mg
Use this code for Naropin.
AHA: 4Q,18

J2796 Injection, romiplostim, 10 mcg
Use this code for Nplate.
AHA: 4Q,18

J2797 Injection, rolapitant, 0.5 mg
Use this code for Varubi.
AHA: 1Q,19; 4Q,18

J2798 Injection, risperidone, (Perseris), 0.5 mg
AHA: 4Q,19

J2800 Injection, methocarbamol, up to 10 ml
Use this code for Robaxin.
AHA: 4Q,18

J2805 Injection, sincalide, 5 mcg
Use this code for Kinevac.
AHA: 4Q,18

J2810 Injection, theophylline, per 40 mg
AHA: 4Q,18

J2820 Injection, sargramostim (GM-CSF), 50 mcg
Use this code for Leukine.
AHA: 4Q,18

J2840 Injection, sebelipase alfa, 1 mg
Use this code for Kanuma.
AHA: 4Q,18

J2850 Injection, secretin, synthetic, human, 1 mcg
AHA: 4Q,18

J2860 Injection, siltuximab, 10 mg
Use this code for Sylvant.
AHA: 4Q,18; 1Q,16

J2910 Injection, aurothioglucose, up to 50 mg
Use this code for Solganal.
AHA: 4Q,18

J2916 Injection, sodium ferric gluconate complex in sucrose injection, 12.5 mg
CMS: 100-03,110.10
AHA: 4Q,18

J2920 Injection, methylprednisolone sodium succinate, up to 40 mg
Use this code for Solu-Medrol, A-methaPred.
AHA: 4Q,18

J2930 Injection, methylprednisolone sodium succinate, up to 125 mg
Use this code for Solu-Medrol, A-methaPred.
AHA: 4Q,18

J2940 Injection, somatrem, 1 mg
Use this code for Protropin.
AHA: 4Q,18

J2941 Injection, somatropin, 1 mg
Use this code for Humatrope, Genotropin Nutropin, Biotropin, Genotropin, Genotropin Miniquick, Norditropin, Nutropin, Nutropin AQ, Saizen, Saizen Somatropin RDNA Origin, Serostim, Serostim RDNA Origin, Zorbtive.
CMS: 100-02,15,50.5
AHA: 4Q,18

J2950 Injection, promazine HCl, up to 25 mg
Use this code for Sparine, Prozine-50.
AHA: 4Q,18

J2993 Injection, reteplase, 18.1 mg
Use this code for Retavase.
AHA: 3Q,21; 4Q,18

J2995 Injection, streptokinase, per 250,000 IU
Use this code for Streptase.
AHA: 3Q,21; 4Q,18

J2997 Injection, alteplase recombinant, 1 mg
Use this code for Activase, Cathflo.
AHA: 3Q,21; 4Q,18

● **J2998** Injection, plasminogen, human-tvmh, 1 mg
Use this code for Ryplazim.
AHA: 3Q,22

J3000 Injection, streptomycin, up to 1 g
Use this code for Streptomycin Sulfate.
AHA: 4Q,18

Special Coverage Instructions | Noncovered by Medicare | Carrier Discretion | ☑ Quantity Alert | ● New Code | ○ Recycled/Reinstated | ▲ Revised Code

© 2022 Optum, Inc. | A2–Z3 ASC Pmt | CMS: IOM | AHA: Coding Clinic | DMEPOS Paid | ⊘ SNF Excluded | J Codes — 101

Drugs Administered Other Than Oral Method

J3010 — J3310

J3010 Injection, fentanyl citrate, 0.1 mg [N][N1][✓]
Use this code for Sublimaze.
CMS: 100-04,20,180; 100-04,32,411.3
AHA: 4Q,18

J3030 Injection, sumatriptan succinate, 6 mg (code may be used for Medicare when drug administered under the direct supervision of a physician, not for use when drug is self-administered) [N][N1][✓]
Use this code for Imitrex.
CMS: 100-02,15,50.5
AHA: 4Q,18

J3031 Injection, fremanezumab-vfrm, 1 mg (code may be used for Medicare when drug administered under the direct supervision of a physician, not for use when drug is self-administered) [K2]
Use this code for Ajovy.
AHA: 4Q,19

J3032 Injection, eptinezumab-jjmr, 1 mg [K2]
Use this code for Vyepti.
AHA: 4Q,20

J3060 Injection, taliglucerase alfa, 10 units [K][K2][✓]
Use this code for Elelyso.
AHA: 4Q,18

J3070 Injection, pentazocine, 30 mg [K][N1][✓]
Use this code for Talwin.
AHA: 4Q,18

J3090 Injection, tedizolid phosphate, 1 mg [K][K2][✓]
Use this code for Sivextro.
AHA: 4Q,18; 1Q,16

J3095 Injection, telavancin, 10 mg [K][K2][✓]
Use this code for VIBATIV.
AHA: 4Q,18

J3101 Injection, tenecteplase, 1 mg [K][K2][✓]
Use this code for TNKase.
AHA: 3Q,21; 3Q,20; 4Q,18

J3105 Injection, terbutaline sulfate, up to 1 mg [N][N1][✓]
For terbutaline in inhalation solution, see K0525 and K0526.
AHA: 4Q,18

J3110 Injection, teriparatide, 10 mcg [B][✓]
Use this code for Forteo.
CMS: 100-02,15,50.5; 100-04,10,90.1
AHA: 4Q,18

J3111 Injection, romosozumab-aqqg, 1 mg [K2]
Use this code for Evenity.
CMS: 100-04,10,90.1

J3121 Injection, testosterone enanthate, 1 mg [N][N1][✓]
Use this code for Delatstryl.
AHA: 4Q,18

J3145 Injection, testosterone undecanoate, 1 mg [K][K2][✓]
Use this code for Aveed.
AHA: 4Q,18

J3230 Injection, chlorpromazine HCl, up to 50 mg [N][N1][✓]
Use this code for Thorazine.
AHA: 4Q,18

J3240 Injection, thyrotropin alpha, 0.9 mg, provided in 1.1 mg vial [K][K2][✓]
Use this code for Thyrogen.
AHA: 4Q,18

J3241 Injection, teprotumumab-trbw, 10 mg [K2]
Use this code for Tepezza.
AHA: 4Q,20

J3243 Injection, tigecycline, 1 mg [K][N1][✓]
Use this code for Tygacil.
AHA: 4Q,18

● **J3244** Injection, tigecycline (Accord) not therapeutically equivalent to J3243, 1 mg
Use this code for tigecycline manufactured by Accord.

J3245 Injection, tildrakizumab, 1 mg [K2]
Use this code for Ilumya.
AHA: 4Q,18

J3246 Injection, tirofiban HCl, 0.25 mg [K][K2][✓]
Use this code for Aggrastat.
AHA: 4Q,18

J3250 Injection, trimethobenzamide HCl, up to 200 mg [N][N1][✓]
Use this code for Tigan, Tiject-20, Arrestin.
AHA: 4Q,18

J3260 Injection, tobramycin sulfate, up to 80 mg [N][N1][✓]
Use this code for Nebcin.
AHA: 4Q,18

J3262 Injection, tocilizumab, 1 mg [K][K2][✓]
Use this code for ACTEMRA.
AHA: 4Q,18

J3265 Injection, torsemide, 10 mg/ml [N][N1][✓]
Use this code for Demadex, Torsemide.
AHA: 4Q,18

J3280 Injection, thiethylperazine maleate, up to 10 mg [EI][✓]
AHA: 4Q,18

J3285 Injection, treprostinil, 1 mg [K][K2][✓]
Use this code for Remodulin.
CMS: 100-04,20,180; 100-04,32,411.3
AHA: 4Q,18

● **J3299** Injection, triamcinolone acetonide (Xipere), 1 mg [K2]
AHA: 3Q,22

J3300 Injection, triamcinolone acetonide, preservative free, 1 mg [K][N1][✓]
Use this code for TRIVARIS, TRIESENCE.
AHA: 4Q,18

J3301 Injection, triamcinolone acetonide, not otherwise specified, 10 mg [N][N1][✓]
Use this code for Kenalog-10, Kenalog-40, Tri-Kort, Kenaject-40, Cenacort A-40, Triam-A, Trilog.
AHA: 4Q,18; 3Q,17

J3302 Injection, triamcinolone diacetate, per 5 mg [N][N1][✓]
Use this code for Aristocort, Aristocort Intralesional, Aristocort Forte, Amcort, Trilone, Cenacort Forte.
AHA: 4Q,18

J3303 Injection, triamcinolone hexacetonide, per 5 mg [N][N1][✓]
Use this code for Aristospan Intralesional, Aristospan Intra-articular.
AHA: 4Q,18

J3304 Injection, triamcinolone acetonide, preservative-free, extended-release, microsphere formulation, 1 mg [K2]
Use this code for Zilretta.
AHA: 1Q,19; 4Q,18

J3305 Injection, trimetrexate glucuronate, per 25 mg [EI][✓]
Use this code for Neutrexin.
AHA: 4Q,18

J3310 Injection, perphenazine, up to 5 mg [N][N1][✓]
Use this code for Trilafon.
AHA: 4Q,18

Special Coverage Instructions | Noncovered by Medicare | Carrier Discretion | ✓ Quantity Alert | ● New Code | ○ Recycled/Reinstated | ▲ Revised Code

102 — J Codes | [A] Age Edit | [M] Maternity Edit | ♀ Female Only | ♂ Male Only | [A]-[Y] OPPS Status Indicators | © 2022 Optum, Inc.

J3315 — J3490 — Drugs Administered Other Than Oral Method

J3315 Injection, triptorelin pamoate, 3.75 mg
Use this code for Trelstar Depot, Trelstar Depot Plus Debioclip Kit, Trelstar LA.
AHA: 4Q,18

J3316 Injection, triptorelin, extended-release, 3.75 mg
Use this code for Triptodur.
AHA: 1Q,19; 4Q,18

J3320 Injection, spectinomycin dihydrochloride, up to 2 g
Use this code for Trobicin.
AHA: 4Q,18

J3350 Injection, urea, up to 40 g
AHA: 4Q,18

J3355 Injection, urofollitropin, 75 IU
Use this code for Metrodin, Bravelle, Fertinex.
CMS: 100-02,15,50.5
AHA: 4Q,18

J3357 Ustekinumab, for subcutaneous injection, 1 mg
Use this code for STELARA.
CMS: 100-02,15,50.5
AHA: 4Q,18; 1Q,17; 4Q,16

J3358 Ustekinumab, for intravenous injection, 1 mg
Use this code for Stelara.
AHA: 4Q,18; 1Q,18

J3360 Injection, diazepam, up to 5 mg
Use this code for Diastat, Dizac, Valium.
CMS: 100-04,8,60.2.1
AHA: 4Q,18

J3364 Injection, urokinase, 5,000 IU vial
Use this code for Kinlytic.
AHA: 3Q,21; 4Q,18

J3365 Injection, IV, urokinase, 250,000 IU vial
Use this code for Kinlytic.
AHA: 3Q,21; 4Q,18

J3370 Injection, vancomycin HCl, 500 mg
Use this code for Vancocin.
AHA: 4Q,18

● **J3371** Injection, vancomycin HCl (Mylan) not therapeutically equivalent to J3370, 500 mg
Use this code for vancomycin HCl manufactured by Mylan.

● **J3372** Injection, vancomycin HCl (Xellia) not therapeutically equivalent to J3370, 500 mg
Use this code for vancomycin HCl manufactured by Xellia.

J3380 Injection, vedolizumab, 1 mg
Use this code for Entyvio.
AHA: 4Q,18; 1Q,16

J3385 Injection, velaglucerase alfa, 100 units
Use this code for VPRIV.
AHA: 4Q,18

J3396 Injection, verteporfin, 0.1 mg
Use this code for Visudyne.
CMS: 100-03,80.2; 100-03,80.2.1; 100-03,80.3; 100-03,80.3.1; 100-04,32,300; 100-04,32,300.1; 100-04,32,300.2
AHA: 1Q,20; 4Q,18

J3397 Injection, vestronidase alfa-vjbk, 1 mg
Use this code for Mepsevii.
CMS: 100-04,4,260.1; 100-04,4,260.1.1
AHA: 1Q,19; 4Q,18

J3398 Injection, voretigene neparvovec-rzyl, 1 billion vector genomes
Use this code for Luxturna.
AHA: 1Q,19; 4Q,18

J3399 Injection, onasemnogene abeparvovec-xioi, per treatment, up to 5×10^{15} vector genomes
Use this code for Zolgensma.
AHA: 2Q,20

J3400 Injection, triflupromazine HCl, up to 20 mg
AHA: 4Q,18

J3410 Injection, hydroxyzine HCl, up to 25 mg
Use this code for Vistaril, Vistaject-25, Hyzine, Hyzine-50.
AHA: 4Q,18

J3411 Injection, thiamine HCl, 100 mg
AHA: 4Q,18

J3415 Injection, pyridoxine HCl, 100 mg
AHA: 4Q,18

J3420 Injection, vitamin B-12 cyanocobalamin, up to 1,000 mcg
Use this code for Sytobex, Redisol, Rubramin PC, Betalin 12, Berubigen, Cobex, Cobal, Crystal B12, Cyano, Cyanocobalamin, Hydroxocobalamin, Hydroxycobal, Nutri-Twelve.
AHA: 4Q,18

J3430 Injection, phytonadione (vitamin K), per 1 mg
Use this code for AquaMephyton, Konakion, Menadione, Phytonadione.
AHA: 4Q,18

J3465 Injection, voriconazole, 10 mg
AHA: 4Q,18

J3470 Injection, hyaluronidase, up to 150 units
AHA: 4Q,18

J3471 Injection, hyaluronidase, ovine, preservative free, per 1 USP unit (up to 999 USP units)
AHA: 4Q,18

J3472 Injection, hyaluronidase, ovine, preservative free, per 1,000 USP units
AHA: 4Q,18

J3473 Injection, hyaluronidase, recombinant, 1 USP unit
AHA: 4Q,18

J3475 Injection, magnesium sulfate, per 500 mg
Use this code for Mag Sul, Sulfa Mag.
AHA: 4Q,18

J3480 Injection, potassium chloride, per 2 mEq
AHA: 4Q,18

J3485 Injection, zidovudine, 10 mg
Use this code for Retrovir, Zidovudine.
AHA: 4Q,18

J3486 Injection, ziprasidone mesylate, 10 mg
Use this code for Geodon.
AHA: 4Q,18

J3489 Injection, zoledronic acid, 1 mg
Use this code for Reclast and Zometa.
AHA: 4Q,18

J3490 Unclassified drugs
CMS: 100-02,15,50.5; 100-03,1,110.22; 100-03,110.22; 100-04,10,90.1; 100-04,32,280.1; 100-04,32,280.2; 100-04,32,400; 100-04,32,400.1; 100-04,32,400.2; 100-04,32,400.2.1; 100-04,32,400.2.2; 100-04,32,400.2.3; 100-04,32,400.2.4; 100-04,32,400.3; 100-04,32,400.4; 100-04,32,400.5; 100-04,4,260.1; 100-04,4,260.1.1; 100-04,8,60.2.1.1; 100-04,8,60.2.3
AHA: 3Q,21; 1Q,17

Drugs Administered Other Than Oral Method

J3520 — Edetate disodium, per 150 mg
Use this code for Endrate, Disotate, Meritate, Chealamide, E.D.T.A. This drug is used in chelation therapy, a treatment for atherosclerosis that is not covered by Medicare.

J3530 — Nasal vaccine inhalation

J3535 — Drug administered through a metered dose inhaler

J3570 — Laetrile, amygdalin, vitamin B-17
The FDA has found Laetrile to have no safe or effective therapeutic purpose.

J3590 — Unclassified biologics
CMS: 100-02,15,50.5; 100-03,1,110.22; 100-03,110.22; 100-04,10,90.1; 100-04,32,280.1; 100-04,32,280.2; 100-04,32,400; 100-04,32,400.1; 100-04,32,400.2; 100-04,32,400.2.1; 100-04,32,400.2.2; 100-04,32,400.2.3; 100-04,32,400.2.4; 100-04,32,400.3; 100-04,32,400.4; 100-04,32,400.5
AHA: 1Q,17; 4Q,16

J3591 — Unclassified drug or biological used for ESRD on dialysis
CMS: 100-04,4,260.1; 100-04,4,260.1.1; 100-04,8,20
AHA: 1Q,19

J7030 — Infusion, normal saline solution, 1,000 cc

J7040 — Infusion, normal saline solution, sterile (500 ml=1 unit)

J7042 — 5% dextrose/normal saline (500 ml = 1 unit)

J7050 — Infusion, normal saline solution, 250 cc

J7060 — 5% dextrose/water (500 ml = 1 unit)

J7070 — Infusion, D-5-W, 1,000 cc

J7100 — Infusion, dextran 40, 500 ml
Use this code for Gentran, 10% LMD, Rheomacrodex.

J7110 — Infusion, dextran 75, 500 ml
Use this code for Gentran 75.

J7120 — Ringers lactate infusion, up to 1,000 cc

J7121 — 5% dextrose in lactated ringers infusion, up to 1000 cc

J7131 — Hypertonic saline solution, 1 ml

J7168 — Prothrombin complex concentrate (human), Kcentra, per IU of Factor IX activity
AHA: 3Q,21

J7169 — Injection, coagulation Factor Xa (recombinant), inactivated-zhzo (Andexxa), 10 mg
AHA: 2Q,20

J7170 — Injection, emicizumab-kxwh, 0.5 mg
Use this code for Hemlibra.
AHA: 1Q,19; 4Q,18

J7175 — Injection, Factor X, (human), 1 IU
Use this code for Coagadex.
AHA: 4Q,18; 1Q,17

J7177 — Injection, human fibrinogen concentrate (Fibryga), 1 mg
CMS: 100-04,4,260.1; 100-04,4,260.1.1
AHA: 1Q,19; 4Q,18

J7178 — Injection, human fibrinogen concentrate, not otherwise specified, 1 mg
Use this code for RiaSTAP.
AHA: 4Q,18

J7179 — Injection, von Willebrand factor (recombinant), (Vonvendi), 1 IU VWF:RCo
AHA: 4Q,18; 1Q,17

J7180 — Injection, Factor XIII (antihemophilic factor, human), 1 IU
Use this code for Corifact.
AHA: 4Q,18

J7181 — Injection, Factor XIII A-subunit, (recombinant), per IU
AHA: 4Q,18

J7182 — Injection, Factor VIII, (antihemophilic factor, recombinant), (NovoEight), per IU
AHA: 4Q,18

J7183 — Injection, von Willebrand factor complex (human), Wilate, 1 IU VWF:RCO
AHA: 4Q,18

J7185 — Injection, Factor VIII (antihemophilic factor, recombinant) (Xyntha), per IU
AHA: 4Q,18

J7186 — Injection, antihemophilic Factor VIII/von Willebrand factor complex (human), per Factor VIII IU
Use this code for Alphanate.
CMS: 100-04,17,80.4.1
AHA: 4Q,18

J7187 — Injection, von Willebrand factor complex (Humate-P), per IU VWF:RCO
CMS: 100-04,17,80.4.1
AHA: 4Q,18

J7188 — Injection, Factor VIII (antihemophilic factor, recombinant) (Obizur), per IU
AHA: 4Q,18; 1Q,16

J7189 — Factor VIIa (antihemophilic factor, recombinant), (NovoSeven RT), 1 mcg
CMS: 100-04,17,80.4.1

J7190 — Factor VIII (antihemophilic factor, human) per IU
Use this code for Koate-DVI, Monarc-M, Monoclate-P.
CMS: 100-04,17,80.4; 100-04,17,80.4.1

J7191 — Factor VIII (antihemophilic factor (porcine)), per IU
CMS: 100-04,17,80.4; 100-04,17,80.4.1

J7192 — Factor VIII (antihemophilic factor, recombinant) per IU, not otherwise specified
Use this code for Advate rAHF-PFM, Antihemophilic Factor Human Method M Monoclonal Purified, Bioclate, Kogenate FS, Recombinate, Refacto.
CMS: 100-04,17,80.4; 100-04,17,80.4.1

J7193 — Factor IX (antihemophilic factor, purified, nonrecombinant) per IU
Use this code for AlphaNine SD, Mononine.
CMS: 100-04,17,80.4; 100-04,17,80.4.1

J7194 — Factor IX complex, per IU
Use this code for Konyne-80, Profilnine SD, Proplex T, Proplex T, Bebulin VH, factor IX+ complex, Profilnine SD.
CMS: 100-04,17,80.4; 100-04,17,80.4.1

J7195 — Injection, Factor IX (antihemophilic factor, recombinant) per IU, not otherwise specified
Use this code for Antithrombate III, Benefix, Thrombate III.
CMS: 100-04,17,80.4; 100-04,17,80.4.1
AHA: 4Q,18

J7196 — Injection, antithrombin recombinant, 50 IU
Use this code for ATryn.
AHA: 4Q,18

J7197 — Antithrombin III (human), per IU
Use this code for Thrombate III, ATnativ.
CMS: 100-04,17,80.4.1

2023 HCPCS Level II

J7198 — Antiinhibitor, per IU
Medicare jurisdiction: local contractor. Use this code for Autoplex T, Feiba VH AICC.
CMS: 100-03,110.3; 100-04,17,80.4; 100-04,17,80.4.1

J7199 — Hemophilia clotting factor, not otherwise classified
Medicare jurisdiction: local contractor.
CMS: 100-04,17,80.4; 100-04,17,80.4.1

J7200 — Injection, Factor IX, (antihemophilic factor, recombinant), Rixubis, per IU
AHA: 4Q,18

J7201 — Injection, Factor IX, Fc fusion protein, (recombinant), Alprolix, 1 IU
AHA: 4Q,18

J7202 — Injection, Factor IX, albumin fusion protein, (recombinant), Idelvion, 1 IU
AHA: 4Q,18; 4Q,16

J7203 — Injection Factor IX, (antihemophilic factor, recombinant), glycoPEGylated, (Rebinyn), 1 IU
AHA: 1Q,19; 4Q,18

J7204 — Injection, Factor VIII, antihemophilic factor (recombinant), (Esperoct), glycopegylated-exei, per IU
AHA: 2Q,20

J7205 — Injection, Factor VIII Fc fusion protein (recombinant), per IU
Use this code for Eloctate.
AHA: 4Q,18; 1Q,16

J7207 — Injection, Factor VIII, (antihemophilic factor, recombinant), PEGylated, 1 IU
Use this code for Adynovate.
AHA: 4Q,18

J7208 — Injection, Factor VIII, (antihemophilic factor, recombinant), PEGylated-aucl, (Jivi), 1 IU
AHA: 3Q,19

J7209 — Injection, Factor VIII, (antihemophilic factor, recombinant), (Nuwiq), 1 IU
AHA: 4Q,18

J7210 — Injection, Factor VIII, (antihemophilic factor, recombinant), (Afstyla), 1 IU
AHA: 4Q,18; 1Q,18

J7211 — Injection, Factor VIII, (antihemophilic factor, recombinant), (Kovaltry), 1 IU
AHA: 4Q,18; 1Q,18

J7212 — Factor VIIa (antihemophilic factor, recombinant)-jncw (Sevenfact), 1 mcg
AHA: 1Q,21

J7294 — Segesterone acetate and ethinyl estradiol 0.15 mg, 0.013 mg per 24 hours; yearly vaginal system, ea
Use this code for Annovera vaginal ring.
AHA: 4Q,21

J7295 — Ethinyl estradiol and etonogestrel 0.015 mg, 0.12 mg per 24 hours; monthly vaginal ring, ea
Use this code for NuvaRing vaginal ring.
AHA: 4Q,21

J7296 — Levonorgestrel-releasing intrauterine contraceptive system, (Kyleena), 19.5 mg
AHA: 1Q,18

J7297 — Levonorgestrel-releasing intrauterine contraceptive system (Liletta), 52 mg

J7298 — Levonorgestrel-releasing intrauterine contraceptive system (Mirena), 52 mg

J7300 — Intrauterine copper contraceptive
Use this code for Paragard T380A.

J7301 — Levonorgestrel-releasing intrauterine contraceptive system (Skyla), 13.5 mg

J7304 — Contraceptive supply, hormone containing patch, each

J7306 — Levonorgestrel (contraceptive) implant system, including implants and supplies

J7307 — Etonogestrel (contraceptive) implant system, including implant and supplies
Use this code for Implanon and Nexplanon.

J7308 — Aminolevulinic acid HCl for topical administration, 20%, single unit dosage form (354 mg)
Use this code for Levulan Kerastick.
AHA: 1Q,20

J7309 — Methyl aminolevulinate (MAL) for topical administration, 16.8%, 1 g
Use this code for Metvixia.
AHA: 1Q,20

J7310 — Ganciclovir, 4.5 mg, long-acting implant
Use this code for Vitrasert.

J7311 — Injection, fluocinolone acetonide, intravitreal implant (Retisert), 0.01 mg

J7312 — Injection, dexamethasone, intravitreal implant, 0.1 mg
Use this code for OZURDEX.
AHA: 4Q,18

J7313 — Injection, fluocinolone acetonide, intravitreal implant (Iluvien), 0.01 mg
AHA: 4Q,18; 1Q,16

J7314 — Injection, fluocinolone acetonide, intravitreal implant (Yutiq), 0.01 mg
AHA: 4Q,19

J7315 — Mitomycin, opthalmic, 0.2 mg
Use this code for Mitosol.

J7316 — Injection, ocriplasmin, 0.125 mg
Use this code for Jetrea.
AHA: 4Q,18

J7318 — Hyaluronan or derivative, Durolane, for intra-articular injection, 1 mg
AHA: 1Q,19; 4Q,18

J7320 — Hyaluronan or derivative, GenVisc 850, for intra-articular injection, 1 mg
AHA: 4Q,18

J7321 — Hyaluronan or derivative, Hyalgan, Supartz or Visco-3, for intra-articular injection, per dose
AHA: 1Q,21; 2Q,20; 4Q,18

J7322 — Hyaluronan or derivative, Hymovis, for intra-articular injection, 1 mg
AHA: 4Q,18

J7323 — Hyaluronan or derivative, Euflexxa, for intra-articular injection, per dose
AHA: 4Q,18

J7324 — Hyaluronan or derivative, Orthovisc, for intra-articular injection, per dose
AHA: 4Q,18

J7325 — Hyaluronan or derivative, Synvisc or Synvisc-One, for intra-articular injection, 1 mg
AHA: 4Q,18

Special Coverage Instructions | Noncovered by Medicare | Carrier Discretion | ☑ Quantity Alert | ● New Code | ○ Recycled/Reinstated | ▲ Revised Code

© 2022 Optum, Inc. | A2–Z3 ASC Pmt | CMS: IOM | AHA: Coding Clinic | DMEPOS Paid | SNF Excluded

Drugs Administered Other Than Oral Method

J7326 Hyaluronan or derivative, Gel-One, for intra-articular injection, per dose K K2 ✓
AHA: 4Q,18

J7327 Hyaluronan or derivative, Monovisc, for intra-articular injection, per dose K K2 ✓
AHA: 4Q,18

J7328 Hyaluronan or derivative, GELSYN-3, for intra-articular injection, 0.1 mg G K2 ✓
AHA: 4Q,18; 1Q,16

J7329 Hyaluronan or derivative, Trivisc, for intra-articular injection, 1 mg K2
CMS: 100-04,4,260.1; 100-04,4,260.1.1
AHA: 1Q,19; 4Q,18

J7330 Autologous cultured chondrocytes, implant B ✓
Medicare jurisdiction: local contractor. Use this code for Carticel.

J7331 Hyaluronan or derivative, SYNOJOYNT, for intra-articular injection, 1 mg K2
AHA: 4Q,19

J7332 Hyaluronan or derivative, Triluron, for intra-articular injection, 1 mg
AHA: 4Q,19

J7336 Capsaicin 8% patch, per sq cm K K2 ✓
Use this code for Qutenza.

J7340 Carbidopa 5 mg/levodopa 20 mg enteral suspension, 100 ml K K2 ✓
Use this code for Duopa.

J7342 Instillation, ciprofloxacin otic suspension, 6 mg G K2 ✓
Use this code for Otipro.

J7345 Aminolevulinic acid HCl for topical administration, 10% gel, 10 mg G K2
Use this code for Ameluz.
AHA: 1Q,20; 1Q,18; 4Q,17

J7351 Injection, bimatoprost, intracameral implant, 1 mcg K2
Use this code for Durysta.
AHA: 4Q,20

J7352 Afamelanotide implant, 1 mg K2
Use this code for Scenesse.
AHA: 1Q,21

J7402 Mometasone furoate sinus implant, (Sinuva), 10 mcg K2
AHA: 1Q,21

J7500 Azathioprine, oral, 50 mg N N1 ✓
Use this code for Azasan, Imuran.
CMS: 100-04,17,80.3

J7501 Azathioprine, parenteral, 100 mg K K2 ✓
CMS: 100-04,17,80.3

J7502 Cyclosporine, oral, 100 mg N N1 ✓
Use this code for Neoral, Sandimmune, Gengraf, Sangcya.
CMS: 100-04,17,80.3

J7503 Tacrolimus, extended release, (Envarsus XR), oral, 0.25 mg G N1 ✓

J7504 Lymphocyte immune globulin, antithymocyte globulin, equine, parenteral, 250 mg K K2 ✓
Use this code for Atgam.
CMS: 100-03,260.7; 100-04,17,80.3

J7505 Muromonab-CD3, parenteral, 5 mg K N1 ✓
Use this code for Orthoclone OKT3.
CMS: 100-04,17,80.3

J7507 Tacrolimus, immediate release, oral, 1 mg N N1 ✓
Use this code for Prograf.
CMS: 100-04,17,80.3

J7508 Tacrolimus, extended release, (Astagraf XL), oral, 0.1 mg N N1 ✓

J7509 Methylprednisolone, oral, per 4 mg N N1 ✓
Use this code for Medrol, Methylpred.
CMS: 100-04,17,80.3

J7510 Prednisolone, oral, per 5 mg N N1 ✓
Use this code for Delta-Cortef, Cotolone, Pediapred, Prednoral, Prelone.
CMS: 100-04,17,80.3

J7511 Lymphocyte immune globulin, antithymocyte globulin, rabbit, parenteral, 25 mg K K2 ✓
Use this code for Thymoglobulin.
CMS: 100-04,17,80.3

J7512 Prednisone, immediate release or delayed release, oral, 1 mg N N1 ✓

J7513 Daclizumab, parenteral, 25 mg EI ✓
Use this code for Zenapax.

J7515 Cyclosporine, oral, 25 mg N N1 ✓
Use this code for Neoral, Sandimmune, Gengraf, Sangcya.
CMS: 100-04,17,80.3

J7516 Cyclosporine, parenteral, 250 mg N N1 ✓
Use this code for Neoral, Sandimmune, Gengraf, Sangcya.
CMS: 100-04,17,80.3

J7517 Mycophenolate mofetil, oral, 250 mg N N1 ✓
Use this code for CellCept.
CMS: 100-04,17,80.3

J7518 Mycophenolic acid, oral, 180 mg N N1 ✓
Use this code for Myfortic Delayed Release.
CMS: 100-04,17,80.3.1

J7520 Sirolimus, oral, 1 mg N N1 ✓
Use this code for Rapamune.
CMS: 100-04,17,80.3

J7525 Tacrolimus, parenteral, 5 mg K K2 ✓
Use this code for Prograf.
CMS: 100-04,17,80.3

J7527 Everolimus, oral, 0.25 mg N N1 ✓
Use this code for Zortress, Afinitor.

J7599 Immunosuppressive drug, not otherwise classified N N1 ✓
Determine if an alternative HCPCS Level II or a CPT code better describes the service being reported. This code should be used only if a more specific code is unavailable.
CMS: 100-04,17,80.3

Inhalation Drugs

J7604 Acetylcysteine, inhalation solution, compounded product, administered through DME, unit dose form, per g M ✓

J7605 Arformoterol, inhalation solution, FDA-approved final product, noncompounded, administered through DME, unit dose form, 15 mcg M ✓
CMS: 100-02,15,50.5

J7606 Formoterol fumarate, inhalation solution, FDA-approved final product, noncompounded, administered through DME, unit dose form, 20 mcg M ✓
Use this code for PERFOROMIST.
CMS: 100-02,15,50.5

Drugs Administered Other Than Oral Method

J7607 — J7660

J7607 Levalbuterol, inhalation solution, compounded product, administered through DME, concentrated form, 0.5 mg
CMS: 100-03,200.2

J7608 Acetylcysteine, inhalation solution, FDA-approved final product, noncompounded, administered through DME, unit dose form, per g
Use this code for Acetadote, Mucomyst, Mucosil.

J7609 Albuterol, inhalation solution, compounded product, administered through DME, unit dose, 1 mg

J7610 Albuterol, inhalation solution, compounded product, administered through DME, concentrated form, 1 mg

J7611 Albuterol, inhalation solution, FDA-approved final product, noncompounded, administered through DME, concentrated form, 1 mg
Use this code for Accuneb, Proventil, Respirol, Ventolin.

J7612 Levalbuterol, inhalation solution, FDA-approved final product, noncompounded, administered through DME, concentrated form, 0.5 mg
Use this code for Xopenex HFA.
CMS: 100-03,200.2

J7613 Albuterol, inhalation solution, FDA-approved final product, noncompounded, administered through DME, unit dose, 1 mg
Use this code for Accuneb, Proventil, Respirol, Ventolin.

J7614 Levalbuterol, inhalation solution, FDA-approved final product, noncompounded, administered through DME, unit dose, 0.5 mg
Use this code for Xopenex.
CMS: 100-03,200.2

J7615 Levalbuterol, inhalation solution, compounded product, administered through DME, unit dose, 0.5 mg
CMS: 100-03,200.2

J7620 Albuterol, up to 2.5 mg and ipratropium bromide, up to 0.5 mg, FDA-approved final product, noncompounded, administered through DME

J7622 Beclomethasone, inhalation solution, compounded product, administered through DME, unit dose form, per mg
Use this code for Beclovent, Beconase.

J7624 Betamethasone, inhalation solution, compounded product, administered through DME, unit dose form, per mg

J7626 Budesonide, inhalation solution, FDA-approved final product, noncompounded, administered through DME, unit dose form, up to 0.5 mg
Use this code for Pulmicort, Pulmicort Flexhaler, Pulmicort Respules, Vanceril.

J7627 Budesonide, inhalation solution, compounded product, administered through DME, unit dose form, up to 0.5 mg

J7628 Bitolterol mesylate, inhalation solution, compounded product, administered through DME, concentrated form, per mg

J7629 Bitolterol mesylate, inhalation solution, compounded product, administered through DME, unit dose form, per mg

J7631 Cromolyn sodium, inhalation solution, FDA-approved final product, noncompounded, administered through DME, unit dose form, per 10 mg
Use this code for Intal, Nasalcrom.

J7632 Cromolyn sodium, inhalation solution, compounded product, administered through DME, unit dose form, per 10 mg

J7633 Budesonide, inhalation solution, FDA-approved final product, noncompounded, administered through DME, concentrated form, per 0.25 mg
Use this code for Pulmicort, Pulmicort Flexhaler, Pulmicort Respules, Vanceril.

J7634 Budesonide, inhalation solution, compounded product, administered through DME, concentrated form, per 0.25 mg

J7635 Atropine, inhalation solution, compounded product, administered through DME, concentrated form, per mg

J7636 Atropine, inhalation solution, compounded product, administered through DME, unit dose form, per mg

J7637 Dexamethasone, inhalation solution, compounded product, administered through DME, concentrated form, per mg

J7638 Dexamethasone, inhalation solution, compounded product, administered through DME, unit dose form, per mg

J7639 Dornase alfa, inhalation solution, FDA-approved final product, noncompounded, administered through DME, unit dose form, per mg
Use this code for Pulmozyme.
CMS: 100-02,15,50.5

J7640 Formoterol, inhalation solution, compounded product, administered through DME, unit dose form, 12 mcg

J7641 Flunisolide, inhalation solution, compounded product, administered through DME, unit dose, per mg
Use this code for Aerobid, Flunisolide.

J7642 Glycopyrrolate, inhalation solution, compounded product, administered through DME, concentrated form, per mg

J7643 Glycopyrrolate, inhalation solution, compounded product, administered through DME, unit dose form, per mg

J7644 Ipratropium bromide, inhalation solution, FDA-approved final product, noncompounded, administered through DME, unit dose form, per mg
Use this code for Atrovent.

J7645 Ipratropium bromide, inhalation solution, compounded product, administered through DME, unit dose form, per mg

J7647 Isoetharine HCl, inhalation solution, compounded product, administered through DME, concentrated form, per mg

J7648 Isoetharine HCl, inhalation solution, FDA-approved final product, noncompounded, administered through DME, concentrated form, per mg
Use this code for Beta-2.

J7649 Isoetharine HCl, inhalation solution, FDA-approved final product, noncompounded, administered through DME, unit dose form, per mg

J7650 Isoetharine HCl, inhalation solution, compounded product, administered through DME, unit dose form, per mg

J7657 Isoproterenol HCl, inhalation solution, compounded product, administered through DME, concentrated form, per mg

J7658 Isoproterenol HCl, inhalation solution, FDA-approved final product, noncompounded, administered through DME, concentrated form, per mg
Use this code for Isuprel HCl.

J7659 Isoproterenol HCl, inhalation solution, FDA-approved final product, noncompounded, administered through DME, unit dose form, per mg
Use this code for Isuprel HCl.

J7660 Isoproterenol HCl, inhalation solution, compounded product, administered through DME, unit dose form, per mg

Chemotherapy Drugs

J7665 — Mannitol, administered through an inhaler, 5 mg
Use this code for ARIDOL.

J7667 — Metaproterenol sulfate, inhalation solution, compounded product, concentrated form, per 10 mg

J7668 — Metaproterenol sulfate, inhalation solution, FDA-approved final product, noncompounded, administered through DME, concentrated form, per 10 mg
Use this code for Alupent.

J7669 — Metaproterenol sulfate, inhalation solution, FDA-approved final product, noncompounded, administered through DME, unit dose form, per 10 mg
Use this code for Alupent.

J7670 — Metaproterenol sulfate, inhalation solution, compounded product, administered through DME, unit dose form, per 10 mg

J7674 — Methacholine chloride administered as inhalation solution through a nebulizer, per 1 mg

J7676 — Pentamidine isethionate, inhalation solution, compounded product, administered through DME, unit dose form, per 300 mg

J7677 — Revefenacin inhalation solution, FDA-approved final product, noncompounded, administered through DME, 1 mcg
Use this code for Yupelri.

J7680 — Terbutaline sulfate, inhalation solution, compounded product, administered through DME, concentrated form, per mg
Use this code for Brethine.

J7681 — Terbutaline sulfate, inhalation solution, compounded product, administered through DME, unit dose form, per mg
Use this code for Brethine.

J7682 — Tobramycin, inhalation solution, FDA-approved final product, noncompounded, unit dose form, administered through DME, per 300 mg
Use this code for Tobi.
CMS: 100-02,15,50.5

J7683 — Triamcinolone, inhalation solution, compounded product, administered through DME, concentrated form, per mg
Use this code for Azmacort.

J7684 — Triamcinolone, inhalation solution, compounded product, administered through DME, unit dose form, per mg
Use this code for Azmacort.

J7685 — Tobramycin, inhalation solution, compounded product, administered through DME, unit dose form, per 300 mg

J7686 — Treprostinil, inhalation solution, FDA-approved final product, noncompounded, administered through DME, unit dose form, 1.74 mg
Use this code for Tyvaso.
CMS: 100-02,15,50.5

J7699 — NOC drugs, inhalation solution administered through DME
CMS: 100-02,15,50.5

J7799 — NOC drugs, other than inhalation drugs, administered through DME
CMS: 100-04,20,180; 100-04,32,411.4; 100-04,32,411.5; 100-04,32,411.6

J7999 — Compounded drug, not otherwise classified
CMS: 100-04,20,180; 100-04,32,411.4; 100-04,32,411.5; 100-04,32,411.6
AHA: 1Q,17; 4Q,16; 1Q,16

J8498 — Antiemetic drug, rectal/suppository, not otherwise specified

J8499 — Prescription drug, oral, nonchemotherapeutic, NOS
CMS: 100-02,15,50.5

J Codes Chemotherapy Drugs J8501-J9999

Oral Chemotherapy Drugs

J8501 — Aprepitant, oral, 5 mg
Use this code for Emend.
CMS: 100-02,15,50.5.4; 100-03,110.18; 100-04,17,80.2.1; 100-04,17,80.2.4

J8510 — Busulfan, oral, 2 mg
Use this code for Busulfex, Myleran.
CMS: 100-04,17,80.1.1

J8515 — Cabergoline, oral, 0.25 mg
Use this code for Dostinex.

J8520 — Capecitabine, oral, 150 mg
Use this code for Xeloda.
CMS: 100-04,17,80.1.1

J8521 — Capecitabine, oral, 500 mg
Use this code for Xeloda.
CMS: 100-04,17,80.1.1

J8530 — Cyclophosphamide, oral, 25 mg
Use this code for Cytoxan.
CMS: 100-04,17,80.1.1

J8540 — Dexamethasone, oral, 0.25 mg
Use this code for Decadron.

J8560 — Etoposide, oral, 50 mg
Use this code for VePesid.
CMS: 100-04,17,80.1.1

J8562 — Fludarabine phosphate, oral, 10 mg
Use this code for Oforta.

J8565 — Gefitinib, oral, 250 mg
Use this code for Iressa.
CMS: 100-04,17,80.1.1

J8597 — Antiemetic drug, oral, not otherwise specified

J8600 — Melphalan, oral, 2 mg
Use this code for Alkeran.
CMS: 100-04,17,80.1.1

J8610 — Methotrexate, oral, 2.5 mg
Use this code for Trexall, RHEUMATREX.
CMS: 100-04,17,80.1.1

J8650 — Nabilone, oral, 1 mg
Use this code for Cesamet.

J8655 — Netupitant 300 mg and palonosetron 0.5 mg, oral
Use this code for Akynzeo.

J8670 — Rolapitant, oral, 1 mg
Use this code for Varubi.

J8700 — Temozolomide, oral, 5 mg
Use this code for Temodar.

J8705 — Topotecan, oral, 0.25 mg
Use this code for Hycamtin.

J8999 — Prescription drug, oral, chemotherapeutic, NOS
Determine if an alternative HCPCS Level II or a CPT code better describes the service being reported. This code should be used only if a more specific code is unavailable.
CMS: 100-04,17,80.1.1; 100-04,17,80.1.2

Injectable Chemotherapy Drugs

These codes cover the cost of the chemotherapy drug only, not the administration.

J9000 — Injection, doxorubicin HCl, 10 mg
Use this code for Adriamycin PFS, Adriamycin RDF, Rubex.
CMS: 100-04,20,180; 100-04,32,411.3
AHA: 4Q,18

2023 HCPCS Level II

J9015 — Injection, aldesleukin, per single use vial
Use this code for Proleukin, IL-2, Interleukin.
AHA: 4Q,18

J9017 — Injection, arsenic trioxide, 1 mg
Use this code for Trisenox.
AHA: 4Q,18

J9019 — Injection, asparaginase (Erwinaze), 1,000 IU
AHA: 4Q,18

J9020 — Injection, asparaginase, not otherwise specified, 10,000 units
Use this code for Elspar.
AHA: 4Q,18

J9021 — Injection, asparaginase, recombinant, (Rylaze), 0.1 mg
Use this code for Rylaze.
AHA: 1Q,22

J9022 — Injection, atezolizumab, 10 mg
Use this code for Tecentriq.
AHA: 4Q,18; 1Q,18

J9023 — Injection, avelumab, 10 mg
Use this code for Bavencio.
AHA: 4Q,18; 1Q,18

J9025 — Injection, azacitidine, 1 mg
Use this code for Vidaza.
AHA: 4Q,18

J9027 — Injection, clofarabine, 1 mg
Use this code for Clolar.
AHA: 4Q,18

J9030 — BCG live intravesical instillation, 1 mg
Use this code for Pacis, TICE BCG.
AHA: 3Q,19

J9032 — Injection, belinostat, 10 mg
Use this code for Beleodaq.
AHA: 4Q,18; 1Q,16

J9033 — Injection, bendamustine HCl (Treanda), 1 mg
AHA: 4Q,18

J9034 — Injection, bendamustine HCl (Bendeka), 1 mg
AHA: 4Q,18; 1Q,17

J9035 — Injection, bevacizumab, 10 mg
Use this code for Avastin.
CMS: 100-03,110.17
AHA: 4Q,18

J9036 — Injection, bendamustine HCl, (Belrapzo/bendamustine), 1 mg
AHA: 3Q,19

J9037 — Injection, belantamab mafodontin-blmf, 0.5 mg
Use this code for Blenrep.
AHA: 1Q,21

J9039 — Injection, blinatumomab, 1 mcg
Use this code for Blincyto.
CMS: 100-04,20,180; 100-04,32,411.3
AHA: 4Q,18; 1Q,16

J9040 — Injection, bleomycin sulfate, 15 units
Use this code for Blenoxane.
CMS: 100-04,20,180; 100-04,32,411.3
AHA: 4Q,18

▲ **J9041** — Injection, bortezomib, 0.1 mg
AHA: 4Q,18

J9042 — Injection, brentuximab vedotin, 1 mg
Use this code for Adcentris.
AHA: 4Q,18

J9043 — Injection, cabazitaxel, 1 mg
Use this code for Jevtana.
AHA: 4Q,18

J9044 — ~~Injection, bortezomib, not otherwise specified, 0.1 mg~~
To report, see ~J9041, J9046, J9048, J9049

J9045 — Injection, carboplatin, 50 mg
Use this code for Paraplatin.
AHA: 4Q,18

● **J9046** — Injection, bortezomib (Dr. Reddy's), not therapeutically equivalent to J9041, 0.1 mg
Use this code for bortezomib manufactured by Dr. Reddy's.

J9047 — Injection, carfilzomib, 1 mg
Use this code for Kyprolis.
AHA: 4Q,18

● **J9048** — Injection, bortezomib (Fresenius Kabi), not therapeutically equivalent to J9041, 0.1 mg
Use this code for bortezomib manufactured by Fresenius Kabi.

● **J9049** — Injection, bortezomib (Hospira), not therapeutically equivalent to J9041, 0.1 mg
Use this code for bortezomib manufactured by Hospira.

J9050 — Injection, carmustine, 100 mg
Use this code for BiCNU.
AHA: 4Q,18

J9055 — Injection, cetuximab, 10 mg
Use this code for Erbitux.
CMS: 100-03,110.17
AHA: 4Q,18

J9057 — Injection, copanlisib, 1 mg
Use this code for Aliqopa.
AHA: 1Q,19; 4Q,18

J9060 — Injection, cisplatin, powder or solution, 10 mg
Use this code for Plantinol AQ.
AHA: 4Q,18

J9061 — Injection, amivantamab-vmjw, 2 mg
Use this code for Rybrevant.
AHA: 1Q,22

J9065 — Injection, cladribine, per 1 mg
Use this code for Leustatin.
CMS: 100-04,20,180; 100-04,32,411.3
AHA: 4Q,18

J9070 — Cyclophosphamide, 100 mg
Use this code for Endoxan-Asta.
AHA: 4Q,18

● **J9071** — Injection, cyclophosphamide, (AuroMedics), 5 mg
AHA: 2Q,22

J9098 — Injection, cytarabine liposome, 10 mg
Use this code for Depocyt.
AHA: 4Q,18

J9100 — Injection, cytarabine, 100 mg
Use this code for Cytosar-U, Ara-C, Tarabin CFS.
CMS: 100-04,20,180; 100-04,32,411.3
AHA: 4Q,18

J9118 — Injection, calaspargase pegol-mknl, 10 units
Use this code for Asparla.
AHA: 4Q,19

Chemotherapy Drugs

J9119 Injection, cemiplimab-rwlc, 1 mg [K2]
Use this code for Libtayo.
AHA: 4Q,19

J9120 Injection, dactinomycin, 0.5 mg [K][K2][✓][⊘]
Use this code for Cosmegen.
AHA: 4Q,18

J9130 Dacarbazine, 100 mg [N][N1][✓][⊘]
Use this code for DTIC-Dome.
AHA: 4Q,18

J9144 Injection, daratumumab, 10 mg and hyaluronidase-fihj [K2]
Use this code for Darzalex Faspro.
AHA: 1Q,21

J9145 Injection, daratumumab, 10 mg [G][K2][✓]
Use this code for Darzalex.
AHA: 4Q,18

J9150 Injection, daunorubicin, 10 mg [K][K2][✓][⊘]
Use this code for Cerubidine.
AHA: 4Q,18

J9151 Injection, daunorubicin citrate, liposomal formulation, 10 mg [EI][✓][⊘]
Use this code for Daunoxome.
AHA: 4Q,18

J9153 Injection, liposomal, 1 mg daunorubicin and 2.27 mg cytarabine [K2]
Use this code for Vyxeos.
AHA: 1Q,19; 4Q,18

J9155 Injection, degarelix, 1 mg [K][K2][✓]
CMS: 100-02,15,50.5
AHA: 4Q,18

J9160 Injection, denileukin diftitox, 300 mcg [EI][✓][⊘]
Use this code for Ontak.
AHA: 4Q,18

J9165 Injection, diethylstilbestrol diphosphate, 250 mg [EI][✓]
AHA: 4Q,18

J9171 Injection, docetaxel, 1 mg [K][N1][✓][⊘]
Use this code for Taxotere.
AHA: 4Q,18

J9173 Injection, durvalumab, 10 mg [K2]
Use this code for Imfinzi.
AHA: 1Q,19; 4Q,18

J9175 Injection, Elliotts' B solution, 1 ml [N][N1][✓]
AHA: 4Q,18

J9176 Injection, elotuzumab, 1 mg [G][K2][✓]
Use this code for Empliciti.
AHA: 4Q,18

J9177 Injection, enfortumab vedotin-ejfv, 0.25 mg [K2]
Use this code for PADCEV.
AHA: 2Q,20

J9178 Injection, epirubicin HCl, 2 mg [N][N1][✓][⊘]
Use this code for Ellence.
AHA: 4Q,18

J9179 Injection, eribulin mesylate, 0.1 mg [K][K2][✓]
Use this code for Halaven.
AHA: 4Q,18

J9181 Injection, etoposide, 10 mg [N][N1][✓][⊘]
Use this code for VePesid, Toposar.
AHA: 4Q,18

J9185 Injection, fludarabine phosphate, 50 mg [K][N1][✓][⊘]
Use this code for Fludara.
AHA: 4Q,18

J9190 Injection, fluorouracil, 500 mg [N][N1][✓]
Use this code for Adrucil.
CMS: 100-04,20,180; 100-04,32,411.3
AHA: 4Q,18

J9198 Injection, gemcitabine HCl, (Infugem), 100 mg [K2]
AHA: 2Q,20

J9200 Injection, floxuridine, 500 mg [N][N1][✓][⊘]
Use this code for FUDR.
CMS: 100-04,20,180
AHA: 4Q,18

J9201 Injection, gemcitabine HCl, not otherwise specified, 200 mg [N][N1][✓][⊘]
Use this code for Gemzar.
AHA: 4Q,18

J9202 Goserelin acetate implant, per 3.6 mg [K][K2][✓]
Use this code for Zoladex.
AHA: 4Q,18

J9203 Injection, gemtuzumab ozogamicin, 0.1 mg [G][K2]
Use this code for Mylotarg.
AHA: 4Q,18; 1Q,18; 4Q,17

J9204 Injection, mogamulizumab-kpkc, 1 mg [K2]
Use this code for Poteligeo.
AHA: 4Q,19

J9205 Injection, irinotecan liposome, 1 mg [G][K2][✓]
Use this code for Onivyde.
AHA: 4Q,18

J9206 Injection, irinotecan, 20 mg [N][N1][✓][⊘]
Use this code for Camptosar.
CMS: 100-03,110.17
AHA: 4Q,18

J9207 Injection, ixabepilone, 1 mg [K][K2][✓][⊘]
Use this code for IXEMPRA.
AHA: 4Q,18

J9208 Injection, ifosfamide, 1 g [N][N1][✓][⊘]
Use this code for IFEX, Mitoxana.
AHA: 4Q,18

J9209 Injection, mesna, 200 mg [N][N1][✓]
Use this code for Mesnex.
AHA: 4Q,18

J9210 Injection, emapalumab-lzsg, 1 mg [K2]
Use this code for Gamifant.
AHA: 4Q,19

J9211 Injection, idarubicin HCl, 5 mg [K][N1][✓][⊘]
Use this code for Idamycin.
AHA: 4Q,18

J9212 Injection, interferon alfacon-1, recombinant, 1 mcg [N][✓]
Use this code for Infergen.
AHA: 4Q,18

J9213 Injection, interferon, alfa-2a, recombinant, 3 million units [N][✓]
Use this code for Roferon-A.
AHA: 4Q,18

J9214 Injection, interferon, alfa-2b, recombinant, 1 million units [K][K2][✓]
Use this code for Intron A, Rebetron Kit.
CMS: 100-02,15,50.5
AHA: 4Q,18

2023 HCPCS Level II J9302

Chemotherapy Drugs

J9215 Injection, interferon, alfa-N3, (human leukocyte derived), 250,000 IU
Use this code for Alferon N.
AHA: 4Q,18

J9216 Injection, interferon, gamma 1-b, 3 million units
Use this code for Actimmune.
CMS: 100-02,15,50.5
AHA: 4Q,18

J9217 Leuprolide acetate (for depot suspension), 7.5 mg
Use this code for Lupron Depot, Eligard.
AHA: 2Q,19; 4Q,18

J9218 Leuprolide acetate, per 1 mg
Use this code for Lupron.
CMS: 100-02,15,50.5
AHA: 2Q,19; 4Q,18

J9219 Leuprolide acetate implant, 65 mg
Use this code for Lupron Implant, Viadur.
AHA: 4Q,18

J9223 Injection, lurbinectedin, 0.1 mg
Use this code for Zepzelca.
AHA: 1Q,21

J9225 Histrelin implant (Vantas), 50 mg
AHA: 4Q,18

J9226 Histrelin implant (Supprelin LA), 50 mg
AHA: 4Q,18

J9227 Injection, isatuximab-irfc, 10 mg
Use this code for Sarclisa.
AHA: 4Q,20

J9228 Injection, ipilimumab, 1 mg
Use this code for YERVOY.
AHA: 4Q,18

J9229 Injection, inotuzumab ozogamicin, 0.1 mg
Use this code for Besponsa.
AHA: 1Q,19; 4Q,18

J9230 Injection, mechlorethamine HCl, (nitrogen mustard), 10 mg
Use this code for Mustargen.
AHA: 4Q,18

J9245 Injection, melphalan HCl, not otherwise specified, 50 mg
AHA: 2Q,20; 4Q,18

J9246 Injection, melphalan (Evomela), 1 mg
AHA: 2Q,20

J9247 Injection, melphalan flufenamide, 1 mg
Use this code for Pepaxto.
AHA: 4Q,21

J9250 Methotrexate sodium, 5 mg
Use this code for Folex, Folex PFS, Methotrexate LPF.
AHA: 4Q,18

J9260 Methotrexate sodium, 50 mg
Use this code for Folex, Folex PFS, Methotrexate LPF.
AHA: 4Q,18

J9261 Injection, nelarabine, 50 mg
Use this code for Arranon.
AHA: 4Q,18

J9262 Injection, omacetaxine mepesuccinate, 0.01 mg
Use this code for Synribo.
CMS: 100-02,15,50.5
AHA: 4Q,18

J9263 Injection, oxaliplatin, 0.5 mg
Use this code for Eloxatin.
AHA: 4Q,18

J9264 Injection, paclitaxel protein-bound particles, 1 mg
Use this code for Abraxane.
AHA: 4Q,18

J9266 Injection, pegaspargase, per single dose vial
Use this code for Oncaspar.
AHA: 4Q,18

J9267 Injection, paclitaxel, 1 mg
Use this code for Taxol.
AHA: 4Q,18

J9268 Injection, pentostatin, 10 mg
Use this code for Nipent.
AHA: 4Q,18

J9269 Injection, tagraxofusp-erzs, 10 mcg
Use this code for Elzonris.
AHA: 4Q,19

J9270 Injection, plicamycin, 2.5 mg
Use this code for Mithacin.
AHA: 4Q,18

J9271 Injection, pembrolizumab, 1 mg
Use this code for Keytruda.
AHA: 4Q,18; 1Q,16

J9272 Injection, dostarlimab-gxly, 10 mg
Use this code for Jemperli.
AHA: 1Q,22

● **J9273** Injection, tisotumab vedotin-tftv, 1 mg
Use this code for Tivdak.
AHA: 2Q,22

● **J9274** Injection, tebentafusp-tebn, 1 mcg
Use this code for Kimmtrak.

J9280 Injection, mitomycin, 5 mg
Use this code for Mutamycin.
AHA: 4Q,18; 4Q,17; 4Q,16

J9281 Mitomycin pyelocalyceal instillation, 1 mg
Use this code for Jelmyto.
AHA: 1Q,21

J9285 Injection, olaratumab, 10 mg
Use this code for Lartruvo.
AHA: 4Q,18; 1Q,18

J9293 Injection, mitoxantrone HCl, per 5 mg
Use this code for Navantrone.
AHA: 4Q,18

J9295 Injection, necitumumab, 1 mg
Use this code for Portrazza.
AHA: 4Q,18

● **J9298** Injection, nivolumab and relatlimab-rmbw, 3 mg/1 mg
Use this code for Opdualag.

J9299 Injection, nivolumab, 1 mg
Use this code for Opdivo.
AHA: 4Q,18; 1Q,16

J9301 Injection, obinutuzumab, 10 mg
Use this code for Gazyva.
AHA: 4Q,18

J9302 Injection, ofatumumab, 10 mg
Use this code for Arzerra.
AHA: 4Q,18

Special Coverage Instructions | Noncovered by Medicare | Carrier Discretion | ☑ Quantity Alert ● New Code ○ Recycled/Reinstated ▲ Revised Code

© 2022 Optum, Inc. | A2-Z3 ASC Pmt | CMS: IOM | AHA: Coding Clinic | DMEPOS Paid | ⊘ SNF Excluded | J Codes — 111

Chemotherapy Drugs

J9303 — J9395

J9303 Injection, panitumumab, 10 mg
Use this code for Vectibix.
AHA: 4Q,18

J9304 Injection, pemetrexed (Pemfexy), 10 mg
AHA: 4Q,20

J9305 Injection, pemetrexed, NOS, 10 mg
AHA: 4Q,20; 4Q,18

J9306 Injection, pertuzumab, 1 mg
Use this code for Perjeta.
AHA: 4Q,18

J9307 Injection, pralatrexate, 1 mg
Use this code for FOLOTYN.
AHA: 4Q,18

J9308 Injection, ramucirumab, 5 mg
Use this code for Cyramza.
AHA: 4Q,18; 1Q,16

J9309 Injection, polatuzumab vedotin-piiq, 1 mg
Use this code for Polivy.

J9311 Injection, rituximab 10 mg and hyaluronidase
Use this code for Rituxin Hycela.
AHA: 1Q,19; 4Q,18

J9312 Injection, rituximab, 10 mg
Use this code for Rituxin.
AHA: 1Q,19; 4Q,18

J9313 Injection, moxetumomab pasudotox-tdfk, 0.01 mg
Use this code for Lumoxiti.
AHA: 4Q,19

J9316 Injection, pertuzumab, trastuzumab, and hyaluronidase-zzxf, per 10 mg
Use this code for PHESGO.
AHA: 1Q,21

J9317 Injection, sacituzumab govitecan-hziy, 2.5 mg
Use this code for Trodelvy.
AHA: 1Q,21

J9318 Injection, romidepsin, nonlyophilized, 0.1 mg

J9319 Injection, romidepsin, lyophilized, 0.1 mg
Use this code for Istodax.
AHA: 4Q,21

J9320 Injection, streptozocin, 1 g
Use this code for Zanosar.
AHA: 4Q,18

J9325 Injection, talimogene laherparepvec, per 1 million plaque forming units
Use this code for Imlygic.
AHA: 2Q,19; 4Q,18

J9328 Injection, temozolomide, 1 mg
Use this code for Temodar.
AHA: 4Q,18

J9330 Injection, temsirolimus, 1 mg
Use this code for TORISEL.
AHA: 4Q,18

● **J9331** Injection, sirolimus protein-bound particles, 1 mg
AHA: 3Q,22

● **J9332** Injection, efgartigimod alfa-fcab, 2 mg
Use this code for Vyvgart.
AHA: 3Q,22

J9340 Injection, thiotepa, 15 mg
Use this code for Thioplex.
AHA: 4Q,18

J9348 Injection, naxitamab-gqgk, 1 mg
AHA: 3Q,21

J9349 Injection, tafasitamab-cxix, 2 mg
Use this code for Monjuvi.
AHA: 1Q,21

J9351 Injection, topotecan, 0.1 mg
Use this code for Hycamtin.
AHA: 4Q,18

J9352 Injection, trabectedin, 0.1 mg
Use this code for Yondelis.
AHA: 4Q,18

J9353 Injection, margetuximab-cmkb, 5 mg
AHA: 3Q,21

J9354 Injection, ado-trastuzumab emtansine, 1 mg
Use this code for Kadcyla.
AHA: 4Q,18

J9355 Injection, trastuzumab, excludes biosimilar, 10 mg
Use this code for Herceptin.
AHA: 3Q,19; 4Q,18

J9356 Injection, trastuzumab, 10 mg and hyaluronidase-oysk
Use this code for Herceptin Hylecta.
AHA: 3Q,19

J9357 Injection, valrubicin, intravesical, 200 mg
Use this code for Valstar.
AHA: 4Q,18

J9358 Injection, fam-trastuzumab deruxtecan-nxki, 1 mg
Use this code for Enhertu.
AHA: 2Q,20

● **J9359** Injection, loncastuximab tesirine-lpyl, 0.075 mg
Use this code for Zylonta.
AHA: 2Q,22

J9360 Injection, vinblastine sulfate, 1 mg
Use this code for Velban.
CMS: 100-04,20,180; 100-04,32,411.3
AHA: 4Q,18

J9370 Vincristine sulfate, 1 mg
Use this code for Oncovin, Vincasar PFS.
CMS: 100-04,20,180; 100-04,32,411.3
AHA: 4Q,18

J9371 Injection, vincristine sulfate liposome, 1 mg
Use this code for Marqibo kit.
AHA: 4Q,18

J9390 Injection, vinorelbine tartrate, 10 mg
Use this code for Navelbine.
AHA: 4Q,18

● **J9393** Injection, fulvestrant (Teva) not therapeutically equivalent to J9395, 25 mg
Use this code for fulvestrant manufactured by Teva.

● **J9394** Injection, fulvestrant (Fresenius Kabi) not therapeutically equivalent to J9395, 25 mg
Use this code for fulvestrant manufactured by Fresenius Kabi.

J9395 Injection, fulvestrant, 25 mg
Use this code for Faslodex.
AHA: 4Q,18

J9400 Injection, ziv-aflibercept, 1 mg
Use this code for Zaltrap.
AHA: 4Q,18

J9600 Injection, porfimer sodium, 75 mg
Use this code for Photofrin.
AHA: 1Q,20; 4Q,18

J9999 Not otherwise classified, antineoplastic drugs
Determine if an alternative HCPCS Level II or a CPT code better describes the service being reported. This code should be used only if a more specific code is unavailable.
CMS: 100-02,15,50.5; 100-04,32,400; 100-04,32,400.1; 100-04,32,400.2; 100-04,32,400.2.1; 100-04,32,400.2.2; 100-04,32,400.2.3; 100-04,32,400.2.4; 100-04,32,400.3; 100-04,32,400.4; 100-04,32,400.5; 100-04,32,411.3; 100-04,4,260.1; 100-04,4,260.1.1
AHA: 1Q,17

2023 HCPCS Level II

Temporary Codes K0001-K1027

The K codes were established for use by the DME Medicare Administrative Contractors (DME MACs). The K codes are developed when the currently existing permanent national codes for supplies and certain product categories do not include the codes needed to implement a DME MAC medical review policy.

Wheelchairs and Accessories

Code	Description	Indicators
K0001	Standard wheelchair	Y (RR)
K0002	Standard hemi (low seat) wheelchair	Y (RR)
K0003	Lightweight wheelchair	Y (RR)
K0004	High strength, lightweight wheelchair	Y (RR)
K0005	Ultralightweight wheelchair	Y ☑ (NU, RR, UE)
K0006	Heavy-duty wheelchair	Y (RR)
K0007	Extra heavy-duty wheelchair	Y (RR)
K0008	Custom manual wheelchair/base	Y
K0009	Other manual wheelchair/base	Y
K0010	Standard-weight frame motorized/power wheelchair	Y (RR)
K0011	Standard-weight frame motorized/power wheelchair with programmable control parameters for speed adjustment, tremor dampening, acceleration control and braking CMS: 100-04,20,30.9	Y (RR)
K0012	Lightweight portable motorized/power wheelchair	Y (RR)
K0013	Custom motorized/power wheelchair base	Y
K0014	Other motorized/power wheelchair base	Y
K0015	Detachable, nonadjustable height armrest, each	Y ☑ (RR)
K0017	Detachable, adjustable height armrest, base, replacement only, each	Y ☑ (NU, RR, UE)
K0018	Detachable, adjustable height armrest, upper portion, replacement only, each	Y ☑ (NU, RR, UE)
K0019	Arm pad, replacement only, each	Y ☑ (NU, RR, UE)
K0020	Fixed, adjustable height armrest, pair	Y ☑ (NU, RR, UE)
K0037	High mount flip-up footrest, each	Y ☑ (NU, RR, UE)
K0038	Leg strap, each	Y ☑ (NU, RR, UE)
K0039	Leg strap, H style, each	Y ☑ (NU, RR, UE)
K0040	Adjustable angle footplate, each	Y ☑ (NU, RR, UE)
K0041	Large size footplate, each	Y ☑ (NU, RR, UE)
K0042	Standard size footplate, replacement only, each	Y ☑ (NU, RR, UE)
K0043	Footrest, lower extension tube, replacement only, each	Y ☑ (NU, RR, UE)
K0044	Footrest, upper hanger bracket, replacement only, each	Y ☑ (NU, RR, UE)
K0045	Footrest, complete assembly, replacement only, each	Y ☑ (NU, RR, UE)
K0046	Elevating legrest, lower extension tube, replacement only, each	Y ☑ (NU, RR, UE)
K0047	Elevating legrest, upper hanger bracket, replacement only, each	Y ☑ (NU, RR, UE)
K0050	Ratchet assembly, replacement only	Y ☑ (NU, RR, UE)
K0051	Cam release assembly, footrest or legrest, replacement only, each	Y ☑ (NU, RR, UE)
K0052	Swingaway, detachable footrests, replacement only, each	Y ☑ (NU, RR, UE)
K0053	Elevating footrests, articulating (telescoping), each	Y ☑ (NU, RR, UE)
K0056	Seat height less than 17 in or equal to or greater than 21 in for a high-strength, lightweight, or ultralightweight wheelchair	Y ☑ (NU, RR, UE)
K0065	Spoke protectors, each	Y ☑ (NU, RR, UE)
K0069	Rear wheel assembly, complete, with solid tire, spokes or molded, replacement only, each	Y ☑ (NU, RR, UE)
K0070	Rear wheel assembly, complete, with pneumatic tire, spokes or molded, replacement only, each	Y ☑ (RR)
K0071	Front caster assembly, complete, with pneumatic tire, replacement only, each	Y ☑ (NU, RR, UE)
K0072	Front caster assembly, complete, with semi-pneumatic tire, replacement only, each	Y ☑ (NU, RR, UE)
K0073	Caster pin lock, each	Y ☑ (NU, RR, UE)
K0077	Front caster assembly, complete, with solid tire, replacement only, each	Y ☑ (NU, RR, UE)
K0098	Drive belt for power wheelchair, replacement only	Y ☑ (NU, RR, UE)
K0105	IV hanger, each	Y ☑ (NU, RR, UE)
K0108	Wheelchair component or accessory, not otherwise specified	Y
K0195	Elevating legrests, pair (for use with capped rental wheelchair base)	Y (RR)

Equipment, Replacement, Repair, Rental

Code	Description	Indicators
K0455	Infusion pump used for uninterrupted parenteral administration of medication, (e.g., epoprostenol or treprostinol)	Y (RR)
K0462	Temporary replacement for patient-owned equipment being repaired, any type CMS: 100-04,20,40.1	Y
K0552	Supplies for external noninsulin drug infusion pump, syringe type cartridge, sterile, each	Y ☑
~~K0553~~	~~Supply allowance for therapeutic continuous glucose monitor (CGM), includes all supplies and accessories, 1 month supply = 1 unit of service~~	
~~K0554~~	~~Receiver (monitor), dedicated, for use with therapeutic glucose continuous monitor system~~	
K0601	Replacement battery for external infusion pump owned by patient, silver oxide, 1.5 volt, each	Y ☑ (NU)
K0602	Replacement battery for external infusion pump owned by patient, silver oxide, 3 volt, each	Y ☑ (NU)
K0603	Replacement battery for external infusion pump owned by patient, alkaline, 1.5 volt, each	Y ☑ (NU)
K0604	Replacement battery for external infusion pump owned by patient, lithium, 3.6 volt, each	Y ☑ (NU)
K0605	Replacement battery for external infusion pump owned by patient, lithium, 4.5 volt, each	Y ☑ (NU)
K0606	Automatic external defibrillator, with integrated electrocardiogram analysis, garment type	Y (RR)
K0607	Replacement battery for automated external defibrillator, garment type only, each	Y ☑ (RR)
K0608	Replacement garment for use with automated external defibrillator, each	Y ☑ (NU, RR, UE)
K0609	Replacement electrodes for use with automated external defibrillator, garment type only, each	Y ☑ (KF)

Special Coverage Instructions | Noncovered by Medicare | Carrier Discretion | ☑ Quantity Alert | ● New Code | ○ Recycled/Reinstated | ▲ Revised Code

© 2022 Optum, Inc. | A2-Z3 ASC Pmt | CMS: IOM | AHA: Coding Clinic | DMEPOS Paid | ⊘ SNF Excluded

Code	Description
K0669	Wheelchair accessory, wheelchair seat or back cushion, does not meet specific code criteria or no written coding verification from DME PDAC Y
K0672	Addition to lower extremity orthotic, removable soft interface, all components, replacement only, each A ☑
K0730	Controlled dose inhalation drug delivery system Y (RR)
K0733	Power wheelchair accessory, 12 to 24 amp hour sealed lead acid battery, each (e.g., gel cell, absorbed glassmat) Y (NU, RR, UE)
K0738	Portable gaseous oxygen system, rental; home compressor used to fill portable oxygen cylinders; includes portable containers, regulator, flowmeter, humidifier, cannula or mask, and tubing Y (RR) CMS: 100-04,20,130.6
K0739	Repair or nonroutine service for durable medical equipment other than oxygen equipment requiring the skill of a technician, labor component, per 15 minutes Y ☑
K0740	Repair or nonroutine service for oxygen equipment requiring the skill of a technician, labor component, per 15 minutes E ☑
K0743	Suction pump, home model, portable, for use on wounds Y
K0744	Absorptive wound dressing for use with suction pump, home model, portable, pad size 16 sq in or less A ☑
K0745	Absorptive wound dressing for use with suction pump, home model, portable, pad size more than 16 sq in but less than or equal to 48 sq in A ☑
K0746	Absorptive wound dressing for use with suction pump, home model, portable, pad size greater than 48 sq in A

Power Operated Vehicle and Accessories

Code	Description
K0800	Power operated vehicle, group 1 standard, patient weight capacity up to and including 300 pounds Y (NU, RR, UE) CMS: 100-04,12,30.6.15.4
K0801	Power operated vehicle, group 1 heavy-duty, patient weight capacity 301 to 450 pounds Y (NU, RR, UE) CMS: 100-04,12,30.6.15.4
K0802	Power operated vehicle, group 1 very heavy-duty, patient weight capacity 451 to 600 pounds Y (NU, RR, UE) CMS: 100-04,12,30.6.15.4
K0806	Power operated vehicle, group 2 standard, patient weight capacity up to and including 300 pounds Y (NU, RR, UE) CMS: 100-04,12,30.6.15.4
K0807	Power operated vehicle, group 2 heavy-duty, patient weight capacity 301 to 450 pounds Y (NU, RR, UE) CMS: 100-04,12,30.6.15.4
K0808	Power operated vehicle, group 2 very heavy-duty, patient weight capacity 451 to 600 pounds Y (NU, RR, UE) CMS: 100-04,12,30.6.15.4
K0812	Power operated vehicle, not otherwise classified Y CMS: 100-04,12,30.6.15.4

Power Wheelchairs

Code	Description
K0813	Power wheelchair, group 1 standard, portable, sling/solid seat and back, patient weight capacity up to and including 300 pounds Y (RR)
K0814	Power wheelchair, group 1 standard, portable, captain's chair, patient weight capacity up to and including 300 pounds Y (RR)
K0815	Power wheelchair, group 1 standard, sling/solid seat and back, patient weight capacity up to and including 300 pounds Y (RR)
K0816	Power wheelchair, group 1 standard, captain's chair, patient weight capacity up to and including 300 pounds Y (RR)
K0820	Power wheelchair, group 2 standard, portable, sling/solid seat/back, patient weight capacity up to and including 300 pounds Y (RR)
K0821	Power wheelchair, group 2 standard, portable, captain's chair, patient weight capacity up to and including 300 pounds Y (RR)
K0822	Power wheelchair, group 2 standard, sling/solid seat/back, patient weight capacity up to and including 300 pounds Y (RR)
K0823	Power wheelchair, group 2 standard, captain's chair, patient weight capacity up to and including 300 pounds Y (RR)
K0824	Power wheelchair, group 2 heavy-duty, sling/solid seat/back, patient weight capacity 301 to 450 pounds Y (RR)
K0825	Power wheelchair, group 2 heavy-duty, captain's chair, patient weight capacity 301 to 450 pounds Y (RR)
K0826	Power wheelchair, group 2 very heavy-duty, sling/solid seat/back, patient weight capacity 451 to 600 pounds Y (RR)
K0827	Power wheelchair, group 2 very heavy-duty, captain's chair, patient weight capacity 451 to 600 pounds Y (RR)
K0828	Power wheelchair, group 2 extra heavy-duty, sling/solid seat/back, patient weight capacity 601 pounds or more Y (RR)
K0829	Power wheelchair, group 2 extra heavy-duty, captain's chair, patient weight 601 pounds or more Y (RR)
K0830	Power wheelchair, group 2 standard, seat elevator, sling/solid seat/back, patient weight capacity up to and including 300 pounds Y
K0831	Power wheelchair, group 2 standard, seat elevator, captain's chair, patient weight capacity up to and including 300 pounds Y
K0835	Power wheelchair, group 2 standard, single power option, sling/solid seat/back, patient weight capacity up to and including 300 pounds Y (RR)
K0836	Power wheelchair, group 2 standard, single power option, captain's chair, patient weight capacity up to and including 300 pounds Y (RR)
K0837	Power wheelchair, group 2 heavy-duty, single power option, sling/solid seat/back, patient weight capacity 301 to 450 pounds Y (RR)
K0838	Power wheelchair, group 2 heavy-duty, single power option, captain's chair, patient weight capacity 301 to 450 pounds Y (RR)
K0839	Power wheelchair, group 2 very heavy-duty, single power option sling/solid seat/back, patient weight capacity 451 to 600 pounds Y (RR)
K0840	Power wheelchair, group 2 extra heavy-duty, single power option, sling/solid seat/back, patient weight capacity 601 pounds or more Y (RR)
K0841	Power wheelchair, group 2 standard, multiple power option, sling/solid seat/back, patient weight capacity up to and including 300 pounds Y (RR)

Code	Description
K0842	Power wheelchair, group 2 standard, multiple power option, captain's chair, patient weight capacity up to and including 300 pounds Y ♿ (RR)
K0843	Power wheelchair, group 2 heavy-duty, multiple power option, sling/solid seat/back, patient weight capacity 301 to 450 pounds Y ♿ (RR)
K0848	Power wheelchair, group 3 standard, sling/solid seat/back, patient weight capacity up to and including 300 pounds **CMS:** 100-04,20,30.9
K0849	Power wheelchair, group 3 standard, captain's chair, patient weight capacity up to and including 300 pounds Y ♿ (RR) **CMS:** 100-04,20,30.9
K0850	Power wheelchair, group 3 heavy-duty, sling/solid seat/back, patient weight capacity 301 to 450 pounds Y ♿ (RR) **CMS:** 100-04,20,30.9
K0851	Power wheelchair, group 3 heavy-duty, captain's chair, patient weight capacity 301 to 450 pounds Y ♿ (RR) **CMS:** 100-04,20,30.9
K0852	Power wheelchair, group 3 very heavy-duty, sling/solid seat/back, patient weight capacity 451 to 600 pounds Y ♿ (RR) **CMS:** 100-04,20,30.9
K0853	Power wheelchair, group 3 very heavy-duty, captain's chair, patient weight capacity 451 to 600 pounds Y ♿ (RR) **CMS:** 100-04,20,30.9
K0854	Power wheelchair, group 3 extra heavy-duty, sling/solid seat/back, patient weight capacity 601 pounds or more **CMS:** 100-04,20,30.9
K0855	Power wheelchair, group 3 extra heavy-duty, captain's chair, patient weight capacity 601 pounds or more Y ♿ (RR) **CMS:** 100-04,20,30.9
K0856	Power wheelchair, group 3 standard, single power option, sling/solid seat/back, patient weight capacity up to and including 300 pounds Y ♿ (RR) **CMS:** 100-04,20,30.9
K0857	Power wheelchair, group 3 standard, single power option, captain's chair, patient weight capacity up to and including 300 pounds Y ♿ (RR) **CMS:** 100-04,20,30.9
K0858	Power wheelchair, group 3 heavy-duty, single power option, sling/solid seat/back, patient weight 301 to 450 pounds **CMS:** 100-04,20,30.9
K0859	Power wheelchair, group 3 heavy-duty, single power option, captain's chair, patient weight capacity 301 to 450 pounds Y ♿ (RR) **CMS:** 100-04,20,30.9
K0860	Power wheelchair, group 3 very heavy-duty, single power option, sling/solid seat/back, patient weight capacity 451 to 600 pounds Y ♿ (RR) **CMS:** 100-04,20,30.9
K0861	Power wheelchair, group 3 standard, multiple power option, sling/solid seat/back, patient weight capacity up to and including 300 pounds Y ♿ (RR) **CMS:** 100-04,20,30.9
K0862	Power wheelchair, group 3 heavy-duty, multiple power option, sling/solid seat/back, patient weight capacity 301 to 450 pounds Y ♿ (RR) **CMS:** 100-04,20,30.9
K0863	Power wheelchair, group 3 very heavy-duty, multiple power option, sling/solid seat/back, patient weight capacity 451 to 600 pounds Y ♿ (RR) **CMS:** 100-04,20,30.9
K0864	Power wheelchair, group 3 extra heavy-duty, multiple power option, sling/solid seat/back, patient weight capacity 601 pounds or more Y ♿ (RR) **CMS:** 100-04,20,30.9
K0868	Power wheelchair, group 4 standard, sling/solid seat/back, patient weight capacity up to and including 300 pounds Y
K0869	Power wheelchair, group 4 standard, captain's chair, patient weight capacity up to and including 300 pounds Y
K0870	Power wheelchair, group 4 heavy-duty, sling/solid seat/back, patient weight capacity 301 to 450 pounds Y
K0871	Power wheelchair, group 4 very heavy-duty, sling/solid seat/back, patient weight capacity 451 to 600 pounds Y
K0877	Power wheelchair, group 4 standard, single power option, sling/solid seat/back, patient weight capacity up to and including 300 pounds Y
K0878	Power wheelchair, group 4 standard, single power option, captain's chair, patient weight capacity up to and including 300 pounds Y
K0879	Power wheelchair, group 4 heavy-duty, single power option, sling/solid seat/back, patient weight capacity 301 to 450 pounds Y
K0880	Power wheelchair, group 4 very heavy-duty, single power option, sling/solid seat/back, patient weight 451 to 600 pounds Y
K0884	Power wheelchair, group 4 standard, multiple power option, sling/solid seat/back, patient weight capacity up to and including 300 pounds Y
K0885	Power wheelchair, group 4 standard, multiple power option, captain's chair, patient weight capacity up to and including 300 pounds Y
K0886	Power wheelchair, group 4 heavy-duty, multiple power option, sling/solid seat/back, patient weight capacity 301 to 450 pounds Y
K0890	Power wheelchair, group 5 pediatric, single power option, sling/solid seat/back, patient weight capacity up to and including 125 pounds Y
K0891	Power wheelchair, group 5 pediatric, multiple power option, sling/solid seat/back, patient weight capacity up to and including 125 pounds Y
K0898	Power wheelchair, not otherwise classified Y
K0899	Power mobility device, not coded by DME PDAC or does not meet criteria Y **CMS:** 100-04,12,30.6.15.4

Other DME

Code	Description
K0900	Customized durable medical equipment, other than wheelchair Y
K1001	Electronic positional obstructive sleep apnea treatment, with sensor, includes all components and accessories, any type
▲ K1002	Cranial electrotherapy stimulation (CES) system, any type (RR)
K1003	Whirlpool tub, walk in, portable
K1004	Low frequency ultrasonic diathermy treatment device for home use, includes all components and accessories
K1005	Disposable collection and storage bag for breast milk, any size, any type, each

Temporary Codes

K1006 — K1034

Code	Description
K1006	Suction pump, home model, portable or stationary, electric, any type, for use with external urine management system
K1007	Bilateral hip, knee, ankle, foot (HKAFO) device, powered, includes pelvic component, single or double upright(s), knee joints any type, with or without ankle joints any type, includes all components and accessories, motors, microprocessors, sensors
K1009	Speech volume modulation system, any type, including all components and accessories
K1013	Enema tube, with or without adapter, any type, replacement only, each
K1014	Addition, endoskeletal knee-shin system, 4 bar linkage or multiaxial, fluid swing and stance phase control
K1015	Foot, adductus positioning device, adjustable
K1016	Transcutaneous electrical nerve stimulator for electrical stimulation of the trigeminal nerve (RR)
K1017	Monthly supplies for use of device coded at K1016
K1018	External upper limb tremor stimulator of the peripheral nerves of the wrist (RR)
▲ **K1019**	Replacement supplies and accessories for external upper limb tremor stimulator of the peripheral nerves of the wrist
K1020	Noninvasive vagus nerve stimulator (RR)
K1021	Exsufflation belt, includes all supplies and accessories
K1022	Addition to lower extremity prosthesis, endoskeletal, knee disarticulation, above knee, hip disarticulation, positional rotation unit, any type
K1023	Distal transcutaneous electrical nerve stimulator, stimulates peripheral nerves of the upper arm
K1024	Nonpneumatic compression controller with sequential calibrated gradient pressure (RR)
K1025	Nonpneumatic sequential compression garment, full arm (RR)
K1026	Mechanical allergen particle barrier/inhalation filter, cream, nasal, topical
K1027	Oral device/appliance used to reduce upper airway collapsibility, without fixed mechanical hinge, custom fabricated, includes fitting and adjustment
● **K1028**	Power source and control electronics unit for oral device/appliance for neuromuscular electrical stimulation of the tongue muscle for the reduction of snoring and obstructive sleep apnea, controlled by phone application
● **K1029**	Oral device/appliance for neuromuscular electrical stimulation of the tongue muscle, used in conjunction with the power source and control electronics unit, controlled by phone application, 90-day supply
● **K1030**	External recharging system for battery (internal) for use with implanted cardiac contractility modulation generator, replacement only
● **K1031**	Nonpneumatic compression controller without calibrated gradient pressure (RR)
● **K1032**	Nonpneumatic sequential compression garment, full leg (RR)
● **K1033**	Nonpneumatic sequential compression garment, half leg (RR)
● **K1034**	Provision of COVID-19 test, nonprescription self-administered and self-collected use, FDA approved, authorized or cleared, one test count **AHA:** 3Q,22

Orthotic Procedures and Devices L0112-L4631

L codes include orthotic and prosthetic procedures and devices, as well as scoliosis equipment, orthopedic shoes, and prosthetic implants.

Cervical

L0112 Cranial cervical orthosis, congenital torticollis type, with or without soft interface material, adjustable range of motion joint, custom fabricated

L0113 Cranial cervical orthosis, torticollis type, with or without joint, with or without soft interface material, prefabricated, includes fitting and adjustment

L0120 Cervical, flexible, nonadjustable, prefabricated, off-the-shelf (foam collar)

L0130 Cervical, flexible, thermoplastic collar, molded to patient

L0140 Cervical, semi-rigid, adjustable (plastic collar)

L0150 Cervical, semi-rigid, adjustable molded chin cup (plastic collar with mandibular/occipital piece)

L0160 Cervical, semi-rigid, wire frame occipital/mandibular support, prefabricated, off-the-shelf

L0170 Cervical, collar, molded to patient model

L0172 Cervical, collar, semi-rigid thermoplastic foam, two piece, prefabricated, off-the-shelf

L0174 Cervical, collar, semi-rigid, thermoplastic foam, two piece with thoracic extension, prefabricated, off-the-shelf

Multiple Post Collar

L0180 Cervical, multiple post collar, occipital/mandibular supports, adjustable

L0190 Cervical, multiple post collar, occipital/mandibular supports, adjustable cervical bars (SOMI, Guilford, Taylor types)

L0200 Cervical, multiple post collar, occipital/mandibular supports, adjustable cervical bars, and thoracic extension

Thoracic

L0220 Thoracic, rib belt, custom fabricated

L0450 Thoracic-lumbar-sacral orthosis (TLSO), flexible, provides trunk support, upper thoracic region, produces intracavitary pressure to reduce load on the intervertebral disks with rigid stays or panel(s), includes shoulder straps and closures, prefabricated, off-the-shelf

TLSO brace with adjustable straps and pads (L0450). The model at right and similar devices such as the Boston brace are molded polymer over foam and may be bivalve (front and back components)

Thoracic lumbar sacral othosis (TLSO)

L0452 Thoracic-lumbar-sacral orthosis (TLSO), flexible, provides trunk support, upper thoracic region, produces intracavitary pressure to reduce load on the intervertebral disks with rigid stays or panel(s), includes shoulder straps and closures, custom fabricated

L0454 Thoracic-lumbar-sacral orthosis (TLSO), flexible, provides trunk support, extends from sacrococcygeal junction to above T-9 vertebra, restricts gross trunk motion in the sagittal plane, produces intracavitary pressure to reduce load on the intervertebral disks with rigid stays or panel(s), includes shoulder straps and closures, prefabricated item that has been trimmed, bent, molded, assembled, or otherwise customized to fit a specific patient by an individual with expertise

L0455 Thoracic-lumbar-sacral orthosis (TLSO), flexible, provides trunk support, extends from sacrococcygeal junction to above T-9 vertebra, restricts gross trunk motion in the sagittal plane, produces intracavitary pressure to reduce load on the intervertebral disks with rigid stays or panel(s), includes shoulder straps and closures, prefabricated, off-the-shelf

L0456 Thoracic-lumbar-sacral orthosis (TLSO), flexible, provides trunk support, thoracic region, rigid posterior panel and soft anterior apron, extends from the sacrococcygeal junction and terminates just inferior to the scapular spine, restricts gross trunk motion in the sagittal plane, produces intracavitary pressure to reduce load on the intervertebral disks, includes straps and closures, prefabricated item that has been trimmed, bent, molded, assembled, or otherwise customized to fit a specific patient by an individual with expertise

L0457 Thoracic-lumbar-sacral orthosis (TLSO), flexible, provides trunk support, thoracic region, rigid posterior panel and soft anterior apron, extends from the sacrococcygeal junction and terminates just inferior to the scapular spine, restricts gross trunk motion in the sagittal plane, produces intracavitary pressure to reduce load on the intervertebral disks, includes straps and closures, prefabricated, off-the-shelf

L0458 Thoracic-lumbar-sacral orthosis (TLSO), triplanar control, modular segmented spinal system, two rigid plastic shells, posterior extends from the sacrococcygeal junction and terminates just inferior to the scapular spine, anterior extends from the symphysis pubis to the xiphoid, soft liner, restricts gross trunk motion in the sagittal, coronal, and transverse planes, lateral strength is provided by overlapping plastic and stabilizing closures, includes straps and closures, prefabricated, includes fitting and adjustment

L0460 Thoracic-lumbar-sacral orthosis (TLSO), triplanar control, modular segmented spinal system, two rigid plastic shells, posterior extends from the sacrococcygeal junction and terminates just inferior to the scapular spine, anterior extends from the symphysis pubis to the sternal notch, soft liner, restricts gross trunk motion in the sagittal, coronal, and transverse planes, lateral strength is provided by overlapping plastic and stabilizing closures, includes straps and closures, prefabricated item that has been trimmed, bent, molded, assembled, or otherwise customized to fit a specific patient by an individual with expertise

L0462 Thoracic-lumbar-sacral orthosis (TLSO), triplanar control, modular segmented spinal system, three rigid plastic shells, posterior extends from the sacrococcygeal junction and terminates just inferior to the scapular spine, anterior extends from the symphysis pubis to the sternal notch, soft liner, restricts gross trunk motion in the sagittal, coronal, and transverse planes, lateral strength is provided by overlapping plastic and stabilizing closures, includes straps and closures, prefabricated, includes fitting and adjustment

L0464 Thoracic-lumbar-sacral orthosis (TLSO), triplanar control, modular segmented spinal system, four rigid plastic shells, posterior extends from sacrococcygeal junction and terminates just inferior to scapular spine, anterior extends from symphysis pubis to the sternal notch, soft liner, restricts gross trunk motion in sagittal, coronal, and transverse planes, lateral strength is provided by overlapping plastic and stabilizing closures, includes straps and closures, prefabricated, includes fitting and adjustment

L0466 Thoracic-lumbar-sacral orthosis (TLSO), sagittal control, rigid posterior frame and flexible soft anterior apron with straps, closures and padding, restricts gross trunk motion in sagittal plane, produces intracavitary pressure to reduce load on intervertebral disks, prefabricated item that has been trimmed, bent, molded, assembled, or otherwise customized to fit a specific patient by an individual with expertise

L0467 Thoracic-lumbar-sacral orthosis (TLSO), sagittal control, rigid posterior frame and flexible soft anterior apron with straps, closures and padding, restricts gross trunk motion in sagittal plane, produces intracavitary pressure to reduce load on intervertebral disks, prefabricated, off-the-shelf

L0468 Thoracic-lumbar-sacral orthosis (TLSO), sagittal-coronal control, rigid posterior frame and flexible soft anterior apron with straps, closures and padding, extends from sacrococcygeal junction over scapulae, lateral strength provided by pelvic, thoracic, and lateral frame pieces, restricts gross trunk motion in sagittal, and coronal planes, produces intracavitary pressure to reduce load on intervertebral disks, prefabricated item that has been trimmed, bent, molded, assembled, or otherwise customized to fit a specific patient by an individual with expertise

L0469 Thoracic-lumbar-sacral orthosis (TLSO), sagittal-coronal control, rigid posterior frame and flexible soft anterior apron with straps, closures and padding, extends from sacrococcygeal junction over scapulae, lateral strength provided by pelvic, thoracic, and lateral frame pieces, restricts gross trunk motion in sagittal and coronal planes, produces intracavitary pressure to reduce load on intervertebral disks, prefabricated, off-the-shelf

L0470 Thoracic-lumbar-sacral orthosis (TLSO), triplanar control, rigid posterior frame and flexible soft anterior apron with straps, closures and padding extends from sacrococcygeal junction to scapula, lateral strength provided by pelvic, thoracic, and lateral frame pieces, rotational strength provided by subclavicular extensions, restricts gross trunk motion in sagittal, coronal, and transverse planes, provides intracavitary pressure to reduce load on the intervertebral disks, includes fitting and shaping the frame, prefabricated, includes fitting and adjustment

L0472 Thoracic-lumbar-sacral orthosis (TLSO), triplanar control, hyperextension, rigid anterior and lateral frame extends from symphysis pubis to sternal notch with two anterior components (one pubic and one sternal), posterior and lateral pads with straps and closures, limits spinal flexion, restricts gross trunk motion in sagittal, coronal, and transverse planes, includes fitting and shaping the frame, prefabricated, includes fitting and adjustment

L0480 Thoracic-lumbar-sacral orthosis (TLSO), triplanar control, one-piece rigid plastic shell without interface liner, with multiple straps and closures, posterior extends from sacrococcygeal junction and terminates just inferior to scapular spine, anterior extends from symphysis pubis to sternal notch, anterior or posterior opening, restricts gross trunk motion in sagittal, coronal, and transverse planes, includes a carved plaster or CAD-CAM model, custom fabricated

L0482 Thoracic-lumbar-sacral orthosis (TLSO), triplanar control, one-piece rigid plastic shell with interface liner, multiple straps and closures, posterior extends from sacrococcygeal junction and terminates just inferior to scapular spine, anterior extends from symphysis pubis to sternal notch, anterior or posterior opening, restricts gross trunk motion in sagittal, coronal, and transverse planes, includes a carved plaster or CAD-CAM model, custom fabricated

L0484 Thoracic-lumbar-sacral orthosis (TLSO), triplanar control, two-piece rigid plastic shell without interface liner, with multiple straps and closures, posterior extends from sacrococcygeal junction and terminates just inferior to scapular spine, anterior extends from symphysis pubis to sternal notch, lateral strength is enhanced by overlapping plastic, restricts gross trunk motion in the sagittal, coronal, and transverse planes, includes a carved plaster or CAD-CAM model, custom fabricated

L0486 Thoracic-lumbar-sacral orthosis (TLSO), triplanar control, two-piece rigid plastic shell with interface liner, multiple straps and closures, posterior extends from sacrococcygeal junction and terminates just inferior to scapular spine, anterior extends from symphysis pubis to sternal notch, lateral strength is enhanced by overlapping plastic, restricts gross trunk motion in the sagittal, coronal, and transverse planes, includes a carved plaster or CAD-CAM model, custom fabricated

L0488 Thoracic-lumbar-sacral orthosis (TLSO), triplanar control, one-piece rigid plastic shell with interface liner, multiple straps and closures, posterior extends from sacrococcygeal junction and terminates just inferior to scapular spine, anterior extends from symphysis pubis to sternal notch, anterior or posterior opening, restricts gross trunk motion in sagittal, coronal, and transverse planes, prefabricated, includes fitting and adjustment

L0490 Thoracic-lumbar-sacral orthosis (TLSO), sagittal-coronal control, one-piece rigid plastic shell, with overlapping reinforced anterior, with multiple straps and closures, posterior extends from sacrococcygeal junction and terminates at or before the T-9 vertebra, anterior extends from symphysis pubis to xiphoid, anterior opening, restricts gross trunk motion in sagittal and coronal planes, prefabricated, includes fitting and adjustment

L0491 — Thoracic-lumbar-sacral orthosis (TLSO), sagittal-coronal control, modular segmented spinal system, two rigid plastic shells, posterior extends from the sacrococcygeal junction and terminates just inferior to the scapular spine, anterior extends from the symphysis pubis to the xiphoid, soft liner, restricts gross trunk motion in the sagittal and coronal planes, lateral strength is provided by overlapping plastic and stabilizing closures, includes straps and closures, prefabricated, includes fitting and adjustment

L0492 — Thoracic-lumbar-sacral orthosis (TLSO), sagittal-coronal control, modular segmented spinal system, three rigid plastic shells, posterior extends from the sacrococcygeal junction and terminates just inferior to the scapular spine, anterior extends from the symphysis pubis to the xiphoid, soft liner, restricts gross trunk motion in the sagittal and coronal planes, lateral strength is provided by overlapping plastic and stabilizing closures, includes straps and closures, prefabricated, includes fitting and adjustment

Cervical-Thoracic-Lumbar-Sacral Orthoses

L0621 — Sacroiliac orthosis (SO), flexible, provides pelvic-sacral support, reduces motion about the sacroiliac joint, includes straps, closures, may include pendulous abdomen design, prefabricated, off-the-shelf

L0622 — Sacroiliac orthosis (SO), flexible, provides pelvic-sacral support, reduces motion about the sacroiliac joint, includes straps, closures, may include pendulous abdomen design, custom fabricated

L0623 — Sacroiliac orthosis (SO), provides pelvic-sacral support, with rigid or semi-rigid panels over the sacrum and abdomen, reduces motion about the sacroiliac joint, includes straps, closures, may include pendulous abdomen design, prefabricated, off-the-shelf

L0624 — Sacroiliac orthosis (SO), provides pelvic-sacral support, with rigid or semi-rigid panels placed over the sacrum and abdomen, reduces motion about the sacroiliac joint, includes straps, closures, may include pendulous abdomen design, custom fabricated

L0625 — Lumbar orthosis (LO), flexible, provides lumbar support, posterior extends from L-1 to below L-5 vertebra, produces intracavitary pressure to reduce load on the intervertebral discs, includes straps, closures, may include pendulous abdomen design, shoulder straps, stays, prefabricated, off-the-shelf

L0626 — Lumbar orthosis (LO), sagittal control, with rigid posterior panel(s), posterior extends from L-1 to below L-5 vertebra, produces intracavitary pressure to reduce load on the intervertebral discs, includes straps, closures, may include padding, stays, shoulder straps, pendulous abdomen design, prefabricated item that has been trimmed, bent, molded, assembled, or otherwise customized to fit a specific patient by an individual with expertise

L0627 — Lumbar orthosis (LO), sagittal control, with rigid anterior and posterior panels, posterior extends from L-1 to below L-5 vertebra, produces intracavitary pressure to reduce load on the intervertebral discs, includes straps, closures, may include padding, shoulder straps, pendulous abdomen design, prefabricated item that has been trimmed, bent, molded, assembled, or otherwise customized to fit a specific patient by an individual with expertise

L0628 — Lumbar-sacral orthosis (LSO), flexible, provides lumbo-sacral support, posterior extends from sacrococcygeal junction to T-9 vertebra, produces intracavitary pressure to reduce load on the intervertebral discs, includes straps, closures, may include stays, shoulder straps, pendulous abdomen design, prefabricated, off-the-shelf

L0629 — Lumbar-sacral orthosis (LSO), flexible, provides lumbo-sacral support, posterior extends from sacrococcygeal junction to T-9 vertebra, produces intracavitary pressure to reduce load on the intervertebral discs, includes straps, closures, may include stays, shoulder straps, pendulous abdomen design, custom fabricated

L0630 — Lumbar-sacral orthosis (LSO), sagittal control, with rigid posterior panel(s), posterior extends from sacrococcygeal junction to T-9 vertebra, produces intracavitary pressure to reduce load on the intervertebral discs, includes straps, closures, may include padding, stays, shoulder straps, pendulous abdomen design, prefabricated item that has been trimmed, bent, molded, assembled, or otherwise customized to fit a specific patient by an individual with expertise

L0631 — Lumbar-sacral orthosis (LSO), sagittal control, with rigid anterior and posterior panels, posterior extends from sacrococcygeal junction to T-9 vertebra, produces intracavitary pressure to reduce load on the intervertebral discs, includes straps, closures, may include padding, shoulder straps, pendulous abdomen design, prefabricated item that has been trimmed, bent, molded, assembled, or otherwise customized to fit a specific patient by an individual with expertise

L0632 — Lumbar-sacral orthosis (LSO), sagittal control, with rigid anterior and posterior panels, posterior extends from sacrococcygeal junction to T-9 vertebra, produces intracavitary pressure to reduce load on the intervertebral discs, includes straps, closures, may include padding, shoulder straps, pendulous abdomen design, custom fabricated

L0633 — Lumbar-sacral orthosis (LSO), sagittal-coronal control, with rigid posterior frame/panel(s), posterior extends from sacrococcygeal junction to T-9 vertebra, lateral strength provided by rigid lateral frame/panels, produces intracavitary pressure to reduce load on intervertebral discs, includes straps, closures, may include padding, stays, shoulder straps, pendulous abdomen design, prefabricated item that has been trimmed, bent, molded, assembled, or otherwise customized to fit a specific patient by an individual with expertise

L0634 — Lumbar-sacral orthosis (LSO), sagittal-coronal control, with rigid posterior frame/panel(s), posterior extends from sacrococcygeal junction to T-9 vertebra, lateral strength provided by rigid lateral frame/panel(s), produces intracavitary pressure to reduce load on intervertebral discs, includes straps, closures, may include padding, stays, shoulder straps, pendulous abdomen design, custom fabricated

L0635 — Lumbar-sacral orthosis (LSO), sagittal-coronal control, lumbar flexion, rigid posterior frame/panel(s), lateral articulating design to flex the lumbar spine, posterior extends from sacrococcygeal junction to T-9 vertebra, lateral strength provided by rigid lateral frame/panel(s), produces intracavitary pressure to reduce load on intervertebral discs, includes straps, closures, may include padding, anterior panel, pendulous abdomen design, prefabricated, includes fitting and adjustment

L0636 — Lumbar-sacral orthosis (LSO), sagittal-coronal control, lumbar flexion, rigid posterior frame/panels, lateral articulating design to flex the lumbar spine, posterior extends from sacrococcygeal junction to T-9 vertebra, lateral strength provided by rigid lateral frame/panels, produces intracavitary pressure to reduce load on intervertebral discs, includes straps, closures, may include padding, anterior panel, pendulous abdomen design, custom fabricated

Code	Description
L0637	Lumbar-sacral orthosis (LSO), sagittal-coronal control, with rigid anterior and posterior frame/panels, posterior extends from sacrococcygeal junction to T-9 vertebra, lateral strength provided by rigid lateral frame/panels, produces intracavitary pressure to reduce load on intervertebral discs, includes straps, closures, may include padding, shoulder straps, pendulous abdomen design, prefabricated item that has been trimmed, bent, molded, assembled, or otherwise customized to fit a specific patient by an individual with expertise
L0638	Lumbar-sacral orthosis (LSO), sagittal-coronal control, with rigid anterior and posterior frame/panels, posterior extends from sacrococcygeal junction to T-9 vertebra, lateral strength provided by rigid lateral frame/panels, produces intracavitary pressure to reduce load on intervertebral discs, includes straps, closures, may include padding, shoulder straps, pendulous abdomen design, custom fabricated
L0639	Lumbar-sacral orthosis (LSO), sagittal-coronal control, rigid shell(s)/panel(s), posterior extends from sacrococcygeal junction to T-9 vertebra, anterior extends from symphysis pubis to xyphoid, produces intracavitary pressure to reduce load on the intervertebral discs, overall strength is provided by overlapping rigid material and stabilizing closures, includes straps, closures, may include soft interface, pendulous abdomen design, prefabricated item that has been trimmed, bent, molded, assembled, or otherwise customized to fit a specific patient by an individual with expertise
L0640	Lumbar-sacral orthosis (LSO), sagittal-coronal control, rigid shell(s)/panel(s), posterior extends from sacrococcygeal junction to T-9 vertebra, anterior extends from symphysis pubis to xyphoid, produces intracavitary pressure to reduce load on the intervertebral discs, overall strength is provided by overlapping rigid material and stabilizing closures, includes straps, closures, may include soft interface, pendulous abdomen design, custom fabricated
L0641	Lumbar orthosis (LO), sagittal control, with rigid posterior panel(s), posterior extends from L-1 to below L-5 vertebra, produces intracavitary pressure to reduce load on the intervertebral discs, includes straps, closures, may include padding, stays, shoulder straps, pendulous abdomen design, prefabricated, off-the-shelf
L0642	Lumbar orthosis (LO), sagittal control, with rigid anterior and posterior panels, posterior extends from L-1 to below L-5 vertebra, produces intracavitary pressure to reduce load on the intervertebral discs, includes straps, closures, may include padding, shoulder straps, pendulous abdomen design, prefabricated, off-the-shelf
L0643	Lumbar-sacral orthosis (LSO), sagittal control, with rigid posterior panel(s), posterior extends from sacrococcygeal junction to T-9 vertebra, produces intracavitary pressure to reduce load on the intervertebral discs, includes straps, closures, may include padding, stays, shoulder straps, pendulous abdomen design, prefabricated, off-the-shelf
L0648	Lumbar-sacral orthosis (LSO), sagittal control, with rigid anterior and posterior panels, posterior extends from sacrococcygeal junction to T-9 vertebra, produces intracavitary pressure to reduce load on the intervertebral discs, includes straps, closures, may include padding, shoulder straps, pendulous abdomen design, prefabricated, off-the-shelf
L0649	Lumbar-sacral orthosis (LSO), sagittal-coronal control, with rigid posterior frame/panel(s), posterior extends from sacrococcygeal junction to T-9 vertebra, lateral strength provided by rigid lateral frame/panels, produces intracavitary pressure to reduce load on intervertebral discs, includes straps, closures, may include padding, stays, shoulder straps, pendulous abdomen design, prefabricated, off-the-shelf
L0650	Lumbar-sacral orthosis (LSO), sagittal-coronal control, with rigid anterior and posterior frame/panel(s), posterior extends from sacrococcygeal junction to T-9 vertebra, lateral strength provided by rigid lateral frame/panel(s), produces intracavitary pressure to reduce load on intervertebral discs, includes straps, closures, may include padding, shoulder straps, pendulous abdomen design, prefabricated, off-the-shelf
L0651	Lumbar-sacral orthosis (LSO), sagittal-coronal control, rigid shell(s)/panel(s), posterior extends from sacrococcygeal junction to T-9 vertebra, anterior extends from symphysis pubis to xyphoid, produces intracavitary pressure to reduce load on the intervertebral discs, overall strength is provided by overlapping rigid material and stabilizing closures, includes straps, closures, may include soft interface, pendulous abdomen design, prefabricated, off-the-shelf
L0700	Cervical-thoracic-lumbar-sacral orthosis (CTLSO), anterior-posterior-lateral control, molded to patient model, (Minerva type)
L0710	Cervical-thoracic-lumbar-sacral orthosis (CTLSO), anterior-posterior-lateral control, molded to patient model, with interface material, (Minerva type)

Halo Procedure

Code	Description
L0810	Halo procedure, cervical halo incorporated into jacket vest
L0820	Halo procedure, cervical halo incorporated into plaster body jacket
L0830	Halo procedure, cervical halo incorporated into Milwaukee type orthotic
L0859	Addition to halo procedure, magnetic resonance image compatible systems, rings and pins, any material
L0861	Addition to halo procedure, replacement liner/interface material

Additions to Spinal Orthoses

Code	Description
L0970	Thoracic-lumbar-sacral orthosis (TLSO), corset front
L0972	Lumbar-sacral orthosis (LSO), corset front
L0974	Thoracic-lumbar-sacral orthosis (TLSO), full corset
L0976	Lumbar-sacral orthosis (LSO), full corset
L0978	Axillary crutch extension
L0980	Peroneal straps, prefabricated, off-the-shelf, pair
L0982	Stocking supporter grips, prefabricated, off-the-shelf, set of four (4)
L0984	Protective body sock, prefabricated, off-the-shelf, each
L0999	Addition to spinal orthosis, not otherwise specified

Determine if an alternative HCPCS Level II or a CPT code better describes the service being reported. This code should be used only if a more specific code is unavailable.

Orthotic Devices - Scoliosis Procedures

The orthotic care of scoliosis differs from other orthotic care in that the treatment is more dynamic in nature and uses continual modification of the orthosis to the patient's changing condition. This coding structure uses the proper names - or eponyms - of the procedures because they have historic and universal acceptance in the profession. It should be recognized that variations to the basic procedures described by the founders/developers are accepted in various medical and orthotic practices throughout the country. All procedures include model of patient when indicated.

2023 HCPCS Level II

Code	Description
L1000	Cervical-thoracic-lumbar-sacral orthosis (CTLSO) (Milwaukee), inclusive of furnishing initial orthotic, including model

A variety of configurations are available for the Milwaukee brace (L1000)

Milwaukee-style braces, cervical thoracic lumbar sacral orthosis (CTSLO)

Code	Description
L1001	Cervical-thoracic-lumbar-sacral orthosis (CTLSO), immobilizer, infant size, prefabricated, includes fitting and adjustment
L1005	Tension based scoliosis orthosis and accessory pads, includes fitting and adjustment
L1010	Addition to cervical-thoracic-lumbar-sacral orthosis (CTLSO) or scoliosis orthosis, axilla sling
L1020	Addition to cervical-thoracic-lumbar-sacral orthosis (CTLSO) or scoliosis orthosis, kyphosis pad
L1025	Addition to cervical-thoracic-lumbar-sacral orthosis (CTLSO) or scoliosis orthosis, kyphosis pad, floating
L1030	Addition to cervical-thoracic-lumbar-sacral orthosis (CTLSO) or scoliosis orthosis, lumbar bolster pad
L1040	Addition to cervical-thoracic-lumbar-sacral orthosis (CTLSO) or scoliosis orthosis, lumbar or lumbar rib pad
L1050	Addition to cervical-thoracic-lumbar-sacral orthosis (CTLSO) or scoliosis orthosis, sternal pad
L1060	Addition to cervical-thoracic-lumbar-sacral orthosis (CTLSO) or scoliosis orthosis, thoracic pad
L1070	Addition to cervical-thoracic-lumbar-sacral orthosis (CTLSO) or scoliosis orthosis, trapezius sling
L1080	Addition to cervical-thoracic-lumbar-sacral orthosis (CTLSO) or scoliosis orthosis, outrigger
L1085	Addition to cervical-thoracic-lumbar-sacral orthosis (CTLSO) or scoliosis orthosis, outrigger, bilateral with vertical extensions
L1090	Addition to cervical-thoracic-lumbar-sacral orthosis (CTLSO) or scoliosis orthosis, lumbar sling
L1100	Addition to cervical-thoracic-lumbar-sacral orthosis (CTLSO) or scoliosis orthosis, ring flange, plastic or leather
L1110	Addition to cervical-thoracic-lumbar-sacral orthosis (CTLSO) or scoliosis orthosis, ring flange, plastic or leather, molded to patient model
L1120	Addition to cervical-thoracic-lumbar-sacral orthosis (CTLSO), scoliosis orthosis, cover for upright, each

Thoracic-Lumbar-Sacral Orthosis (TLSO) (Low Profile)

Code	Description
L1200	Thoracic-lumbar-sacral orthosis (TLSO), inclusive of furnishing initial orthosis only
L1210	Addition to thoracic-lumbar-sacral orthosis (TLSO), (low profile), lateral thoracic extension
L1220	Addition to thoracic-lumbar-sacral orthosis (TLSO), (low profile), anterior thoracic extension
L1230	Addition to thoracic-lumbar-sacral orthosis (TLSO), (low profile), Milwaukee type superstructure
L1240	Addition to thoracic-lumbar-sacral orthosis (TLSO), (low profile), lumbar derotation pad
L1250	Addition to thoracic-lumbar-sacral orthosis (TLSO), (low profile), anterior ASIS pad
L1260	Addition to thoracic-lumbar-sacral orthosis (TLSO), (low profile), anterior thoracic derotation pad
L1270	Addition to thoracic-lumbar-sacral orthosis (TLSO), (low profile), abdominal pad **AHA:** 2Q,19
L1280	Addition to thoracic-lumbar-sacral orthosis (TLSO), (low profile), rib gusset (elastic), each
L1290	Addition to thoracic-lumbar-sacral orthosis (TLSO), (low profile), lateral trochanteric pad

Other Scoliosis Procedures

Code	Description
L1300	Other scoliosis procedure, body jacket molded to patient model
L1310	Other scoliosis procedure, postoperative body jacket
L1499	Spinal orthosis, not otherwise specified Determine if an alternative HCPCS Level II or a CPT code better describes the service being reported. This code should be used only if a more specific code is unavailable.

Hip Orthoses (HO) - Flexible

Code	Description
L1600	Hip orthosis (HO), abduction control of hip joints, flexible, Frejka type with cover, prefabricated item that has been trimmed, bent, molded, assembled, or otherwise customized to fit a specific patient by an individual with expertise
L1610	Hip orthosis (HO), abduction control of hip joints, flexible, (Frejka cover only), prefabricated item that has been trimmed, bent, molded, assembled, or otherwise customized to fit a specific patient by an individual with expertise
L1620	Hip orthosis (HO), abduction control of hip joints, flexible, (Pavlik harness), prefabricated item that has been trimmed, bent, molded, assembled, or otherwise customized to fit a specific patient by an individual with expertise
L1630	Hip orthosis (HO), abduction control of hip joints, semi-flexible (Von Rosen type), custom fabricated
L1640	Hip orthosis (HO), abduction control of hip joints, static, pelvic band or spreader bar, thigh cuffs, custom fabricated
L1650	Hip orthosis (HO), abduction control of hip joints, static, adjustable, (Ilfled type), prefabricated, includes fitting and adjustment
L1652	Hip orthosis (HO), bilateral thigh cuffs with adjustable abductor spreader bar, adult size, prefabricated, includes fitting and adjustment, any type
L1660	Hip orthosis (HO), abduction control of hip joints, static, plastic, prefabricated, includes fitting and adjustment

Orthotic Devices and Procedures

L1680 — L1920

Code	Description
L1680	Hip orthosis (HO), abduction control of hip joints, dynamic, pelvic control, adjustable hip motion control, thigh cuffs (Rancho hip action type), custom fabricated
L1685	Hip orthosis (HO), abduction control of hip joint, postoperative hip abduction type, custom fabricated
L1686	Hip orthosis (HO), abduction control of hip joint, postoperative hip abduction type, prefabricated, includes fitting and adjustment
L1690	Combination, bilateral, lumbo-sacral, hip, femur orthosis providing adduction and internal rotation control, prefabricated, includes fitting and adjustment

Legg Perthes

Code	Description
L1700	Legg Perthes orthosis, (Toronto type), custom fabricated
L1710	Legg Perthes orthosis, (Newington type), custom fabricated
L1720	Legg Perthes orthosis, trilateral, (Tachdijan type), custom fabricated
L1730	Legg Perthes orthosis, (Scottish Rite type), custom fabricated
L1755	Legg Perthes orthosis, (Patten bottom type), custom fabricated

Knee Orthosis

Code	Description
L1810	Knee orthosis (KO), elastic with joints, prefabricated item that has been trimmed, bent, molded, assembled, or otherwise customized to fit a specific patient by an individual with expertise
L1812	Knee orthosis (KO), elastic with joints, prefabricated, off-the-shelf
L1820	Knee orthosis (KO), elastic with condylar pads and joints, with or without patellar control, prefabricated, includes fitting and adjustment
L1830	Knee orthosis (KO), immobilizer, canvas longitudinal, prefabricated, off-the-shelf
L1831	Knee orthosis (KO), locking knee joint(s), positional orthosis, prefabricated, includes fitting and adjustment
L1832	Knee orthosis (KO), adjustable knee joints (unicentric or polycentric), positional orthosis, rigid support, prefabricated item that has been trimmed, bent, molded, assembled, or otherwise customized to fit a specific patient by an individual with expertise
L1833	Knee orthosis (KO), adjustable knee joints (unicentric or polycentric), positional orthosis, rigid support, prefabricated, off-the shelf
L1834	Knee orthosis (KO), without knee joint, rigid, custom fabricated
L1836	Knee orthosis (KO), rigid, without joint(s), includes soft interface material, prefabricated, off-the-shelf
L1840	Knee orthosis (KO), derotation, medial-lateral, anterior cruciate ligament, custom fabricated
L1843	Knee orthosis (KO), single upright, thigh and calf, with adjustable flexion and extension joint (unicentric or polycentric), medial-lateral and rotation control, with or without varus/valgus adjustment, prefabricated item that has been trimmed, bent, molded, assembled, or otherwise customized to fit a specific patient by an individual with expertise
L1844	Knee orthosis (KO), single upright, thigh and calf, with adjustable flexion and extension joint (unicentric or polycentric), medial-lateral and rotation control, with or without varus/valgus adjustment, custom fabricated
L1845	Knee orthosis (KO), double upright, thigh and calf, with adjustable flexion and extension joint (unicentric or polycentric), medial-lateral and rotation control, with or without varus/valgus adjustment, prefabricated item that has been trimmed, bent, molded, assembled, or otherwise customized to fit a specific patient by an individual with expertise
L1846	Knee orthosis (KO), double upright, thigh and calf, with adjustable flexion and extension joint (unicentric or polycentric), medial-lateral and rotation control, with or without varus/valgus adjustment, custom fabricated
L1847	Knee orthosis (KO), double upright with adjustable joint, with inflatable air support chamber(s), prefabricated item that has been trimmed, bent, molded, assembled, or otherwise customized to fit a specific patient by an individual with expertise
L1848	Knee orthosis (KO), double upright with adjustable joint, with inflatable air support chamber(s), prefabricated, off-the-shelf
L1850	Knee orthosis (KO), Swedish type, prefabricated, off-the-shelf
L1851	Knee orthosis (KO), single upright, thigh and calf, with adjustable flexion and extension joint (unicentric or polycentric), medial-lateral and rotation control, with or without varus/valgus adjustment, prefabricated, off-the-shelf
L1852	Knee orthosis (KO), double upright, thigh and calf, with adjustable flexion and extension joint (unicentric or polycentric), medial-lateral and rotation control, with or without varus/valgus adjustment, prefabricated, off-the-shelf
L1860	Knee orthosis (KO), modification of supracondylar prosthetic socket, custom fabricated (SK)

Ankle-Foot Orthosis (AFO)

Code	Description
L1900	Ankle-foot orthosis (AFO), spring wire, dorsiflexion assist calf band, custom fabricated
L1902	Ankle orthosis (AO), ankle gauntlet or similar, with or without joints, prefabricated, off-the-shelf
L1904	Ankle orthosis (AO), ankle gauntlet or similar, with or without joints, custom fabricated
L1906	Ankle foot orthosis (AFO), multiligamentous ankle support, prefabricated, off-the-shelf
L1907	Ankle orthosis (AO), supramalleolar with straps, with or without interface/pads, custom fabricated
L1910	Ankle-foot orthosis (AFO), posterior, single bar, clasp attachment to shoe counter, prefabricated, includes fitting and adjustment
L1920	Ankle-foot orthosis (AFO), single upright with static or adjustable stop (Phelps or Perlstein type), custom fabricated

2023 HCPCS Level II · L2106

L1930 Ankle-foot orthosis (AFO), plastic or other material, prefabricated, includes fitting and adjustment

Ankle foot orthotic (AFO), plastic or other material (L1930)
Flexible carbon component
Foot component may fit inside shoe

L1932 Ankle-foot orthosis (AFO), rigid anterior tibial section, total carbon fiber or equal material, prefabricated, includes fitting and adjustment

L1940 Ankle-foot orthosis (AFO), plastic or other material, custom fabricated

L1945 Ankle-foot orthosis (AFO), plastic, rigid anterior tibial section (floor reaction), custom fabricated

Rigid tibial anterior floor reaction; ankle-foot orthosis (AFO) (L1945)
Spiral; ankle foot orthosis (AFO) (L1950)

L1950 Ankle-foot orthosis (AFO), spiral, (Institute of Rehabilitative Medicine type), plastic, custom fabricated

L1951 Ankle-foot orthosis (AFO), spiral, (Institute of rehabilitative Medicine type), plastic or other material, prefabricated, includes fitting and adjustment

L1960 Ankle-foot orthosis (AFO), posterior solid ankle, plastic, custom fabricated

L1970 Ankle-foot orthosis (AFO), plastic with ankle joint, custom fabricated

L1971 Ankle-foot orthosis (AFO), plastic or other material with ankle joint, prefabricated, includes fitting and adjustment

L1980 Ankle-foot orthosis (AFO), single upright free plantar dorsiflexion, solid stirrup, calf band/cuff (single bar 'BK' orthosis), custom fabricated

L1990 Ankle-foot orthosis (AFO), double upright free plantar dorsiflexion, solid stirrup, calf band/cuff (double bar 'BK' orthosis), custom fabricated

Knee-Ankle-Foot Orthosis (KAFO) - Or Any Combination

L2000 Knee-ankle-foot orthosis (KAFO), single upright, free knee, free ankle, solid stirrup, thigh and calf bands/cuffs (single bar 'AK' orthosis), custom fabricated

L2005 Knee-ankle-foot orthosis (KAFO), any material, single or double upright, stance control, automatic lock and swing phase release, any type activation, includes ankle joint, any type, custom fabricated

L2006 Knee ankle foot device, any material, single or double upright, swing and stance phase microprocessor control with adjustability, includes all components (e.g., sensors, batteries, charger), any type activation, with or without ankle joint(s), custom fabricated

L2010 Knee-ankle-foot orthosis (KAFO), single upright, free ankle, solid stirrup, thigh and calf bands/cuffs (single bar 'AK' orthosis), without knee joint, custom fabricated

L2020 Knee-ankle-foot orthosis (KAFO), double upright, free ankle, solid stirrup, thigh and calf bands/cuffs (double bar 'AK' orthosis), custom fabricated

L2030 Knee-ankle-foot orthosis (KAFO), double upright, free ankle, solid stirrup, thigh and calf bands/cuffs, (double bar 'AK' orthosis), without knee joint, custom fabricated

L2034 Knee-ankle-foot orthosis (KAFO), full plastic, single upright, with or without free motion knee, medial-lateral rotation control, with or without free motion ankle, custom fabricated

L2035 Knee-ankle-foot orthosis (KAFO), full plastic, static (pediatric size), without free motion ankle, prefabricated, includes fitting and adjustment

L2036 Knee-ankle-foot orthosis (KAFO), full plastic, double upright, with or without free motion knee, with or without free motion ankle, custom fabricated

L2037 Knee-ankle-foot orthosis (KAFO), full plastic, single upright, with or without free motion knee, with or without free motion ankle, custom fabricated

L2038 Knee-ankle-foot orthosis (KAFO), full plastic, with or without free motion knee, multi-axis ankle, custom fabricated

Torsion Control: Hip-Knee-Ankle-Foot Orthosis (HKAFO)

L2040 Hip-knee-ankle-foot orthosis (HKAFO), torsion control, bilateral rotation straps, pelvic band/belt, custom fabricated

L2050 Hip-knee-ankle-foot orthosis (HKAFO), torsion control, bilateral torsion cables, hip joint, pelvic band/belt, custom fabricated

L2060 Hip-knee-ankle-foot orthosis (HKAFO), torsion control, bilateral torsion cables, ball bearing hip joint, pelvic band/ belt, custom fabricated

L2070 Hip-knee-ankle-foot orthosis (HKAFO), torsion control, unilateral rotation straps, pelvic band/belt, custom fabricated

L2080 Hip-knee-ankle-foot orthosis (HKAFO), torsion control, unilateral torsion cable, hip joint, pelvic band/belt, custom fabricated

L2090 Hip-knee-ankle-foot orthosis (HKAFO), torsion control, unilateral torsion cable, ball bearing hip joint, pelvic band/ belt, custom fabricated

L2106 Ankle-foot orthosis (AFO), fracture orthosis, tibial fracture cast orthosis, thermoplastic type casting material, custom fabricated

Code	Description
L2108	Ankle-foot orthosis (AFO), fracture orthosis, tibial fracture cast orthosis, custom fabricated
L2112	Ankle-foot orthosis (AFO), fracture orthosis, tibial fracture orthosis, soft, prefabricated, includes fitting and adjustment
L2114	Ankle-foot orthosis (AFO), fracture orthosis, tibial fracture orthosis, semi-rigid, prefabricated, includes fitting and adjustment
L2116	Ankle-foot orthosis (AFO), fracture orthosis, tibial fracture orthosis, rigid, prefabricated, includes fitting and adjustment
L2126	Knee-ankle-foot orthosis (KAFO), fracture orthosis, femoral fracture cast orthosis, thermoplastic type casting material, custom fabricated
L2128	Knee-ankle-foot orthosis (KAFO), fracture orthosis, femoral fracture cast orthosis, custom fabricated
L2132	Knee-ankle-foot orthosis (KAFO), fracture orthosis, femoral fracture cast orthosis, soft, prefabricated, includes fitting and adjustment
L2134	Knee-ankle-foot orthosis (KAFO), fracture orthosis, femoral fracture cast orthosis, semi-rigid, prefabricated, includes fitting and adjustment
L2136	Knee-ankle-foot orthosis (KAFO), fracture orthosis, femoral fracture cast orthosis, rigid, prefabricated, includes fitting and adjustment

Additions to Fracture Orthosis

Code	Description
L2180	Addition to lower extremity fracture orthosis, plastic shoe insert with ankle joints
L2182	Addition to lower extremity fracture orthosis, drop lock knee joint
L2184	Addition to lower extremity fracture orthosis, limited motion knee joint
L2186	Addition to lower extremity fracture orthosis, adjustable motion knee joint, Lerman type
L2188	Addition to lower extremity fracture orthosis, quadrilateral brim
L2190	Addition to lower extremity fracture orthosis, waist belt
L2192	Addition to lower extremity fracture orthosis, hip joint, pelvic band, thigh flange, and pelvic belt

Additions to Lower Extremity Orthosis: Shoe-Ankle-Shin-Knee

Code	Description
L2200	Addition to lower extremity, limited ankle motion, each joint
L2210	Addition to lower extremity, dorsiflexion assist (plantar flexion resist), each joint
L2220	Addition to lower extremity, dorsiflexion and plantar flexion assist/resist, each joint
L2230	Addition to lower extremity, split flat caliper stirrups and plate attachment
L2232	Addition to lower extremity orthosis, rocker bottom for total contact ankle-foot orthosis (AFO), for custom fabricated orthosis only
L2240	Addition to lower extremity, round caliper and plate attachment
L2250	Addition to lower extremity, foot plate, molded to patient model, stirrup attachment
L2260	Addition to lower extremity, reinforced solid stirrup (Scott-Craig type)
L2265	Addition to lower extremity, long tongue stirrup
L2270	Addition to lower extremity, varus/valgus correction (T) strap, padded/lined or malleolus pad
L2275	Addition to lower extremity, varus/valgus correction, plastic modification, padded/lined
L2280	Addition to lower extremity, molded inner boot
L2300	Addition to lower extremity, abduction bar (bilateral hip involvement), jointed, adjustable
L2310	Addition to lower extremity, abduction bar, straight
L2320	Addition to lower extremity, nonmolded lacer, for custom fabricated orthosis only
L2330	Addition to lower extremity, lacer molded to patient model, for custom fabricated orthosis only
L2335	Addition to lower extremity, anterior swing band
L2340	Addition to lower extremity, pretibial shell, molded to patient model
L2350	Addition to lower extremity, prosthetic type, (BK) socket, molded to patient model, (used for PTB, AFO orthoses)
L2360	Addition to lower extremity, extended steel shank
L2370	Addition to lower extremity, Patten bottom
L2375	Addition to lower extremity, torsion control, ankle joint and half solid stirrup
L2380	Addition to lower extremity, torsion control, straight knee joint, each joint
L2385	Addition to lower extremity, straight knee joint, heavy-duty, each joint
L2387	Addition to lower extremity, polycentric knee joint, for custom fabricated knee-ankle-foot orthosis (KAFO), each joint
L2390	Addition to lower extremity, offset knee joint, each joint
L2395	Addition to lower extremity, offset knee joint, heavy-duty, each joint
L2397	Addition to lower extremity orthosis, suspension sleeve

Additions to Straight Knee or Offset Knee Joints

Code	Description
L2405	Addition to knee joint, drop lock, each
L2415	Addition to knee lock with integrated release mechanism (bail, cable, or equal), any material, each joint
L2425	Addition to knee joint, disc or dial lock for adjustable knee flexion, each joint
L2430	Addition to knee joint, ratchet lock for active and progressive knee extension, each joint
L2492	Addition to knee joint, lift loop for drop lock ring

Additions: Thigh/Weight Bearing - Gluteal/Ischial Weight Bearing

Code	Description
L2500	Addition to lower extremity, thigh/weight bearing, gluteal/ischial weight bearing, ring
L2510	Addition to lower extremity, thigh/weight bearing, quadri-lateral brim, molded to patient model
L2520	Addition to lower extremity, thigh/weight bearing, quadri-lateral brim, custom fitted
L2525	Addition to lower extremity, thigh/weight bearing, ischial containment/narrow M-L brim molded to patient model

Code	Description
L2526	Addition to lower extremity, thigh/weight bearing, ischial containment/narrow M-L brim, custom fitted
L2530	Addition to lower extremity, thigh/weight bearing, lacer, nonmolded
L2540	Addition to lower extremity, thigh/weight bearing, lacer, molded to patient model
L2550	Addition to lower extremity, thigh/weight bearing, high roll cuff

Additions: Pelvic and Thoracic Control

Code	Description
L2570	Addition to lower extremity, pelvic control, hip joint, Clevis type two-position joint, each
L2580	Addition to lower extremity, pelvic control, pelvic sling
L2600	Addition to lower extremity, pelvic control, hip joint, Clevis type, or thrust bearing, free, each
L2610	Addition to lower extremity, pelvic control, hip joint, Clevis or thrust bearing, lock, each
L2620	Addition to lower extremity, pelvic control, hip joint, heavy-duty, each
L2622	Addition to lower extremity, pelvic control, hip joint, adjustable flexion, each
L2624	Addition to lower extremity, pelvic control, hip joint, adjustable flexion, extension, abduction control, each
L2627	Addition to lower extremity, pelvic control, plastic, molded to patient model, reciprocating hip joint and cables
L2628	Addition to lower extremity, pelvic control, metal frame, reciprocating hip joint and cables
L2630	Addition to lower extremity, pelvic control, band and belt, unilateral
L2640	Addition to lower extremity, pelvic control, band and belt, bilateral
L2650	Addition to lower extremity, pelvic and thoracic control, gluteal pad, each
L2660	Addition to lower extremity, thoracic control, thoracic band
L2670	Addition to lower extremity, thoracic control, paraspinal uprights
L2680	Addition to lower extremity, thoracic control, lateral support uprights

Additions: General

Code	Description
L2750	Addition to lower extremity orthosis, plating chrome or nickel, per bar
L2755	Addition to lower extremity orthosis, high strength, lightweight material, all hybrid lamination/prepreg composite, per segment, for custom fabricated orthosis only
L2760	Addition to lower extremity orthosis, extension, per extension, per bar (for lineal adjustment for growth)
L2768	Orthotic side bar disconnect device, per bar
L2780	Addition to lower extremity orthosis, noncorrosive finish, per bar
L2785	Addition to lower extremity orthosis, drop lock retainer, each
L2795	Addition to lower extremity orthosis, knee control, full kneecap
L2800	Addition to lower extremity orthosis, knee control, knee cap, medial or lateral pull, for use with custom fabricated orthosis only
L2810	Addition to lower extremity orthosis, knee control, condylar pad
L2820	Addition to lower extremity orthosis, soft interface for molded plastic, below knee section
L2830	Addition to lower extremity orthosis, soft interface for molded plastic, above knee section
L2840	Addition to lower extremity orthosis, tibial length sock, fracture or equal, each
L2850	Addition to lower extremity orthosis, femoral length sock, fracture or equal, each
L2861	Addition to lower extremity joint, knee or ankle, concentric adjustable torsion style mechanism for custom fabricated orthotics only, each
L2999	Lower extremity orthoses, not otherwise specified Determine if an alternative HCPCS Level II or a CPT code better describes the service being reported. This code should be used only if a more specific code is unavailable.

Orthopedic Footwear

Inserts

Code	Description
L3000	Foot insert, removable, molded to patient model, UCB type, Berkeley shell, each
L3001	Foot, insert, removable, molded to patient model, Spenco, each
L3002	Foot insert, removable, molded to patient model, Plastazote or equal, each
L3003	Foot insert, removable, molded to patient model, silicone gel, each
L3010	Foot insert, removable, molded to patient model, longitudinal arch support, each
L3020	Foot insert, removable, molded to patient model, longitudinal/metatarsal support, each
L3030	Foot insert, removable, formed to patient foot, each
L3031	Foot, insert/plate, removable, addition to lower extremity orthosis, high strength, lightweight material, all hybrid lamination/prepreg composite, each

Arch Support, Removable, Premolded

Code	Description
L3040	Foot, arch support, removable, premolded, longitudinal, each
L3050	Foot, arch support, removable, premolded, metatarsal, each
L3060	Foot, arch support, removable, premolded, longitudinal/metatarsal, each

Arch Support, Nonremovable, Attached to Shoe

Code	Description
L3070	Foot, arch support, nonremovable, attached to shoe, longitudinal, each
L3080	Foot, arch support, nonremovable, attached to shoe, metatarsal, each
L3090	Foot, arch support, nonremovable, attached to shoe, longitudinal/metatarsal, each
L3100	Hallus-valgus night dynamic splint, prefabricated, off-the-shelf

Abduction and Rotation Bars

L3140 Foot, abduction rotation bar, including shoes

A Denis-Browne style splint is a bar that can be applied by a strap or mounted on a shoe. This type of splint generally corrects congenital conditions such as genu varus

The angle may be adjusted on a plate on the sole of the shoe

Denis-Browne splint

L3150 Foot, abduction rotation bar, without shoes
L3160 Foot, adjustable shoe-styled positioning device
L3170 Foot, plastic, silicone or equal, heel stabilizer, prefabricated, off-the-shelf, each

Orthopedic Shoes and Boots

L3201 Orthopedic shoe, Oxford with supinator or pronator, infant
L3202 Orthopedic shoe, Oxford with supinator or pronator, child
L3203 Orthopedic shoe, Oxford with supinator or pronator, junior
L3204 Orthopedic shoe, hightop with supinator or pronator, infant
L3206 Orthopedic shoe, hightop with supinator or pronator, child
L3207 Orthopedic shoe, hightop with supinator or pronator, junior
L3208 Surgical boot, each, infant
L3209 Surgical boot, each, child
L3211 Surgical boot, each, junior
L3212 Benesch boot, pair, infant
L3213 Benesch boot, pair, child
L3214 Benesch boot, pair, junior
L3215 Orthopedic footwear, ladies shoe, Oxford, each
L3216 Orthopedic footwear, ladies shoe, depth inlay, each
L3217 Orthopedic footwear, ladies shoe, hightop, depth inlay, each
L3219 Orthopedic footwear, mens shoe, Oxford, each
L3221 Orthopedic footwear, mens shoe, depth inlay, each
L3222 Orthopedic footwear, mens shoe, hightop, depth inlay, each
L3224 Orthopedic footwear, woman's shoe, Oxford, used as an integral part of a brace (orthosis)
L3225 Orthopedic footwear, man's shoe, Oxford, used as an integral part of a brace (orthosis)
L3230 Orthopedic footwear, custom shoe, depth inlay, each
L3250 Orthopedic footwear, custom molded shoe, removable inner mold, prosthetic shoe, each
L3251 Foot, shoe molded to patient model, silicone shoe, each
L3252 Foot, shoe molded to patient model, Plastazote (or similar), custom fabricated, each
L3253 Foot, molded shoe, Plastazote (or similar), custom fitted, each
L3254 Nonstandard size or width
L3255 Nonstandard size or length
L3257 Orthopedic footwear, additional charge for split size
L3260 Surgical boot/shoe, each
L3265 Plastazote sandal, each

Shoe Modification - Lifts

L3300 Lift, elevation, heel, tapered to metatarsals, per in
L3310 Lift, elevation, heel and sole, neoprene, per in
L3320 Lift, elevation, heel and sole, cork, per in
L3330 Lift, elevation, metal extension (skate)
L3332 Lift, elevation, inside shoe, tapered, up to one-half in
L3334 Lift, elevation, heel, per in

Shoe Modification - Wedges

L3340 Heel wedge, SACH
L3350 Heel wedge
L3360 Sole wedge, outside sole
L3370 Sole wedge, between sole
L3380 Clubfoot wedge
L3390 Outflare wedge
L3400 Metatarsal bar wedge, rocker
L3410 Metatarsal bar wedge, between sole
L3420 Full sole and heel wedge, between sole

Shoe Modifications - Heels

L3430 Heel, counter, plastic reinforced
L3440 Heel, counter, leather reinforced
L3450 Heel, SACH cushion type
L3455 Heel, new leather, standard
L3460 Heel, new rubber, standard
L3465 Heel, Thomas with wedge
L3470 Heel, Thomas extended to ball
L3480 Heel, pad and depression for spur
L3485 Heel, pad, removable for spur

Miscellaneous Shoe Additions

L3500 Orthopedic shoe addition, insole, leather
L3510 Orthopedic shoe addition, insole, rubber

Code	Description
L3520	Orthopedic shoe addition, insole, felt covered with leather
L3530	Orthopedic shoe addition, sole, half
L3540	Orthopedic shoe addition, sole, full
L3550	Orthopedic shoe addition, toe tap, standard
L3560	Orthopedic shoe addition, toe tap, horseshoe
L3570	Orthopedic shoe addition, special extension to instep (leather with eyelets)
L3580	Orthopedic shoe addition, convert instep to Velcro closure
L3590	Orthopedic shoe addition, convert firm shoe counter to soft counter
L3595	Orthopedic shoe addition, March bar

Transfer or Replacement

Code	Description
L3600	Transfer of an orthosis from one shoe to another, caliper plate, existing
L3610	Transfer of an orthosis from one shoe to another, caliper plate, new
L3620	Transfer of an orthosis from one shoe to another, solid stirrup, existing
L3630	Transfer of an orthosis from one shoe to another, solid stirrup, new
L3640	Transfer of an orthosis from one shoe to another, Dennis Browne splint (Riveton), both shoes
L3649	Orthopedic shoe, modification, addition or transfer, not otherwise specified

Determine if an alternative HCPCS Level II or a CPT code better describes the service being reported. This code should be used only if a more specific code is unavailable.

Shoulder Orthosis (SO)

Code	Description
L3650	Shoulder orthosis (SO), figure of eight design abduction restrainer, prefabricated, off-the-shelf
L3660	Shoulder orthosis (SO), figure of eight design abduction restrainer, canvas and webbing, prefabricated, off-the-shelf
L3670	Shoulder orthosis (SO), acromio/clavicular (canvas and webbing type), prefabricated, off-the-shelf
L3671	Shoulder orthosis (SO), shoulder joint design, without joints, may include soft interface, straps, custom fabricated, includes fitting and adjustment
L3674	Shoulder orthosis (SO), abduction positioning (airplane design), thoracic component and support bar, with or without nontorsion joint/turnbuckle, may include soft interface, straps, custom fabricated, includes fitting and adjustment
L3675	Shoulder orthosis (SO), vest type abduction restrainer, canvas webbing type or equal, prefabricated, off-the-shelf
L3677	Shoulder orthosis (SO), shoulder joint design, without joints, may include soft interface, straps, prefabricated item that has been trimmed, bent, molded, assembled, or otherwise customized to fit a specific patient by an individual with expertise
L3678	Shoulder orthosis (SO), shoulder joint design, without joints, may include soft interface, straps, prefabricated, off-the-shelf

Elbow Orthosis (EO)

Code	Description
L3702	Elbow orthosis (EO), without joints, may include soft interface, straps, custom fabricated, includes fitting and adjustment
L3710	Elbow orthosis (EO), elastic with metal joints, prefabricated, off-the-shelf
L3720	Elbow orthosis (EO), double upright with forearm/arm cuffs, free motion, custom fabricated
L3730	Elbow orthosis (EO), double upright with forearm/arm cuffs, extension/ flexion assist, custom fabricated
L3740	Elbow orthosis (EO), double upright with forearm/arm cuffs, adjustable position lock with active control, custom fabricated
L3760	Elbow orthosis (EO), with adjustable position locking joint(s), prefabricated, item that has been trimmed, bent, molded, assembled, or otherwise customized to fit a specific patient by an individual with expertise
L3761	Elbow orthosis (EO), with adjustable position locking joint(s), prefabricated, off-the-shelf
L3762	Elbow orthosis (EO), rigid, without joints, includes soft interface material, prefabricated, off-the-shelf
L3763	Elbow-wrist-hand orthosis (EWHO), rigid, without joints, may include soft interface, straps, custom fabricated, includes fitting and adjustment
L3764	Elbow-wrist-hand orthosis (EWHO), includes one or more nontorsion joints, elastic bands, turnbuckles, may include soft interface, straps, custom fabricated, includes fitting and adjustment
L3765	Elbow-wrist-hand-finger orthosis (EWHFO), rigid, without joints, may include soft interface, straps, custom fabricated, includes fitting and adjustment
L3766	Elbow-wrist-hand-finger orthosis (EWHFO), includes one or more nontorsion joints, elastic bands, turnbuckles, may include soft interface, straps, custom fabricated, includes fitting and adjustment

Wrist-Hand-Finger Orthosis (WHFO)

Code	Description
L3806	Wrist-hand-finger orthosis (WHFO), includes one or more nontorsion joint(s), turnbuckles, elastic bands/springs, may include soft interface material, straps, custom fabricated, includes fitting and adjustment
L3807	Wrist-hand-finger orthosis (WHFO), without joint(s), prefabricated item that has been trimmed, bent, molded, assembled, or otherwise customized to fit a specific patient by an individual with expertise
L3808	Wrist-hand-finger orthosis (WHFO), rigid without joints, may include soft interface material; straps, custom fabricated, includes fitting and adjustment
L3809	Wrist-hand-finger orthosis (WHFO), without joint(s), prefabricated, off-the-shelf, any type

Additions to Upper Extremity Orthosis

Code	Description
L3891	Addition to upper extremity joint, wrist or elbow, concentric adjustable torsion style mechanism for custom fabricated orthotics only, each

Dynamic Flexor Hinge, Reciprocal Wrist Extension/Flexion, Finger Flexion/Extension

Code	Description
L3900	Wrist-hand-finger orthosis (WHFO), dynamic flexor hinge, reciprocal wrist extension/ flexion, finger flexion/extension, wrist or finger driven, custom fabricated

L3901 Wrist-hand-finger orthosis (WHFO), dynamic flexor hinge, reciprocal wrist extension/ flexion, finger flexion/extension, cable driven, custom fabricated

External Power

L3904 Wrist-hand-finger orthosis (WHFO), external powered, electric, custom fabricated

Other Upper Extremity Orthoses

L3905 Wrist-hand orthosis (WHO), includes one or more nontorsion joints, elastic bands, turnbuckles, may include soft interface, straps, custom fabricated, includes fitting and adjustment

L3906 Wrist-hand orthosis (WHO), without joints, may include soft interface, straps, custom fabricated, includes fitting and adjustment

L3908 Wrist-hand orthosis (WHO), wrist extension control cock-up, nonmolded, prefabricated, off-the-shelf

L3912 Hand-finger orthosis (HFO), flexion glove with elastic finger control, prefabricated, off-the-shelf

L3913 Hand-finger orthosis (HFO), without joints, may include soft interface, straps, custom fabricated, includes fitting and adjustment

L3915 Wrist-hand orthosis (WHO), includes one or more nontorsion joint(s), elastic bands, turnbuckles, may include soft interface, straps, prefabricated item that has been trimmed, bent, molded, assembled, or otherwise customized to fit a specific patient by an individual with expertise

L3916 Wrist-hand orthosis (WHO), includes one or more nontorsion joint(s), elastic bands, turnbuckles, may include soft interface, straps, prefabricated, off-the-shelf

L3917 Hand orthosis (HO), metacarpal fracture orthosis, prefabricated item that has been trimmed, bent, molded, assembled, or otherwise customized to fit a specific patient by an individual with expertise

L3918 Hand orthosis (HO), metacarpal fracture orthosis, prefabricated, off-the-shelf

L3919 Hand orthosis (HO), without joints, may include soft interface, straps, custom fabricated, includes fitting and adjustment

L3921 Hand-finger orthosis (HFO), includes one or more nontorsion joints, elastic bands, turnbuckles, may include soft interface, straps, custom fabricated, includes fitting and adjustment

L3923 Hand-finger orthosis (HFO), without joints, may include soft interface, straps, prefabricated item that has been trimmed, bent, molded, assembled, or otherwise customized to fit a specific patient by an individual with expertise

L3924 Hand-finger orthosis (HFO), without joints, may include soft interface, straps, prefabricated, off-the-shelf

L3925 Finger orthosis (FO), proximal interphalangeal (PIP)/distal interphalangeal (DIP), nontorsion joint/spring, extension/flexion, may include soft interface material, prefabricated, off-the-shelf

L3927 Finger orthosis (FO), proximal interphalangeal (PIP)/distal interphalangeal (DIP), without joint/spring, extension/flexion (e.g., static or ring type), may include soft interface material, prefabricated, off-the-shelf

L3929 Hand-finger orthosis (HFO), includes one or more nontorsion joint(s), turnbuckles, elastic bands/springs, may include soft interface material, straps, prefabricated item that has been trimmed, bent, molded, assembled, or otherwise customized to fit a specific patient by an individual with expertise

L3930 Hand-finger orthosis (HFO), includes one or more nontorsion joint(s), turnbuckles, elastic bands/springs, may include soft interface material, straps, prefabricated, off-the-shelf

L3931 Wrist-hand-finger orthosis (WHFO), includes one or more nontorsion joint(s), turnbuckles, elastic bands/springs, may include soft interface material, straps, prefabricated, includes fitting and adjustment

L3933 Finger orthosis (FO), without joints, may include soft interface, custom fabricated, includes fitting and adjustment

L3935 Finger orthosis (FO), nontorsion joint, may include soft interface, custom fabricated, includes fitting and adjustment

L3956 Addition of joint to upper extremity orthosis, any material; per joint

Shoulder, Elbow, Wrist, Hand Orthosis

L3960 Shoulder-elbow-wrist-hand orthosis (SEWHO), abduction positioning, airplane design, prefabricated, includes fitting and adjustment

L3961 Shoulder-elbow-wrist-hand orthosis (SEWHO), shoulder cap design, without joints, may include soft interface, straps, custom fabricated, includes fitting and adjustment

L3962 Shoulder-elbow-wrist-hand orthosis (SEWHO), abduction positioning, Erb's palsy design, prefabricated, includes fitting and adjustment

L3967 Shoulder-elbow-wrist-hand orthosis (SEWHO), abduction positioning (airplane design), thoracic component and support bar, without joints, may include soft interface, straps, custom fabricated, includes fitting and adjustment

Additions to Mobile Arm Supports

L3971 Shoulder-elbow-wrist-hand orthotic (SEWHO), shoulder cap design, includes one or more nontorsion joints, elastic bands, turnbuckles, may include soft interface, straps, custom fabricated, includes fitting and adjustment

L3973 Shoulder-elbow-wrist-hand orthosis (SEWHO), abduction positioning (airplane design), thoracic component and support bar, includes one or more nontorsion joints, elastic bands, turnbuckles, may include soft interface, straps, custom fabricated, includes fitting and adjustment

L3975 Shoulder-elbow-wrist-hand-finger orthosis (SEWHO), shoulder cap design, without joints, may include soft interface, straps, custom fabricated, includes fitting and adjustment

L3976 Shoulder-elbow-wrist-hand-finger orthosis (SEWHO), abduction positioning (airplane design), thoracic component and support bar, without joints, may include soft interface, straps, custom fabricated, includes fitting and adjustment

L3977 Shoulder-elbow-wrist-hand-finger orthosis (SEWHO), shoulder cap design, includes one or more nontorsion joints, elastic bands, turnbuckles, may include soft interface, straps, custom fabricated, includes fitting and adjustment

L3978 Shoulder-elbow-wrist-hand-finger orthosis (SEWHO), abduction positioning (airplane design), thoracic component and support bar, includes one or more nontorsion joints, elastic bands, turnbuckles, may include soft interface, straps, custom fabricated, includes fitting and adjustment

Fracture Orthotic

Code	Description
L3980	Upper extremity fracture orthosis, humeral, prefabricated, includes fitting and adjustment
L3981	Upper extremity fracture orthosis, humeral, prefabricated, includes shoulder cap design, with or without joints, forearm section, may include soft interface, straps, includes fitting and adjustments
L3982	Upper extremity fracture orthosis, radius/ulnar, prefabricated, includes fitting and adjustment
L3984	Upper extremity fracture orthosis, wrist, prefabricated, includes fitting and adjustment
L3995	Addition to upper extremity orthosis, sock, fracture or equal, each
L3999	Upper limb orthosis, not otherwise specified

Repairs

Code	Description
L4000	Replace girdle for spinal orthosis (cervical-thoracic-lumbar-sacral orthosis (CTLSO) or spinal orthosis SO)
L4002	Replacement strap, any orthosis, includes all components, any length, any type
L4010	Replace trilateral socket brim
L4020	Replace quadrilateral socket brim, molded to patient model
L4030	Replace quadrilateral socket brim, custom fitted
L4040	Replace molded thigh lacer, for custom fabricated orthosis only
L4045	Replace nonmolded thigh lacer, for custom fabricated orthosis only
L4050	Replace molded calf lacer, for custom fabricated orthosis only
L4055	Replace nonmolded calf lacer, for custom fabricated orthosis only
L4060	Replace high roll cuff
L4070	Replace proximal and distal upright for KAFO
L4080	Replace metal bands KAFO, proximal thigh
L4090	Replace metal bands KAFO-AFO, calf or distal thigh
L4100	Replace leather cuff KAFO, proximal thigh
L4110	Replace leather cuff KAFO-AFO, calf or distal thigh
L4130	Replace pretibial shell
L4205	Repair of orthotic device, labor component, per 15 minutes
L4210	Repair of orthotic device, repair or replace minor parts

Miscellaneous Lower Limb Supports

Code	Description
L4350	Ankle control orthosis, stirrup style, rigid, includes any type interface (e.g., pneumatic, gel), prefabricated, off-the-shelf
L4360	Walking boot, pneumatic and/or vacuum, with or without joints, with or without interface material, prefabricated item that has been trimmed, bent, molded, assembled, or otherwise customized to fit a specific patient by an individual with expertise
L4361	Walking boot, pneumatic and/or vacuum, with or without joints, with or without interface material, prefabricated, off-the-shelf
L4370	Pneumatic full leg splint, prefabricated, off-the-shelf
L4386	Walking boot, nonpneumatic, with or without joints, with or without interface material, prefabricated item that has been trimmed, bent, molded, assembled, or otherwise customized to fit a specific patient by an individual with expertise
L4387	Walking boot, nonpneumatic, with or without joints, with or without interface material, prefabricated, off-the-shelf
L4392	Replacement, soft interface material, static AFO
L4394	Replace soft interface material, foot drop splint
L4396	Static or dynamic ankle foot orthosis, including soft interface material, adjustable for fit, for positioning, may be used for minimal ambulation, prefabricated item that has been trimmed, bent, molded, assembled, or otherwise customized to fit a specific patient by an individual with expertise
L4397	Static or dynamic ankle foot orthosis, including soft interface material, adjustable for fit, for positioning, may be used for minimal ambulation, prefabricated, off-the-shelf
L4398	Foot drop splint, recumbent positioning device, prefabricated, off-the-shelf
L4631	Ankle-foot orthosis (AFO), walking boot type, varus/valgus correction, rocker bottom, anterior tibial shell, soft interface, custom arch support, plastic or other material, includes straps and closures, custom fabricated

Prosthetic Procedures L5000-L9900

The codes in this section are considered as "base" or "basic procedures or prosthetics" and may be modified by listing items/procedures or special materials from the "additions" sections and adding them to the base procedure.

Partial Foot

Code	Description
L5000	Partial foot, shoe insert with longitudinal arch, toe filler
L5010	Partial foot, molded socket, ankle height, with toe filler
L5020	Partial foot, molded socket, tibial tubercle height, with toe filler

Ankle

Code	Description
L5050	Ankle, Symes, molded socket, SACH foot
L5060	Ankle, Symes, metal frame, molded leather socket, articulated ankle/foot (SACH)

Below Knee

Code	Description
L5100	Below knee (BK), molded socket, shin, SACH foot
L5105	Below knee (BK), plastic socket, joints and thigh lacer, SACH foot

Knee Disarticulation

Code	Description
L5150	Knee disarticulation (or through knee), molded socket, external knee joints, shin, SACH foot
L5160	Knee disarticulation (or through knee), molded socket, bent knee configuration, external knee joints, shin, SACH foot

Above Knee

Code	Description
L5200	Above knee (AK), molded socket, single axis constant friction knee, shin, SACH foot
L5210	Above knee (AK), short prosthesis, no knee joint (stubbies), with foot blocks, no ankle joints, each
L5220	Above knee (AK), short prosthesis, no knee joint (stubbies), with articulated ankle/foot, dynamically aligned, each
L5230	Above knee (AK), for proximal femoral focal deficiency, constant friction knee, shin, SACH foot

Hip Disarticulation

L5250 Hip disarticulation, Canadian type; molded socket, hip joint, single axis constant friction knee, shin, SACH foot

L5270 Hip disarticulation, tilt table type; molded socket, locking hip joint, single axis constant friction knee, shin, SACH foot

Hemipelvectomy

L5280 Hemipelvectomy, Canadian type; molded socket, hip joint, single axis constant friction knee, shin, SACH foot

L5301 Below knee (BK), molded socket, shin, SACH foot, endoskeletal system

L5312 Knee disarticulation (or through knee), molded socket, single axis knee, pylon, SACH foot, endoskeletal system

L5321 Above knee (AK), molded socket, open end, SACH foot, endoskeletal system, single axis knee

L5331 Hip disarticulation, Canadian type, molded socket, endoskeletal system, hip joint, single axis knee, SACH foot

L5341 Hemipelvectomy, Canadian type, molded socket, endoskeletal system, hip joint, single axis knee, SACH foot

Immediate Postsurgical or Early Fitting Procedures

L5400 Immediate postsurgical or early fitting, application of initial rigid dressing, including fitting, alignment, suspension, and one cast change, below knee (BK)

Above-the-knee test socket

Below-the-knee early fitting rigid dressing (L5400)

Test sockets are often made of clear plastic so the prosthetist can visualize the fit against the residual limb

L5410 Immediate postsurgical or early fitting, application of initial rigid dressing, including fitting, alignment and suspension, below knee (BK), each additional cast change and realignment

L5420 Immediate postsurgical or early fitting, application of initial rigid dressing, including fitting, alignment and suspension and one cast change above knee (AK) or knee disarticulation

L5430 Immediate postsurgical or early fitting, application of initial rigid dressing, including fitting, alignment and suspension, above knee (AK) or knee disarticulation, each additional cast change and realignment

L5450 Immediate postsurgical or early fitting, application of nonweight bearing rigid dressing, below knee (BK)

L5460 Immediate postsurgical or early fitting, application of nonweight bearing rigid dressing, above knee (AK)

Initial Prosthesis

L5500 Initial, below knee (BK) PTB type socket, nonalignable system, pylon, no cover, SACH foot, plaster socket, direct formed

L5505 Initial, above knee (AK), knee disarticulation, ischial level socket, nonalignable system, pylon, no cover, SACH foot, plaster socket, direct formed

Preparatory Prosthesis

L5510 Preparatory, below knee (BK) PTB type socket, nonalignable system, pylon, no cover, SACH foot, plaster socket, molded to model

L5520 Preparatory, below knee (BK) PTB type socket, nonalignable system, pylon, no cover, SACH foot, thermoplastic or equal, direct formed

L5530 Preparatory, below knee (BK) PTB type socket, nonalignable system, pylon, no cover, SACH foot, thermoplastic or equal, molded to model

L5535 Preparatory, below knee (BK) PTB type socket, nonalignable system, no cover, SACH foot, prefabricated, adjustable open end socket

L5540 Preparatory, below knee (BK) PTB type socket, nonalignable system, pylon, no cover, SACH foot, laminated socket, molded to model

L5560 Preparatory, above knee (AK), knee disarticulation, ischial level socket, nonalignable system, pylon, no cover, SACH foot, plaster socket, molded to model

L5570 Preparatory, above knee (AK), knee disarticulation, ischial level socket, nonalignable system, pylon, no cover, SACH foot, thermoplastic or equal, direct formed

L5580 Preparatory, above knee (AK), knee disarticulation, ischial level socket, nonalignable system, pylon, no cover, SACH foot, thermoplastic or equal, molded to model

L5585 Preparatory, above knee (AK), knee disarticulation, ischial level socket, nonalignable system, pylon, no cover, SACH foot, prefabricated adjustable open end socket

L5590 Preparatory, above knee (AK), knee disarticulation, ischial level socket, nonalignable system, pylon, no cover, SACH foot, laminated socket, molded to model

L5595 Preparatory, hip disarticulation/hemipelvectomy, pylon, no cover, SACH foot, thermoplastic or equal, molded to patient model

L5600 Preparatory, hip disarticulation/hemipelvectomy, pylon, no cover, SACH foot, laminated socket, molded to patient model

Additions

Additions: Lower Extremity

L5610 Addition to lower extremity, endoskeletal system, above knee (AK), hydracadence system

L5611 Addition to lower extremity, endoskeletal system, above knee (AK), knee disarticulation, four-bar linkage, with friction swing phase control

L5613 Addition to lower extremity, endoskeletal system, above knee (AK), knee disarticulation, four-bar linkage, with hydraulic swing phase control

L5614 Addition to lower extremity, exoskeletal system, above knee (AK), knee disarticulation, four-bar linkage, with pneumatic swing phase control

Code	Description
L5616	Addition to lower extremity, endoskeletal system, above knee (AK), universal multiplex system, friction swing phase control
L5617	Addition to lower extremity, quick change self-aligning unit, above knee (AK) or below knee (BK), each

Additions: Test Sockets

Code	Description
L5618	Addition to lower extremity, test socket, Symes
L5620	Addition to lower extremity, test socket, below knee (BK)
L5622	Addition to lower extremity, test socket, knee disarticulation
L5624	Addition to lower extremity, test socket, above knee (AK)
L5626	Addition to lower extremity, test socket, hip disarticulation
L5628	Addition to lower extremity, test socket, hemipelvectomy
L5629	Addition to lower extremity, below knee, acrylic socket

Additions: Socket Variations

Code	Description
L5630	Addition to lower extremity, Symes type, expandable wall socket
L5631	Addition to lower extremity, above knee (AK) or knee disarticulation, acrylic socket
L5632	Addition to lower extremity, Symes type, PTB brim design socket
L5634	Addition to lower extremity, Symes type, posterior opening (Canadian) socket
L5636	Addition to lower extremity, Symes type, medial opening socket
L5637	Addition to lower extremity, below knee (BK), total contact
L5638	Addition to lower extremity, below knee (BK), leather socket
L5639	Addition to lower extremity, below knee (BK), wood socket
L5640	Addition to lower extremity, knee disarticulation, leather socket
L5642	Addition to lower extremity, above knee (AK), leather socket
L5643	Addition to lower extremity, hip disarticulation, flexible inner socket, external frame
L5644	Addition to lower extremity, above knee (AK), wood socket
L5645	Addition to lower extremity, below knee (BK), flexible inner socket, external frame
L5646	Addition to lower extremity, below knee (BK), air, fluid, gel or equal, cushion socket
L5647	Addition to lower extremity, below knee (BK), suction socket
L5648	Addition to lower extremity, above knee (AK), air, fluid, gel or equal, cushion socket
L5649	Addition to lower extremity, ischial containment/narrow M-L socket
L5650	Additions to lower extremity, total contact, above knee (AK) or knee disarticulation socket
L5651	Addition to lower extremity, above knee (AK), flexible inner socket, external frame
L5652	Addition to lower extremity, suction suspension, above knee (AK) or knee disarticulation socket
L5653	Addition to lower extremity, knee disarticulation, expandable wall socket

Additions: Socket Insert and Suspension

Code	Description
L5654	Addition to lower extremity, socket insert, Symes, (Kemblo, Pelite, Aliplast, Plastazote or equal)
L5655	Addition to lower extremity, socket insert, below knee (BK) (Kemblo, Pelite, Aliplast, Plastazote or equal)
L5656	Addition to lower extremity, socket insert, knee disarticulation (Kemblo, Pelite, Aliplast, Plastazote or equal)
L5658	Addition to lower extremity, socket insert, above knee (AK) (Kemblo, Pelite, Aliplast, Plastazote or equal)
L5661	Addition to lower extremity, socket insert, multidurometer Symes
L5665	Addition to lower extremity, socket insert, multidurometer, below knee (BK)
L5666	Addition to lower extremity, below knee (BK), cuff suspension
L5668	Addition to lower extremity, below knee (BK), molded distal cushion
L5670	Addition to lower extremity, below knee (BK), molded supracondylar suspension (PTS or similar)

As the suspension sleeve is donned, air is driven out through a valve

The valve is closed upon donning and a suction fit is formed around the residual limb

Code	Description
L5671	Addition to lower extremity, below knee (BK)/above knee (AK) suspension locking mechanism (shuttle, lanyard, or equal), excludes socket insert
L5672	Addition to lower extremity, below knee (BK), removable medial brim suspension
L5673	Addition to lower extremity, below knee (BK)/above knee (AK), custom fabricated from existing mold or prefabricated, socket insert, silicone gel, elastomeric or equal, for use with locking mechanism
L5676	Additions to lower extremity, below knee (BK), knee joints, single axis, pair

Code	Description
L5677	Additions to lower extremity, below knee (BK), knee joints, polycentric, pair
L5678	Additions to lower extremity, below knee (BK), joint covers, pair
L5679	Addition to lower extremity, below knee (BK)/above knee (AK), custom fabricated from existing mold or prefabricated, socket insert, silicone gel, elastomeric or equal, not for use with locking mechanism
L5680	Addition to lower extremity, below knee (BK), thigh lacer, nonmolded
L5681	Addition to lower extremity, below knee (BK)/above knee (AK), custom fabricated socket insert for congenital or atypical traumatic amputee, silicone gel, elastomeric or equal, for use with or without locking mechanism, initial only (for other than initial, use code L5673 or L5679)
L5682	Addition to lower extremity, below knee (BK), thigh lacer, gluteal/ischial, molded
L5683	Addition to lower extremity, below knee (BK)/above knee (AK), custom fabricated socket insert for other than congenital or atypical traumatic amputee, silicone gel, elastomeric or equal, for use with or without locking mechanism, initial only (for other than initial, use code L5673 or L5679)
L5684	Addition to lower extremity, below knee, fork strap
L5685	Addition to lower extremity prosthesis, below knee, suspension/sealing sleeve, with or without valve, any material, each
L5686	Addition to lower extremity, below knee (BK), back check (extension control)
L5688	Addition to lower extremity, below knee (BK), waist belt, webbing
L5690	Addition to lower extremity, below knee (BK), waist belt, padded and lined
L5692	Addition to lower extremity, above knee (AK), pelvic control belt, light
L5694	Addition to lower extremity, above knee (AK), pelvic control belt, padded and lined
L5695	Addition to lower extremity, above knee (AK), pelvic control, sleeve suspension, neoprene or equal, each
L5696	Addition to lower extremity, above knee (AK) or knee disarticulation, pelvic joint
L5697	Addition to lower extremity, above knee (AK) or knee disarticulation, pelvic band
L5698	Addition to lower extremity, above knee (AK) or knee disarticulation, Silesian bandage
L5699	All lower extremity prostheses, shoulder harness

Replacements

Code	Description
L5700	Replacement, socket, below knee (BK), molded to patient model
L5701	Replacement, socket, above knee (AK)/knee disarticulation, including attachment plate, molded to patient model
L5702	Replacement, socket, hip disarticulation, including hip joint, molded to patient model
L5703	Ankle, Symes, molded to patient model, socket without solid ankle cushion heel (SACH) foot, replacement only
L5704	Custom shaped protective cover, below knee (BK)
L5705	Custom shaped protective cover, above knee (AK)
L5706	Custom shaped protective cover, knee disarticulation
L5707	Custom shaped protective cover, hip disarticulation

Additions: Exoskeletal Knee-Shin System

Code	Description
L5710	Addition, exoskeletal knee-shin system, single axis, manual lock
L5711	Additions exoskeletal knee-shin system, single axis, manual lock, ultra-light material
L5712	Addition, exoskeletal knee-shin system, single axis, friction swing and stance phase control (safety knee)
L5714	Addition, exoskeletal knee-shin system, single axis, variable friction swing phase control
L5716	Addition, exoskeletal knee-shin system, polycentric, mechanical stance phase lock
L5718	Addition, exoskeletal knee-shin system, polycentric, friction swing and stance phase control
L5722	Addition, exoskeletal knee-shin system, single axis, pneumatic swing, friction stance phase control
L5724	Addition, exoskeletal knee-shin system, single axis, fluid swing phase control
L5726	Addition, exoskeletal knee-shin system, single axis, external joints, fluid swing phase control
L5728	Addition, exoskeletal knee-shin system, single axis, fluid swing and stance phase control
L5780	Addition, exoskeletal knee-shin system, single axis, pneumatic/hydra pneumatic swing phase control
L5781	Addition to lower limb prosthesis, vacuum pump, residual limb volume management and moisture evacuation system
L5782	Addition to lower limb prosthesis, vacuum pump, residual limb volume management and moisture evacuation system, heavy-duty

Component Modification

Code	Description
L5785	Addition, exoskeletal system, below knee (BK), ultra-light material (titanium, carbon fiber or equal)
L5790	Addition, exoskeletal system, above knee (AK), ultra-light material (titanium, carbon fiber or equal)
L5795	Addition, exoskeletal system, hip disarticulation, ultra-light material (titanium, carbon fiber or equal)

Additions: Endoskeletal Knee-Shin System

Code	Description
L5810	Addition, endoskeletal knee-shin system, single axis, manual lock
L5811	Addition, endoskeletal knee-shin system, single axis, manual lock, ultra-light material
L5812	Addition, endoskeletal knee-shin system, single axis, friction swing and stance phase control (safety knee)
L5814	Addition, endoskeletal knee-shin system, polycentric, hydraulic swing phase control, mechanical stance phase lock
L5816	Addition, endoskeletal knee-shin system, polycentric, mechanical stance phase lock
L5818	Addition, endoskeletal knee-shin system, polycentric, friction swing and stance phase control
L5822	Addition, endoskeletal knee-shin system, single axis, pneumatic swing, friction stance phase control
L5824	Addition, endoskeletal knee-shin system, single axis, fluid swing phase control

2023 HCPCS Level II

L5826 Addition, endoskeletal knee-shin system, single axis, hydraulic swing phase control, with miniature high activity frame

L5828 Addition, endoskeletal knee-shin system, single axis, fluid swing and stance phase control

L5830 Addition, endoskeletal knee-shin system, single axis, pneumatic/swing phase control

L5840 Addition, endoskeletal knee-shin system, four-bar linkage or multiaxial, pneumatic swing phase control

L5845 Addition, endoskeletal knee-shin system, stance flexion feature, adjustable

L5848 Addition to endoskeletal knee-shin system, fluid stance extension, dampening feature, with or without adjustability

L5850 Addition, endoskeletal system, above knee (AK) or hip disarticulation, knee extension assist

L5855 Addition, endoskeletal system, hip disarticulation, mechanical hip extension assist

L5856 Addition to lower extremity prosthesis, endoskeletal knee-shin system, microprocessor control feature, swing and stance phase, includes electronic sensor(s), any type

L5857 Addition to lower extremity prosthesis, endoskeletal knee-shin system, microprocessor control feature, swing phase only, includes electronic sensor(s), any type

L5858 Addition to lower extremity prosthesis, endoskeletal knee-shin system, microprocessor control feature, stance phase only, includes electronic sensor(s), any type

L5859 Addition to lower extremity prosthesis, endoskeletal knee-shin system, powered and programmable flexion/extension assist control, includes any type motor(s)

L5910 Addition, endoskeletal system, below knee (BK), alignable system

L5920 Addition, endoskeletal system, above knee (AK) or hip disarticulation, alignable system

L5925 Addition, endoskeletal system, above knee (AK), knee disarticulation or hip disarticulation, manual lock

L5930 Addition, endoskeletal system, high activity knee control frame

L5940 Addition, endoskeletal system, below knee (BK), ultra-light material (titanium, carbon fiber or equal)

L5950 Addition, endoskeletal system, above knee (AK), ultra-light material (titanium, carbon fiber or equal)

L5960 Addition, endoskeletal system, hip disarticulation, ultra-light material (titanium, carbon fiber or equal)

L5961 Addition, endoskeletal system, polycentric hip joint, pneumatic or hydraulic control, rotation control, with or without flexion and/or extension control

L5962 Addition, endoskeletal system, below knee (BK), flexible protective outer surface covering system

L5964 Addition, endoskeletal system, above knee (AK), flexible protective outer surface covering system

L5966 Addition, endoskeletal system, hip disarticulation, flexible protective outer surface covering system

L5968 Addition to lower limb prosthesis, multiaxial ankle with swing phase active dorsiflexion feature

L5969 Addition, endoskeletal ankle-foot or ankle system, power assist, includes any type motor(s)

L5970 All lower extremity prostheses, foot, external keel, SACH foot

L5971 All lower extremity prostheses, solid ankle cushion heel (SACH) foot, replacement only

L5972 All lower extremity prostheses, foot, flexible keel

L5973 Endoskeletal ankle foot system, microprocessor controlled feature, dorsiflexion and/or plantar flexion control, includes power source

L5974 All lower extremity prostheses, foot, single axis ankle/foot

Foot prosthesis (L5974)
Energy storing foot (L5976) Carbon

L5975 All lower extremity prostheses, combination single axis ankle and flexible keel foot

L5976 All lower extremity prostheses, energy storing foot (Seattle Carbon Copy II or equal)

L5978 All lower extremity prostheses, foot, multiaxial ankle/foot

Foot prosthesis, multi-axial ankle (L5978)

L5979 All lower extremity prostheses, multiaxial ankle, dynamic response foot, one-piece system

L5980 All lower extremity prostheses, flex-foot system

L5981 All lower extremity prostheses, flex-walk system or equal

L5982 All exoskeletal lower extremity prostheses, axial rotation unit

L5984 All endoskeletal lower extremity prostheses, axial rotation unit, with or without adjustability

---

Special Coverage Instructions   Noncovered by Medicare   Carrier Discretion   ☑ Quantity Alert   ● New Code   ○ Recycled/Reinstated   ▲ Revised Code

© 2022 Optum, Inc.   A2–Z3 ASC Pmt   CMS: IOM   AHA: Coding Clinic   DMEPOS Paid   SNF Excluded

Prosthetic Devices and Procedures

Code	Description
L5985	All endoskeletal lower extremity prostheses, dynamic prosthetic pylon
L5986	All lower extremity prostheses, multiaxial rotation unit (MCP or equal)
L5987	All lower extremity prostheses, shank foot system with vertical loading pylon
L5988	Addition to lower limb prosthesis, vertical shock reducing pylon feature
L5990	Addition to lower extremity prosthesis, user adjustable heel height
L5999	Lower extremity prosthesis, not otherwise specified Determine if an alternative HCPCS Level II or a CPT code better describes the service being reported. This code should be used only if a more specific code is unavailable.

Partial Hand

Code	Description
L6000	Partial hand, thumb remaining
L6010	Partial hand, little and/or ring finger remaining
L6020	Partial hand, no finger remaining
L6026	Transcarpal/metacarpal or partial hand disarticulation prosthesis, external power, self-suspended, inner socket with removable forearm section, electrodes and cables, two batteries, charger, myoelectric control of terminal device, excludes terminal device(s)

Wrist Disarticulation

Code	Description
L6050	Wrist disarticulation, molded socket, flexible elbow hinges, triceps pad
L6055	Wrist disarticulation, molded socket with expandable interface, flexible elbow hinges, triceps pad

Below Elbow

Code	Description
L6100	Below elbow, molded socket, flexible elbow hinge, triceps pad
L6110	Below elbow, molded socket (Muenster or Northwestern suspension types)
L6120	Below elbow, molded double wall split socket, step-up hinges, half cuff
L6130	Below elbow, molded double wall split socket, stump activated locking hinge, half cuff

Elbow Disarticulation

Code	Description
L6200	Elbow disarticulation, molded socket, outside locking hinge, forearm
L6205	Elbow disarticulation, molded socket with expandable interface, outside locking hinges, forearm

Above Elbow

Code	Description
L6250	Above elbow, molded double wall socket, internal locking elbow, forearm

Shoulder Disarticulation

Code	Description
L6300	Shoulder disarticulation, molded socket, shoulder bulkhead, humeral section, internal locking elbow, forearm
L6310	Shoulder disarticulation, passive restoration (complete prosthesis)
L6320	Shoulder disarticulation, passive restoration (shoulder cap only)

Interscapular Thoracic

Code	Description
L6350	Interscapular thoracic, molded socket, shoulder bulkhead, humeral section, internal locking elbow, forearm
L6360	Interscapular thoracic, passive restoration (complete prosthesis)
L6370	Interscapular thoracic, passive restoration (shoulder cap only)

Immediate and Early Postsurgical Procedures

Code	Description
L6380	Immediate postsurgical or early fitting, application of initial rigid dressing, including fitting alignment and suspension of components, and one cast change, wrist disarticulation or below elbow
L6382	Immediate postsurgical or early fitting, application of initial rigid dressing including fitting alignment and suspension of components, and one cast change, elbow disarticulation or above elbow
L6384	Immediate postsurgical or early fitting, application of initial rigid dressing including fitting alignment and suspension of components, and one cast change, shoulder disarticulation or interscapular thoracic
L6386	Immediate postsurgical or early fitting, each additional cast change and realignment
L6388	Immediate postsurgical or early fitting, application of rigid dressing only

Molded Socket

Code	Description
L6400	Below elbow, molded socket, endoskeletal system, including soft prosthetic tissue shaping
L6450	Elbow disarticulation, molded socket, endoskeletal system, including soft prosthetic tissue shaping
L6500	Above elbow, molded socket, endoskeletal system, including soft prosthetic tissue shaping
L6550	Shoulder disarticulation, molded socket, endoskeletal system, including soft prosthetic tissue shaping
L6570	Interscapular thoracic, molded socket, endoskeletal system, including soft prosthetic tissue shaping

Preparatory Socket

Code	Description
L6580	Preparatory, wrist disarticulation or below elbow, single wall plastic socket, friction wrist, flexible elbow hinges, figure of eight harness, humeral cuff, Bowden cable control, USMC or equal pylon, no cover, molded to patient model
L6582	Preparatory, wrist disarticulation or below elbow, single wall socket, friction wrist, flexible elbow hinges, figure of eight harness, humeral cuff, Bowden cable control, USMC or equal pylon, no cover, direct formed
L6584	Preparatory, elbow disarticulation or above elbow, single wall plastic socket, friction wrist, locking elbow, figure of eight harness, fair lead cable control, USMC or equal pylon, no cover, molded to patient model
L6586	Preparatory, elbow disarticulation or above elbow, single wall socket, friction wrist, locking elbow, figure of eight harness, fair lead cable control, USMC or equal pylon, no cover, direct formed
L6588	Preparatory, shoulder disarticulation or interscapular thoracic, single wall plastic socket, shoulder joint, locking elbow, friction wrist, chest strap, fair lead cable control, USMC or equal pylon, no cover, molded to patient model
L6590	Preparatory, shoulder disarticulation or interscapular thoracic, single wall socket, shoulder joint, locking elbow, friction wrist, chest strap, fair lead cable control, USMC or equal pylon, no cover, direct formed

Additions: Upper Limb

The following procedures/modifications/components may be added to other base procedures. The items in this section should reflect the additional complexity of each modification procedure, in addition to the base procedure, at the time of the original order.

Code	Description
L6600	Upper extremity additions, polycentric hinge, pair
L6605	Upper extremity additions, single pivot hinge, pair
L6610	Upper extremity additions, flexible metal hinge, pair
L6611	Addition to upper extremity prosthesis, external powered, additional switch, any type
L6615	Upper extremity addition, disconnect locking wrist unit
L6616	Upper extremity addition, additional disconnect insert for locking wrist unit, each
L6620	Upper extremity addition, flexion/extension wrist unit, with or without friction
L6621	Upper extremity prosthesis addition, flexion/extension wrist with or without friction, for use with external powered terminal device
L6623	Upper extremity addition, spring assisted rotational wrist unit with latch release
L6624	Upper extremity addition, flexion/extension and rotation wrist unit
L6625	Upper extremity addition, rotation wrist unit with cable lock
L6628	Upper extremity addition, quick disconnect hook adapter, Otto Bock or equal
L6629	Upper extremity addition, quick disconnect lamination collar with coupling piece, Otto Bock or equal
L6630	Upper extremity addition, stainless steel, any wrist
L6632	Upper extremity addition, latex suspension sleeve, each
L6635	Upper extremity addition, lift assist for elbow
L6637	Upper extremity addition, nudge control elbow lock
L6638	Upper extremity addition to prosthesis, electric locking feature, only for use with manually powered elbow
L6640	Upper extremity additions, shoulder abduction joint, pair
L6641	Upper extremity addition, excursion amplifier, pulley type
L6642	Upper extremity addition, excursion amplifier, lever type
L6645	Upper extremity addition, shoulder flexion-abduction joint, each
L6646	Upper extremity addition, shoulder joint, multipositional locking, flexion, adjustable abduction friction control, for use with body powered or external powered system
L6647	Upper extremity addition, shoulder lock mechanism, body powered actuator
L6648	Upper extremity addition, shoulder lock mechanism, external powered actuator
L6650	Upper extremity addition, shoulder universal joint, each
L6655	Upper extremity addition, standard control cable, extra
L6660	Upper extremity addition, heavy-duty control cable
L6665	Upper extremity addition, Teflon, or equal, cable lining
L6670	Upper extremity addition, hook to hand, cable adapter
L6672	Upper extremity addition, harness, chest or shoulder, saddle type
L6675	Upper extremity addition, harness, (e.g., figure of eight type), single cable design
L6676	Upper extremity addition, harness, (e.g., figure of eight type), dual cable design
L6677	Upper extremity addition, harness, triple control, simultaneous operation of terminal device and elbow
L6680	Upper extremity addition, test socket, wrist disarticulation or below elbow
L6682	Upper extremity addition, test socket, elbow disarticulation or above elbow
L6684	Upper extremity addition, test socket, shoulder disarticulation or interscapular thoracic
L6686	Upper extremity addition, suction socket
L6687	Upper extremity addition, frame type socket, below elbow or wrist disarticulation
L6688	Upper extremity addition, frame type socket, above elbow or elbow disarticulation
L6689	Upper extremity addition, frame type socket, shoulder disarticulation
L6690	Upper extremity addition, frame type socket, interscapular-thoracic
L6691	Upper extremity addition, removable insert, each
L6692	Upper extremity addition, silicone gel insert or equal, each
L6693	Upper extremity addition, locking elbow, forearm counterbalance
L6694	Addition to upper extremity prosthesis, below elbow/above elbow, custom fabricated from existing mold or prefabricated, socket insert, silicone gel, elastomeric or equal, for use with locking mechanism
L6695	Addition to upper extremity prosthesis, below elbow/above elbow, custom fabricated from existing mold or prefabricated, socket insert, silicone gel, elastomeric or equal, not for use with locking mechanism
L6696	Addition to upper extremity prosthesis, below elbow/above elbow, custom fabricated socket insert for congenital or atypical traumatic amputee, silicone gel, elastomeric or equal, for use with or without locking mechanism, initial only (for other than initial, use code L6694 or L6695)
L6697	Addition to upper extremity prosthesis, below elbow/above elbow, custom fabricated socket insert for other than congenital or atypical traumatic amputee, silicone gel, elastomeric or equal, for use with or without locking mechanism, initial only (for other than initial, use code L6694 or L6695)
L6698	Addition to upper extremity prosthesis, below elbow/above elbow, lock mechanism, excludes socket insert

Terminal Device

Code	Description
L6703	Terminal device, passive hand/mitt, any material, any size

Prosthetic Devices and Procedures

L6704 — L7007

Code	Description
L6704	Terminal device, sport/recreational/work attachment, any material, any size
L6706	Terminal device, hook, mechanical, voluntary opening, any material, any size, lined or unlined
L6707	Terminal device, hook, mechanical, voluntary closing, any material, any size, lined or unlined
L6708	Terminal device, hand, mechanical, voluntary opening, any material, any size
L6709	Terminal device, hand, mechanical, voluntary closing, any material, any size
L6711	Terminal device, hook, mechanical, voluntary opening, any material, any size, lined or unlined, pediatric
L6712	Terminal device, hook, mechanical, voluntary closing, any material, any size, lined or unlined, pediatric
L6713	Terminal device, hand, mechanical, voluntary opening, any material, any size, pediatric
L6714	Terminal device, hand, mechanical, voluntary closing, any material, any size, pediatric
L6715	Terminal device, multiple articulating digit, includes motor(s), initial issue or replacement
L6721	Terminal device, hook or hand, heavy-duty, mechanical, voluntary opening, any material, any size, lined or unlined
L6722	Terminal device, hook or hand, heavy-duty, mechanical, voluntary closing, any material, any size, lined or unlined

Addition to Terminal Device

Code	Description
L6805	Addition to terminal device, modifier wrist unit
L6810	Addition to terminal device, precision pinch device
L6880	Electric hand, switch or myoelectric controlled, independently articulating digits, any grasp pattern or combination of grasp patterns, includes motor(s)
L6881	Automatic grasp feature, addition to upper limb electric prosthetic terminal device
L6882	Microprocessor control feature, addition to upper limb prosthetic terminal device

Replacement Socket

Code	Description
L6883	Replacement socket, below elbow/wrist disarticulation, molded to patient model, for use with or without external power
L6884	Replacement socket, above elbow/elbow disarticulation, molded to patient model, for use with or without external power
L6885	Replacement socket, shoulder disarticulation/interscapular thoracic, molded to patient model, for use with or without external power

Hand Restoration

Code	Description
L6890	Addition to upper extremity prosthesis, glove for terminal device, any material, prefabricated, includes fitting and adjustment
L6895	Addition to upper extremity prosthesis, glove for terminal device, any material, custom fabricated
L6900	Hand restoration (casts, shading and measurements included), partial hand, with glove, thumb or one finger remaining
L6905	Hand restoration (casts, shading and measurements included), partial hand, with glove, multiple fingers remaining
L6910	Hand restoration (casts, shading and measurements included), partial hand, with glove, no fingers remaining
L6915	Hand restoration (shading and measurements included), replacement glove for above

External Power

Code	Description
L6920	Wrist disarticulation, external power, self-suspended inner socket, removable forearm shell, Otto Bock or equal switch, cables, two batteries and one charger, switch control of terminal device
L6925	Wrist disarticulation, external power, self-suspended inner socket, removable forearm shell, Otto Bock or equal electrodes, cables, two batteries and one charger, myoelectronic control of terminal device
L6930	Below elbow, external power, self-suspended inner socket, removable forearm shell, Otto Bock or equal switch, cables, two batteries and one charger, switch control of terminal device
L6935	Below elbow, external power, self-suspended inner socket, removable forearm shell, Otto Bock or equal electrodes, cables, two batteries and one charger, myoelectronic control of terminal device
L6940	Elbow disarticulation, external power, molded inner socket, removable humeral shell, outside locking hinges, forearm, Otto Bock or equal switch, cables, two batteries and one charger, switch control of terminal device
L6945	Elbow disarticulation, external power, molded inner socket, removable humeral shell, outside locking hinges, forearm, Otto Bock or equal electrodes, cables, two batteries and one charger, myoelectronic control of terminal device
L6950	Above elbow, external power, molded inner socket, removable humeral shell, internal locking elbow, forearm, Otto Bock or equal switch, cables, two batteries and one charger, switch control of terminal device
L6955	Above elbow, external power, molded inner socket, removable humeral shell, internal locking elbow, forearm, Otto Bock or equal electrodes, cables, two batteries and one charger, myoelectronic control of terminal device
L6960	Shoulder disarticulation, external power, molded inner socket, removable shoulder shell, shoulder bulkhead, humeral section, mechanical elbow, forearm, Otto Bock or equal switch, cables, two batteries and one charger, switch control of terminal device
L6965	Shoulder disarticulation, external power, molded inner socket, removable shoulder shell, shoulder bulkhead, humeral section, mechanical elbow, forearm, Otto Bock or equal electrodes, cables, two batteries and one charger, myoelectronic control of terminal device
L6970	Interscapular-thoracic, external power, molded inner socket, removable shoulder shell, shoulder bulkhead, humeral section, mechanical elbow, forearm, Otto Bock or equal switch, cables, two batteries and one charger, switch control of terminal device
L6975	Interscapular-thoracic, external power, molded inner socket, removable shoulder shell, shoulder bulkhead, humeral section, mechanical elbow, forearm, Otto Bock or equal electrodes, cables, two batteries and one charger, myoelectronic control of terminal device

Electric Hand and Accessories

Code	Description
L7007	Electric hand, switch or myoelectric controlled, adult

2023 HCPCS Level II   L8040

L7008	Electric hand, switch or myoelectric, controlled, pediatric
L7009	Electric hook, switch or myoelectric controlled, adult
L7040	Prehensile actuator, switch controlled
L7045	Electric hook, switch or myoelectric controlled, pediatric

Electronic Elbow and Accessories

L7170	Electronic elbow, Hosmer or equal, switch controlled
L7180	Electronic elbow, microprocessor sequential control of elbow and terminal device
L7181	Electronic elbow, microprocessor simultaneous control of elbow and terminal device
L7185	Electronic elbow, adolescent, Variety Village or equal, switch controlled
L7186	Electronic elbow, child, Variety Village or equal, switch controlled
L7190	Electronic elbow, adolescent, Variety Village or equal, myoelectronically controlled
L7191	Electronic elbow, child, Variety Village or equal, myoelectronically controlled

Electronic Wrist and Accessories

| L7259 | Electronic wrist rotator, any type |

Battery Components

L7360	Six volt battery, each
L7362	Battery charger, six volt, each
L7364	Twelve volt battery, each
L7366	Battery charger, 12 volt, each
L7367	Lithium ion battery, rechargeable, replacement
L7368	Lithium ion battery charger, replacement only

Additions to Upper Extremity Prosthesis

L7400	Addition to upper extremity prosthesis, below elbow/wrist disarticulation, ultra-light material (titanium, carbon fiber or equal)
L7401	Addition to upper extremity prosthesis, above elbow disarticulation, ultra-light material (titanium, carbon fiber or equal)
L7402	Addition to upper extremity prosthesis, shoulder disarticulation/interscapular thoracic, ultra-light material (titanium, carbon fiber or equal)
L7403	Addition to upper extremity prosthesis, below elbow/wrist disarticulation, acrylic material
L7404	Addition to upper extremity prosthesis, above elbow disarticulation, acrylic material
L7405	Addition to upper extremity prosthesis, shoulder disarticulation/interscapular thoracic, acrylic material
L7499	Upper extremity prosthesis, not otherwise specified

Repairs

L7510	Repair of prosthetic device, repair or replace minor parts
	Medicare jurisdiction: local contractor if repair of implanted prosthetic device.
L7520	Repair prosthetic device, labor component, per 15 minutes
	Medicare jurisdiction: local contractor if repair of implanted prosthetic device.

Prosthesis Supplies

| L7600 | Prosthetic donning sleeve, any material, each |
| L7700 | Gasket or seal, for use with prosthetic socket insert, any type, each |

Male Prosthetic

| L7900 | Male vacuum erection system |
| L7902 | Tension ring, for vacuum erection device, any type, replacement only, each |

Breast Prosthesis

L8000	Breast prosthesis, mastectomy bra, without integrated breast prosthesis form, any size, any type
L8001	Breast prosthesis, mastectomy bra, with integrated breast prosthesis form, unilateral, any size, any type
L8002	Breast prosthesis, mastectomy bra, with integrated breast prosthesis form, bilateral, any size, any type
L8010	Breast prosthesis, mastectomy sleeve
L8015	External breast prosthesis garment, with mastectomy form, post mastectomy
L8020	Breast prosthesis, mastectomy form
L8030	Breast prosthesis, silicone or equal, without integral adhesive
L8031	Breast prosthesis, silicone or equal, with integral adhesive
L8032	Nipple prosthesis, prefabricated, reusable, any type, each
L8033	Nipple prosthesis, custom fabricated, reusable, any material, any type, each
L8035	Custom breast prosthesis, post mastectomy, molded to patient model
L8039	Breast prosthesis, not otherwise specified

Face and Ear Prosthesis

| L8040 | Nasal prosthesis, provided by a nonphysician (KM, KN) |
| | CMS: 100-04,20,30.9 |

Nasal prosthesis (L8040)
Orbital and midfacial prosthesis (L8041-L8042)
Prosthesis

Facial prosthetics are typically custom manufactured from polymers and carefully matched to the original features. The maxilla, zygoma, frontal, and nasal bones are often involved, either singly or in combination (L8040-L8044)

Frontal bone
Nasal bone
Maxilla
Zygoma
(L8043–L8044)

Prosthetic Devices and Procedures

L8041 Midfacial prosthesis, provided by a nonphysician [A] [&] (KM, KN)
CMS: 100-04,20,30.9

L8042 Orbital prosthesis, provided by a nonphysician [A] [&] (KM, KN)
CMS: 100-04,20,30.9

L8043 Upper facial prosthesis, provided by a nonphysician [A] [&] (KM, KN)
CMS: 100-04,20,30.9

L8044 Hemi-facial prosthesis, provided by a nonphysician [A] [&] (KM, KN)
CMS: 100-04,20,30.9

L8045 Auricular prosthesis, provided by a nonphysician [A] [&] (KM, KN)
CMS: 100-04,20,30.9

L8046 Partial facial prosthesis, provided by a nonphysician [A] [&] (KM, KN)
CMS: 100-04,20,30.9

L8047 Nasal septal prosthesis, provided by a nonphysician [A] [&] (KM, KN)
CMS: 100-04,20,30.9

L8048 Unspecified maxillofacial prosthesis, by report, provided by a nonphysician [A]

L8049 Repair or modification of maxillofacial prosthesis, labor component, 15 minute increments, provided by a nonphysician [A]

Trusses

L8300 Truss, single with standard pad [A] [&]
L8310 Truss, double with standard pads [A] [&]
L8320 Truss, addition to standard pad, water pad [A] [&]
L8330 Truss, addition to standard pad, scrotal pad [♂] [A] [&]

Prosthetic Socks

L8400 Prosthetic sheath, below knee, each [A] [✓] [&]
L8410 Prosthetic sheath, above knee, each [A] [✓] [&]
L8415 Prosthetic sheath, upper limb, each [A] [✓] [&]
L8417 Prosthetic sheath/sock, including a gel cushion layer, below knee (BK) or above knee (AK), each [A] [✓] [&]
L8420 Prosthetic sock, multiple ply, below knee (BK), each [A] [✓] [&]
L8430 Prosthetic sock, multiple ply, above knee (AK), each [A] [✓] [&]
L8435 Prosthetic sock, multiple ply, upper limb, each [A] [✓] [&]
L8440 Prosthetic shrinker, below knee (BK), each [A] [✓] [&]
L8460 Prosthetic shrinker, above knee (AK), each [A] [✓] [&]
L8465 Prosthetic shrinker, upper limb, each [A] [✓] [&]
L8470 Prosthetic sock, single ply, fitting, below knee (BK), each [A] [✓] [&]
L8480 Prosthetic sock, single ply, fitting, above knee (AK), each [A] [✓] [&]
L8485 Prosthetic sock, single ply, fitting, upper limb, each [A] [✓] [&]
L8499 Unlisted procedure for miscellaneous prosthetic services [A]
Determine if an alternative HCPCS Level II or a CPT code better describes the service being reported. This code should be used only if a more specific code is unavailable.

Larynx and Trachea Prothetics and Accessories

L8500 Artificial larynx, any type [A] [&]
L8501 Tracheostomy speaking valve [&]
L8505 Artificial larynx replacement battery/accessory, any type [A]

L8507 Tracheo-esophageal voice prosthesis, patient inserted, any type, each [A] [&]

L8509 Tracheo-esophageal voice prosthesis, inserted by a licensed health care provider, any type [A]

L8510 Voice amplifier [A]

L8511 Insert for indwelling tracheo-esophageal prosthesis, with or without valve, replacement only, each [A] [✓] [&]

L8512 Gelatin capsules or equivalent, for use with tracheo-esophageal voice prosthesis, replacement only, per 10 [A] [✓] [&]

L8513 Cleaning device used with tracheoesophageal voice prosthesis, pipet, brush, or equal, replacement only, each [A] [✓] [&]

L8514 Tracheo-esophageal puncture dilator, replacement only, each [A] [✓] [&]

L8515 Gelatin capsule, application device for use with tracheo-esophageal voice prosthesis, each [A] [✓] [&]

Breast Implant

L8600 Implantable breast prosthesis, silicone or equal [♀] [N] [N1] [&]
Medicare covers implants inserted in post-mastectomy reconstruction in a breast cancer patient. Always report concurrent to the implant procedure.
CMS: 100-04,4,190

Bulking Agents

L8603 Injectable bulking agent, collagen implant, urinary tract, 2.5 ml syringe, includes shipping and necessary supplies [N] [N1] [✓] [&]
CMS: 100-04,4,190

L8604 Injectable bulking agent, dextranomer/hyaluronic acid copolymer implant, urinary tract, 1 ml, includes shipping and necessary supplies [N] [N1] [✓]

L8605 Injectable bulking agent, dextranomer/hyaluronic acid copolymer implant, anal canal, 1 ml, includes shipping and necessary supplies [N] [N1]

L8606 Injectable bulking agent, synthetic implant, urinary tract, 1 ml syringe, includes shipping and necessary supplies [N] [N1] [&]

L8607 Injectable bulking agent for vocal cord medialization, 0.1 ml, includes shipping and necessary supplies [N] [N1] [&]

Eye and Ear Implants and Accessories

L8608 Miscellaneous external component, supply or accessory for use with the Argus II Retinal Prosthesis System

L8609 Artificial cornea [N] [N1] [&]

L8610 Ocular implant [N] [N1] [&]
CMS: 100-04,4,190

2023 HCPCS Level II

L8612 Aqueous shunt
CMS: 100-04,4,190

L8613 Ossicula implant
CMS: 100-04,4,190

L8614 Cochlear device, includes all internal and external components
A cochlear implant is covered by Medicare when the patient has bilateral sensorineural deafness.
CMS: 100-04,14,40.8; 100-04,4,190; 100-04,4,60.4.2

L8615 Headset/headpiece for use with cochlear implant device, replacement

L8616 Microphone for use with cochlear implant device, replacement

L8617 Transmitting coil for use with cochlear implant device, replacement

L8618 Transmitter cable for use with cochlear implant device or auditory osseointegrated device, replacement

L8619 Cochlear implant, external speech processor and controller, integrated system, replacement
Medicare jurisdiction: local contractor.

L8621 Zinc air battery for use with cochlear implant device and auditory osseointegrated sound processors, replacement, each

L8622 Alkaline battery for use with cochlear implant device, any size, replacement, each

L8623 Lithium ion battery for use with cochlear implant device speech processor, other than ear level, replacement, each

L8624 Lithium ion battery for use with cochlear implant or auditory osseointegrated device speech processor, ear level, replacement, each

L8625 External recharging system for battery for use with cochlear implant or auditory osseointegrated device, replacement only, each

L8627 Cochlear implant, external speech processor, component, replacement

L8628 Cochlear implant, external controller component, replacement

L8629 Transmitting coil and cable, integrated, for use with cochlear implant device, replacement

Upper Extremity Implants

L8630 Metacarpophalangeal joint implant
CMS: 100-04,4,190

Bone is cut at the MP joint (arthroplasty)

Bone may be hollowed out in both metacarpal and phalangeal sides in preparation for a prosthesis

Prosthetic joint implant

Prosthesis in place

Metacarpophalangeal prosthetic implant

L8631 Metacarpal phalangeal joint replacement, two or more pieces, metal (e.g., stainless steel or cobalt chrome), ceramic-like material (e.g., pyrocarbon), for surgical implantation (all sizes, includes entire system)

Lower Extremity Implants

L8641 Metatarsal joint implant
CMS: 100-04,4,190

L8642 Hallux implant
CMS: 100-04,4,190

Interphalangeal Implants

L8658 Interphalangeal joint spacer, silicone or equal, each
CMS: 100-04,4,190

L8659 Interphalangeal finger joint replacement, two or more pieces, metal (e.g., stainless steel or cobalt chrome), ceramic-like material (e.g., pyrocarbon) for surgical implantation, any size

Cardiovascular Implant

L8670 Vascular graft material, synthetic, implant
CMS: 100-04,4,190

Neurostimulator and Accessories

L8679 Implantable neurostimulator, pulse generator, any type

L8680 Implantable neurostimulator electrode, each

L8681 Patient programmer (external) for use with implantable programmable neurostimulator pulse generator, replacement only

Prosthetic Devices and Procedures

Code	Description
L8682	Implantable neurostimulator radiofrequency receiver N N1
L8683	Radiofrequency transmitter (external) for use with implantable neurostimulator radiofrequency receiver A
L8684	Radiofrequency transmitter (external) for use with implantable sacral root neurostimulator receiver for bowel and bladder management, replacement A
L8685	Implantable neurostimulator pulse generator, single array, rechargeable, includes extension EI
L8686	Implantable neurostimulator pulse generator, single array, nonrechargeable, includes extension EI
L8687	Implantable neurostimulator pulse generator, dual array, rechargeable, includes extension EI
L8688	Implantable neurostimulator pulse generator, dual array, nonrechargeable, includes extension EI
L8689	External recharging system for battery (internal) for use with implantable neurostimulator, replacement only A

Miscellaneous Prosthetics and Accessories

Code	Description
L8690	Auditory osseointegrated device, includes all internal and external components N N1
	CMS: 100-04,14,40.8; 100-04,4,60.4.2
L8691	Auditory osseointegrated device, external sound processor, excludes transducer/actuator, replacement only, each A
L8692	Auditory osseointegrated device, external sound processor, used without osseointegration, body worn, includes headband or other means of external attachment EI
L8693	Auditory osseointegrated device abutment, any length, replacement only A
L8694	Auditory osseointegrated device, transducer/actuator, replacement only, each A
L8695	External recharging system for battery (external) for use with implantable neurostimulator, replacement only A
L8696	Antenna (external) for use with implantable diaphragmatic/phrenic nerve stimulation device, replacement, each A
L8698	Miscellaneous component, supply or accessory for use with total artificial heart system
L8699	Prosthetic implant, not otherwise specified N N1
	Determine if an alternative HCPCS Level II or a CPT code better describes the service being reported. This code should be used only if a more specific code is unavailable.
	CMS: 100-04,4,190
L8701	Powered upper extremity range of motion assist device, elbow, wrist, hand with single or double upright(s), includes microprocessor, sensors, all components and accessories, custom fabricated
L8702	Powered upper extremity range of motion assist device, elbow, wrist, hand, finger, single or double upright(s), includes microprocessor, sensors, all components and accessories, custom fabricated
L9900	Orthotic and prosthetic supply, accessory, and/or service component of another HCPCS L code N N1

2023 HCPCS Level II — M0250

MIPS Value Pathways M0001-M0005

- **M0001** Advancing Cancer Care MIPS Value Pathways
- **M0002** Optimal Care for Kidney Health MIPS Value Pathways
- **M0003** Optimal Care for Patients with Episodic Neurological Conditions MIPS Value Pathways
- **M0004** Supportive Care for Neurodegenerative Conditions MIPS Value Pathways
- **M0005** Promoting Wellness MIPS Value Pathways

Medical Services M0075-M0301

Other Medical Services

M codes include office services, cellular therapy, prolotherapy, intragastric hypothermia, IV chelation therapy, and fabric wrapping of an abdominal aneurysm.

M0075 Cellular therapy
The therapeutic efficacy of injecting foreign proteins has not been established.

M0076 Prolotherapy
The therapeutic efficacy of prolotherapy and joint sclerotherapy has not been established.

M0100 Intragastric hypothermia using gastric freezing
Code with caution: This procedure is considered obsolete.

M0201 COVID-19 vaccine administration inside a patient's home; reported only once per individual home, per date of service, when only COVID-19 vaccine administration is performed at the patient's home
AHA: 3Q,21

M0220 Injection, tixagevimab and cilgavimab, for the pre-exposure prophylaxis only, for certain adults and pediatric individuals (12 years of age and older weighing at least 40kg) with no known SARS-CoV-2 exposure, who either have moderate to severely compromised immune systems or for whom vaccination with any available COVID-19 vaccine is not recommended due to a history of severe adverse reaction to a COVID-19 vaccine(s) and/or COVID-19 vaccine component(s), includes injection and post administration monitoring
AHA: 2Q,22

M0221 Injection, tixagevimab and cilgavimab, for the pre-exposure prophylaxis only, for certain adults and pediatric individuals (12 years of age and older weighing at least 40kg) with no known SARS-CoV-2 exposure, who either have moderate to severely compromised immune systems or for whom vaccination with any available COVID-19 vaccine is not recommended due to a history of severe adverse reaction to a COVID-19 vaccine(s) and/or COVID-19 vaccine component(s), includes injection and post administration monitoring in the home or residence; this includes a beneficiary's home that has been made provider-based to the hospital during the COVID-19 public health emergency
AHA: 2Q,22

M0222 Intravenous injection, bebtelovimab, includes injection and post administration monitoring
AHA: 2Q,22

M0223 Intravenous injection, bebtelovimab, includes injection and post administration monitoring in the home or residence; this includes a beneficiary's home that has been made provider-based to the hospital during the COVID-19 public health emergency
AHA: 2Q,22

M0240 Intravenous infusion or subcutaneous injection, casirivimab and imdevimab, includes infusion or injection and post administration monitoring, subsequent repeat doses
Use this code for casirivimab and imdevimab 600 mg administered as post exposure prophylaxis. Report also Q0240 for drug.
AHA: 4Q,21; 3Q,21

M0241 Intravenous infusion or subcutaneous injection, casirivimab and imdevimab, includes infusion or injection, and post administration monitoring in the home or residence. This includes a beneficiary's home that has been made provider-based to the hospital during the covid-19 public health emergency, subsequent repeat doses
Use this code for casirivimab and imdevimab 600 mg administered as post exposure prophylaxis. Report also Q0240 for drug.
AHA: 4Q,21; 3Q,21

M0243 Intravenous infusion or subcutaneous injection, casirivimab and imdevimab, includes infusion or injection, and post administration monitoring
Use this code for administration of Casirivimab and Imdevimab (REGN-COV2), Regeneron. Report also Q0243 for drug.
AHA: 2Q,22; 1Q,21; 4Q,20

M0244 Intravenous infusion or subcutaneous injection, casirivimab and imdevimab, includes infusion or injection and post administration monitoring in the home or residence; this includes a beneficiary's home that has been made provider-based to the hospital during the COVID-19 public health emergency
Use this code for administration of casirivimab and imdevimab in the home setting. Report also Q0243 for drug.
AHA: 3Q,21

M0245 Intravenous infusion, bamlanivimab and etesevimab, includes infusion and post administration monitoring
Use this code for administration of bamlanivimab (LY-CoV555) and etesevimab (LY-CoV016). Report also Q0245 for drug.
AHA: 1Q,21

M0246 Intravenous infusion, bamlanivimab and etesevimab, includes infusion and post administration monitoring in the home or residence; this includes a beneficiary's home that has been made provider-based to the hospital during the COVID-19 public health emergency
Use this code for administration of bamlanivimab and etesevimab in the home setting. Report also Q0245 for drug.
AHA: 3Q,21

M0247 Intravenous infusion, sotrovimab, includes infusion and post administration monitoring
AHA: 3Q,21

M0248 Intravenous infusion, sotrovimab, includes infusion and post administration monitoring in the home or residence; this includes a beneficiary's home that has been made provider-based to the hospital during the COVID-19 public health emergency
AHA: 3Q,21

M0249 Intravenous infusion, tocilizumab, for hospitalized adults and pediatric patients (2 years of age and older) with COVID-19 who are receiving systemic corticosteroids and require supplemental oxygen, non-invasive or invasive mechanical ventilation, or extracorporeal membrane oxygenation (ECMO) only, includes infusion and post administration monitoring, first dose
AHA: 4Q,21

M0250 Intravenous infusion, tocilizumab, for hospitalized adults and pediatric patients (2 years of age and older) with COVID-19 who are receiving systemic corticosteroids and require supplemental oxygen, non-invasive or invasive mechanical ventilation, or extracorporeal membrane oxygenation (ECMO) only, includes infusion and post administration monitoring, second dose
AHA: 4Q,21

M0300

2023 HCPCS Level II

Medical Services

Cardiovascular Services

M0300 IV chelation therapy (chemical endarterectomy) [EI]
Chelation therapy is considered experimental in the United States.
CMS: 100-03*; 100-03,20.22

M0301 Fabric wrapping of abdominal aneurysm [EI]
Code with caution: This procedure has largely been replaced with more effective treatment modalities. Submit documentation.

Quality Measures M1003-M1149

Quality Measures

▲ **M1003** TB screening performed and results interpreted within 12 months prior to initiation of first-time biologic and/or immune response modifier therapy

M1004 Documentation of medical reason for not screening for TB or interpreting results (i.e., patient positive for TB and documentation of past treatment; patient who has recently completed a course of anti-TB therapy)

M1005 TB screening not performed or results not interpreted, reason not given

M1006 Disease activity not assessed, reason not given

M1007 >=50% of total number of a patient's outpatient RA encounters assessed

M1008 <50% of total number of a patient's outpatient RA encounters assessed

M1009 Discharge/discontinuation of the episode of care documented in the medical record

M1010 Discharge/discontinuation of the episode of care documented in the medical record

M1011 Discharge/discontinuation of the episode of care documented in the medical record

M1012 Discharge/discontinuation of the episode of care documented in the medical record

M1013 Discharge/discontinuation of the episode of care documented in the medical record

M1014 Discharge/discontinuation of the episode of care documented in the medical record

M1016 Female patients unable to bear children

~~M1017~~ ~~Patient admitted to palliative care services~~

M1018 Patients with an active diagnosis or history of cancer (except basal cell and squamous cell skin carcinoma), patients who are heavy tobacco smokers, lung cancer screening patients

M1019 Adolescent patients 12 to 17 years of age with major depression or dysthymia who reached remission at 12 months as demonstrated by a 12 month (+/-60 days) PHQ-9 or PHQ-9M score of less than 5

M1020 Adolescent patients 12 to 17 years of age with major depression or dysthymia who did not reach remission at 12 months as demonstrated by a 12 month (+/-60 days) PHQ-9 or PHQ-9M score of less than 5. Either PHQ-9 or PHQ-9M score was not assessed or is greater than or equal to 5

M1021 Patient had only urgent care visits during the performance period

M1027 Imaging of the head (CT or MRI) was obtained

M1028 Documentation of patients with primary headache diagnosis and imaging other than CT or MRI obtained

M1029 Imaging of the head (CT or MRI) was not obtained, reason not given

M1032 Adults currently taking pharmacotherapy for OUD

M1034 Adults who have at least 180 days of continuous pharmacotherapy with a medication prescribed for OUD without a gap of more than seven days

M1035 Adults who are deliberately phased out of medication assisted treatment (MAT) prior to 180 days of continuous treatment

M1036 Adults who have not had at least 180 days of continuous pharmacotherapy with a medication prescribed for OUD without a gap of more than seven days

M1037 Patients with a diagnosis of lumbar spine region cancer at the time of the procedure

M1038 Patients with a diagnosis of lumbar spine region fracture at the time of the procedure

M1039 Patients with a diagnosis of lumbar spine region infection at the time of the procedure

M1040 Patients with a diagnosis of lumbar idiopathic or congenital scoliosis

M1041 Patient had cancer, acute fracture or infection related to the lumbar spine or patient had neuromuscular, idiopathic or congenital lumbar scoliosis

M1043 Functional status was not measured by the Oswestry Disability Index (ODI version 2.1a) at 1 year (9 to 15 months) postoperatively

M1045 Functional status measured by the Oxford Knee Score (OKS) at one year (9 to 15 months) postoperatively was greater than or equal to 37 or knee injury and osteoarthritis outcome score joint replacement (KOOS, JR.) was greater than or equal to 71

M1046 Functional status measured by the Oxford Knee Score (OKS) at one year (9 to 15 months) postoperatively was less than 37 or the knee injury and osteoarthritis outcome score joint replacement (KOOS, JR.) was less than 71 postoperatively

M1049 Functional status was not measured by the Oswestry Disability Index (ODI version 2.1a) at 3 months (6 to 20 weeks) postoperatively

M1051 Patient had cancer, acute fracture or infection related to the lumbar spine or patient had neuromuscular, idiopathic or congenital lumbar scoliosis

▲ **M1052** Leg pain was not measured by the visual analog scale (VAS) or numeric pain scale at one year (9 to 15 months) postoperatively

M1054 Patient had only urgent care visits during the performance period

M1055 Aspirin or another antiplatelet therapy used

M1056 Prescribed anticoagulant medication during the performance period, history of GI bleeding, history of intracranial bleeding, bleeding disorder and specific provider documented reasons: allergy to aspirin or antiplatelets, use of nonsteroidal antiinflammatory agents, drug-drug interaction, uncontrolled hypertension > 180/110 mm Hg or gastroesophageal reflux disease

M1057 Aspirin or another antiplatelet therapy not used, reason not given

M1058 Patient was a permanent nursing home resident at any time during the performance period

M1059 Patient was in hospice or receiving palliative care at any time during the performance period

M1060 Patient died prior to the end of the performance period

M1067 Hospice services for patient provided any time during the measurement period

M1068 Adults who are not ambulatory

M1069 Patient screened for future fall risk

Special Coverage Instructions | Noncovered by Medicare | Carrier Discretion | ☑ Quantity Alert | ● New Code | ○ Recycled/Reinstated | ▲ Revised Code

144 — M Codes | A Age Edit | M Maternity Edit | ♀ Female Only | ♂ Male Only | A-Y OPPS Status Indicators | © 2022 Optum, Inc.

2023 HCPCS Level II

Code	Description
M1070	Patient not screened for future fall risk, reason not given
~~M1071~~	~~Patient had any additional spine procedures performed on the same date as the lumbar discectomy/laminotomy~~
M1106	The start of an episode of care documented in the medical record
M1107	Documentation stating patient has a diagnosis of a degenerative neurological condition such as ALS, MS, or Parkinson's diagnosed at any time before or during the episode of care
M1108	Ongoing care not clinically indicated because the patient needed a home program only, referral to another provider or facility, or consultation only, as documented in the medical record
M1109	Ongoing care not medically possible because the patient was discharged early due to specific medical events, documented in the medical record, such as the patient became hospitalized or scheduled for surgery
M1110	Ongoing care not possible because the patient self-discharged early (e.g., financial or insurance reasons, transportation problems, or reason unknown)
M1111	The start of an episode of care documented in the medical record
M1112	Documentation stating patient has a diagnosis of a degenerative neurological condition such as ALS, MS, or Parkinson's diagnosed at any time before or during the episode of care
M1113	Ongoing care not clinically indicated because the patient needed a home program only, referral to another provider or facility, or consultation only, as documented in the medical record
M1114	Ongoing care not medically possible because the patient was discharged early due to specific medical events, documented in the medical record, such as the patient became hospitalized or scheduled for surgery
M1115	Ongoing care not possible because the patient self-discharged early (e.g., financial or insurance reasons, transportation problems, or reason unknown)
M1116	The start of an episode of care documented in the medical record
M1117	Documentation stating patient has a diagnosis of a degenerative neurological condition such as ALS, MS, or Parkinson's diagnosed at any time before or during the episode of care
M1118	Ongoing care not clinically indicated because the patient needed a home program only, referral to another provider or facility, or consultation only, as documented in the medical record
M1119	Ongoing care not medically possible because the patient was discharged early due to specific medical events, documented in the medical record, such as the patient became hospitalized or scheduled for surgery
M1120	Ongoing care not possible because the patient self-discharged early (e.g., financial or insurance reasons, transportation problems, or reason unknown)
M1121	The start of an episode of care documented in the medical record
M1122	Documentation stating patient has a diagnosis of a degenerative neurological condition such as ALS, MS, or Parkinson's diagnosed at any time before or during the episode of care
M1123	Ongoing care not clinically indicated because the patient needed a home program only, referral to another provider or facility, or consultation only, as documented in the medical record
M1124	Ongoing care not medically possible because the patient was discharged early due to specific medical events, documented in the medical record, such as the patient became hospitalized or scheduled for surgery
M1125	Ongoing care not possible because the patient self-discharged early (e.g., financial or insurance reasons, transportation problems, or reason unknown)
M1126	The start of an episode of care documented in the medical record
M1127	Documentation stating patient has a diagnosis of a degenerative neurological condition such as ALS, MS, or Parkinson's diagnosed at any time before or during the episode of care
M1128	Ongoing care not clinically indicated because the patient needed a home program only, referral to another provider or facility, or consultation only, as documented in the medical record
M1129	Ongoing care not medically possible because the patient was discharged early due to specific medical events, documented in the medical record, such as the patient became hospitalized or scheduled for surgery
M1130	Ongoing care not possible because the patient self-discharged early (e.g., financial or insurance reasons, transportation problems, or reason unknown)
M1131	Documentation stating patient has a diagnosis of a degenerative neurological condition such as ALS, MS, or Parkinson's diagnosed at any time before or during the episode of care
M1132	Ongoing care not clinically indicated because the patient needed a home program only, referral to another provider or facility, or consultation only, as documented in the medical record
M1133	Ongoing care not medically possible because the patient was discharged early due to specific medical events, documented in the medical record, such as the patient became hospitalized or scheduled for surgery
M1134	Ongoing care not possible because the patient self-discharged early (e.g., financial or insurance reasons, transportation problems, or reason unknown)
M1135	The start of an episode of care documented in the medical record
M1141	Functional status was not measured by the Oxford Knee Score (OKS) or the knee injury and osteoarthritis outcome score joint replacement (KOOS, JR.) at one year (9 to 15 months) postoperatively
M1142	Emergent cases
M1143	Initiated episode of rehabilitation therapy, medical, or chiropractic care for neck impairment
~~M1145~~	~~Most favored nation (MFN) model drug add-on amount, per dose; (do not bill with line items that have the JW modifier)~~
M1146	Ongoing care not clinically indicated because the patient needed a home program only, referral to another provider or facility, or consultation only, as documented in the medical record
M1147	Ongoing care not medically possible because the patient was discharged early due to specific medical events, documented in the medical record, such as the patient became hospitalized or scheduled for surgery
M1148	Ongoing care not possible because the patient self-discharged early (e.g., financial or insurance reasons, transportation problems, or reason unknown)
M1149	Patient unable to complete the neck FS PROM at initial evaluation and/or discharge due to blindness, illiteracy, severe mental incapacity or language incompatibility, and an adequate proxy is not available
● M1150	Left ventricular ejection fraction (LVEF) less than or equal to 40% or documentation of moderately or severely depressed left ventricular systolic function
● M1151	Patients with a history of heart transplant or with a left ventricular assist device (LVAD)

Medical Services

M1152 — M1195

- **M1152** Patients with a history of heart transplant or with a left ventricular assist device (LVAD)
- **M1153** Patient with diagnosis of osteoporosis on date of encounter
- **M1154** Hospice services provided to patient any time during the measurement period
- **M1155** Patient had anaphylaxis due to the pneumococcal vaccine any time during or before the measurement period
- **M1156** Patient received active chemotherapy any time during the measurement period
- **M1157** Patient received bone marrow transplant any time during the measurement period
- **M1158** Patient had history of immunocompromising conditions prior to or during the measurement period
- **M1159** Hospice services provided to patient any time during the measurement period
- **M1160** Patient had anaphylaxis due to the meningococcal vaccine any time on or before the patient's 13th birthday
- **M1161** Patient had anaphylaxis due to the tetanus, diphtheria or pertussis vaccine any time on or before the patient's 13th birthday
- **M1162** Patient had encephalitis due to the tetanus, diphtheria or pertussis vaccine any time on or before the patient's 13th birthday
- **M1163** Patient had anaphylaxis due to the HPV vaccine any time on or before the patient's 13th birthday
- **M1164** Patients with dementia any time during the patient's history through the end of the measurement period
- **M1165** Patients who use hospice services any time during the measurement period
- **M1166** Pathology report for tissue specimens produced from wide local excisions or re-excisions
- **M1167** In hospice or using hospice services during the measurement period
- **M1168** Patient received an influenza vaccine on or between July 1 of the year prior to the measurement period and June 30 of the measurement period
- **M1169** Documentation of medical reason(s) for not administering influenza vaccine (e.g., prior anaphylaxis due to the influenza vaccine)
- **M1170** Patient did not receive an influenza vaccine on or between July 1 of the year prior to the measurement period and June 30 of the measurement period
- **M1171** Patient received at least 1 TD vaccine or 1 TDaP vaccine between 9 years prior to the encounter and the end of the measurement period
- **M1172** Documentation of medical reason(s) for not administering TD or TDaP vaccine (e.g., prior anaphylaxis due to the TD or TDaP vaccine or history of encephalopathy within 7 days after a previous dose of a TD-containing vaccine)
- **M1173** Patient did not receive at least 1 TD vaccine or 1 TDaP vaccine between 9 years prior to the encounter and the end of the measurement period
- **M1174** Patient received at least 1 dose of the herpes zoster live vaccine or 2 doses of the herpes zoster recombinant vaccine (at least 28 days apart) anytime on or after the patient's 50th birthday before or during the measurement period
- **M1175** Documentation of medical reason(s) for not administering zoster vaccine (e.g., prior anaphylaxis due to the zoster vaccine)
- **M1176** Patient did not receive at least one dose of the herpes zoster live vaccine or two doses of the herpes zoster recombinant vaccine (at least 28 days apart) anytime on or after the patient's 50th birthday before or during the measurement period
- **M1177** Patient received any pneumococcal conjugate or polysaccharide vaccine on or after their 60th birthday and before the end of the measurement period
- **M1178** Documentation of medical reason(s) for not administering pneumococcal vaccine (e.g., prior anaphylaxis due to the pneumococcal vaccine)
- **M1179** Patient did not receive any pneumococcal conjugate or polysaccharide vaccine, on or after their 60th birthday and before or during measurement period
- **M1180** Patients on immune checkpoint inhibitor therapy
- **M1181** Grade 2 or above diarrhea and/or Grade 2 or above colitis
- **M1182** Patients not eligible due to pre-existing inflammatory bowel disease (IBD) (e.g., ulcerative colitis, Crohn's disease)
- **M1183** Documentation of immune checkpoint inhibitor therapy held and corticosteroids or immunosuppressants prescribed or administered
- **M1184** Documentation of medical reason(s) for not prescribing or administering corticosteroid or immunosuppressant treatment (e.g., allergy, intolerance, infectious etiology, pancreatic insufficiency, hyperthyroidism, prior bowel surgical interventions, celiac disease, receiving other medication, awaiting diagnostic workup results for alternative etiologies, other medical reasons/contraindication)
- **M1185** Documentation of immune checkpoint inhibitor therapy not held and/or corticosteroids or immunosuppressants prescribed or administered was not performed, reason not given
- **M1186** Patients who have an order for or are receiving hospice or palliative care
- **M1187** Patients with a diagnosis of end stage renal disease (ESRD)
- **M1188** Patients with a diagnosis of chronic kidney disease (CKD) Stage 5
- **M1189** Documentation of a kidney health evaluation defined by an estimated glomerular filtration rate (EGFR) and urine albumin-creatinine ratio (UACR) performed
- **M1190** Documentation of a kidney health evaluation was not performed or defined by an estimated glomerular filtration rate (EGFR) and urine albumin-creatinine ratio (UACR)
- **M1191** Hospice services provided to patient any time during the measurement period
- **M1192** Patients with an existing diagnosis of squamous cell carcinoma of the esophagus
- **M1193** Surgical pathology reports that contain impression or conclusion of or recommendation for testing of MMR by immunohistochemistry, MSI by DNA-based testing status, or both
- **M1194** Documentation of medical reason(s) surgical pathology reports did not contain impression or conclusion of or recommendation for testing of MMR by immunohistochemistry, MSI by DNA-based testing status, or both tests were not included (e.g., patient will not be treated with checkpoint inhibitor therapy, no residual carcinoma is present in the sample [tissue exhausted or status post neoadjuvant treatment], insufficient tumor for testing)
- **M1195** Surgical pathology reports that do not contain impression or conclusion of or recommendation for testing of MMR by immunohistochemistry, MSI by DNA-based testing status, or both, reason not given

2023 HCPCS Level II   M1210

- **M1196** Initial (index visit) numeric rating scale (NRS), visual rating scale (VRS), or ItchyQuant assessment score of greater than or equal to 4
- **M1197** Itch severity assessment score is reduced by 2 or more points from the initial (index) assessment score to the follow-up visit score
- **M1198** Itch severity assessment score was not reduced by at least 2 points from initial (index) score to the follow-up visit score or assessment was not completed during the follow-up encounter
- **M1199** Patients receiving RRT
- **M1200** Ace inhibitor (ACE-I) or ARB therapy prescribed during the measurement period
- **M1201** Documentation of medical reason(s) for not prescribing ACE inhibitor (ACE-I) or ARB therapy during the measurement period (e.g., pregnancy, history of angioedema to ACE-I, other allergy to ACE-I and ARB, hyperkalemia or history of hyperkalemia while on ACE-I or ARB therapy, acute kidney injury due to ACE-I or ARB therapy), other medical reasons)
- **M1202** Documentation of patient reason(s) for not prescribing ACE inhibitor or ARB therapy during the measurement period, (e.g., patient declined, other patient reasons)
- **M1203** Ace inhibitor or ARB therapy not prescribed during the measurement period, reason not given
- **M1204** Initial (index visit) numeric rating scale (NRS), visual rating scale (VRS), or ItchyQuant assessment score of greater than or equal to 4
- **M1205** Itch severity assessment score is reduced by 2 or more points from the initial (index) assessment score to the follow-up visit score
- **M1206** Itch severity assessment score was not reduced by at least 2 points from initial (index) score to the follow-up visit score or assessment was not completed during the follow-up encounter
- **M1207** Number of patients screened for food insecurity, housing instability, transportation needs, utility difficulties, and interpersonal safety
- **M1208** Number of patients not screened for food insecurity, housing instability, transportation needs, utility difficulties, and interpersonal safety
- **M1209** At least two orders for high-risk medications from the same drug class, (Table 4), not ordered
- **M1210** At least two orders for high-risk medications from the same drug class, (Table 4), not ordered

Pathology and Laboratory Services P2028-P9615

P codes include chemistry, toxicology, and microbiology tests, screening Papanicolaou procedures, and various blood products.

Chemistry and Toxicology Tests

P2028 Cephalin floculation, blood [A]
Code with caution: This test is considered obsolete. Submit documentation.

P2029 Congo red, blood [A]
Code with caution: This test is considered obsolete. Submit documentation.

P2031 Hair analysis (excluding arsenic) [E1]

P2033 Thymol turbidity, blood [A]
Code with caution: This test is considered obsolete. Submit documentation.

P2038 Mucoprotein, blood (seromucoid) (medical necessity procedure) [A]
Code with caution: This test is considered obsolete. Submit documentation.

Pathology Screening Tests

P3000 Screening Papanicolaou smear, cervical or vaginal, up to three smears, by technician under physician supervision [A] ♀ [A]
One Pap test is covered by Medicare every two years, unless the physician suspects cervical abnormalities and shortens the interval. See also G0123-G0124.
CMS: 100-02,15,280.4; 100-03,210.2.1; 100-04,18,10.1.2; 100-04,18,30.2.1; 100-04,18,30.5; 100-04,18,30.6

P3001 Screening Papanicolaou smear, cervical or vaginal, up to three smears, requiring interpretation by physician [A] ♀ [B] ○
One Pap test is covered by Medicare every two years, unless the physician suspects cervical abnormalities and shortens the interval. See also G0123-G0124.
CMS: 100-02,15,280.4; 100-03,210.2.1; 100-04,18,10.1.2; 100-04,18,30.2.1; 100-04,18,30.5; 100-04,18,30.6

Microbiology Tests

P7001 Culture, bacterial, urine; quantitative, sensitivity study [E1]

Miscellaneous

P9010 Blood (whole), for transfusion, per unit [R] ☑
CMS: 100-01,3,20.5; 100-01,3,20.5.2; 100-01,3,20.5.3; 100-02,1,10; 100-04,3,40.2.2

P9011 Blood, split unit [R] ☑
CMS: 100-01,3,20.5; 100-01,3,20.5.2; 100-01,3,20.5.3; 100-02,1,10; 100-04,3,40.2.2; 100-04,4,231.4

P9012 Cryoprecipitate, each unit [R] ☑
CMS: 100-02,1,10; 100-04,3,40.2.2

P9016 Red blood cells, leukocytes reduced, each unit [R] ☑
CMS: 100-02,1,10; 100-04,3,40.2.2

P9017 Fresh frozen plasma (single donor), frozen within 8 hours of collection, each unit [R] ☑
CMS: 100-02,1,10; 100-04,3,40.2.2

P9019 Platelets, each unit [R] ☑
CMS: 100-02,1,10; 100-04,3,40.2.2

P9020 Platelet rich plasma, each unit [R] ☑
CMS: 100-04,3,40.2.2

P9021 Red blood cells, each unit [R] ☑
CMS: 100-01,3,20.5; 100-01,3,20.5.2; 100-01,3,20.5.3; 100-02,1,10; 100-04,3,40.2.2

P9022 Red blood cells, washed, each unit [R] ☑
CMS: 100-01,3,20.5; 100-01,3,20.5.2; 100-01,3,20.5.3; 100-02,1,10; 100-04,3,40.2.2

P9023 Plasma, pooled multiple donor, solvent/detergent treated, frozen, each unit [R] ☑
CMS: 100-02,1,10; 100-04,3,40.2.2

P9025 Plasma, cryoprecipitate reduced, pathogen reduced, each unit
AHA: 4Q,21

P9026 Cryoprecipitated fibrinogen complex, pathogen reduced, each unit
AHA: 4Q,21

P9031 Platelets, leukocytes reduced, each unit [R] ☑
CMS: 100-02,1,10; 100-04,3,40.2.2

P9032 Platelets, irradiated, each unit [R] ☑
CMS: 100-02,1,10; 100-04,3,40.2.2

P9033 Platelets, leukocytes reduced, irradiated, each unit [R] ☑
CMS: 100-02,1,10; 100-04,3,40.2.2

P9034 Platelets, pheresis, each unit [R] ☑
CMS: 100-02,1,10; 100-04,3,40.2.2

P9035 Platelets, pheresis, leukocytes reduced, each unit [R] ☑
CMS: 100-02,1,10; 100-04,3,40.2.2

P9036 Platelets, pheresis, irradiated, each unit [R] ☑
CMS: 100-02,1,10; 100-04,3,40.2.2

P9037 Platelets, pheresis, leukocytes reduced, irradiated, each unit [R] ☑
CMS: 100-02,1,10; 100-04,3,40.2.2

P9038 Red blood cells, irradiated, each unit [R] ☑
CMS: 100-01,3,20.5; 100-01,3,20.5.2; 100-01,3,20.5.3; 100-02,1,10; 100-04,3,40.2.2

P9039 Red blood cells, deglycerolized, each unit [R] ☑
CMS: 100-02,1,10; 100-04,3,40.2.2

P9040 Red blood cells, leukocytes reduced, irradiated, each unit [R] ☑
CMS: 100-02,1,10; 100-04,3,40.2.2

P9041 Infusion, albumin (human), 5%, 50 ml [K] [K2] ☑
CMS: 100-02,1,10; 100-04,3,40.2.2

P9043 Infusion, plasma protein fraction (human), 5%, 50 ml [R] ☑
CMS: 100-02,1,10; 100-04,3,40.2.2

P9044 Plasma, cryoprecipitate reduced, each unit [R] ☑
CMS: 100-02,1,10; 100-04,3,40.2.2

P9045 Infusion, albumin (human), 5%, 250 ml [K] [K2] ☑
CMS: 100-02,1,10; 100-04,3,40.2.2

P9046 Infusion, albumin (human), 25%, 20 ml [K] [K2] ☑
CMS: 100-02,1,10; 100-04,3,40.2.2

P9047 Infusion, albumin (human), 25%, 50 ml [K] [K2] ☑
CMS: 100-02,1,10; 100-04,3,40.2.2

P9048 Infusion, plasma protein fraction (human), 5%, 250 ml [R] ☑
CMS: 100-02,1,10; 100-04,3,40.2.2

P9050 Granulocytes, pheresis, each unit [E1] ☑
CMS: 100-02,1,10; 100-03,110.5; 100-04,3,40.2.2

P9051 Whole blood or red blood cells, leukocytes reduced, CMV-negative, each unit [R] ☑
CMS: 100-02,1,10; 100-04,3,40.2.2

P9052 Platelets, HLA-matched leukocytes reduced, apheresis/pheresis, each unit [R] ☑
CMS: 100-02,1,10; 100-04,3,40.2.2

P9053 Platelets, pheresis, leukocytes reduced, CMV-negative, irradiated, each unit [R] ☑
CMS: 100-02,1,10; 100-04,3,40.2.2

P9054 Whole blood or red blood cells, leukocytes reduced, frozen, deglycerol, washed, each unit [R] ☑
CMS: 100-02,1,10; 100-04,3,40.2.2

P9055 Platelets, leukocytes reduced, CMV-negative, apheresis/pheresis, each unit [R] [✓]
CMS: 100-02,1,10; 100-04,3,40.2.2

P9056 Whole blood, leukocytes reduced, irradiated, each unit [R] [✓]
CMS: 100-02,1,10; 100-04,3,40.2.2

P9057 Red blood cells, frozen/deglycerolized/washed, leukocytes reduced, irradiated, each unit [R] [✓]
CMS: 100-02,1,10; 100-04,3,40.2.2

P9058 Red blood cells, leukocytes reduced, CMV-negative, irradiated, each unit [R] [✓]
CMS: 100-02,1,10; 100-04,3,40.2.2

P9059 Fresh frozen plasma between 8-24 hours of collection, each unit [R] [✓]
CMS: 100-02,1,10; 100-04,3,40.2.2

P9060 Fresh frozen plasma, donor retested, each unit [R] [✓]
CMS: 100-02,1,10; 100-04,3,40.2.2

P9070 Plasma, pooled multiple donor, pathogen reduced, frozen, each unit [R]

P9071 Plasma (single donor), pathogen reduced, frozen, each unit [R]

P9073 Platelets, pheresis, pathogen-reduced, each unit [R]
AHA: 1Q,18

P9099 Blood component or product not otherwise classified

P9100 Pathogen(s) test for platelets [S]
AHA: 1Q,18

P9603 Travel allowance, one way in connection with medically necessary laboratory specimen collection drawn from homebound or nursing homebound patient; prorated miles actually travelled [A] [✓]
CMS: 100-04,16,60; 100-04,16,60.2

P9604 Travel allowance, one way in connection with medically necessary laboratory specimen collection drawn from homebound or nursing homebound patient; prorated trip charge [A] [✓]
CMS: 100-04,16,60; 100-04,16,60.2

P9612 Catheterization for collection of specimen, single patient, all places of service [A]
CMS: 100-04,16,60

P9615 Catheterization for collection of specimen(s) (multiple patients) [N]
CMS: 100-04,16,60; 100-04,16,60.1.4

Q Codes (Temporary) Q0035-Q9992

Temporary Q codes are used to pay health care providers for supplies, drugs, and biologicals to which no permanent code has been assigned.

Q0035 Cardiokymography

Covered only in conjunction with electrocardiographic stress testing in male patients with atypical angina or nonischemic chest pain, or female patients with angina.

Q0081 Infusion therapy, using other than chemotherapeutic drugs, per visit

Q0083 Chemotherapy administration by other than infusion technique only (e.g., subcutaneous, intramuscular, push), per visit

Q0084 Chemotherapy administration by infusion technique only, per visit

Q0085 Chemotherapy administration by both infusion technique and other technique(s) (e.g. subcutaneous, intramuscular, push), per visit

Q0091 Screening Papanicolaou smear; obtaining, preparing and conveyance of cervical or vaginal smear to laboratory

One pap test is covered by Medicare every two years for low risk patients and every one year for high risk patients. Q0091 can be reported with an E/M code when a separately identifiable E/M service is provided.

CMS: 100-02,13,220; 100-02,13,220.1; 100-02,13,220.3; 100-02,15,280.4; 100-03,210.2.1; 100-04,18,10.1.2; 100-04,18,30.2.1; 100-04,18,30.5; 100-04,18,30.6; 1004-04,13,220.1

Q0092 Set-up portable x-ray equipment
CMS: 100-04,13,90.4

Q0111 Wet mounts, including preparations of vaginal, cervical or skin specimens

Q0112 All potassium hydroxide (KOH) preparations

Q0113 Pinworm examinations

Q0114 Fern test

Q0115 Postcoital direct, qualitative examinations of vaginal or cervical mucous

Q0138 Injection, ferumoxytol, for treatment of iron deficiency anemia, 1 mg (non-ESRD use)
Use this code for Feraheme.

Q0139 Injection, ferumoxytol, for treatment of iron deficiency anemia, 1 mg (for ESRD on dialysis)
Use this code for Feraheme.

Q0144 Azithromycin dihydrate, oral, capsules/powder, 1 g
Use this code for Zithromax, Zithromax Z-PAK.

Q0161 Chlorpromazine HCl, 5 mg, oral, FDA-approved prescription antiemetic, for use as a complete therapeutic substitute for an IV antiemetic at the time of chemotherapy treatment, not to exceed a 48-hour dosage regimen
CMS: 100-02,15,50.5.4; 100-03,110.18; 100-04,17,80.2.1

Q0162 Ondansetron 1 mg, oral, FDA-approved prescription antiemetic, for use as a complete therapeutic substitute for an IV antiemetic at the time of chemotherapy treatment, not to exceed a 48-hour dosage regimen
Use this code for Zofran, Zuplenz.
CMS: 100-02,15,50.5.4; 100-03,110.18; 100-04,17,80.2.1

Q0163 Diphenhydramine HCl, 50 mg, oral, FDA-approved prescription antiemetic, for use as a complete therapeutic substitute for an IV antiemetic at time of chemotherapy treatment not to exceed a 48-hour dosage regimen

See also J1200. Medicare covers at the time of chemotherapy if regimen doesn't exceed 48 hours. Submit on the same claim as the chemotherapy. Use this code for Truxadryl.
CMS: 100-02,15,50.5.4; 100-03,110.18; 100-04,17,80.2.1
AHA: 4Q,19

Q0164 Prochlorperazine maleate, 5 mg, oral, FDA-approved prescription antiemetic, for use as a complete therapeutic substitute for an IV antiemetic at the time of chemotherapy treatment, not to exceed a 48-hour dosage regimen

Medicare covers at the time of chemotherapy if regimen doesn't exceed 48 hours. Submit on the same claim as the chemotherapy. Use this code for Compazine.
CMS: 100-02,15,50.5.4; 100-03,110.18; 100-04,17,80.2.1

Q0166 Granisetron HCl, 1 mg, oral, FDA-approved prescription antiemetic, for use as a complete therapeutic substitute for an IV antiemetic at the time of chemotherapy treatment, not to exceed a 24-hour dosage regimen

Medicare covers at the time of chemotherapy if regimen doesn't exceed 48 hours. Submit on the same claim as the chemotherapy. Use this code for Kytril.
CMS: 100-02,15,50.5.4; 100-03,110.18; 100-04,17,80.2.1

Q0167 Dronabinol, 2.5 mg, oral, FDA-approved prescription antiemetic, for use as a complete therapeutic substitute for an IV antiemetic at the time of chemotherapy treatment, not to exceed a 48-hour dosage regimen

Medicare covers at the time of chemotherapy if regimen doesn't exceed 48 hours. Submit on the same claim as the chemotherapy. Use this code for Marinol.
CMS: 100-02,15,50.5.4; 100-03,110.18; 100-04,17,80.2.1

Q0169 Promethazine HCl, 12.5 mg, oral, FDA-approved prescription antiemetic, for use as a complete therapeutic substitute for an IV antiemetic at the time of chemotherapy treatment, not to exceed a 48-hour dosage regimen

Medicare covers at the time of chemotherapy if regimen doesn't exceed 48 hours. Submit on the same claim as the chemotherapy. Use this code for Phenergan, Amergan.
CMS: 100-02,15,50.5.4; 100-03,110.18; 100-04,17,80.2.1

Q0173 Trimethobenzamide HCl, 250 mg, oral, FDA-approved prescription antiemetic, for use as a complete therapeutic substitute for an IV antiemetic at the time of chemotherapy treatment, not to exceed a 48-hour dosage regimen

Medicare covers at the time of chemotherapy if regimen doesn't exceed 48 hours. Submit on the same claim as the chemotherapy. Use this code for Tebamide, T-Gen, Ticon, Tigan, Triban, Thimazide.
CMS: 100-02,15,50.5.4; 100-03,110.18; 100-04,17,80.2.1

Q0174 Thiethylperazine maleate, 10 mg, oral, FDA-approved prescription antiemetic, for use as a complete therapeutic substitute for an IV antiemetic at the time of chemotherapy treatment, not to exceed a 48-hour dosage regimen

Medicare covers at the time of chemotherapy if regimen doesn't exceed 48 hours. Submit on the same claim as the chemotherapy.
CMS: 100-02,15,50.5.4; 100-03,110.18; 100-04,17,80.2.1

Q0175 Perphenazine, 4 mg, oral, FDA-approved prescription antiemetic, for use as a complete therapeutic substitute for an IV antiemetic at the time of chemotherapy treatment, not to exceed a 48-hour dosage regimen

Medicare covers at the time of chemotherapy if regimen doesn't exceed 48 hours. Submit on the same claim as the chemotherapy. Use this code for Trilifon.
CMS: 100-02,15,50.5.4; 100-03,110.18; 100-04,17,80.2.1

2023 HCPCS Level II

Q Codes (Temporary)

Q0177 Hydroxyzine pamoate, 25 mg, oral, FDA-approved prescription antiemetic, for use as a complete therapeutic substitute for an IV antiemetic at the time of chemotherapy treatment, not to exceed a 48-hour dosage regimen [N] [N1] ☑
Medicare covers at the time of chemotherapy if regimen doesn't exceed 48 hours. Submit on the same claim as the chemotherapy. Use this code for Vistaril.
CMS: 100-02,15,50.5.4; 100-03,110.18; 100-04,17,80.2.1

Q0180 Dolasetron mesylate, 100 mg, oral, FDA-approved prescription antiemetic, for use as a complete therapeutic substitute for an IV antiemetic at the time of chemotherapy treatment, not to exceed a 24-hour dosage regimen [N] [N1] ☑
Medicare covers at the time of chemotherapy if regimen doesn't exceed 24 hours. Submit on the same claim as the chemotherapy. Use this code for Anzemet.
CMS: 100-02,15,50.5.4; 100-03,110.18; 100-04,17,80.2.1

Q0181 Unspecified oral dosage form, FDA-approved prescription antiemetic, for use as a complete therapeutic substitute for an IV antiemetic at the time of chemotherapy treatment, not to exceed a 48-hour dosage regimen [N] [N1] ☑
Medicare covers at the time of chemotherapy if regimen doesn't exceed 48-hours. Submit on the same claim as the chemotherapy.
CMS: 100-02,15,50.5.4; 100-03,110.18; 100-04,17,80.2.1
AHA: 4Q,19

Q0220 Injection, tixagevimab and cilgavimab, for the pre-exposure prophylaxis only, for certain adults and pediatric individuals (12 years of age and older weighing at least 40kg) with no known SARS-CoV-2 exposure, who either have moderate to severely compromised immune systems or for whom vaccination with any available COVID-19 vaccine is not recommended due to a history of severe adverse reaction to a COVID-19 vaccine(s) and/or COVID-19 vaccine component(s), 300 mg
Use this code for tixagevimab and cilgavimab (Evusheld) 300 mg administered as pre-exposure prophylaxis. Report also M0220 or M0221 for administration.

● **Q0221** Injection, tixagevimab and cilgavimab, for the pre-exposure prophylaxis only, for certain adults and pediatric individuals (12 years of age and older weighing at least 40kg) with no known SARS-CoV-2 exposure, who either have moderate to severely compromised immune systems or for whom vaccination with any available COVID-19 vaccine is not recommended due to a history of severe adverse reaction to a COVID-19 vaccine(s) and/or COVID-19 vaccine component(s), 600 mg
AHA: 2Q,22

● **Q0222** Injection, bebtelovimab, 175 mg
AHA: 2Q,22

Q0240 Injection, casirivimab and imdevimab, 600 mg [L1]
Use this code for casirivimab and imdevimab 600 mg administered as post exposure prophylaxis. Report also M0240 or M0241 for administration.
AHA: 4Q,21; 3Q,21

Q0243 Injection, casirivimab and imdevimab, 2400 mg [L1]
Use this code for Casirivimab and Imdevimab (REGN-COV2), Regeneron.
AHA: 1Q,21; 4Q,20

Q0244 Injection, casirivimab and imdevimab, 1200 mg [L1]
AHA: 4Q,21

Q0245 Injection, bamlanivimab and etesevimab, 2100 mg [L1]
Use this code for Eli Lilly's bamlanivimab (LY-CoV555) 700 mg and etesevimab (LY-CoV016) 1400 mg, administered together.
AHA: 1Q,21

Q0247 Injection, sotrovimab, 500 mg [L1]
AHA: 3Q,21

Q0249 Injection, tocilizumab, for hospitalized adults and pediatric patients (2 years of age and older) with COVID-19 who are receiving systemic corticosteroids and require supplemental oxygen, non-invasive or invasive mechanical ventilation, or extracorporeal membrane oxygenation (ECMO) only, 1 mg [L1]
AHA: 4Q,21

Q0477 Power module patient cable for use with electric or electric/pneumatic ventricular assist device, replacement only [A] &

Q0478 Power adapter for use with electric or electric/pneumatic ventricular assist device, vehicle type [A] &

Q0479 Power module for use with electric or electric/pneumatic ventricular assist device, replacement only [A] &

Q0480 Driver for use with pneumatic ventricular assist device, replacement only [A] &
CMS: 100-04,32,320.3.4

Q0481 Microprocessor control unit for use with electric ventricular assist device, replacement only [A] &
CMS: 100-04,32,320.3.4

Q0482 Microprocessor control unit for use with electric/pneumatic combination ventricular assist device, replacement only [A] &
CMS: 100-04,32,320.3.4

Q0483 Monitor/display module for use with electric ventricular assist device, replacement only [A] &
CMS: 100-04,32,320.3.4

Q0484 Monitor/display module for use with electric or electric/pneumatic ventricular assist device, replacement only [A] &
CMS: 100-04,32,320.3.4

Q0485 Monitor control cable for use with electric ventricular assist device, replacement only [A] &
CMS: 100-04,32,320.3.4

Q0486 Monitor control cable for use with electric/pneumatic ventricular assist device, replacement only [A] &
CMS: 100-04,32,320.3.4

Q0487 Leads (pneumatic/electrical) for use with any type electric/pneumatic ventricular assist device, replacement only [A] &
CMS: 100-04,32,320.3.4

Q0488 Power pack base for use with electric ventricular assist device, replacement only [A]
CMS: 100-04,32,320.3.4

Q0489 Power pack base for use with electric/pneumatic ventricular assist device, replacement only [A] &
CMS: 100-04,32,320.3.4

Q0490 Emergency power source for use with electric ventricular assist device, replacement only [A] &
CMS: 100-04,32,320.3.4

Q0491 Emergency power source for use with electric/pneumatic ventricular assist device, replacement only [A] &
CMS: 100-04,32,320.3.4

Q0492 Emergency power supply cable for use with electric ventricular assist device, replacement only [A] &
CMS: 100-04,32,320.3.4

Q0493 Emergency power supply cable for use with electric/pneumatic ventricular assist device, replacement only [A] &
CMS: 100-04,32,320.3.4

Q0494 Emergency hand pump for use with electric or electric/pneumatic ventricular assist device, replacement only [A] &
CMS: 100-04,32,320.3.4

Q Codes (Temporary)

Q0495 — Q2049

Code	Description
Q0495	Battery/power pack charger for use with electric or electric/pneumatic ventricular assist device, replacement only A ♿ **CMS:** 100-04,32,320.3.4
Q0496	Battery, other than lithium-ion, for use with electric or electric/pneumatic ventricular assist device, replacement only A ♿ **CMS:** 100-04,32,320.3.4
Q0497	Battery clips for use with electric or electric/pneumatic ventricular assist device, replacement only A ♿ **CMS:** 100-04,32,320.3.4
Q0498	Holster for use with electric or electric/pneumatic ventricular assist device, replacement only A ♿ **CMS:** 100-04,32,320.3.4
Q0499	Belt/vest/bag for use to carry external peripheral components of any type ventricular assist device, replacement only A ♿ **CMS:** 100-04,32,320.3.4
Q0500	Filters for use with electric or electric/pneumatic ventricular assist device, replacement only A ☑ ♿ The base unit for this code is for each filter. **CMS:** 100-04,32,320.3.4
Q0501	Shower cover for use with electric or electric/pneumatic ventricular assist device, replacement only A ♿ **CMS:** 100-04,32,320.3.4
Q0502	Mobility cart for pneumatic ventricular assist device, replacement only A ♿ **CMS:** 100-04,32,320.3.4
Q0503	Battery for pneumatic ventricular assist device, replacement only, each A ♿ **CMS:** 100-04,32,320.3.4
Q0504	Power adapter for pneumatic ventricular assist device, replacement only, vehicle type A ♿ **CMS:** 100-04,32,320.3.4
Q0506	Battery, lithium-ion, for use with electric or electric/pneumatic ventricular assist device, replacement only A ♿ **CMS:** 100-04,32,320.3.4
Q0507	Miscellaneous supply or accessory for use with an external ventricular assist device A **CMS:** 100-04,32,320.3.4
Q0508	Miscellaneous supply or accessory for use with an implanted ventricular assist device A **CMS:** 100-04,32,320.3.4
Q0509	Miscellaneous supply or accessory for use with any implanted ventricular assist device for which payment was not made under Medicare Part A A **CMS:** 100-04,32,320.3.4
Q0510	Pharmacy supply fee for initial immunosuppressive drug(s), first month following transplant B ☑
Q0511	Pharmacy supply fee for oral anticancer, oral antiemetic, or immunosuppressive drug(s); for the first prescription in a 30-day period B ☑
Q0512	Pharmacy supply fee for oral anticancer, oral antiemetic, or immunosuppressive drug(s); for a subsequent prescription in a 30-day period B ☑
Q0513	Pharmacy dispensing fee for inhalation drug(s); per 30 days B ☑
Q0514	Pharmacy dispensing fee for inhalation drug(s); per 90 days B ☑
Q0515	Injection, sermorelin acetate, 1 mcg E1 ☑
Q1004	New technology, intraocular lens, category 4 as defined in Federal Register notice E1
Q1005	New technology, intraocular lens, category 5 as defined in Federal Register notice E1
Q2004	Irrigation solution for treatment of bladder calculi, for example renacidin, per 500 ml N N1 ☑
Q2009	Injection, fosphenytoin, 50 mg phenytoin equivalent K N1 ☑ Use this code for Cerebyx.
Q2017	Injection, teniposide, 50 mg K K2 ☑ Use this code for Vumon.
Q2026	Injection, Radiesse, 0.1 ml E1 K2 ☑ **CMS:** 100-03,250.5; 100-04,32,260.1; 100-04,32,260.1.1; 100-04,32,260.2.1; 100-04,32,260.2.2
Q2028	Injection, sculptra, 0.5 mg E1 K2 ☑ **CMS:** 100-04,32,260.1.1; 100-04,32,260.2.2
Q2034	Influenza virus vaccine, split virus, for intramuscular use (Agriflu) L L1 ☑
Q2035	Influenza virus vaccine, split virus, when administered to individuals 3 years of age and older, for intramuscular use (AFLURIA) A L L1 ☑ **CMS:** 100-02,15,50.4.4.2
Q2036	Influenza virus vaccine, split virus, when administered to individuals 3 years of age and older, for intramuscular use (FLULAVAL) A L L1 ☑ **CMS:** 100-02,15,50.4.4.2
Q2037	Influenza virus vaccine, split virus, when administered to individuals 3 years of age and older, for intramuscular use (FLUVIRIN) A L L1 ☑ **CMS:** 100-02,15,50.4.4.2
Q2038	Influenza virus vaccine, split virus, when administered to individuals 3 years of age and older, for intramuscular use (Fluzone) A L L1 ☑ **CMS:** 100-02,15,50.4.4.2
Q2039	Influenza virus vaccine, not otherwise specified A L L1 ☑ **CMS:** 100-02,15,50.4.4.2 **AHA:** 4Q,17
Q2041	Axicabtagene ciloleucel, up to 200 million autologous anti-CD19 CAR positive T cells, including leukapheresis and dose preparation procedures, per therapeutic dose G Use this code for Yescarta. **CMS:** 100-04,32,400; 100-04,32,400.1; 100-04,32,400.2; 100-04,32,400.2.1; 100-04,32,400.2.2; 100-04,32,400.2.3; 100-04,32,400.2.4; 100-04,32,400.3; 100-04,32,400.4; 100-04,32,400.5; 100-04,32,66.2 **AHA:** 2Q,19; 2Q,18; 1Q,18
Q2042	Tisagenlecleucel, up to 600 million CAR-positive viable T cells, including leukapheresis and dose preparation procedures, per therapeutic dose Use this code for Kymriah. **CMS:** 100-04,32,400; 100-04,32,400.1; 100-04,32,400.2; 100-04,32,400.2.1; 100-04,32,400.2.2; 100-04,32,400.2.3; 100-04,32,400.2.4; 100-04,32,400.3; 100-04,32,400.4; 100-04,32,400.5; 100-04,32,66.2 **AHA:** 2Q,19; 1Q,19
Q2043	Sipuleucel-T, minimum of 50 million autologous CD54+ cells activated with PAP-GM-CSF, including leukapheresis and all other preparatory procedures, per infusion ♂ K K2 ☑ Use this code for PROVENGE. **CMS:** 100-03,1,110.22; 100-03,110.22; 100-04,32,280.1; 100-04,32,280.2; 100-04,32,280.4; 100-04,32,280.5
Q2049	Injection, doxorubicin HCl, liposomal, imported Lipodox, 10 mg K K2 ☑

Special Coverage Instructions | Noncovered by Medicare | Carrier Discretion | ☑ Quantity Alert ● New Code ○ Recycled/Reinstated ▲ Revised Code

152 — Q Codes (Temporary) A Age Edit M Maternity Edit ♀ Female Only ♂ Male Only A–Y OPPS Status Indicators © 2022 Optum, Inc.

Q2050 Injection, doxorubicin HCl, liposomal, not otherwise specified, 10 mg

Q2052 Services, supplies and accessories used in the home under the Medicare intravenous immune globulin (IVIG) demonstration

Q2053 Brexucabtagene autoleucel, up to 200 million autologous anti-CD19 CAR positive viable T cells, including leukapheresis and dose preparation procedures, per therapeutic dose
Use this code for Tecartus.
CMS: 100-04,32,400; 100-04,32,400.1; 100-04,32,400.2; 100-04,32,400.2.1; 100-04,32,400.2.2; 100-04,32,400.2.3; 100-04,32,400.2.4; 100-04,32,400.3; 100-04,32,400.4; 100-04,32,400.5
AHA: 1Q,21

Q2054 Lisocabtagene maraleucel, up to 110 million autologous anti-CD19 CAR-positive viable T cells, including leukapheresis and dose preparation procedures, per therapeutic dose
Use this code for Breyanzi.
CMS: 100-04,32,400.2.2; 100-04,32,400.2.3; 100-04,32,400.2.4; 100-04,32,400.3; 100-04,32,400.4
AHA: 4Q,21

Q2055 Idecabtagene vicleucel, up to 460 million autologous B-cell maturation antigen (BCMA) directed CAR-positive T cells, including leukapheresis and dose preparation procedures, per therapeutic dose
Use this code for Abecma.
CMS: 100-04,32,400.2.2; 100-04,32,400.2.3; 100-04,32,400.2.4; 100-04,32,400.3; 100-04,32,400.4
AHA: 1Q,22

● **Q2056** Ciltacabtagene autoleucel, up to 100 million autologous B-cell maturation antigen (BCMA) directed CAR-positive T cells, including leukapheresis and dose preparation procedures, per therapeutic dose
Use this code for Carvykti.

Q3001 Radioelements for brachytherapy, any type, each

Q3014 Telehealth originating site facility fee
CMS: 100-04,12,190.5; 100-04,12,190.6; 100-04,39,30.5

Q3027 Injection, interferon beta-1a, 1 mcg for intramuscular use
Use this code for Avonex.
CMS: 100-02,15,50.5

Q3028 Injection, interferon beta-1a, 1 mcg for subcutaneous use
Use this code for Rebif.
CMS: 100-02,15,50.5

Q3031 Collagen skin test

Q4001 Casting supplies, body cast adult, with or without head, plaster
CMS: 100-04,20,170

Q4002 Cast supplies, body cast adult, with or without head, fiberglass
CMS: 100-04,20,170

Q4003 Cast supplies, shoulder cast, adult (11 years +), plaster
CMS: 100-04,20,170

Q4004 Cast supplies, shoulder cast, adult (11 years +), fiberglass
CMS: 100-04,20,170

Q4005 Cast supplies, long arm cast, adult (11 years +), plaster
CMS: 100-04,20,170

Q4006 Cast supplies, long arm cast, adult (11 years +), fiberglass
CMS: 100-04,20,170

Q4007 Cast supplies, long arm cast, pediatric (0-10 years), plaster
CMS: 100-04,20,170

Q4008 Cast supplies, long arm cast, pediatric (0-10 years), fiberglass
CMS: 100-04,20,170

Q4009 Cast supplies, short arm cast, adult (11 years +), plaster
CMS: 100-04,20,170

Q4010 Cast supplies, short arm cast, adult (11 years +), fiberglass
CMS: 100-04,20,170

Q4011 Cast supplies, short arm cast, pediatric (0-10 years), plaster
CMS: 100-04,20,170

Q4012 Cast supplies, short arm cast, pediatric (0-10 years), fiberglass
CMS: 100-04,20,170

Q4013 Cast supplies, gauntlet cast (includes lower forearm and hand), adult (11 years +), plaster
CMS: 100-04,20,170

Q4014 Cast supplies, gauntlet cast (includes lower forearm and hand), adult (11 years +), fiberglass
CMS: 100-04,20,170

Q4015 Cast supplies, gauntlet cast (includes lower forearm and hand), pediatric (0-10 years), plaster
CMS: 100-04,20,170

Q4016 Cast supplies, gauntlet cast (includes lower forearm and hand), pediatric (0-10 years), fiberglass
CMS: 100-04,20,170

Q4017 Cast supplies, long arm splint, adult (11 years +), plaster
CMS: 100-04,20,170

Q4018 Cast supplies, long arm splint, adult (11 years +), fiberglass
CMS: 100-04,20,170

Q4019 Cast supplies, long arm splint, pediatric (0-10 years), plaster
CMS: 100-04,20,170

Q4020 Cast supplies, long arm splint, pediatric (0-10 years), fiberglass
CMS: 100-04,20,170

Q4021 Cast supplies, short arm splint, adult (11 years +), plaster
CMS: 100-04,20,170

Q4022 Cast supplies, short arm splint, adult (11 years +), fiberglass
CMS: 100-04,20,170

Q4023 Cast supplies, short arm splint, pediatric (0-10 years), plaster
CMS: 100-04,20,170

Q4024 Cast supplies, short arm splint, pediatric (0-10 years), fiberglass
CMS: 100-04,20,170

Q Codes (Temporary)

Q4025 — Q4114

Q4025 Cast supplies, hip spica (one or both legs), adult (11 years +), plaster
CMS: 100-04,20,170

Q4026 Cast supplies, hip spica (one or both legs), adult (11 years +), fiberglass
CMS: 100-04,20,170

Q4027 Cast supplies, hip spica (one or both legs), pediatric (0-10 years), plaster
CMS: 100-04,20,170

Q4028 Cast supplies, hip spica (one or both legs), pediatric (0-10 years), fiberglass
CMS: 100-04,20,170

Q4029 Cast supplies, long leg cast, adult (11 years +), plaster
CMS: 100-04,20,170

Q4030 Cast supplies, long leg cast, adult (11 years +), fiberglass
CMS: 100-04,20,170

Q4031 Cast supplies, long leg cast, pediatric (0-10 years), plaster
CMS: 100-04,20,170

Q4032 Cast supplies, long leg cast, pediatric (0-10 years), fiberglass
CMS: 100-04,20,170

Q4033 Cast supplies, long leg cylinder cast, adult (11 years +), plaster
CMS: 100-04,20,170

Q4034 Cast supplies, long leg cylinder cast, adult (11 years +), fiberglass
CMS: 100-04,20,170

Q4035 Cast supplies, long leg cylinder cast, pediatric (0-10 years), plaster
CMS: 100-04,20,170

Q4036 Cast supplies, long leg cylinder cast, pediatric (0-10 years), fiberglass
CMS: 100-04,20,170

Q4037 Cast supplies, short leg cast, adult (11 years +), plaster
CMS: 100-04,20,170

Q4038 Cast supplies, short leg cast, adult (11 years +), fiberglass
CMS: 100-04,20,170

Q4039 Cast supplies, short leg cast, pediatric (0-10 years), plaster
CMS: 100-04,20,170

Q4040 Cast supplies, short leg cast, pediatric (0-10 years), fiberglass
CMS: 100-04,20,170

Q4041 Cast supplies, long leg splint, adult (11 years +), plaster
CMS: 100-04,20,170

Q4042 Cast supplies, long leg splint, adult (11 years +), fiberglass
CMS: 100-04,20,170

Q4043 Cast supplies, long leg splint, pediatric (0-10 years), plaster
CMS: 100-04,20,170

Q4044 Cast supplies, long leg splint, pediatric (0-10 years), fiberglass
CMS: 100-04,20,170

Q4045 Cast supplies, short leg splint, adult (11 years +), plaster
CMS: 100-04,20,170

Q4046 Cast supplies, short leg splint, adult (11 years +), fiberglass
CMS: 100-04,20,170

Q4047 Cast supplies, short leg splint, pediatric (0-10 years), plaster
CMS: 100-04,20,170

Q4048 Cast supplies, short leg splint, pediatric (0-10 years), fiberglass
CMS: 100-04,20,170

Q4049 Finger splint, static
CMS: 100-04,20,170

Q4050 Cast supplies, for unlisted types and materials of casts
CMS: 100-04,20,170

Q4051 Splint supplies, miscellaneous (includes thermoplastics, strapping, fasteners, padding and other supplies)
CMS: 100-04,20,170

Q4074 Iloprost, inhalation solution, FDA-approved final product, noncompounded, administered through DME, unit dose form, up to 20 mcg
CMS: 100-02,15,50.5

Q4081 Injection, epoetin alfa, 100 units (for ESRD on dialysis)
CMS: 100-04,8,60.4; 100-04,8,60.4.1; 100-04,8,60.4.2; 100-04,8,60.4.4; 100-04,8,60.4.4.1; 100-04,8,60.4.4.2; 100-04,8,60.4.5.1

Q4082 Drug or biological, not otherwise classified, Part B drug competitive acquisition program (CAP)

Q4100 Skin substitute, not otherwise specified
CMS: 100-04,4,260.1; 100-04,4,260.1.1
AHA: 2Q,22; 2Q,18

Q4101 Apligraf, per sq cm
CMS: 100-04,4,260.1; 100-04,4,260.1.1

Q4102 Oasis wound matrix, per sq cm
CMS: 100-04,4,260.1; 100-04,4,260.1.1

Q4103 Oasis burn matrix, per sq cm
CMS: 100-04,4,260.1; 100-04,4,260.1.1

Q4104 Integra bilayer matrix wound dressing (BMWD), per sq cm
CMS: 100-04,4,260.1; 100-04,4,260.1.1

Q4105 Integra dermal regeneration template (DRT) or Integra Omnigraft dermal regeneration matrix, per sq cm
CMS: 100-04,4,260.1; 100-04,4,260.1.1

Q4106 Dermagraft, per sq cm
CMS: 100-04,4,260.1; 100-04,4,260.1.1

Q4107 GRAFTJACKET, per sq cm
CMS: 100-04,4,260.1; 100-04,4,260.1.1

Q4108 Integra matrix, per sq cm
CMS: 100-04,4,260.1; 100-04,4,260.1.1

Q4110 PriMatrix, per sq cm
CMS: 100-04,4,260.1; 100-04,4,260.1.1

Q4111 GammaGraft, per sq cm
CMS: 100-04,4,260.1; 100-04,4,260.1.1

Q4112 Cymetra, injectable, 1 cc

Q4113 GRAFTJACKET XPRESS, injectable, 1 cc

Q4114 Integra flowable wound matrix, injectable, 1 cc

2023 HCPCS Level II

Code	Description
Q4115	AlloSkin, per sq cm CMS: 100-04,4,260.1; 100-04,4,260.1.1
Q4116	AlloDerm, per sq cm CMS: 100-04,4,260.1; 100-04,4,260.1.1
Q4117	HYALOMATRIX, per sq cm CMS: 100-04,4,260.1; 100-04,4,260.1.1
Q4118	MatriStem micromatrix, 1 mg
Q4121	TheraSkin, per sq cm CMS: 100-04,4,260.1; 100-04,4,260.1.1
Q4122	DermACELL, DermACELL AWM or DermACELL AWM Porous, per sq cm CMS: 100-04,4,260.1; 100-04,4,260.1.1
Q4123	AlloSkin RT, per sq cm CMS: 100-04,4,260.1; 100-04,4,260.1.1
Q4124	OASIS ultra tri-layer wound matrix, per sq cm CMS: 100-04,4,260.1; 100-04,4,260.1.1
Q4125	ArthroFlex, per sq cm
Q4126	MemoDerm, DermaSpan, TranZgraft or InteguPly, per sq cm CMS: 100-04,4,260.1; 100-04,4,260.1.1
Q4127	Talymed, per sq cm CMS: 100-04,4,260.1; 100-04,4,260.1.1
▲ Q4128	FlexHD, or AllopatchHD, per sq cm CMS: 100-04,4,260.1; 100-04,4,260.1.1
Q4130	Strattice™, per sq cm
Q4132	Grafix Core and GrafixPL Core, per sq cm CMS: 100-04,4,260.1; 100-04,4,260.1.1
Q4133	Grafix PRIME, GrafixPL PRIME, Stravix and StravixPL, per sq cm CMS: 100-04,4,260.1; 100-04,4,260.1.1
Q4134	HMatrix, per sq cm CMS: 100-04,4,260.1; 100-04,4,260.1.1
Q4135	Mediskin, per sq cm CMS: 100-04,4,260.1; 100-04,4,260.1.1
Q4136	E-Z Derm, per sq cm CMS: 100-04,4,260.1; 100-04,4,260.1.1
Q4137	AmnioExcel, AmnioExcel Plus or BioDExcel, per sq cm CMS: 100-04,4,260.1; 100-04,4,260.1.1
Q4138	BioDFence DryFlex, per sq cm CMS: 100-04,4,260.1; 100-04,4,260.1.1
Q4139	AmnioMatrix or BioDMatrix, injectable, 1 cc
Q4140	BioDFence, per sq cm CMS: 100-04,4,260.1; 100-04,4,260.1.1
Q4141	AlloSkin AC, per sq cm CMS: 100-04,4,260.1; 100-04,4,260.1.1
Q4142	XCM biologic tissue matrix, per sq cm
Q4143	Repriza, per sq cm CMS: 100-04,4,260.1; 100-04,4,260.1.1
Q4145	EpiFix, injectable, 1 mg
Q4146	Tensix, per sq cm CMS: 100-04,4,260.1; 100-04,4,260.1.1
Q4147	Architect, Architect PX, or Architect FX, extracellular matrix, per sq cm CMS: 100-04,4,260.1; 100-04,4,260.1.1
Q4148	Neox Cord 1K, Neox Cord RT, or Clarix Cord 1K, per sq cm CMS: 100-04,4,260.1; 100-04,4,260.1.1
Q4149	Excellagen, 0.1 cc
Q4150	AlloWrap DS or dry, per sq cm CMS: 100-04,4,260.1; 100-04,4,260.1.1
Q4151	AmnioBand or Guardian, per sq cm CMS: 100-04,4,260.1; 100-04,4,260.1.1
Q4152	DermaPure, per sq cm CMS: 100-04,4,260.1; 100-04,4,260.1.1
Q4153	Dermavest and Plurivest, per sq cm CMS: 100-04,4,260.1; 100-04,4,260.1.1
Q4154	Biovance, per sq cm CMS: 100-04,4,260.1; 100-04,4,260.1.1
Q4155	Neox Flo or Clarix Flo 1 mg
Q4156	Neox 100 or Clarix 100, per sq cm CMS: 100-04,4,260.1; 100-04,4,260.1.1
Q4157	Revitalon, per sq cm CMS: 100-04,4,260.1; 100-04,4,260.1.1
Q4158	Kerecis Omega3, per sq cm CMS: 100-04,4,260.1; 100-04,4,260.1.1
Q4159	Affinity, per sq cm CMS: 100-04,4,260.1; 100-04,4,260.1.1
Q4160	Nushield, per sq cm CMS: 100-04,4,260.1; 100-04,4,260.1.1
Q4161	bio-ConneKt wound matrix, per sq cm CMS: 100-04,4,260.1; 100-04,4,260.1.1
Q4162	WoundEx Flow, BioSkin Flow, 0.5 cc
Q4163	WoundEx, BioSkin, per sq cm CMS: 100-04,4,260.1; 100-04,4,260.1.1
Q4164	Helicoll, per sq cm CMS: 100-04,4,260.1; 100-04,4,260.1.1
Q4165	Keramatrix or Kerasorb, per sq cm CMS: 100-04,4,260.1; 100-04,4,260.1.1
Q4166	Cytal, per sq cm CMS: 100-04,4,260.1; 100-04,4,260.1.1 AHA: 1Q,17
Q4167	Truskin, per sq cm CMS: 100-04,4,260.1; 100-04,4,260.1.1
Q4168	AmnioBand, 1 mg AHA: 1Q,17
Q4169	Artacent wound, per sq cm CMS: 100-04,4,260.1; 100-04,4,260.1.1 AHA: 1Q,17
Q4170	Cygnus, per sq cm CMS: 100-04,4,260.1; 100-04,4,260.1.1 AHA: 1Q,17
Q4171	Interfyl, 1 mg AHA: 1Q,17
Q4173	PalinGen or PalinGen XPlus, per sq cm CMS: 100-04,4,260.1; 100-04,4,260.1.1 AHA: 1Q,17
Q4174	PalinGen or ProMatrX, 0.36 mg per 0.25 cc AHA: 1Q,17

Q4175 Miroderm, per sq cm
CMS: 100-04,4,260.1; 100-04,4,260.1.1
AHA: 1Q,17

Q4176 Neopatch or therion, per square centimeter
CMS: 100-04,4,260.1; 100-04,4,260.1.1
AHA: 2Q,20; 1Q,18

Q4177 FlowerAmnioFlo, 0.1 cc
AHA: 1Q,18

Q4178 FlowerAmnioPatch, per sq cm
CMS: 100-04,4,260.1; 100-04,4,260.1.1
AHA: 1Q,18

Q4179 FlowerDerm, per sq cm
CMS: 100-04,4,260.1; 100-04,4,260.1.1
AHA: 1Q,18

Q4180 Revita, per sq cm
CMS: 100-04,4,260.1; 100-04,4,260.1.1
AHA: 1Q,18

Q4181 Amnio Wound, per sq cm
CMS: 100-04,4,260.1; 100-04,4,260.1.1
AHA: 1Q,18

Q4182 Transcyte, per sq cm
CMS: 100-04,4,260.1; 100-04,4,260.1.1
AHA: 1Q,18

Q4183 Surgigraft, per sq cm
CMS: 100-04,4,260.1; 100-04,4,260.1.1
AHA: 1Q,19

Q4184 Cellesta or Cellesta Duo, per sq cm
CMS: 100-04,4,260.1; 100-04,4,260.1.1
AHA: 1Q,19

Q4185 Cellesta Flowable Amnion (25 mg per cc); per 0.5 cc
CMS: 100-04,4,260.1; 100-04,4,260.1.1
AHA: 1Q,19

Q4186 Epifix, per sq cm
CMS: 100-04,4,260.1; 100-04,4,260.1.1
AHA: 1Q,19

Q4187 Epicord, per sq cm
CMS: 100-04,4,260.1; 100-04,4,260.1.1
AHA: 1Q,19

Q4188 AmnioArmor, per sq cm
CMS: 100-04,4,260.1; 100-04,4,260.1.1
AHA: 1Q,19

Q4189 Artacent AC, 1 mg
CMS: 100-04,4,260.1; 100-04,4,260.1.1
AHA: 1Q,19

Q4190 Artacent AC, per sq cm
CMS: 100-04,4,260.1; 100-04,4,260.1.1
AHA: 1Q,19

Q4191 Restorigin, per sq cm
CMS: 100-04,4,260.1; 100-04,4,260.1.1
AHA: 1Q,19

Q4192 Restorigin, 1 cc
CMS: 100-04,4,260.1; 100-04,4,260.1.1
AHA: 1Q,19

Q4193 Coll-e-Derm, per sq cm
CMS: 100-04,4,260.1; 100-04,4,260.1.1
AHA: 1Q,19

Q4194 Novachor, per sq cm
CMS: 100-04,4,260.1; 100-04,4,260.1.1
AHA: 1Q,19

Q4195 PuraPly, per sq cm
CMS: 100-04,4,260.1; 100-04,4,260.1.1
AHA: 1Q,19

Q4196 PuraPly AM, per sq cm
CMS: 100-04,4,260.1; 100-04,4,260.1.1
AHA: 1Q,19

Q4197 PuraPly XT, per sq cm
CMS: 100-04,4,260.1; 100-04,4,260.1.1
AHA: 1Q,19

Q4198 Genesis Amniotic Membrane, per sq cm
CMS: 100-04,4,260.1; 100-04,4,260.1.1
AHA: 1Q,19

Q4199 Cygnus matrix, per sq cm
AHA: 1Q,22

Q4200 SkinTE, per sq cm
CMS: 100-04,4,260.1; 100-04,4,260.1.1
AHA: 1Q,19

Q4201 Matrion, per sq cm
CMS: 100-04,4,260.1; 100-04,4,260.1.1
AHA: 1Q,19

Q4202 Keroxx (2.5 g/cc), 1 cc
CMS: 100-04,4,260.1; 100-04,4,260.1.1
AHA: 1Q,19

Q4203 Derma-Gide, per sq cm
CMS: 100-04,4,260.1; 100-04,4,260.1.1
AHA: 1Q,19

Q4204 XWRAP, per sq cm
CMS: 100-04,4,260.1; 100-04,4,260.1.1
AHA: 1Q,19

Q4205 Membrane Graft or Membrane Wrap, per sq cm
AHA: 4Q,19

Q4206 Fluid Flow or Fluid GF, 1 cc
AHA: 4Q,19

Q4208 Novafix, per sq cm
AHA: 4Q,19

Q4209 SurGraft, per sq cm
AHA: 4Q,19

Q4210 Axolotl Graft or Axolotl DualGraft, per sq cm
AHA: 4Q,19

Q4211 Amnion Bio or AxoBioMembrane, per sq cm
AHA: 4Q,19

Q4212 AlloGen, per cc
AHA: 4Q,19

Q4213 Ascent, 0.5 mg
AHA: 4Q,19

Q4214 Cellesta Cord, per sq cm
AHA: 4Q,19

Q4215 Axolotl Ambient or Axolotl Cryo, 0.1 mg
AHA: 4Q,19

Q4216 Artacent Cord, per sq cm
AHA: 4Q,19

Q4217 WoundFix, BioWound, WoundFix Plus, BioWound Plus, WoundFix Xplus or BioWound Xplus, per sq cm
AHA: 4Q,19

Q4218 SurgiCORD, per sq cm
AHA: 4Q,19

2023 HCPCS Level II   Q5010

Code	Description
Q4219	SurgiGRAFT-DUAL, per sq cm — N1 AHA: 4Q,19
Q4220	BellaCell HD or Surederm, per sq cm — N1 AHA: 4Q,19
Q4221	Amnio Wrap2, per sq cm — N1 AHA: 4Q,19
Q4222	ProgenaMatrix, per sq cm — N1 AHA: 4Q,19
● Q4224	Human Health Factor 10 Amniotic Patch (HHF10-P), per sq cm — N1 AHA: 2Q,22
● Q4225	AmnioBind, per sq cm — N1 AHA: 2Q,22
Q4226	MyOwn Skin, includes harvesting and preparation procedures, per sq cm — N1 AHA: 4Q,19
Q4227	AmnioCore™, per sq cm — N1 AHA: 2Q,20
Q4229	Cogenex Amniotic Membrane, per sq cm — N1 AHA: 2Q,20
Q4230	Cogenex Flowable Amnion, per 0.5 cc — N1 AHA: 2Q,20
Q4231	Corplex P, per cc — N1 AHA: 2Q,20
Q4232	Corplex, per sq cm — N1 AHA: 2Q,20
Q4233	SurFactor or NuDyn, per 0.5 cc — N1 AHA: 2Q,20
Q4234	XCellerate, per sq cm — N1 AHA: 2Q,20
Q4235	AMNIOREPAIR or AltiPly, per sq cm — N1 AHA: 2Q,20
○ Q4236	carePATCH, per sq cm
Q4237	Cryo-Cord, per sq cm — N1 AHA: 2Q,20
Q4238	Derm-Maxx, per sq cm — N1 AHA: 2Q,20
Q4239	Amnio-Maxx or Amnio-Maxx Lite, per sq cm — N1 AHA: 2Q,20
Q4240	CoreCyte, for topical use only, per 0.5 cc — N1 AHA: 2Q,20
Q4241	PolyCyte, for topical use only, per 0.5 cc — N1 AHA: 2Q,20
Q4242	AmnioCyte Plus, per 0.5 cc — N1 AHA: 2Q,20
Q4244	Procenta, per 200 mg — N1 AHA: 2Q,20
Q4245	AmnioText, per cc — N1 AHA: 2Q,20
Q4246	CoreText or ProText, per cc — N1 AHA: 2Q,20
Q4247	Amniotext patch, per sq cm — N1 AHA: 2Q,20
Q4248	Dermacyte Amniotic Membrane Allograft, per sq cm — N1 AHA: 2Q,20
Q4249	AMNIPLY, for topical use only, per sq cm — N1 AHA: 4Q,20
Q4250	AmnioAmp-MP, per sq cm — N1 AHA: 4Q,20
Q4251	Vim, per sq cm — N1 AHA: 4Q,21
Q4252	Vendaje, per sq cm — N1 AHA: 4Q,21
Q4253	Zenith Amniotic Membrane, per sq cm — N1 AHA: 4Q,21
Q4254	Novafix DL, per sq cm — N1 AHA: 4Q,20
Q4255	REGUaRD, for topical use only, per sq cm — N1 AHA: 4Q,20
● Q4256	MLG-Complete, per sq cm — N1 AHA: 2Q,22
● Q4257	Relese, per sq cm — N1 AHA: 2Q,22
● Q4258	Enverse, per sq cm — N1 AHA: 2Q,22
● Q4259	Celera Dual Layer or Celera Dual Membrane, per sq cm — N1 AHA: 3Q,22
● Q4260	Signature APatch, per sq cm — N1 AHA: 3Q,22
● Q4261	TAG, per sq cm — N1 AHA: 3Q,22
● Q4262	Dual Layer Impax Membrane, per sq cm
● Q4263	SurGraft TL, per sq cm
● Q4264	Cocoon Membrane, per sq cm
Q5001	Hospice or home health care provided in patient's home/residence — B CMS: 100-01,3,30.3; 100-04,10,40.2; 100-04,11,10; 100-04,11,130.1; 100-04,11,30.3
Q5002	Hospice or home health care provided in assisted living facility — B CMS: 100-01,3,30.3; 100-04,10,40.2; 100-04,11,10; 100-04,11,130.1; 100-04,11,30.3
Q5003	Hospice care provided in nursing long-term care facility (LTC) or nonskilled nursing facility (NF) — B CMS: 100-01,3,30.3; 100-04,11,10; 100-04,11,130.1; 100-04,11,30.3
Q5004	Hospice care provided in skilled nursing facility (SNF) — B CMS: 100-01,3,30.3; 100-04,11,10; 100-04,11,130.1; 100-04,11,30.3
Q5005	Hospice care provided in inpatient hospital — B CMS: 100-01,3,30.3; 100-04,11,10; 100-04,11,130.1; 100-04,11,30.3
Q5006	Hospice care provided in inpatient hospice facility — B CMS: 100-01,3,30.3; 100-04,11,10; 100-04,11,130.1; 100-04,11,30.3
Q5007	Hospice care provided in long-term care facility — B CMS: 100-01,3,30.3; 100-04,11,10; 100-04,11,130.1; 100-04,11,30.3
Q5008	Hospice care provided in inpatient psychiatric facility — B CMS: 100-01,3,30.3; 100-04,11,10; 100-04,11,130.1; 100-04,11,30.3
Q5009	Hospice or home health care provided in place not otherwise specified (NOS) — B CMS: 100-01,3,30.3; 100-04,10,40.2; 100-04,11,10; 100-04,11,130.1; 100-04,11,30.3
Q5010	Hospice home care provided in a hospice facility — B CMS: 100-01,3,30.3; 100-04,11,10; 100-04,11,130.1; 100-04,11,30.3

Special Coverage Instructions   Noncovered by Medicare   Carrier Discretion   ☑ Quantity Alert   ● New Code   ○ Recycled/Reinstated   ▲ Revised Code

© 2022 Optum, Inc.   A2-Z3 ASC Pmt   CMS: IOM   AHA: Coding Clinic   DMEPOS Paid   SNF Excluded   Q Codes (Temporary) — 157

Q5101   2023 HCPCS Level II

Q Codes (Temporary)

Q5101 Injection, filgrastim-sndz, biosimilar, (Zarxio), 1 mcg [G][K2]
AHA: 4Q,18; 2Q,18; 1Q,18; 2Q,16

Q5103 Injection, infliximab-dyyb, biosimilar, (Inflectra), 10 mg [G][K2]
AHA: 4Q,18; 2Q,18; 1Q,18

Q5104 Injection, infliximab-abda, biosimilar, (Renflexis), 10 mg [G][K2]
AHA: 4Q,18; 2Q,18; 1Q,18

Q5105 Injection, epoetin alfa-epbx, biosimilar, (Retacrit) (for ESRD on dialysis), 100 units [N1]
CMS: 100-04,8,60.4.2
AHA: 4Q,18; 2Q,18

Q5106 Injection, epoetin alfa-epbx, biosimilar, (Retacrit) (for non-ESRD use), 1000 units [K2]
AHA: 4Q,18; 2Q,18

Q5107 Injection, bevacizumab-awwb, biosimilar, (Mvasi), 10 mg [K2]
CMS: 100-04,4,260.1; 100-04,4,260.1.1
AHA: 4Q,19; 1Q,19; 4Q,18

Q5108 Injection, pegfilgrastim-jmdb, biosimilar, (Fulphila), 0.5 mg [K2]
CMS: 100-04,4,260.1; 100-04,4,260.1.1
AHA: 1Q,19; 4Q,18; 3Q,18

Q5109 Injection, infliximab-qbtx, biosimilar, (Ixifi), 10 mg [K2]
CMS: 100-04,4,260.1; 100-04,4,260.1.1
AHA: 1Q,19; 4Q,18

Q5110 Injection, filgrastim-aafi, biosimilar, (Nivestym), 1 mcg [K2]
CMS: 100-04,4,260.1; 100-04,4,260.1.1
AHA: 1Q,19; 4Q,18; 3Q,18

Q5111 Injection, pegfilgrastim-cbqv, biosimilar, (Udenyca), 0.5 mg [K2]
CMS: 100-04,4,260.1; 100-04,4,260.1.1
AHA: 1Q,19; 4Q,18

Q5112 Injection, trastuzumab-dttb, biosimilar, (Ontruzant), 10 mg [K2]
AHA: 3Q,19

Q5113 Injection, trastuzumab-pkrb, biosimilar, (Herzuma), 10 mg [K2]
AHA: 3Q,19

Q5114 Injection, Trastuzumab-dkst, biosimilar, (Ogivri), 10 mg [K2]
AHA: 3Q,19

Q5115 Injection, rituximab-abbs, biosimilar, (Truxima), 10 mg [K2]
AHA: 3Q,19

Q5116 Injection, trastuzumab-qyyp, biosimilar, (Trazimera), 10 mg [K2]
AHA: 4Q,19

Q5117 Injection, trastuzumab-anns, biosimilar, (Kanjinti), 10 mg [K2]
AHA: 4Q,19

Q5118 Injection, bevacizumab-bvzr, biosimilar, (Zirabev), 10 mg [K2]
AHA: 4Q,19

Q5119 Injection, rituximab-pvvr, biosimilar, (RUXIENCE), 10 mg [K2]
AHA: 2Q,20

Q5120 Injection, pegfilgrastim-bmez, biosimilar, (ZIEXTENZO), 0.5 mg [K2]
AHA: 2Q,20

Q5121 Injection, infliximab-axxq, biosimilar, (AVSOLA), 10 mg [K2]
AHA: 2Q,20

Q5122 Injection, pegfilgrastim-apgf, biosimilar, (Nyvepria), 0.5 mg [K2]
AHA: 1Q,21

Q5123 Injection, rituximab-arrx, biosimilar, (Riabni), 10 mg [K2]
AHA: 3Q,21

● **Q5124** Injection, ranibizumab-nuna, biosimilar, (Byooviz), 0.1 mg
AHA: 2Q,22

● **Q5125** Injection, filgrastim-ayow, biosimilar, (Releuko), 1 mcg [K2]

● **Q5126** Injection, bevacizumab-maly, biosimilar, (Alymsys), 10 mg

▲ **Q9001** Assessment by chaplain services

▲ **Q9002** Counseling, individual, by chaplain services

▲ **Q9003** Counseling, group, by chaplain services

Q9004 Department of Veterans Affairs Whole Health Partner Services

Q9950 Injection, sulfur hexafluoride lipid microspheres, per ml [N][N1]
Use this code for Lumason.
CMS: 100-03,1,220.2

Q9951 Low osmolar contrast material, 400 or greater mg/ml iodine concentration, per ml [N][N1][✓]
CMS: 100-03,1,220.2

Q9953 Injection, iron-based magnetic resonance contrast agent, per ml [N][N1][✓]
CMS: 100-03,1,220.2

Q9954 Oral magnetic resonance contrast agent, per 100 ml [N][N1][✓]
CMS: 100-03,1,220.2

Q9955 Injection, perflexane lipid microspheres, per ml [N][N1][✓]

Q9956 Injection, octafluoropropane microspheres, per ml [N][N1][✓]
Use this code for Optison.

Q9957 Injection, perflutren lipid microspheres, per ml [N][N1][✓]
Use this code for Definity.

Q9958 High osmolar contrast material, up to 149 mg/ml iodine concentration, per ml [N][N1][✓]
CMS: 100-03,1,220.2

Q9959 High osmolar contrast material, 150-199 mg/ml iodine concentration, per ml [N][N1][✓]
CMS: 100-03,1,220.2

Q9960 High osmolar contrast material, 200-249 mg/ml iodine concentration, per ml [N][N1][✓]
CMS: 100-03,1,220.2

Q9961 High osmolar contrast material, 250-299 mg/ml iodine concentration, per ml [N][N1][✓]
CMS: 100-03,1,220.2

Q9962 High osmolar contrast material, 300-349 mg/ml iodine concentration, per ml [N][N1][✓]
CMS: 100-03,1,220.2

Q9963 High osmolar contrast material, 350-399 mg/ml iodine concentration, per ml [N][N1][✓]
CMS: 100-03,1,220.2

Q9964 High osmolar contrast material, 400 or greater mg/ml iodine concentration, per ml [N][N1][✓]
CMS: 100-03,1,220.2

Q9965 Low osmolar contrast material, 100-199 mg/ml iodine concentration, per ml [N][N1][✓]
Use this code for Omnipaque 140, Omnipaque 180, Optiray 160, Optiray 140, ULTRAVIST 150.
CMS: 100-03,1,220.2

Q9966 Low osmolar contrast material, 200-299 mg/ml iodine concentration, per ml [N][N1][✓]
Use this code for Omnipaque 240, Optiray 240, ULTRAVIST 240.
CMS: 100-03,1,220.2

Special Coverage Instructions   Noncovered by Medicare   Carrier Discretion   ☑ Quantity Alert   ● New Code   ○ Recycled/Reinstated   ▲ Revised Code

158 — Q Codes (Temporary)   **A** Age Edit   **M** Maternity Edit   ♀ Female Only   ♂ Male Only   **A-Y** OPPS Status Indicators   © 2022 Optum, Inc.

Code	Description
Q9967	Low osmolar contrast material, 300-399 mg/ml iodine concentration, per ml N N1 ☑
	Use this code for Omnipaque 300, Omnipaque 350, Optiray, Optiray 300, Optiray 320, Oxilan 300, Oxilan 350, ULTRAVIST 300, ULTRAVIST 370.
	CMS: 100-03,1,220.2
Q9968	Injection, nonradioactive, noncontrast, visualization adjunct (e.g., methylene blue, isosulfan blue), 1 mg K K2 ☑
Q9969	Tc-99m from nonhighly enriched uranium source, full cost recovery add-on, per study dose K ☑
Q9982	Flutemetamol F18, diagnostic, per study dose, up to 5 mCi G N1
	Use this code for Vizamyl.
	CMS: 100-04,13,60.12; 100-04,32,60.12
Q9983	Florbetaben F18, diagnostic, per study dose, up to 8.1 mCi G N1
	Use this code for Neuraceq.
	CMS: 100-04,13,60.12; 100-04,32,60.12
Q9991	Injection, buprenorphine extended-release (Sublocade), less than or equal to 100 mg K2
	AHA: 2Q,18
Q9992	Injection, buprenorphine extended-release (Sublocade), greater than 100 mg K2
	AHA: 2Q,18

Diagnostic Radiology Services R0070-R0076

R codes are used for the transportation of portable x-ray and/or EKG equipment.

R0070 Transportation of portable x-ray equipment and personnel to home or nursing home, per trip to facility or location, one patient seen B ☑
Only a single, reasonable transportation charge is allowed for each trip the portable x-ray supplier makes to a location. When more than one patient is x-rayed at the same location, prorate the single allowable transport charge among all patients.
CMS: 100-04,13,90.3

R0075 Transportation of portable x-ray equipment and personnel to home or nursing home, per trip to facility or location, more than one patient seen B ☑
Only a single, reasonable transportation charge is allowed for each trip the portable x-ray supplier makes to a location. When more than one patient is x-rayed at the same location, prorate the single allowable transport charge among all patients.
CMS: 100-04,13,90.3

R0076 Transportation of portable EKG to facility or location, per patient B ☑
Only a single, reasonable transportation charge is allowed for each trip the portable EKG supplier makes to a location. When more than one patient is tested at the same location, prorate the single allowable transport charge among all patients.
CMS: 100-04,13,90.3; 100-04,6,20.3

Temporary National Codes (Non-Medicare) S0012-S9999

The S codes are used by the Blue Cross/Blue Shield Association (BCBSA) and the Health Insurance Association of America (HIAA) to report drugs, services, and supplies for which there are no national codes but for which codes are needed by the private sector to implement policies, programs, or claims processing. They are for the purpose of meeting the particular needs of the private sector. These codes are also used by the Medicaid program, but they are not payable by Medicare.

S0012 Butorphanol tartrate, nasal spray, 25 mg
Use this code for Stadol NS.

S0013 Esketamine, nasal spray, 1 mg
Use this code for Spravato.

S0014 Tacrine HCl, 10 mg
Use this code for Cognex.

S0017 Injection, aminocaproic acid, 5 g
Use this code for Amicar.

S0020 Injection, bupivicaine HCl, 30 ml
Use this code for Marcaine, Sensorcaine.

S0021 Injection, cefoperazone sodium, 1 g
Use this code for Cefobid.

S0023 Injection, cimetidine HCl, 300 mg
Use this code for Tagamet HCl.

S0028 Injection, famotidine, 20 mg
Use this code for Pepcid.

S0030 Injection, metronidazole, 500 mg
Use this code for Flagyl IV RTU.

S0032 Injection, nafcillin sodium, 2 g
Use this code for Nallpen, Unipen.

S0034 Injection, ofloxacin, 400 mg
Use this code for Floxin IV.

S0039 Injection, sulfamethoxazole and trimethoprim, 10 ml
Use this code for Bactrim IV, Septra IV, SMZ-TMP, Sulfutrim.

S0040 Injection, ticarcillin disodium and clavulanate potassium, 3.1 g
Use this code for Timentin.

S0073 Injection, aztreonam, 500 mg
Use this code for Azactam.

S0074 Injection, cefotetan disodium, 500 mg
Use this code for Cefotan.

S0077 Injection, clindamycin phosphate, 300 mg
Use this code for Cleocin Phosphate.

S0078 Injection, fosphenytoin sodium, 750 mg
Use this code for Cerebryx.

S0080 Injection, pentamidine isethionate, 300 mg
Use this code for NebuPent, Pentam 300, Pentacarinat. See also code J2545.

S0081 Injection, piperacillin sodium, 500 mg
Use this code for Pipracil.

S0088 Imatinib, 100 mg
Use this code for Gleevec.

S0090 Sildenafil citrate, 25 mg
Use this code for Viagra.

S0091 Granisetron HCl, 1 mg (for circumstances falling under the Medicare statute, use Q0166)
Use this code for Kytril.

S0092 Injection, hydromorphone HCl, 250 mg (loading dose for infusion pump)
Use this code for Dilaudid, Hydromophone. See also J1170.

S0093 Injection, morphine sulfate, 500 mg (loading dose for infusion pump)
Use this code for Duramorph, MS Contin, Morphine Sulfate. See also J2270, J2271, J2275.

S0104 Zidovudine, oral, 100 mg
See also J3485 for Retrovir.

S0106 Bupropion HCl sustained release tablet, 150 mg, per bottle of 60 tablets
Use this code for Wellbutrin SR tablets.

S0108 Mercaptopurine, oral, 50 mg
Use this code for Purinethol oral.

S0109 Methadone, oral, 5 mg
Use this code for Dolophine.

S0117 Tretinoin, topical, 5 g

S0119 Ondansetron, oral, 4 mg (for circumstances falling under the Medicare statute, use HCPCS Q code)
Use this code for Zofran, Zuplenz.

S0122 Injection, menotropins, 75 IU
Use this code for Humegon, Pergonal, Repronex.
CMS: 100-02,15,50.5

S0126 Injection, follitropin alfa, 75 IU
Use this code for Gonal-F.
CMS: 100-02,15,50.5

S0128 Injection, follitropin beta, 75 IU
Use this code for Follistim.
CMS: 100-02,15,50.5

S0132 Injection, ganirelix acetate, 250 mcg
Use this code for Antagon.
CMS: 100-02,15,50.5

S0136 Clozapine, 25 mg
Use this code for Clozaril.

S0137 Didanosine (ddI), 25 mg
Use this code for Videx.

S0138 Finasteride, 5 mg
Use this code for Propecia (oral), Proscar (oral).

S0139 Minoxidil, 10 mg

S0140 Saquinavir, 200 mg
Use this code for Fortovase (oral), Invirase (oral).

S0142 Colistimethate sodium, inhalation solution administered through DME, concentrated form, per mg

S0145 Injection, PEGylated interferon alfa-2A, 180 mcg per ml
Use this code for Pegasys.
CMS: 100-02,15,50.5

S0148 Injection, PEGylated interferon alfa-2B, 10 mcg
CMS: 100-02,15,50.5

S0155 Sterile dilutant for epoprostenol, 50 ml
Use this code for Flolan.

S0156 Exemestane, 25 mg
Use this code for Aromasin.

S0157 Becaplermin gel 0.01%, 0.5 gm
Use this code for Regraex Gel.

S0160 Dextroamphetamine sulfate, 5 mg

S0164 Injection, pantoprazole sodium, 40 mg
Use this code for Protonix IV.

S0166 Injection, olanzapine, 2.5 mg
Use this code for Zyprexa.

2023 HCPCS Level II

Temporary National Codes (Non-Medicare) — S0169 — S0390

Code	Description
S0169	Calcitrol, 0.25 mcg ☑ Use this code for Calcijex.
S0170	Anastrozole, oral, 1 mg ☑ Use this code for Arimidex.
S0171	Injection, bumetanide, 0.5 mg ☑ Use this code for Bumex.
S0172	Chlorambucil, oral, 2 mg ☑ Use this code for Leukeran.
S0174	Dolasetron mesylate, oral 50 mg (for circumstances falling under the Medicare statute, use Q0180) ☑ Use this code for Anzemet.
S0175	Flutamide, oral, 125 mg ☑ Use this code for Eulexin.
S0176	Hydroxyurea, oral, 500 mg ☑ Use this code for Droxia, Hydrea, Mylocel.
S0177	Levamisole HCl, oral, 50 mg ☑ Use this code for Ergamisol.
S0178	Lomustine, oral, 10 mg ☑ Use this code for Ceenu.
S0179	Megestrol acetate, oral, 20 mg ☑ Use this code for Megace.
S0182	Procarbazine HCl, oral, 50 mg ☑ Use this code for Matulane.
S0183	Prochlorperazine maleate, oral, 5 mg (for circumstances falling under the Medicare statute, use Q0164) ☑ Use this code for Compazine.
S0187	Tamoxifen citrate, oral, 10 mg ☑ Use this code for Nolvadex.
S0189	Testosterone pellet, 75 mg ☑
S0190	Mifepristone, oral, 200 mg ♀☑ Use this code for Mifoprex 200 mg oral.
S0191	Misoprostol, oral, 200 mcg ☑
S0194	Dialysis/stress vitamin supplement, oral, 100 capsules ☑
S0197	Prenatal vitamins, 30-day supply ♀☑
S0199	Medically induced abortion by oral ingestion of medication including all associated services and supplies (e.g., patient counseling, office visits, confirmation of pregnancy by HCG, ultrasound to confirm duration of pregnancy, ultrasound to confirm completion of abortion) except drugs ♀
S0201	Partial hospitalization services, less than 24 hours, per diem
S0207	Paramedic intercept, nonhospital-based ALS service (nonvoluntary), nontransport
S0208	Paramedic intercept, hospital-based ALS service (nonvoluntary), nontransport
S0209	Wheelchair van, mileage, per mile ☑
S0215	Nonemergency transportation; mileage, per mile ☑ See also codes A0021-A0999 for transportation.
S0220	Medical conference by a physician with interdisciplinary team of health professionals or representatives of community agencies to coordinate activities of patient care (patient is present); approximately 30 minutes ☑
S0221	Medical conference by a physician with interdisciplinary team of health professionals or representatives of community agencies to coordinate activities of patient care (patient is present); approximately 60 minutes ☑
S0250	Comprehensive geriatric assessment and treatment planning performed by assessment team [A]
S0255	Hospice referral visit (advising patient and family of care options) performed by nurse, social worker, or other designated staff CMS: 100-04,11,10
S0257	Counseling and discussion regarding advance directives or end of life care planning and decisions, with patient and/or surrogate (list separately in addition to code for appropriate evaluation and management service)
S0260	History and physical (outpatient or office) related to surgical procedure (list separately in addition to code for appropriate evaluation and management service)
S0265	Genetic counseling, under physician supervision, each 15 minutes ☑
S0270	Physician management of patient home care, standard monthly case rate (per 30 days) ☑
S0271	Physician management of patient home care, hospice monthly case rate (per 30 days) ☑
S0272	Physician management of patient home care, episodic care monthly case rate (per 30 days) ☑
S0273	Physician visit at member's home, outside of a capitation arrangement
S0274	Nurse practitioner visit at member's home, outside of a capitation arrangement
S0280	Medical home program, comprehensive care coordination and planning, initial plan
S0281	Medical home program, comprehensive care coordination and planning, maintenance of plan
S0285	Colonoscopy consultation performed prior to a screening colonoscopy procedure
S0302	Completed early periodic screening diagnosis and treatment (EPSDT) service (list in addition to code for appropriate evaluation and management service)
S0310	Hospitalist services (list separately in addition to code for appropriate evaluation and management service)
S0311	Comprehensive management and care coordination for advanced illness, per calendar month
S0315	Disease management program; initial assessment and initiation of the program
S0316	Disease management program, follow-up/reassessment
S0317	Disease management program; per diem ☑
S0320	Telephone calls by a registered nurse to a disease management program member for monitoring purposes; per month
S0340	Lifestyle modification program for management of coronary artery disease, including all supportive services; first quarter/stage
S0341	Lifestyle modification program for management of coronary artery disease, including all supportive services; second or third quarter/stage
S0342	Lifestyle modification program for management of coronary artery disease, including all supportive services; fourth quarter/stage
S0353	Treatment planning and care coordination management for cancer initial treatment
S0354	Treatment planning and care coordination management for cancer established patient with a change of regimen
S0390	Routine foot care; removal and/or trimming of corns, calluses and/or nails and preventive maintenance in specific medical conditions (e.g., diabetes), per visit

Special Coverage Instructions | Noncovered by Medicare | Carrier Discretion | ☑ Quantity Alert | ● New Code | ○ Recycled/Reinstated | ▲ Revised Code

162 — S Codes | [A] Age Edit | [M] Maternity Edit | ♀ Female Only | ♂ Male Only | [A]-[Y] OPPS Status Indicators | © 2022 Optum, Inc.

2023 HCPCS Level II

Code	Description
S0395	Impression casting of a foot performed by a practitioner other than the manufacturer of the orthotic
S0400	Global fee for extracorporeal shock wave lithotripsy treatment of kidney stone(s)
S0500	Disposable contact lens, per lens ☑
S0504	Single vision prescription lens (safety, athletic, or sunglass), per lens ☑
S0506	Bifocal vision prescription lens (safety, athletic, or sunglass), per lens ☑
S0508	Trifocal vision prescription lens (safety, athletic, or sunglass), per lens ☑
S0510	Nonprescription lens (safety, athletic, or sunglass), per lens ☑
S0512	Daily wear specialty contact lens, per lens ☑
S0514	Color contact lens, per lens ☑
S0515	Scleral lens, liquid bandage device, per lens
S0516	Safety eyeglass frames
S0518	Sunglasses frames
S0580	Polycarbonate lens (list this code in addition to the basic code for the lens)
S0581	Nonstandard lens (list this code in addition to the basic code for the lens)
S0590	Integral lens service, miscellaneous services reported separately
S0592	Comprehensive contact lens evaluation
S0595	Dispensing new spectacle lenses for patient supplied frame
S0596	Phakic intraocular lens for correction of refractive error ☑
S0601	Screening proctoscopy ♂
S0610	Annual gynecological examination, new patient A ♀
S0612	Annual gynecological examination, established patient A ♀
S0613	Annual gynecological examination; clinical breast examination without pelvic evaluation ♀
S0618	Audiometry for hearing aid evaluation to determine the level and degree of hearing loss
S0620	Routine ophthalmological examination including refraction; new patient
S0621	Routine ophthalmological examination including refraction; established patient
S0622	Physical exam for college, new or established patient (list separately in addition to appropriate evaluation and management code)
S0630	Removal of sutures; by a physician other than the physician who originally closed the wound
S0800	Laser in situ keratomileusis (LASIK)
S0810	Photorefractive keratectomy (PRK)
S0812	Phototherapeutic keratectomy (PTK)
S1001	Deluxe item, patient aware (list in addition to code for basic item) CMS: 100-02,15,110
S1002	Customized item (list in addition to code for basic item)
S1015	IV tubing extension set
S1016	Non-PVC (polyvinyl chloride) intravenous administration set, for use with drugs that are not stable in PVC, e.g., Paclitaxel
S1030	Continuous noninvasive glucose monitoring device, purchase (for physician interpretation of data, use CPT code)
S1031	Continuous noninvasive glucose monitoring device, rental, including sensor, sensor replacement, and download to monitor (for physician interpretation of data, use CPT code)
S1034	Artificial pancreas device system (e.g., low glucose suspend [LGS] feature) including continuous glucose monitor, blood glucose device, insulin pump and computer algorithm that communicates with all of the devices
S1035	Sensor; invasive (e.g., subcutaneous), disposable, for use with artificial pancreas device system
S1036	Transmitter; external, for use with artificial pancreas device system
S1037	Receiver (monitor); external, for use with artificial pancreas device system
S1040	Cranial remolding orthotic, pediatric, rigid, with soft interface material, custom fabricated, includes fitting and adjustment(s)
S1091	Stent, noncoronary, temporary, with delivery system (Propel)
S2053	Transplantation of small intestine and liver allografts
S2054	Transplantation of multivisceral organs
S2055	Harvesting of donor multivisceral organs, with preparation and maintenance of allografts; from cadaver donor
S2060	Lobar lung transplantation
S2061	Donor lobectomy (lung) for transplantation, living donor
S2065	Simultaneous pancreas kidney transplantation
S2066	Breast reconstruction with gluteal artery perforator (GAP) flap, including harvesting of the flap, microvascular transfer, closure of donor site and shaping the flap into a breast, unilateral
S2067	Breast reconstruction of a single breast with "stacked" deep inferior epigastric perforator (DIEP) flap(s) and/or gluteal artery perforator (GAP) flap(s), including harvesting of the flap(s), microvascular transfer, closure of donor site(s) and shaping the flap into a breast, unilateral
S2068	Breast reconstruction with deep inferior epigastric perforator (DIEP) flap or superficial inferior epigastric artery (SIEA) flap, including harvesting of the flap, microvascular transfer, closure of donor site and shaping the flap into a breast, unilateral
S2070	Cystourethroscopy, with ureteroscopy and/or pyeloscopy; with endoscopic laser treatment of ureteral calculi (includes ureteral catheterization)
S2079	Laparoscopic esophagomyotomy (Heller type)
S2080	Laser-assisted uvulopalatoplasty (LAUP) AHA: 2Q,22
S2083	Adjustment of gastric band diameter via subcutaneous port by injection or aspiration of saline
S2095	Transcatheter occlusion or embolization for tumor destruction, percutaneous, any method, using yttrium-90 microspheres
S2102	Islet cell tissue transplant from pancreas; allogeneic
S2103	Adrenal tissue transplant to brain
S2107	Adoptive immunotherapy i.e. development of specific antitumor reactivity (e.g., tumor-infiltrating lymphocyte therapy) per course of treatment
S2112	Arthroscopy, knee, surgical for harvesting of cartilage (chondrocyte cells)
S2115	Osteotomy, periacetabular, with internal fixation
S2117	Arthroereisis, subtalar
S2118	Metal-on-metal total hip resurfacing, including acetabular and femoral components
S2120	Low density lipoprotein (LDL) apheresis using heparin-induced extracorporeal LDL precipitation

Temporary National Codes (Non-Medicare) — S2140 — S3850

Code	Description
S2140	Cord blood harvesting for transplantation, allogeneic
S2142	Cord blood-derived stem-cell transplantation, allogeneic
S2150	Bone marrow or blood-derived stem cells (peripheral or umbilical), allogeneic or autologous, harvesting, transplantation, and related complications; including: pheresis and cell preparation/storage; marrow ablative therapy; drugs, supplies, hospitalization with outpatient follow-up; medical/surgical, diagnostic, emergency, and rehabilitative services; and the number of days of pre- and posttransplant care in the global definition
S2152	Solid organ(s), complete or segmental, single organ or combination of organs; deceased or living donor(s), procurement, transplantation, and related complications; including: drugs; supplies; hospitalization with outpatient follow-up; medical/surgical, diagnostic, emergency, and rehabilitative services, and the number of days of pre- and posttransplant care in the global definition
S2202	Echosclerotherapy
S2205	Minimally invasive direct coronary artery bypass surgery involving mini-thoracotomy or mini-sternotomy surgery, performed under direct vision; using arterial graft(s), single coronary arterial graft
S2206	Minimally invasive direct coronary artery bypass surgery involving mini-thoracotomy or mini-sternotomy surgery, performed under direct vision; using arterial graft(s), two coronary arterial grafts
S2207	Minimally invasive direct coronary artery bypass surgery involving mini-thoracotomy or mini-sternotomy surgery, performed under direct vision; using venous graft only, single coronary venous graft
S2208	Minimally invasive direct coronary artery bypass surgery involving mini-thoracotomy or mini-sternotomy surgery, performed under direct vision; using single arterial and venous graft(s), single venous graft
S2209	Minimally invasive direct coronary artery bypass surgery involving mini-thoracotomy or mini-sternotomy surgery, performed under direct vision; using two arterial grafts and single venous graft
S2225	Myringotomy, laser-assisted
S2230	Implantation of magnetic component of semi-implantable hearing device on ossicles in middle ear
S2235	Implantation of auditory brain stem implant
S2260	Induced abortion, 17 to 24 weeks [M ♀]
S2265	Induced abortion, 25 to 28 weeks [M ♀]
S2266	Induced abortion, 29 to 31 weeks [M ♀]
S2267	Induced abortion, 32 weeks or greater [M ♀]
S2300	Arthroscopy, shoulder, surgical; with thermally-induced capsulorrhaphy
S2325	Hip core decompression **AHA:** 3Q,17
S2340	Chemodenervation of abductor muscle(s) of vocal cord
S2341	Chemodenervation of adductor muscle(s) of vocal cord
S2342	Nasal endoscopy for postoperative debridement following functional endoscopic sinus surgery, nasal and/or sinus cavity(s), unilateral or bilateral
S2348	Decompression procedure, percutaneous, of nucleus pulposus of intervertebral disc, using radiofrequency energy, single or multiple levels, lumbar
S2350	Diskectomy, anterior, with decompression of spinal cord and/or nerve root(s), including osteophytectomy; lumbar, single interspace
S2351	Diskectomy, anterior, with decompression of spinal cord and/or nerve root(s), including osteophytectomy; lumbar, each additional interspace (list separately in addition to code for primary procedure)
S2400	Repair, congenital diaphragmatic hernia in the fetus using temporary tracheal occlusion, procedure performed in utero [M ♀]
S2401	Repair, urinary tract obstruction in the fetus, procedure performed in utero [M ♀]
S2402	Repair, congenital cystic adenomatoid malformation in the fetus, procedure performed in utero [M ♀]
S2403	Repair, extralobar pulmonary sequestration in the fetus, procedure performed in utero [M ♀]
S2404	Repair, myelomeningocele in the fetus, procedure performed in utero [M ♀]
S2405	Repair of sacrococcygeal teratoma in the fetus, procedure performed in utero [M ♀]
S2409	Repair, congenital malformation of fetus, procedure performed in utero, not otherwise classified [M ♀]
S2411	Fetoscopic laser therapy for treatment of twin-to-twin transfusion syndrome [M ♀]
S2900	Surgical techniques requiring use of robotic surgical system (list separately in addition to code for primary procedure)
S3000	Diabetic indicator; retinal eye exam, dilated, bilateral
S3005	Performance measurement, evaluation of patient self assessment, depression
S3600	STAT laboratory request (situations other than S3601)
S3601	Emergency STAT laboratory charge for patient who is homebound or residing in a nursing facility
S3620	Newborn metabolic screening panel, includes test kit, postage and the laboratory tests specified by the state for inclusion in this panel (e.g., galactose; hemoglobin, electrophoresis; hydroxyprogesterone, 17-d; phenylalanine (PKU); and thyroxine, total) [A]
S3630	Eosinophil count, blood, direct
S3645	HIV-1 antibody testing of oral mucosal transudate
S3650	Saliva test, hormone level; during menopause [A ♀]
S3652	Saliva test, hormone level; to assess preterm labor risk [M ♀]
S3655	Antisperm antibodies test (immunobead) [M ♀]
S3708	Gastrointestinal fat absorption study
S3722	Dose optimization by area under the curve (AUC) analysis, for infusional 5-fluorouracil
S3800	Genetic testing for amyotrophic lateral sclerosis (ALS)
S3840	DNA analysis for germline mutations of the RET proto-oncogene for susceptibility to multiple endocrine neoplasia type 2
S3841	Genetic testing for retinoblastoma
S3842	Genetic testing for Von Hippel-Lindau disease
S3844	DNA analysis of the connexin 26 gene (GJB2) for susceptibility to congenital, profound deafness
S3845	Genetic testing for alpha-thalassemia
S3846	Genetic testing for hemoglobin E beta-thalassemia
S3849	Genetic testing for Niemann-Pick disease
S3850	Genetic testing for sickle cell anemia

2023 HCPCS Level II

Code	Description
S3852	DNA analysis for APOE epsilon 4 allele for susceptibility to Alzheimer's disease
S3853	Genetic testing for myotonic muscular dystrophy
S3854	Gene expression profiling panel for use in the management of breast cancer treatment
S3861	Genetic testing, sodium channel, voltage-gated, type V, alpha subunit (SCN5A) and variants for suspected Brugada Syndrome
S3865	Comprehensive gene sequence analysis for hypertrophic cardiomyopathy
S3866	Genetic analysis for a specific gene mutation for hypertrophic cardiomyopathy (HCM) in an individual with a known HCM mutation in the family
S3870	Comparative genomic hybridization (CGH) microarray testing for developmental delay, autism spectrum disorder and/or intellectual disability
S3900	Surface electromyography (EMG)
S3902	Ballistocardiogram
S3904	Masters two step
S4005	Interim labor facility global (labor occurring but not resulting in delivery)
S4011	In vitro fertilization; including but not limited to identification and incubation of mature oocytes, fertilization with sperm, incubation of embryo(s), and subsequent visualization for determination of development
S4013	Complete cycle, gamete intrafallopian transfer (GIFT), case rate
S4014	Complete cycle, zygote intrafallopian transfer (ZIFT), case rate
S4015	Complete in vitro fertilization cycle, not otherwise specified, case rate
S4016	Frozen in vitro fertilization cycle, case rate
S4017	Incomplete cycle, treatment cancelled prior to stimulation, case rate
S4018	Frozen embryo transfer procedure cancelled before transfer, case rate
S4020	In vitro fertilization procedure cancelled before aspiration, case rate
S4021	In vitro fertilization procedure cancelled after aspiration, case rate
S4022	Assisted oocyte fertilization, case rate
S4023	Donor egg cycle, incomplete, case rate
S4025	Donor services for in vitro fertilization (sperm or embryo), case rate
S4026	Procurement of donor sperm from sperm bank
S4027	Storage of previously frozen embryos
S4028	Microsurgical epididymal sperm aspiration (MESA)
S4030	Sperm procurement and cryopreservation services; initial visit
S4031	Sperm procurement and cryopreservation services; subsequent visit
S4035	Stimulated intrauterine insemination (IUI), case rate
S4037	Cryopreserved embryo transfer, case rate
S4040	Monitoring and storage of cryopreserved embryos, per 30 days
S4042	Management of ovulation induction (interpretation of diagnostic tests and studies, nonface-to-face medical management of the patient), per cycle
S4981	Insertion of levonorgestrel-releasing intrauterine system
S4989	Contraceptive intrauterine device (e.g., Progestacert IUD), including implants and supplies
S4990	Nicotine patches, legend
S4991	Nicotine patches, nonlegend
S4993	Contraceptive pills for birth control
S4995	Smoking cessation gum
S5000	Prescription drug, generic
S5001	Prescription drug, brand name
S5010	5% dextrose and 0.45% normal saline, 1000 ml
S5012	5% dextrose with potassium chloride, 1000 ml
S5013	5% dextrose/0.45% normal saline with potassium chloride and magnesium sulfate, 1000 ml
S5014	5% dextrose/0.45% normal saline with potassium chloride and magnesium sulfate, 1500 ml
S5035	Home infusion therapy, routine service of infusion device (e.g., pump maintenance)
S5036	Home infusion therapy, repair of infusion device (e.g., pump repair)
S5100	Day care services, adult; per 15 minutes
S5101	Day care services, adult; per half day
S5102	Day care services, adult; per diem
S5105	Day care services, center-based; services not included in program fee, per diem
S5108	Home care training to home care client, per 15 minutes
S5109	Home care training to home care client, per session
S5110	Home care training, family; per 15 minutes
S5111	Home care training, family; per session
S5115	Home care training, nonfamily; per 15 minutes
S5116	Home care training, nonfamily; per session
S5120	Chore services; per 15 minutes
S5121	Chore services; per diem
S5125	Attendant care services; per 15 minutes
S5126	Attendant care services; per diem
S5130	Homemaker service, NOS; per 15 minutes
S5131	Homemaker service, NOS; per diem
S5135	Companion care, adult (e.g., IADL/ADL); per 15 minutes
S5136	Companion care, adult (e.g., IADL/ADL); per diem
S5140	Foster care, adult; per diem
S5141	Foster care, adult; per month
S5145	Foster care, therapeutic, child; per diem
S5146	Foster care, therapeutic, child; per month
S5150	Unskilled respite care, not hospice; per 15 minutes
S5151	Unskilled respite care, not hospice; per diem
S5160	Emergency response system; installation and testing
S5161	Emergency response system; service fee, per month (excludes installation and testing)

Temporary National Codes (Non-Medicare)

S3852 — S5161

Special Coverage Instructions | Noncovered by Medicare | Carrier Discretion | ☑ Quantity Alert | ● New Code | ○ Recycled/Reinstated | ▲ Revised Code

© 2022 Optum, Inc. | A2-Z3 ASC Pmt | CMS: IOM | AHA: Coding Clinic | DMEPOS Paid | SNF Excluded | S Codes — 165

Temporary National Codes (Non-Medicare)

Code	Description
S5162	Emergency response system; purchase only
S5165	Home modifications; per service
S5170	Home delivered meals, including preparation; per meal
S5175	Laundry service, external, professional; per order
S5180	Home health respiratory therapy, initial evaluation
S5181	Home health respiratory therapy, NOS, per diem
S5185	Medication reminder service, nonface-to-face; per month ☑
S5190	Wellness assessment, performed by nonphysician
S5199	Personal care item, NOS, each
S5497	Home infusion therapy, catheter care/maintenance, not otherwise classified; includes administrative services, professional pharmacy services, care coordination, and all necessary supplies and equipment (drugs and nursing visits coded separately), per diem ☑
S5498	Home infusion therapy, catheter care/maintenance, simple (single lumen), includes administrative services, professional pharmacy services, care coordination and all necessary supplies and equipment, (drugs and nursing visits coded separately), per diem ☑
S5501	Home infusion therapy, catheter care/maintenance, complex (more than one lumen), includes administrative services, professional pharmacy services, care coordination, and all necessary supplies and equipment (drugs and nursing visits coded separately), per diem ☑
S5502	Home infusion therapy, catheter care/maintenance, implanted access device, includes administrative services, professional pharmacy services, care coordination and all necessary supplies and equipment (drugs and nursing visits coded separately), per diem (use this code for interim maintenance of vascular access not currently in use) ☑
S5517	Home infusion therapy, all supplies necessary for restoration of catheter patency or declotting
S5518	Home infusion therapy, all supplies necessary for catheter repair
S5520	Home infusion therapy, all supplies (including catheter) necessary for a peripherally inserted central venous catheter (PICC) line insertion
S5521	Home infusion therapy, all supplies (including catheter) necessary for a midline catheter insertion
S5522	Home infusion therapy, insertion of peripherally inserted central venous catheter (PICC), nursing services only (no supplies or catheter included)
S5523	Home infusion therapy, insertion of midline venous catheter, nursing services only (no supplies or catheter included)
S5550	Insulin, rapid onset, 5 units ☑
S5551	Insulin, most rapid onset (Lispro or Aspart); 5 units ☑
S5552	Insulin, intermediate acting (NPH or LENTE); 5 units ☑
S5553	Insulin, long acting; 5 units ☑ CMS: 100-02,15,50.5
S5560	Insulin delivery device, reusable pen; 1.5 ml size ☑
S5561	Insulin delivery device, reusable pen; 3 ml size ☑
S5565	Insulin cartridge for use in insulin delivery device other than pump; 150 units ☑
S5566	Insulin cartridge for use in insulin delivery device other than pump; 300 units ☑
S5570	Insulin delivery device, disposable pen (including insulin); 1.5 ml size ☑ CMS: 100-02,15,50.5
S5571	Insulin delivery device, disposable pen (including insulin); 3 ml size ☑ CMS: 100-02,15,50.5
S8030	Scleral application of tantalum ring(s) for localization of lesions for proton beam therapy
S8035	Magnetic source imaging
S8037	Magnetic resonance cholangiopancreatography (MRCP)
S8040	Topographic brain mapping
S8042	Magnetic resonance imaging (MRI), low-field
S8055	Ultrasound guidance for multifetal pregnancy reduction(s), technical component (only to be used when the physician doing the reduction procedure does not perform the ultrasound, guidance is included in the CPT code for multifetal pregnancy reduction (59866)) Ⓜ ♀
S8080	Scintimammography (radioimmunoscintigraphy of the breast), unilateral, including supply of radiopharmaceutical
S8085	Fluorine-18 fluorodeoxyglucose (F-18 FDG) imaging using dual-head coincidence detection system (nondedicated PET scan)
S8092	Electron beam computed tomography (also known as ultrafast CT, cine CT)
S8096	Portable peak flow meter
S8097	Asthma kit (including but not limited to portable peak expiratory flow meter, instructional video, brochure, and/or spacer) ☑
S8100	Holding chamber or spacer for use with an inhaler or nebulizer; without mask
S8101	Holding chamber or spacer for use with an inhaler or nebulizer; with mask
S8110	Peak expiratory flow rate (physician services)
S8120	Oxygen contents, gaseous, 1 unit equals 1 cubic foot ☑
S8121	Oxygen contents, liquid, 1 unit equals 1 pound ☑
S8130	Interferential current stimulator, 2 channel
S8131	Interferential current stimulator, 4 channel
S8185	Flutter device
S8186	Swivel adaptor
S8189	Tracheostomy supply, not otherwise classified
S8210	Mucus trap
S8265	Haberman feeder for cleft lip/palate
S8270	Enuresis alarm, using auditory buzzer and/or vibration device
S8301	Infection control supplies, not otherwise specified
S8415	Supplies for home delivery of infant Ⓜ ♀
S8420	Gradient pressure aid (sleeve and glove combination), custom made
S8421	Gradient pressure aid (sleeve and glove combination), ready made
S8422	Gradient pressure aid (sleeve), custom made, medium weight
S8423	Gradient pressure aid (sleeve), custom made, heavy weight
S8424	Gradient pressure aid (sleeve), ready made
S8425	Gradient pressure aid (glove), custom made, medium weight
S8426	Gradient pressure aid (glove), custom made, heavy weight
S8427	Gradient pressure aid (glove), ready made

Code	Description
S8428	Gradient pressure aid (gauntlet), ready made
S8429	Gradient pressure exterior wrap
S8430	Padding for compression bandage, roll
S8431	Compression bandage, roll
S8450	Splint, prefabricated, digit (specify digit by use of modifier)

Various types of digit splints (S8450)

- Static finger splint
- Mobile dorsal splint
- Slip-on splint

Code	Description
S8451	Splint, prefabricated, wrist or ankle
S8452	Splint, prefabricated, elbow
S8460	Camisole, postmastectomy
S8490	Insulin syringes (100 syringes, any size)
S8930	Electrical stimulation of auricular acupuncture points; each 15 minutes of personal one-on-one contact with patient
S8940	Equestrian/hippotherapy, per session
S8948	Application of a modality (requiring constant provider attendance) to one or more areas; low-level laser; each 15 minutes
S8950	Complex lymphedema therapy, each 15 minutes
S8990	Physical or manipulative therapy performed for maintenance rather than restoration
S8999	Resuscitation bag (for use by patient on artificial respiration during power failure or other catastrophic event)
S9001	Home uterine monitor with or without associated nursing services
S9007	Ultrafiltration monitor
S9024	Paranasal sinus ultrasound
S9025	Omnicardiogram/cardiointegram

Code	Description
S9034	Extracorporeal shockwave lithotripsy for gall stones (if performed with ERCP, use 43265)
S9055	Procuren or other growth factor preparation to promote wound healing
S9056	Coma stimulation per diem
S9061	Home administration of aerosolized drug therapy (e.g., Pentamidine); administrative services, professional pharmacy services, care coordination, all necessary supplies and equipment (drugs and nursing visits coded separately), per diem
S9083	Global fee urgent care centers
S9088	Services provided in an urgent care center (list in addition to code for service)
S9090	Vertebral axial decompression, per session
S9097	Home visit for wound care
S9098	Home visit, phototherapy services (e.g., Bili-lite), including equipment rental, nursing services, blood draw, supplies, and other services, per diem
S9110	Telemonitoring of patient in their home, including all necessary equipment; computer system, connections, and software; maintenance; patient education and support; per month
S9117	Back school, per visit
S9122	Home health aide or certified nurse assistant, providing care in the home; per hour
S9123	Nursing care, in the home; by registered nurse, per hour (use for general nursing care only, not to be used when CPT codes 99500-99602 can be used)
S9124	Nursing care, in the home; by licensed practical nurse, per hour
S9125	Respite care, in the home, per diem
S9126	Hospice care, in the home, per diem CMS: 100-04,11,10
S9127	Social work visit, in the home, per diem
S9128	Speech therapy, in the home, per diem
S9129	Occupational therapy, in the home, per diem
S9131	Physical therapy; in the home, per diem
S9140	Diabetic management program, follow-up visit to non-MD provider
S9141	Diabetic management program, follow-up visit to MD provider
S9145	Insulin pump initiation, instruction in initial use of pump (pump not included)
S9150	Evaluation by ocularist
S9152	Speech therapy, re-evaluation
S9208	Home management of preterm labor, including administrative services, professional pharmacy services, care coordination, and all necessary supplies or equipment (drugs and nursing visits coded separately), per diem (do not use this code with any home infusion per diem code)
S9209	Home management of preterm premature rupture of membranes (PPROM), including administrative services, professional pharmacy services, care coordination, and all necessary supplies or equipment (drugs and nursing visits coded separately), per diem (do not use this code with any home infusion per diem code)

Code	Description
S9211	Home management of gestational hypertension, includes administrative services, professional pharmacy services, care coordination and all necessary supplies and equipment (drugs and nursing visits coded separately); per diem (do not use this code with any home infusion per diem code)
S9212	Home management of postpartum hypertension, includes administrative services, professional pharmacy services, care coordination, and all necessary supplies and equipment (drugs and nursing visits coded separately), per diem (do not use this code with any home infusion per diem code)
S9213	Home management of preeclampsia, includes administrative services, professional pharmacy services, care coordination, and all necessary supplies and equipment (drugs and nursing services coded separately); per diem (do not use this code with any home infusion per diem code)
S9214	Home management of gestational diabetes, includes administrative services, professional pharmacy services, care coordination, and all necessary supplies and equipment (drugs and nursing visits coded separately); per diem (do not use this code with any home infusion per diem code)
S9325	Home infusion therapy, pain management infusion; administrative services, professional pharmacy services, care coordination, and all necessary supplies and equipment, (drugs and nursing visits coded separately), per diem (do not use this code with S9326, S9327 or S9328)
S9326	Home infusion therapy, continuous (24 hours or more) pain management infusion; administrative services, professional pharmacy services, care coordination and all necessary supplies and equipment (drugs and nursing visits coded separately), per diem
S9327	Home infusion therapy, intermittent (less than 24 hours) pain management infusion; administrative services, professional pharmacy services, care coordination, and all necessary supplies and equipment (drugs and nursing visits coded separately), per diem
S9328	Home infusion therapy, implanted pump pain management infusion; administrative services, professional pharmacy services, care coordination, and all necessary supplies and equipment (drugs and nursing visits coded separately), per diem
S9329	Home infusion therapy, chemotherapy infusion; administrative services, professional pharmacy services, care coordination, and all necessary supplies and equipment (drugs and nursing visits coded separately), per diem (do not use this code with S9330 or S9331)
S9330	Home infusion therapy, continuous (24 hours or more) chemotherapy infusion; administrative services, professional pharmacy services, care coordination, and all necessary supplies and equipment (drugs and nursing visits coded separately), per diem
S9331	Home infusion therapy, intermittent (less than 24 hours) chemotherapy infusion; administrative services, professional pharmacy services, care coordination, and all necessary supplies and equipment (drugs and nursing visits coded separately), per diem
S9335	Home therapy, hemodialysis; administrative services, professional pharmacy services, care coordination, and all necessary supplies and equipment (drugs and nursing services coded separately), per diem
S9336	Home infusion therapy, continuous anticoagulant infusion therapy (e.g., Heparin), administrative services, professional pharmacy services, care coordination and all necessary supplies and equipment (drugs and nursing visits coded separately), per diem
S9338	Home infusion therapy, immunotherapy, administrative services, professional pharmacy services, care coordination, and all necessary supplies and equipment (drugs and nursing visits coded separately), per diem
S9339	Home therapy; peritoneal dialysis, administrative services, professional pharmacy services, care coordination and all necessary supplies and equipment (drugs and nursing visits coded separately), per diem
S9340	Home therapy; enteral nutrition; administrative services, professional pharmacy services, care coordination, and all necessary supplies and equipment (enteral formula and nursing visits coded separately), per diem
S9341	Home therapy; enteral nutrition via gravity; administrative services, professional pharmacy services, care coordination, and all necessary supplies and equipment (enteral formula and nursing visits coded separately), per diem
S9342	Home therapy; enteral nutrition via pump; administrative services, professional pharmacy services, care coordination, and all necessary supplies and equipment (enteral formula and nursing visits coded separately), per diem
S9343	Home therapy; enteral nutrition via bolus; administrative services, professional pharmacy services, care coordination, and all necessary supplies and equipment (enteral formula and nursing visits coded separately), per diem
S9345	Home infusion therapy, antihemophilic agent infusion therapy (e.g., Factor VIII); administrative services, professional pharmacy services, care coordination, and all necessary supplies and equipment (drugs and nursing visits coded separately), per diem
S9346	Home infusion therapy, alpha-1-proteinase inhibitor (e.g., Prolastin); administrative services, professional pharmacy services, care coordination, and all necessary supplies and equipment (drugs and nursing visits coded separately), per diem
S9347	Home infusion therapy, uninterrupted, long-term, controlled rate intravenous or subcutaneous infusion therapy (e.g., epoprostenol); administrative services, professional pharmacy services, care coordination, and all necessary supplies and equipment (drugs and nursing visits coded separately), per diem
S9348	Home infusion therapy, sympathomimetic/inotropic agent infusion therapy (e.g., Dobutamine); administrative services, professional pharmacy services, care coordination, all necessary supplies and equipment (drugs and nursing visits coded separately), per diem
S9349	Home infusion therapy, tocolytic infusion therapy; administrative services, professional pharmacy services, care coordination, and all necessary supplies and equipment (drugs and nursing visits coded separately), per diem
S9351	Home infusion therapy, continuous or intermittent antiemetic infusion therapy; administrative services, professional pharmacy services, care coordination, and all necessary supplies and equipment (drugs and visits coded separately), per diem
S9353	Home infusion therapy, continuous insulin infusion therapy; administrative services, professional pharmacy services, care coordination, and all necessary supplies and equipment (drugs and nursing visits coded separately), per diem
S9355	Home infusion therapy, chelation therapy; administrative services, professional pharmacy services, care coordination, and all necessary supplies and equipment (drugs and nursing visits coded separately), per diem

Code	Description
S9357	Home infusion therapy, enzyme replacement intravenous therapy; (e.g., Imiglucerase); administrative services, professional pharmacy services, care coordination, and all necessary supplies and equipment (drugs and nursing visits coded separately), per diem ☑
S9359	Home infusion therapy, antitumor necrosis factor intravenous therapy; (e.g., Infliximab); administrative services, professional pharmacy services, care coordination, and all necessary supplies and equipment (drugs and nursing visits coded separately), per diem ☑
S9361	Home infusion therapy, diuretic intravenous therapy; administrative services, professional pharmacy services, care coordination, and all necessary supplies and equipment (drugs and nursing visits coded separately), per diem ☑
S9363	Home infusion therapy, antispasmotic therapy; administrative services, professional pharmacy services, care coordination, and all necessary supplies and equipment (drugs and nursing visits coded separately), per diem ☑
S9364	Home infusion therapy, total parenteral nutrition (TPN); administrative services, professional pharmacy services, care coordination, and all necessary supplies and equipment including standard TPN formula (lipids, specialty amino acid formulas, drugs other than in standard formula and nursing visits coded separately), per diem (do not use with home infusion codes S9365-S9368 using daily volume scales) ☑
S9365	Home infusion therapy, total parenteral nutrition (TPN); one liter per day, administrative services, professional pharmacy services, care coordination, and all necessary supplies and equipment including standard TPN formula (lipids, specialty amino acid formulas, drugs other than in standard formula and nursing visits coded separately), per diem ☑
S9366	Home infusion therapy, total parenteral nutrition (TPN); more than one liter but no more than two liters per day, administrative services, professional pharmacy services, care coordination, and all necessary supplies and equipment including standard TPN formula (lipids, specialty amino acid formulas, drugs other than in standard formula and nursing visits coded separately), per diem ☑
S9367	Home infusion therapy, total parenteral nutrition (TPN); more than two liters but no more than three liters per day, administrative services, professional pharmacy services, care coordination, and all necessary supplies and equipment including standard TPN formula (lipids, specialty amino acid formulas, drugs other than in standard formula and nursing visits coded separately), per diem ☑
S9368	Home infusion therapy, total parenteral nutrition (TPN); more than three liters per day, administrative services, professional pharmacy services, care coordination, and all necessary supplies and equipment including standard TPN formula (lipids, specialty amino acid formulas, drugs other than in standard formula and nursing visits coded separately), per diem ☑
S9370	Home therapy, intermittent antiemetic injection therapy; administrative services, professional pharmacy services, care coordination, and all necessary supplies and equipment (drugs and nursing visits coded separately), per diem ☑
S9372	Home therapy; intermittent anticoagulant injection therapy (e.g., Heparin); administrative services, professional pharmacy services, care coordination, and all necessary supplies and equipment (drugs and nursing visits coded separately), per diem (do not use this code for flushing of infusion devices with Heparin to maintain patency) ☑
S9373	Home infusion therapy, hydration therapy; administrative services, professional pharmacy services, care coordination, and all necessary supplies and equipment (drugs and nursing visits coded separately), per diem (do not use with hydration therapy codes S9374-S9377 using daily volume scales) ☑
S9374	Home infusion therapy, hydration therapy; 1 liter per day, administrative services, professional pharmacy services, care coordination, and all necessary supplies and equipment (drugs and nursing visits coded separately), per diem ☑
S9375	Home infusion therapy, hydration therapy; more than 1 liter but no more than 2 liters per day, administrative services, professional pharmacy services, care coordination, and all necessary supplies and equipment (drugs and nursing visits coded separately), per diem ☑
S9376	Home infusion therapy, hydration therapy; more than 2 liters but no more than 3 liters per day, administrative services, professional pharmacy services, care coordination, and all necessary supplies and equipment (drugs and nursing visits coded separately), per diem ☑
S9377	Home infusion therapy, hydration therapy; more than 3 liters per day, administrative services, professional pharmacy services, care coordination, and all necessary supplies (drugs and nursing visits coded separately), per diem ☑
S9379	Home infusion therapy, infusion therapy, not otherwise classified; administrative services, professional pharmacy services, care coordination, and all necessary supplies and equipment (drugs and nursing visits coded separately), per diem ☑
S9381	Delivery or service to high risk areas requiring escort or extra protection, per visit
S9401	Anticoagulation clinic, inclusive of all services except laboratory tests, per session
S9430	Pharmacy compounding and dispensing services
S9432	Medical foods for noninborn errors of metabolism
S9433	Medical food nutritionally complete, administered orally, providing 100% of nutritional intake
S9434	Modified solid food supplements for inborn errors of metabolism
S9435	Medical foods for inborn errors of metabolism
S9436	Childbirth preparation/Lamaze classes, nonphysician provider, per session M ♀ ☑
S9437	Childbirth refresher classes, nonphysician provider, per session M ♀
S9438	Cesarean birth classes, nonphysician provider, per session M ♀ ☑
S9439	VBAC (vaginal birth after cesarean) classes, nonphysician provider, per session M ♀ ☑
S9441	Asthma education, nonphysician provider, per session ☑
S9442	Birthing classes, nonphysician provider, per session M ♀ ☑
S9443	Lactation classes, nonphysician provider, per session M ♀ ☑
S9444	Parenting classes, nonphysician provider, per session ☑
S9445	Patient education, not otherwise classified, nonphysician provider, individual, per session ☑
S9446	Patient education, not otherwise classified, nonphysician provider, group, per session ☑
S9447	Infant safety (including CPR) classes, nonphysician provider, per session ☑

Code	Description
S9449	Weight management classes, nonphysician provider, per session
S9451	Exercise classes, nonphysician provider, per session
S9452	Nutrition classes, nonphysician provider, per session
S9453	Smoking cessation classes, nonphysician provider, per session
S9454	Stress management classes, nonphysician provider, per session
S9455	Diabetic management program, group session
S9460	Diabetic management program, nurse visit
S9465	Diabetic management program, dietitian visit
S9470	Nutritional counseling, dietitian visit
S9472	Cardiac rehabilitation program, nonphysician provider, per diem
S9473	Pulmonary rehabilitation program, nonphysician provider, per diem
S9474	Enterostomal therapy by a registered nurse certified in enterostomal therapy, per diem
S9475	Ambulatory setting substance abuse treatment or detoxification services, per diem
S9476	Vestibular rehabilitation program, nonphysician provider, per diem
S9480	Intensive outpatient psychiatric services, per diem
S9482	Family stabilization services, per 15 minutes
S9484	Crisis intervention mental health services, per hour
S9485	Crisis intervention mental health services, per diem
S9490	Home infusion therapy, corticosteroid infusion; administrative services, professional pharmacy services, care coordination, and all necessary supplies and equipment (drugs and nursing visits coded separately), per diem
S9494	Home infusion therapy, antibiotic, antiviral, or antifungal therapy; administrative services, professional pharmacy services, care coordination, and all necessary supplies and equipment (drugs and nursing visits coded separately), per diem (do not use this code with home infusion codes for hourly dosing schedules S9497-S9504)
S9497	Home infusion therapy, antibiotic, antiviral, or antifungal therapy; once every 3 hours; administrative services, professional pharmacy services, care coordination, and all necessary supplies and equipment (drugs and nursing visits coded separately), per diem
S9500	Home infusion therapy, antibiotic, antiviral, or antifungal therapy; once every 24 hours; administrative services, professional pharmacy services, care coordination, and all necessary supplies and equipment (drugs and nursing visits coded separately), per diem
S9501	Home infusion therapy, antibiotic, antiviral, or antifungal therapy; once every 12 hours; administrative services, professional pharmacy services, care coordination, and all necessary supplies and equipment (drugs and nursing visits coded separately), per diem
S9502	Home infusion therapy, antibiotic, antiviral, or antifungal therapy; once every 8 hours, administrative services, professional pharmacy services, care coordination, and all necessary supplies and equipment (drugs and nursing visits coded separately), per diem
S9503	Home infusion therapy, antibiotic, antiviral, or antifungal; once every 6 hours; administrative services, professional pharmacy services, care coordination, and all necessary supplies and equipment (drugs and nursing visits coded separately), per diem
S9504	Home infusion therapy, antibiotic, antiviral, or antifungal; once every 4 hours; administrative services, professional pharmacy services, care coordination, and all necessary supplies and equipment (drugs and nursing visits coded separately), per diem
S9529	Routine venipuncture for collection of specimen(s), single homebound, nursing home, or skilled nursing facility patient
S9537	Home therapy; hematopoietic hormone injection therapy (e.g., erythropoietin, G-CSF, GM-CSF); administrative services, professional pharmacy services, care coordination, and all necessary supplies and equipment (drugs and nursing visits coded separately), per diem
S9538	Home transfusion of blood product(s); administrative services, professional pharmacy services, care coordination and all necessary supplies and equipment (blood products, drugs, and nursing visits coded separately), per diem
S9542	Home injectable therapy, not otherwise classified, including administrative services, professional pharmacy services, care coordination, and all necessary supplies and equipment (drugs and nursing visits coded separately), per diem
S9558	Home injectable therapy; growth hormone, including administrative services, professional pharmacy services, care coordination, and all necessary supplies and equipment (drugs and nursing visits coded separately), per diem
S9559	Home injectable therapy, interferon, including administrative services, professional pharmacy services, care coordination, and all necessary supplies and equipment (drugs and nursing visits coded separately), per diem
S9560	Home injectable therapy; hormonal therapy (e.g., leuprolide, goserelin), including administrative services, professional pharmacy services, care coordination, and all necessary supplies and equipment (drugs and nursing visits coded separately), per diem
S9562	Home injectable therapy, palivizumab, including administrative services, professional pharmacy services, care coordination, and all necessary supplies and equipment (drugs and nursing visits coded separately), per diem
S9590	Home therapy, irrigation therapy (e.g., sterile irrigation of an organ or anatomical cavity); including administrative services, professional pharmacy services, care coordination, and all necessary supplies and equipment (drugs and nursing visits coded separately), per diem
S9810	Home therapy; professional pharmacy services for provision of infusion, specialty drug administration, and/or disease state management, not otherwise classified, per hour (do not use this code with any per diem code)
S9900	Services by a Journal-listed Christian Science practitioner for the purpose of healing, per diem
S9901	Services by a Journal-listed Christian Science nurse, per hour
S9960	Ambulance service, conventional air services, nonemergency transport, one way (fixed wing)
S9961	Ambulance service, conventional air service, nonemergency transport, one way (rotary wing)
S9970	Health club membership, annual
S9975	Transplant related lodging, meals and transportation, per diem

2023 HCPCS Level II

Temporary National Codes (Non-Medicare)

Code	Description
S9976	Lodging, per diem, not otherwise classified
S9977	Meals, per diem, not otherwise specified
S9981	Medical records copying fee, administrative
S9982	Medical records copying fee, per page ☑
S9986	Not medically necessary service (patient is aware that service not medically necessary)
S9988	Services provided as part of a Phase I clinical trial
S9989	Services provided outside of the United States of America (list in addition to code(s) for services(s))
S9990	Services provided as part of a Phase II clinical trial
S9991	Services provided as part of a Phase III clinical trial
S9992	Transportation costs to and from trial location and local transportation costs (e.g., fares for taxicab or bus) for clinical trial participant and one caregiver/companion
S9994	Lodging costs (e.g., hotel charges) for clinical trial participant and one caregiver/companion
S9996	Meals for clinical trial participant and one caregiver/companion
S9999	Sales tax

National T Codes Established for State Medicaid Agencies
T1000-T5999

The T codes are designed for use by Medicaid state agencies to establish codes for items for which there are no permanent national codes but for which codes are necessary to administer the Medicaid program (T codes are not accepted by Medicare but can be used by private insurers). This range of codes describes nursing and home health-related services, substance abuse treatment, and certain training-related procedures.

Code	Description
T1000	Private duty/independent nursing service(s), licensed, up to 15 minutes ☑
T1001	Nursing assessment/evaluation
T1002	RN services, up to 15 minutes ☑
T1003	LPN/LVN services, up to 15 minutes ☑
T1004	Services of a qualified nursing aide, up to 15 minutes ☑
T1005	Respite care services, up to 15 minutes ☑
T1006	Alcohol and/or substance abuse services, family/couple counseling
T1007	Alcohol and/or substance abuse services, treatment plan development and/or modification
T1009	Child sitting services for children of the individual receiving alcohol and/or substance abuse services
T1010	Meals for individuals receiving alcohol and/or substance abuse services (when meals not included in the program)
T1012	Alcohol and/or substance abuse services, skills development
T1013	Sign language or oral interpretive services, per 15 minutes ☑
T1014	Telehealth transmission, per minute, professional services bill separately
T1015	Clinic visit/encounter, all-inclusive
T1016	Case management, each 15 minutes ☑
T1017	Targeted case management, each 15 minutes ☑
T1018	School-based individualized education program (IEP) services, bundled
T1019	Personal care services, per 15 minutes, not for an inpatient or resident of a hospital, nursing facility, ICF/MR or IMD, part of the individualized plan of treatment (code may not be used to identify services provided by home health aide or certified nurse assistant) ☑
T1020	Personal care services, per diem, not for an inpatient or resident of a hospital, nursing facility, ICF/MR or IMD, part of the individualized plan of treatment (code may not be used to identify services provided by home health aide or certified nurse assistant)
T1021	Home health aide or certified nurse assistant, per visit
T1022	Contracted home health agency services, all services provided under contract, per day
T1023	Screening to determine the appropriateness of consideration of an individual for participation in a specified program, project or treatment protocol, per encounter
T1024	Evaluation and treatment by an integrated, specialty team contracted to provide coordinated care to multiple or severely handicapped children, per encounter A
T1025	Intensive, extended multidisciplinary services provided in a clinic setting to children with complex medical, physical, mental and psychosocial impairments, per diem A
T1026	Intensive, extended multidisciplinary services provided in a clinic setting to children with complex medical, physical, medical and psychosocial impairments, per hour A
T1027	Family training and counseling for child development, per 15 minutes ☑
T1028	Assessment of home, physical and family environment, to determine suitability to meet patient's medical needs
T1029	Comprehensive environmental lead investigation, not including laboratory analysis, per dwelling
T1030	Nursing care, in the home, by registered nurse, per diem ☑
T1031	Nursing care, in the home, by licensed practical nurse, per diem ☑
● T1032	Services performed by a doula birth worker, per 15 minutes
● T1033	Services performed by a doula birth worker, per diem
T1040	Medicaid certified community behavioral health clinic services, per diem
T1041	Medicaid certified community behavioral health clinic services, per month
T1502	Administration of oral, intramuscular and/or subcutaneous medication by health care agency/professional, per visit ☑
T1503	Administration of medication, other than oral and/or injectable, by a health care agency/professional, per visit ☑
T1505	Electronic medication compliance management device, includes all components and accessories, not otherwise classified
T1999	Miscellaneous therapeutic items and supplies, retail purchases, not otherwise classified; identify product in "remarks"
T2001	Nonemergency transportation; patient attendant/escort
T2002	Nonemergency transportation; per diem ☑
T2003	Nonemergency transportation; encounter/trip
T2004	Nonemergency transport; commercial carrier, multipass
T2005	Nonemergency transportation; stretcher van
T2007	Transportation waiting time, air ambulance and nonemergency vehicle, one-half (1/2) hour increments ☑
T2010	Preadmission screening and resident review (PASRR) Level I identification screening, per screen ☑
T2011	Preadmission screening and resident review (PASRR) Level II evaluation, per evaluation
T2012	Habilitation, educational; waiver, per diem ☑
T2013	Habilitation, educational, waiver; per hour ☑
T2014	Habilitation, prevocational, waiver; per diem ☑
T2015	Habilitation, prevocational, waiver; per hour ☑
T2016	Habilitation, residential, waiver; per diem ☑
T2017	Habilitation, residential, waiver; 15 minutes ☑
T2018	Habilitation, supported employment, waiver; per diem ☑
T2019	Habilitation, supported employment, waiver; per 15 minutes ☑
T2020	Day habilitation, waiver; per diem ☑
T2021	Day habilitation, waiver; per 15 minutes ☑
T2022	Case management, per month ☑
T2023	Targeted case management; per month ☑
T2024	Service assessment/plan of care development, waiver
T2025	Waiver services; not otherwise specified (NOS)
T2026	Specialized childcare, waiver; per diem ☑
T2027	Specialized childcare, waiver; per 15 minutes ☑
T2028	Specialized supply, not otherwise specified, waiver

Special Coverage Instructions · Noncovered by Medicare · Carrier Discretion · ☑ Quantity Alert · ● New Code · ○ Recycled/Reinstated · ▲ Revised Code

Code	Description
T2029	Specialized medical equipment, not otherwise specified, waiver
T2030	Assisted living, waiver; per month
T2031	Assisted living; waiver, per diem
T2032	Residential care, not otherwise specified (NOS), waiver; per month
T2033	Residential care, not otherwise specified (NOS), waiver; per diem
T2034	Crisis intervention, waiver; per diem
T2035	Utility services to support medical equipment and assistive technology/devices, waiver
T2036	Therapeutic camping, overnight, waiver; each session
T2037	Therapeutic camping, day, waiver; each session
T2038	Community transition, waiver; per service
T2039	Vehicle modifications, waiver; per service
T2040	Financial management, self-directed, waiver; per 15 minutes
T2041	Supports brokerage, self-directed, waiver; per 15 minutes
T2042	Hospice routine home care; per diem CMS: 100-04,11,10
T2043	Hospice continuous home care; per hour CMS: 100-04,11,10
T2044	Hospice inpatient respite care; per diem CMS: 100-04,11,10
T2045	Hospice general inpatient care; per diem CMS: 100-04,11,10
T2046	Hospice long-term care, room and board only; per diem CMS: 100-04,11,10
T2047	Habilitation, prevocational, waiver; per 15 minutes
T2048	Behavioral health; long-term care residential (nonacute care in a residential treatment program where stay is typically longer than 30 days), with room and board, per diem
T2049	Nonemergency transportation; stretcher van, mileage; per mile
● T2050	Financial management, self-directed, waiver; per diem
● T2051	Supports brokerage, self-directed, waiver; per diem
T2101	Human breast milk processing, storage and distribution only ♀
T4521	Adult sized disposable incontinence product, brief/diaper, small, each
T4522	Adult sized disposable incontinence product, brief/diaper, medium, each
T4523	Adult sized disposable incontinence product, brief/diaper, large, each
T4524	Adult sized disposable incontinence product, brief/diaper, extra large, each
T4525	Adult sized disposable incontinence product, protective underwear/pull-on, small size, each
T4526	Adult sized disposable incontinence product, protective underwear/pull-on, medium size, each
T4527	Adult sized disposable incontinence product, protective underwear/pull-on, large size, each
T4528	Adult sized disposable incontinence product, protective underwear/pull-on, extra large size, each
T4529	Pediatric sized disposable incontinence product, brief/diaper, small/medium size, each
T4530	Pediatric sized disposable incontinence product, brief/diaper, large size, each
T4531	Pediatric sized disposable incontinence product, protective underwear/pull-on, small/medium size, each
T4532	Pediatric sized disposable incontinence product, protective underwear/pull-on, large size, each
T4533	Youth sized disposable incontinence product, brief/diaper, each
T4534	Youth sized disposable incontinence product, protective underwear/pull-on, each
T4535	Disposable liner/shield/guard/pad/undergarment, for incontinence, each
T4536	Incontinence product, protective underwear/pull-on, reusable, any size, each
T4537	Incontinence product, protective underpad, reusable, bed size, each
T4538	Diaper service, reusable diaper, each diaper
T4539	Incontinence product, diaper/brief, reusable, any size, each
T4540	Incontinence product, protective underpad, reusable, chair size, each
T4541	Incontinence product, disposable underpad, large, each
T4542	Incontinence product, disposable underpad, small size, each
T4543	Adult sized disposable incontinence product, protective brief/diaper, above extra large, each
T4544	Adult sized disposable incontinence product, protective underwear/pull-on, above extra large, each
T4545	Incontinence product, disposable, penile wrap, each
T5001	Positioning seat for persons with special orthopedic needs
T5999	Supply, not otherwise specified

Coronavirus Services U0001-U0005

U0001 CDC 2019 Novel Coronavirus (2019-nCoV) Real-Time RT-PCR Diagnostic Panel
Use this code for CDC created tests.
AHA: 2Q,20

U0002 2019-nCoV coronavirus, SARS-CoV-2/2019-nCoV (COVID-19), any technique, multiple types or subtypes (includes all targets), non-CDC
Use this code for non-CDC created tests.
AHA: 2Q,20

U0003 Infectious agent detection by nucleic acid (DNA or RNA); severe acute respiratory syndrome coronavirus 2 (SARS-CoV-2) (coronavirus disease [COVID-19]), amplified probe technique, making use of high throughput technologies as described by CMS-2020-01-R
Use this code for testing performed with high throughput technologies.
AHA: 1Q,21; 2Q,20

U0004 2019-nCoV coronavirus, SARS-CoV-2/2019-nCoV (COVID-19), any technique, multiple types or subtypes (includes all targets), non-CDC, making use of high throughput technologies as described by CMS-2020-01-R
Use this code for testing performed with high throughput technologies.
AHA: 1Q,21; 2Q,20

U0005 Infectious agent detection by nucleic acid (DNA or RNA); severe acute respiratory syndrome coronavirus 2 (SARS-CoV-2) (coronavirus disease [COVID-19]), amplified probe technique, CDC or non-CDC, making use of high throughput technologies, completed within 2 calendar days from date of specimen collection (list separately in addition to either HCPCS code U0003 or U0004) as described by CMS-2020-01-R2
AHA: 1Q,21

Vision Services

Vision Services V2020-V2799

These V codes include vision-related supplies, including spectacles, lenses, contact lenses, prostheses, intraocular lenses, and miscellaneous lenses.

Frames

Code	Description	
V2020	Frames, purchases	A ♿
V2025	Deluxe frame CMS: 100-04,1,30.3.5	EI

Single Vision, Glass, or Plastic

Code	Description	
V2100	Sphere, single vision, plano to plus or minus 4.00, per lens	A ☑ ♿

Monofocal spectacles (V2100–V2114)

Trifocal spectacles (V2300–V2314)

Low vision aids mounted to spectacles (V2610)

Telescopic or other compound lens fitted on spectacles as a low vision aid (V2615)

Code	Description	
V2101	Sphere, single vision, plus or minus 4.12 to plus or minus 7.00d, per lens	A ☑ ♿
V2102	Sphere, single vision, plus or minus 7.12 to plus or minus 20.00d, per lens	A ☑ ♿
V2103	Spherocylinder, single vision, plano to plus or minus 4.00d sphere, 0.12 to 2.00d cylinder, per lens	A ☑ ♿
V2104	Spherocylinder, single vision, plano to plus or minus 4.00d sphere, 2.12 to 4.00d cylinder, per lens	A ☑ ♿
V2105	Spherocylinder, single vision, plano to plus or minus 4.00d sphere, 4.25 to 6.00d cylinder, per lens	A ☑ ♿
V2106	Spherocylinder, single vision, plano to plus or minus 4.00d sphere, over 6.00d cylinder, per lens	A ☑ ♿
V2107	Spherocylinder, single vision, plus or minus 4.25 to plus or minus 7.00 sphere, 0.12 to 2.00d cylinder, per lens	A ☑ ♿
V2108	Spherocylinder, single vision, plus or minus 4.25d to plus or minus 7.00d sphere, 2.12 to 4.00d cylinder, per lens	A ☑ ♿
V2109	Spherocylinder, single vision, plus or minus 4.25 to plus or minus 7.00d sphere, 4.25 to 6.00d cylinder, per lens	A ☑ ♿
V2110	Spherocylinder, single vision, plus or minus 4.25 to 7.00d sphere, over 6.00d cylinder, per lens	A ☑ ♿
V2111	Spherocylinder, single vision, plus or minus 7.25 to plus or minus 12.00d sphere, 0.25 to 2.25d cylinder, per lens	A ☑ ♿
V2112	Spherocylinder, single vision, plus or minus 7.25 to plus or minus 12.00d sphere, 2.25d to 4.00d cylinder, per lens	A ☑ ♿
V2113	Spherocylinder, single vision, plus or minus 7.25 to plus or minus 12.00d sphere, 4.25 to 6.00d cylinder, per lens	A ☑ ♿
V2114	Spherocylinder, single vision, sphere over plus or minus 12.00d, per lens	A ☑ ♿
V2115	Lenticular (myodisc), per lens, single vision	A ☑ ♿
V2118	Aniseikonic lens, single vision	A ♿
V2121	Lenticular lens, per lens, single	A ☑ ♿
V2199	Not otherwise classified, single vision lens	A

Bifocal, Glass, or Plastic

Code	Description	
V2200	Sphere, bifocal, plano to plus or minus 4.00d, per lens	A ☑ ♿
V2201	Sphere, bifocal, plus or minus 4.12 to plus or minus 7.00d, per lens	A ☑ ♿
V2202	Sphere, bifocal, plus or minus 7.12 to plus or minus 20.00d, per lens	A ☑ ♿
V2203	Spherocylinder, bifocal, plano to plus or minus 4.00d sphere, 0.12 to 2.00d cylinder, per lens	A ☑ ♿
V2204	Spherocylinder, bifocal, plano to plus or minus 4.00d sphere, 2.12 to 4.00d cylinder, per lens	A ☑ ♿
V2205	Spherocylinder, bifocal, plano to plus or minus 4.00d sphere, 4.25 to 6.00d cylinder, per lens	A ☑ ♿
V2206	Spherocylinder, bifocal, plano to plus or minus 4.00d sphere, over 6.00d cylinder, per lens	A ☑ ♿
V2207	Spherocylinder, bifocal, plus or minus 4.25 to plus or minus 7.00d sphere, 0.12 to 2.00d cylinder, per lens	A ☑ ♿
V2208	Spherocylinder, bifocal, plus or minus 4.25 to plus or minus 7.00d sphere, 2.12 to 4.00d cylinder, per lens	A ☑ ♿
V2209	Spherocylinder, bifocal, plus or minus 4.25 to plus or minus 7.00d sphere, 4.25 to 6.00d cylinder, per lens	A ☑ ♿
V2210	Spherocylinder, bifocal, plus or minus 4.25 to plus or minus 7.00d sphere, over 6.00d cylinder, per lens	A ☑ ♿
V2211	Spherocylinder, bifocal, plus or minus 7.25 to plus or minus 12.00d sphere, 0.25 to 2.25d cylinder, per lens	A ☑ ♿
V2212	Spherocylinder, bifocal, plus or minus 7.25 to plus or minus 12.00d sphere, 2.25 to 4.00d cylinder, per lens	A ☑ ♿
V2213	Spherocylinder, bifocal, plus or minus 7.25 to plus or minus 12.00d sphere, 4.25 to 6.00d cylinder, per lens	A ☑ ♿
V2214	Spherocylinder, bifocal, sphere over plus or minus 12.00d, per lens	A ☑ ♿
V2215	Lenticular (myodisc), per lens, bifocal	A ☑ ♿
V2218	Aniseikonic, per lens, bifocal	A ☑ ♿
V2219	Bifocal seg width over 28mm	A ☑ ♿
V2220	Bifocal add over 3.25d	A ☑ ♿
V2221	Lenticular lens, per lens, bifocal	A ♿
V2299	Specialty bifocal (by report)	A

Pertinent documentation to evaluate medical appropriateness should be included when this code is reported.

Trifocal, Glass, or Plastic

Code	Description	
V2300	Sphere, trifocal, plano to plus or minus 4.00d, per lens	A ☑ ♿
V2301	Sphere, trifocal, plus or minus 4.12 to plus or minus 7.00d per lens	A ☑ ♿
V2302	Sphere, trifocal, plus or minus 7.12 to plus or minus 20.00, per lens	A ☑ ♿
V2303	Spherocylinder, trifocal, plano to plus or minus 4.00d sphere, 0.12 to 2.00d cylinder, per lens	A ☑ ♿
V2304	Spherocylinder, trifocal, plano to plus or minus 4.00d sphere, 2.25 to 4.00d cylinder, per lens	A ☑ ♿
V2305	Spherocylinder, trifocal, plano to plus or minus 4.00d sphere, 4.25 to 6.00 cylinder, per lens	A ☑ ♿

Special Coverage Instructions | **Noncovered by Medicare** | **Carrier Discretion** | ☑ Quantity Alert • New Code ○ Recycled/Reinstated ▲ Revised Code

A Age Edit M Maternity Edit ♀ Female Only ♂ Male Only A-Y OPPS Status Indicators © 2022 Optum, Inc.

2023 HCPCS Level II

Code	Description
V2306	Spherocylinder, trifocal, plano to plus or minus 4.00d sphere, over 6.00d cylinder, per lens
V2307	Spherocylinder, trifocal, plus or minus 4.25 to plus or minus 7.00d sphere, 0.12 to 2.00d cylinder, per lens
V2308	Spherocylinder, trifocal, plus or minus 4.25 to plus or minus 7.00d sphere, 2.12 to 4.00d cylinder, per lens
V2309	Spherocylinder, trifocal, plus or minus 4.25 to plus or minus 7.00d sphere, 4.25 to 6.00d cylinder, per lens
V2310	Spherocylinder, trifocal, plus or minus 4.25 to plus or minus 7.00d sphere, over 6.00d cylinder, per lens
V2311	Spherocylinder, trifocal, plus or minus 7.25 to plus or minus 12.00d sphere, 0.25 to 2.25d cylinder, per lens
V2312	Spherocylinder, trifocal, plus or minus 7.25 to plus or minus 12.00d sphere, 2.25 to 4.00d cylinder, per lens
V2313	Spherocylinder, trifocal, plus or minus 7.25 to plus or minus 12.00d sphere, 4.25 to 6.00d cylinder, per lens
V2314	Spherocylinder, trifocal, sphere over plus or minus 12.00d, per lens
V2315	Lenticular, (myodisc), per lens, trifocal
V2318	Aniseikonic lens, trifocal
V2319	Trifocal seg width over 28 mm
V2320	Trifocal add over 3.25d
V2321	Lenticular lens, per lens, trifocal
V2399	Specialty trifocal (by report)
	Pertinent documentation to evaluate medical appropriateness should be included when this code is reported.

Variable Asphericity Lens, Glass, or Plastic

Code	Description
V2410	Variable asphericity lens, single vision, full field, glass or plastic, per lens
V2430	Variable asphericity lens, bifocal, full field, glass or plastic, per lens
V2499	Variable sphericity lens, other type

Contact Lens

Code	Description
V2500	Contact lens, PMMA, spherical, per lens
V2501	Contact lens, PMMA, toric or prism ballast, per lens
V2502	Contact lens PMMA, bifocal, per lens
V2503	Contact lens, PMMA, color vision deficiency, per lens
V2510	Contact lens, gas permeable, spherical, per lens
V2511	Contact lens, gas permeable, toric, prism ballast, per lens
V2512	Contact lens, gas permeable, bifocal, per lens
V2513	Contact lens, gas permeable, extended wear, per lens
V2520	Contact lens, hydrophilic, spherical, per lens
	Hydrophilic contact lenses are covered by Medicare only for aphakic patients. Local contractor if incident to physician services.
V2521	Contact lens, hydrophilic, toric, or prism ballast, per lens
	Hydrophilic contact lenses are covered by Medicare only for aphakic patients. Local contractor if incident to physician services.
V2522	Contact lens, hydrophilic, bifocal, per lens
	Hydrophilic contact lenses are covered by Medicare only for aphakic patients. Local contractor if incident to physician services.
V2523	Contact lens, hydrophilic, extended wear, per lens
	Hydrophilic contact lenses are covered by Medicare only for aphakic patients.
V2524	Contact lens, hydrophilic, spherical, photochromic additive, per lens
● V2525	Contact lens, hydrophilic, dual focus, per lens
V2530	Contact lens, scleral, gas impermeable, per lens (for contact lens modification, see 92325)
V2531	Contact lens, scleral, gas permeable, per lens (for contact lens modification, see 92325)
V2599	Contact lens, other type
	Local contractor if incident to physician services.

Vision Aids

Code	Description
V2600	Hand held low vision aids and other nonspectacle mounted aids
V2610	Single lens spectacle mounted low vision aids
V2615	Telescopic and other compound lens system, including distance vision telescopic, near vision telescopes and compound microscopic lens system

Prosthetic Eye

Code	Description
V2623	Prosthetic eye, plastic, custom

One type of eye implant — Implant

Reverse angle — Peg

Side view — Previously placed prosthetic receptacle, Implant, Peg, Peg hole drilled into prosthetic

Code	Description
V2624	Polishing/resurfacing of ocular prosthesis
V2625	Enlargement of ocular prosthesis
V2626	Reduction of ocular prosthesis
V2627	Scleral cover shell
	A scleral shell covers the cornea and the anterior sclera. Medicare covers a scleral shell when it is prescribed as an artificial support to a shrunken and sightless eye or as a barrier in the treatment of severe dry eye.
V2628	Fabrication and fitting of ocular conformer
V2629	Prosthetic eye, other type

Intraocular Lenses

V2630 Anterior chamber intraocular lens
The IOL must be FDA-approved for reimbursement. Medicare payment for an IOL is included in the payment for ASC facility services. Medicare jurisdiction: local contractor.

V2631 Iris supported intraocular lens
The IOL must be FDA-approved for reimbursement. Medicare payment for an IOL is included in the payment for ASC facility services. Medicare jurisdiction: local contractor.

V2632 Posterior chamber intraocular lens
The IOL must be FDA-approved for reimbursement. Medicare payment for an IOL is included in the payment for ASC facility services. Medicare jurisdiction: local contractor.
CMS: 100-04,32,120.2

Miscellaneous

V2700 Balance lens, per lens
V2702 Deluxe lens feature
V2710 Slab off prism, glass or plastic, per lens
V2715 Prism, per lens
V2718 Press-on lens, Fresnel prism, per lens
V2730 Special base curve, glass or plastic, per lens
V2744 Tint, photochromatic, per lens
V2745 Addition to lens; tint, any color, solid, gradient or equal, excludes photochromatic, any lens material, per lens
V2750 Antireflective coating, per lens
V2755 U-V lens, per lens
V2756 Eye glass case
V2760 Scratch resistant coating, per lens
V2761 Mirror coating, any type, solid, gradient or equal, any lens material, per lens
V2762 Polarization, any lens material, per lens
V2770 Occluder lens, per lens
V2780 Oversize lens, per lens
V2781 Progressive lens, per lens
V2782 Lens, index 1.54 to 1.65 plastic or 1.60 to 1.79 glass, excludes polycarbonate, per lens
V2783 Lens, index greater than or equal to 1.66 plastic or greater than or equal to 1.80 glass, excludes polycarbonate, per lens
V2784 Lens, polycarbonate or equal, any index, per lens
V2785 Processing, preserving and transporting corneal tissue
Medicare jurisdiction: local contractor.
CMS: 100-04,4,200.1
V2786 Specialty occupational multifocal lens, per lens
V2787 Astigmatism correcting function of intraocular lens
CMS: 100-04,32,120.1; 100-04,32,120.2
V2788 Presbyopia correcting function of intraocular lens
CMS: 100-04,32,120.1; 100-04,32,120.2
V2790 Amniotic membrane for surgical reconstruction, per procedure
Medicare jurisdiction: local contractor.
CMS: 100-04,4,200.4
V2797 Vision supply, accessory and/or service component of another HCPCS vision code

V2799 Vision item or service, miscellaneous
Determine if an alternative HCPCS Level II or a CPT code better describes the service being reported. This code should be used only if a more specific code is unavailable.

Hearing Services V5008-V5364

This range of codes describes hearing tests and related supplies and equipment, speech-language pathology screenings, and repair of augmentative communicative system.

Hearing Services

V5008 Hearing screening
V5010 Assessment for hearing aid
V5011 Fitting/orientation/checking of hearing aid
V5014 Repair/modification of a hearing aid
V5020 Conformity evaluation

Monaural Hearing Aid

V5030 Hearing aid, monaural, body worn, air conduction
V5040 Hearing aid, monaural, body worn, bone conduction
V5050 Hearing aid, monaural, in the ear
V5060 Hearing aid, monaural, behind the ear

Other Hearing Services

V5070 Glasses, air conduction
V5080 Glasses, bone conduction
V5090 Dispensing fee, unspecified hearing aid
V5095 Semi-implantable middle ear hearing prosthesis
V5100 Hearing aid, bilateral, body worn
V5110 Dispensing fee, bilateral

Hearing Aids, Services, and Accessories

V5120 Binaural, body
V5130 Binaural, in the ear
V5140 Binaural, behind the ear
V5150 Binaural, glasses
V5160 Dispensing fee, binaural
V5171 Hearing aid, contralateral routing device, monaural, in the ear (ITE)
V5172 Hearing aid, contralateral routing device, monaural, in the canal (ITC)
V5181 Hearing aid, contralateral routing device, monaural, behind the ear (BTE)
V5190 Hearing aid, contralateral routing, monaural, glasses
V5200 Dispensing fee, contralateral, monaural
V5211 Hearing aid, contralateral routing system, binaural, ITE/ITE
V5212 Hearing aid, contralateral routing system, binaural, ITE/ITC
V5213 Hearing aid, contralateral routing system, binaural, ITE/BTE
V5214 Hearing aid, contralateral routing system, binaural, ITC/ITC
V5215 Hearing aid, contralateral routing system, binaural, ITC/BTE
V5221 Hearing aid, contralateral routing system, binaural, BTE/BTE
V5230 Hearing aid, contralateral routing system, binaural, glasses
V5240 Dispensing fee, contralateral routing system, binaural
V5241 Dispensing fee, monaural hearing aid, any type
V5242 Hearing aid, analog, monaural, CIC (completely in the ear canal)

Code	Description
V5243	Hearing aid, analog, monaural, ITC (in the canal)
V5244	Hearing aid, digitally programmable analog, monaural, CIC
V5245	Hearing aid, digitally programmable, analog, monaural, ITC
V5246	Hearing aid, digitally programmable analog, monaural, ITE (in the ear)
V5247	Hearing aid, digitally programmable analog, monaural, BTE (behind the ear)
V5248	Hearing aid, analog, binaural, CIC
V5249	Hearing aid, analog, binaural, ITC
V5250	Hearing aid, digitally programmable analog, binaural, CIC
V5251	Hearing aid, digitally programmable analog, binaural, ITC
V5252	Hearing aid, digitally programmable, binaural, ITE
V5253	Hearing aid, digitally programmable, binaural, BTE
V5254	Hearing aid, digital, monaural, CIC
V5255	Hearing aid, digital, monaural, ITC
V5256	Hearing aid, digital, monaural, ITE
V5257	Hearing aid, digital, monaural, BTE
V5258	Hearing aid, digital, binaural, CIC
V5259	Hearing aid, digital, binaural, ITC
V5260	Hearing aid, digital, binaural, ITE
V5261	Hearing aid, digital, binaural, BTE
V5262	Hearing aid, disposable, any type, monaural
V5263	Hearing aid, disposable, any type, binaural
V5264	Ear mold/insert, not disposable, any type
V5265	Ear mold/insert, disposable, any type
V5266	Battery for use in hearing device
V5267	Hearing aid or assistive listening device/supplies/accessories, not otherwise specified

Assistive Listening Device

Code	Description
V5268	Assistive listening device, telephone amplifier, any type
V5269	Assistive listening device, alerting, any type
V5270	Assistive listening device, television amplifier, any type
V5271	Assistive listening device, television caption decoder
V5272	Assistive listening device, TDD
V5273	Assistive listening device, for use with cochlear implant
V5274	Assistive listening device, not otherwise specified

Miscellaneous Hearing Services

Code	Description
V5275	Ear impression, each
V5281	Assistive listening device, personal FM/DM system, monaural (1 receiver, transmitter, microphone), any type
V5282	Assistive listening device, personal FM/DM system, binaural (2 receivers, transmitter, microphone), any type
V5283	Assistive listening device, personal FM/DM neck, loop induction receiver
V5284	Assistive listening device, personal FM/DM, ear level receiver
V5285	Assistive listening device, personal FM/DM, direct audio input receiver
V5286	Assistive listening device, personal blue tooth FM/DM receiver
V5287	Assistive listening device, personal FM/DM receiver, not otherwise specified
V5288	Assistive listening device, personal FM/DM transmitter assistive listening device
V5289	Assistive listening device, personal FM/DM adapter/boot coupling device for receiver, any type
V5290	Assistive listening device, transmitter microphone, any type
V5298	Hearing aid, not otherwise classified
V5299	Hearing service, miscellaneous

Determine if an alternative HCPCS Level II or a CPT code better describes the service being reported. This code should be used only if a more specific code is unavailable.

Speech-Language Pathology Services

Code	Description
V5336	Repair/modification of augmentative communicative system or device (excludes adaptive hearing aid)

Medicare jurisdiction: DME regional contractor.

Code	Description
V5362	Speech screening
V5363	Language screening
V5364	Dysphagia screening

Appendix 1 — Table of Drugs and Biologicals

INTRODUCTION AND DIRECTIONS

The HCPCS 2023 Table of Drugs and Biologicals is designed to quickly and easily direct the user to drug names and their corresponding codes. Both generic and brand or trade names are alphabetically listed in the "Drug Name" column of the table. The associated A, C, J, K, Q, or S code is given only for the generic name of the drug. While every effort is made to make the table comprehensive, it is not all-inclusive.

The "Unit Per" column lists the stated amount for the referenced generic drug as provided by CMS. "Up to" listings are inclusive of all quantities up to and including the listed amount. All other listings are for the amount of the drug as listed. The editors recognize that the availability of some drugs in the quantities listed is dependent on many variables beyond the control of the clinical ordering clerk. The availability in your area of regularly used drugs in the most cost-effective quantities should be relayed to your third-party payers.

The "Route of Administration" column addresses the most common methods of delivering the referenced generic drug as described in current pharmaceutical literature. The official definitions for Level II drug codes generally describe administration other than by oral method. Therefore, with a handful of exceptions, oral-delivered options for most drugs are omitted from the Route of Administration column.

Intravenous administration includes all methods, such as gravity infusion, injections, and timed pushes. When several routes of administration are listed, the first listing is simply the first, or most common, method as described in current reference literature. The "VAR" posting denotes various routes of administration and is used for drugs that are commonly administered into joints, cavities, tissues, or topical applications, in addition to other parenteral administrations. Listings posted with "OTH" alert the user to other administration methods, such as suppositories or catheter injections.

Please be reminded that the Table of Drugs and Biologicals, as well as all HCPCS Level II national definitions and listings, constitutes a post-treatment medical reference for billing purposes only. Although the editors have exercised all normal precautions to ensure the accuracy of the table and related material, the use of any of this information to select medical treatment is entirely inappropriate. Do not code directly from the table. Refer to the tabular section for complete information.

See Appendix 3 for abbreviations.

Drug Name	Unit Per	Route	Code
10% LMD	500 ML	IV	J7100
5% DEXTROSE AND .45% NORMAL SALINE	1000 ML	IV	S5010
5% DEXTROSE IN LACTATED RINGERS	1000 CC	IV	J7121
5% DEXTROSE WITH POTASSIUM CHLORIDE	1000 ML	IV	S5012
5% DEXTROSE/.45% NS WITH KCL AND MAG SULFATE	1000ML	IV	S5013
5% DEXTROSE/.45% NS WITH KCL AND MAG SULFATE	1500 ML	IV	S5014
5% DEXTROSE/NORMAL SALINE	5%	VAR	J7042
5% DEXTROSE/WATER	500 ML	IV	J7060
A-HYDROCORT	100 MG	IV, IM, SC	J1720
A-METHAPRED	40 MG	IM, IV	J2920
A-METHAPRED	125 MG	IM, IV	J2930
ABATACEPT	10 MG	IV	J0129
ABCIXIMAB	10 MG	IV	J0130
10% LMD	500 ML	IV	J7100

Drug Name	Unit Per	Route	Code
5% DEXTROSE AND .45% NORMAL SALINE	1000 ML	IV	S5010
5% DEXTROSE IN LACTATED RINGERS	1000 CC	IV	J7121
5% DEXTROSE WITH POTASSIUM CHLORIDE	1000 ML	IV	S5012
5% DEXTROSE/.45% NS WITH KCL AND MAG SULFATE	1000ML	IV	S5013
5% DEXTROSE/.45% NS WITH KCL AND MAG SULFATE	1500 ML	IV	S5014
5% DEXTROSE/NORMAL SALINE	5%	VAR	J7042
5% DEXTROSE/WATER	500 ML	IV	J7060
A-HYDROCORT	100 MG	IV, IM, SC	J1720
A-METHAPRED	40 MG	IM, IV	J2920
A-METHAPRED	125 MG	IM, IV	J2930
ABATACEPT	10 MG	IV	J0129
ABCIXIMAB	10 MG	IV	J0130
ABECMA	UP TO 460 MILLION CELLS	IV	Q2055
ABELCET	10 MG	IV	J0287
ABILIFY	0.25 MG	IM	J0400
ABILIFY MAINTENA KIT	1 MG	IM	J0401
ABLAVAR	1 ML	IV	A9583
ABOBOTULINUMTOXINA	5 UNITS	IM	J0586
ABRAXANE	1 MG	IV	J9264
ACCELULAR PERICARDIAL TISSUE MATRIX NONHUMAN	SQ CM	OTH	C9354
ACCUNEB NONCOMPOUNDED, CONCENTRATED	1 MG	INH	J7611
ACCUNEB NONCOMPOUNDED, UNIT DOSE	1 MG	INH	J7613
ACETADOTE	1 G	INH	J7608
ACETADOTE	100 MG	IV	J0132
ACETAMINOPHEN (B. BRAUN), NOT THERAPEUTICALLY EQUIVALENT TO J0131	10 MG	IV	J0136
ACETAMINOPHEN (FRESENIUS KABI), NOT THERAPEUTICALLY EQUIVALENT TO J0131	10 MG	IV	J0134
ACETAMINOPHEN NOS	10 MG	IV	J0131
ACETAZOLAMIDE SODIUM	500 MG	IM, IV	J1120
ACETYLCYSTEINE COMPOUNDED	PER G	INH	J7604
ACETYLCYSTEINE NONCOMPOUNDED	1 G	INH	J7608
ACTEMRA	1 MG	IV	J3262
ACTEMRA	1 MG	IV	Q0249
ACTHREL	1 MCG	IV	J0795
ACTIMMUNE	3 MU	SC	J9216
ACTIVASE	1 MG	IV	J2997
ACUTECT	STUDY DOSE UP TO 20 MCI	IV	A9504
ACYCLOVIR	5 MG	IV	J0133

Appendix 1 — Table of Drugs and Biologicals

2023 HCPCS Level II

Drug Name	Unit Per	Route	Code
ADAGEN	25 IU	IM	J2504
ADAKVEO	5 MG	IV	J0791
ADALIMUMAB	20 MG	SC	J0135
ADASUVE	1 MG	INH	J2062
ADCETRIS	1 MG	IV	J9042
ADENOCARD	1 MG	IV	J0153
ADENOSINE	1 MG	IV	J0153
ADENSOSCAN	1 MG	IV	J0153
ADO-TRASTUZUMAB EMTANSINE	1 MG	IV	J9354
ADRENALIN	0.1 MG	IM, IV, SC	J0171
ADRENOCORT	1 MG	IM, IV, OTH	J1100
ADRIAMYCIN	10 MG	IV	J9000
ADRUCIL	500 MG	IV	J9190
ADUCANUMAB-AVWA	2 MG	IV	J0172
ADUHELM	2 MG	IV	J0172
ADYNOVATE	1 IU	IV	J7207
AEROBID	1 MG	INH	J7641
AFAMELANOTIDE IMPLANT	1 MG	OTH	J7352
AFFINITY	SQ CM	OTH	Q4159
AFINITOR	0.25 MG	ORAL	J7527
AFLIBERCEPT	1 MG	OTH	J0178
AFLURIA	EA	IM	Q2035
AFSTYLA	1 I.U.	IV	J7210
AGALSIDASE BETA	1 MG	IV	J0180
AGGRASTAT	12.5 MG	IM, IV	J3246
AGRIFLU	UNKNOWN	IM	Q2034
AJOVY	1 MG	SC	J3031
AKYNZEO	300 MG/ 0.5 MG	ORAL	J8655
AKYNZEO	235 MG/ 0.25 MG	IV	J1454
ALATROFLOXACIN MESYLATE	100 MG	IV	J0200
ALBUTEROL AND IPRATROPIUM BROMIDE NONCOMPOUNDED	2.5MG/0.5 MG	INH	J7620
ALBUTEROL COMPOUNDED, CONCENTRATED	1 MG	INH	J7610
ALBUTEROL COMPOUNDED, UNIT DOSE	1 MG	INH	J7609
ALBUTEROL NONCOMPOUNDED, UNIT DOSE	1 MG	INH	J7613
ALBUTEROL, NONCOMPOUNDED, CONCENTRATED FORM	1 MG	INH	J7611
ALDESLEUKIN	1 VIAL	IV	J9015
ALDURAZYME	0.1 MG	IV	J1931
ALEFACEPT	0.5 MG	IV, IM	J0215
ALEMTUZUMAB	1 MG	IV	J0202
ALFERON N	250,000 IU	IM	J9215
ALGLUCERASE	10 U	IV	J0205
ALGLUCOSIDASE ALFA (LUMIZYME)	10 MG	IV	J0221
ALIQOPA	1 MG	IV	J9057
ALKERAN	2 MG	ORAL	J8600
ALLODERM	SQ CM	OTH	Q4116
ALLOGEN	1 CC	OTH	Q4212
ALLOGRAFT, CYMETRA	1 CC	INJ	Q4112
ALLOGRAFT, GRAFTJACKET EXPRESS	1 CC	INJ	Q4113
ALLOPATCHHD	SQ CM	OTH	Q4128

Drug Name	Unit Per	Route	Code
ALLOSKIN	SQ CM	OTH	Q4115
ALLOSKIN AC	SQ CM	OTH	Q4141
ALLOSKIN RT	SQ CM	OTH	Q4123
ALLOWRAP DS OR DRY	SQ CM	OTH	Q4150
ALOXI	25 MCG	IV	J2469
ALPHA 1-PROTENIASE INHIBITOR (HUMAN) (GLASSIA)	10 MG	IV	J0257
ALPHANATE	PER FACTOR VIII IU	IV	J7186
ALPHANINE SD	1 IU	IV	J7193
ALPROLIX	IU	IV	J7201
ALPROSTADIL	1.25 MCG	IV	J0270
ALPROSTADIL	EA	OTH	J0275
ALTEPLASE RECOMBINANT	1 MG	IV	J2997
ALTIPLY	SQ CM	OTH	Q4235
ALUPENT, NONCOMPOUNDED, CONCENTRATED	10 MG	INH	J7668
ALUPENT, NONCOMPOUNDED, UNIT DOSE	10 MG	INH	J7669
ALYMSYS	~~10 MG~~	~~IV~~	~~C9142~~
ALYMSYS	10 MG	IV	Q5126
AMANTADINE HCL (DEMONSTRATION PROJECT)	100 MG	ORAL	G9017
AMANTADINE HYDROCHLORIDE (BRAND NAME) (DEMONSTRTION PROJECT)	100 MG	ORAL	G9033
AMANTADINE HYDROCHLORIDE (GENERIC)	100 MG	ORAL	G9017
AMBISOME	10 MG	IV	J0289
AMCORT	5 MG	IM	J3302
AMELUZ	10 MG	OTH	J7345
AMERGAN	12.5 MG	ORAL	Q0169
AMEVIVE	0.5 MG	IV, IM	J0215
AMICAR	5 G	IV	S0017
AMIFOSTINE	500 MG	IV	J0207
AMIKACIN SULFATE	100 MG	IM, IV	J0278
AMINOCAPRIOC ACID	5 G	IV	S0017
AMINOLEVULINIC ACID HCL	354 MG	OTH	J7308
AMINOLEVULINIC ACID HCL	10 MG	OTH	J7345
AMINOPHYLLINE	250 MG	IV	J0280
AMIODARONE HCL	30 MG	IV	J0282
AMIODARONE HCL	30 MG	IV	J0283
AMITRIPTYLINE HCL	20 MG	IM	J1320
AMIVANTAMAB-VMJW	2 MG	IV	J9061
AMMONIA N-13	STUDY DOSE UP TO 40 MCI	IV	A9526
AMNIO-MAXX	SQ CM	OTH	Q4239
AMNIO-MAXX LITE	SQ CM	OTH	Q4239
AMNIOAMP-MP	SQ CM	OTH	Q4250
AMNIOARMOR	SQ CM	OTH	Q4188
AMNIOBAND	SQ CM	OTH	Q4151
AMNIOBAND	1 MG	OTH	Q4168
AMNIOBIND	SQ CM	OTH	Q4225
AMNIOCORE	SQ CM	OTH	Q4227
AMNIOCYTE PLUS	0.5 CC	OTH	Q4242
AMNIOEXCEL	SQ CM	OTH	Q4137
AMNIOEXCEL PLUS	SQ CM	OTH	Q4137
AMNIOMATRIX	1 CC	OTH	Q4139

Drug Name	Unit Per	Route	Code
AMNION BIO	SQ CM	OTH	Q4211
AMNIOREPAIR	SQ CM	OTH	Q4235
AMNIOTEXT	1 CC	OTH	Q4245
AMNIOTEXT PATCH	SQ CM	OTH	Q4247
AMNIOWOUND	SQ CM	OTH	Q4181
AMNIOWRAP2	SQ CM	OTH	Q4221
AMNIPLY	SQ CM	OTH	Q4249
AMOBARBITAL	125 MG	IM, IV	J0300
AMONDYS 45	10 MG	IV	J1426
AMPHOCIN	50 MG	IV	J0285
AMPHOTEC	10 MG	IV	J0287
AMPHOTERICIN B	50 MG	IV	J0285
AMPHOTERICIN B CHOLESTERYL SULFATE COMPLEX	10 MG	IV	J0288
AMPHOTERICIN B LIPID COMPLEX	10 MG	IV	J0287
AMPHOTERICIN B LIPOSOME	10 MG	IV	J0289
AMPICILLIN SODIUM	500 MG	IM, IV	J0290
AMPICILLIN SODIUM/SULBACTAM SODIUM	1.5 G	IM, IV	J0295
AMVUTTRA	1 MG	SC	J0225
AMYGDALIN	VAR	INJ	J3570
AMYTAL	125 MG	IM, IV	J0300
AMYVID	UP TO 10 MILLICUIRES	IV	A9586
AN-DTPA DIAGNOSTIC	STUDY DOSE UP TO 25 MCI	IV	A9539
AN-DTPA THERAPEUTIC	STUDY DOSE UP TO 25 MCI	INH	A9567
ANASCORP	UP TO 120 MG	IV	J0716
ANASTROZOLE	1 MG	ORAL	S0170
ANAVIP	120 MG	IV	J0841
ANCEF	500 MG	IM, IV	J0690
ANDEXXA	10 MG	IV	J7169
ANECTINE	20 MG	IM, IV	J0330
ANGIOMAX	1 MG	IV	J0583
ANIDULAFUNGIN	1 MG	IV	J0348
ANIFROLUMAB-FNIA	1 MG	IV	C9086
ANIFROLUMAB-FNIA	1 MG	IV	J0491
ANISTREPLASE	30 U	IV	J0350
ANJESO	1 MG	IV	J1738
ANNOVERA VAGINAL RING	0.15 MG/ 0.013 MG	OTH	J7294
ANTAGON	250 MCG	SC	S0132
ANTI-INHIBITOR	1 IU	IV	J7198
ANTI-THYMOCYTE GLOBULIN,EQUINE	250 MG	OTH	J7504
ANTIEMETIC DRUG NOS	VAR	ORAL	J8597
ANTIHEMOPHILIC FACTOR PORCINE	1 IU	IV	J7191
ANTIHEMOPHILIC FACTOR VIII, XYNTHA, RECOMBINANT	1 IU	IV	J7185
ANTIHEMOPHILIC FACTOR VIII/ VON WILLEBRAND FACTOR COMPLEX, HUMAN	PER FACTOR VIII IU	IV	J7186
ANTITHROMBIN RECOMBINANT	50 IU	IV	J7196
ANTIZOL	15 MG	IV	J1451
ANZEMET	10 MG	IV	J1260
ANZEMET	50 MG	ORAL	S0174
ANZEMET	100 MG	ORAL	Q0180

Drug Name	Unit Per	Route	Code
APIS	SQ CM	OTH	A2010
APLIGRAF	SQ CM	OTH	Q4101
APOKYN	1 MG	SC	J0364
APOMORPHINE HYDROCHLORIDE	1 MG	SC	J0364
APREPITANT	1 MG	IV	J0185
APREPITANT	5 MG	ORAL	J8501
APRETUDE	1 MG	IM	J0739
APROTININ	10,000 KIU	IV	J0365
AQUAMEPHYTON	1 MG	IM, SC, IV	J3430
ARA-C	100 MG	SC, IV	J9100
ARALEN	UP TO 250 MG	IM, IV	J0390
ARAMINE	10 MG	IV, IM, SC	J0380
ARANESP, ESRD USE	1 MCG	SC, IV	J0882
ARANESP, NON-ESRD USE	1 MCG	SC, IV	J0881
ARBUTAMINE HCL	1 MG	IV	J0395
ARCALYST	1 MG	SC	J2793
ARCHITECT EXTRACELLULAR MATRIX	SQ CM	OTH	Q4147
AREDIA	30 MG	IV	J2430
ARFORMOTEROL	15 MCG	INH	J7605
ARGATROBAN	1 MG	IV	J0883
ARGATROBAN	1 MG	IV	J0884
ARGATROBAN (ACCORD), NOT THERAPEUTICALLY EQUIVALENT TO J0883 (FOR NON-ESRD USE)	1 MG	IV	J0891
ARGATROBAN (ACCORD), NOT THERAPEUTICALLY EQUIVALENT TO J0884 (FOR ESRD ON DIALYSIS)	1 MG	IV	J0892
ARGATROBAN (AUROMEDICS), NOT THERAPEUTICALLY EQUIVALENT TO J0883 (FOR ESRD ON DIALYSIS)	1 MG	IV	J0899
ARGATROBAN (AUROMEDICS), NOT THERAPEUTICALLY EQUIVALENT TO J0883 (FOR NON-ESRD USE)	1 MG	IV	J0898
ARIDOL	5 MG	INH	J7665
ARIMIDEX	1 MG	ORAL	S0170
ARIPIPRAZOLE	0.25 MG	IM	J0400
ARIPIPRAZOLE LAUROXIL	1 MG	IM	J1943
ARIPIPRAZOLE LAUROXIL	1 MG	IM	J1944
ARIPIPRAZOLE, EXTENDED RELEASE	1 MG	IM	J0401
ARISTADA	1 MG	IM	J1944
ARISTADA INITIO	1 MG	IM	J1943
ARISTOCORT	5 MG	IM	J3302
ARISTOCORTE FORTE	5 MG	IM	J3302
ARISTOCORTE INTRALESIONAL	5 MG	OTH	J3302
ARISTOSPAN	5 MG	VAR	J3303
ARIXTRA	0.5 MG	SC	J1652
AROMASIN	25 MG	ORAL	S0156
ARRANON	50 MG	IV	J9261
ARRESTIN	200 MG	IM	J3250
ARSENIC TRIOXIDE	1 MG	IV	J9017
ARTACENT AC	1 MG	OTH	Q4189
ARTACENT AC	SQ CM	OTH	Q4190
ARTACENT CORD	SQ CM	OTH	Q4216
ARTACENT WOUND	SQ CM	OTH	Q4169
ARTHROFLEX	SQ CM	OTH	Q4125

Appendix 1 — Table of Drugs and Biologicals

2023 HCPCS Level II

Drug Name	Unit Per	Route	Code
ARTISS FIBRIN SEALANT	2 ML	OTH	C9250
ARZERRA	10 MG	IV	J9302
ASCENIV	500 MG	IV	J1554
ASCENT	0.5 MG	OTH	Q4213
ASPARAGINASE	1,000 IU	IM,IV,SC	J9019
ASPARAGINASE, RECOMBINANT	0.1 MG	IM	J9021
ASPARLAS	10 UNITS	IV	J9118
ASTAGRAF XL	0.1 MG	ORAL	J7508
ASTRAMORPH PF	10 MG	OTH	J2274
ATEZOLIZUMAB	10 MG	INF	J9022
ATGAM	250 MG	OTH	J7504
ATIVAN	2 MG	IM, IV	J2060
ATOPICLAIR	ANY SIZE	OTH	A6250
ATROPEN	0.01 MG	IM	J0461
ATROPINE SULFATE	0.01 MG	IM, IV, SC	J0461
ATROPINE, COMPOUNDED, CONCENTRATED	I MG	INH	J7635
ATROPINE, COMPOUNDED, UNIT DOSE	1 MG	INH	J7636
ATROVENT, NONCOMPOUNDED, UNIT DOSE	1 MG	INH	J7644
ATRYN	50 IU	IV	J7196
AUROTHIOGLUCOSE	50 MG	IM	J2910
AUTOPLEX T	1 IU	IV	J7198
~~AVALGLUCOSIDASE ALFA-NGPT~~	~~4 MG~~	~~IV~~	~~C9085~~
AVALGLUCOSIDASE ALFA-NGPT	4 MG	IV	J0219
AVASTIN	0.25 MG	IV	C9257
AVASTIN	10 MG	IV	J9035
AVEED	1 MG	IM	J3145
AVELOX	100 MG	IV	J2280
AVELUMAB	10 MG	INF	J9023
AVONEX	30 MCG	IM	J1826
AVONEX	1 MCG	IM	Q3027
AVSOLA	10 MG	IV	Q5121
AVYCAZ	0.5 G/0.125 G	IV	J0714
AXICABTAGENE CILOLEUCEL	UP TO 200 MILLION CELLS	IV	Q2041
AXOBIOMEMBRANE	SQ CM	OTH	Q4211
AXOLOTL AMBIENT, AXOLOTL CRYO	0.1 MG	OTH	Q4215
AXOLOTL GRAFT, AXOLOTL DUALGRAFT	SQ CM	OTH	Q4210
AXUMIN	1 MCI	IV	A9588
AZACITIDINE	1 MG	SC	J9025
AZACTAM	500 MG	IV	S0073
AZASAN	50 MG	ORAL	J7500
AZATHIOPRINE	50 MG	ORAL	J7500
AZATHIOPRINE	100 MG	OTH	J7501
AZEDRA	1 MCI	IV	A9590
AZITHROMYCIN	1 G	ORAL	Q0144
AZITHROMYCIN	500 MG	IV	J0456
AZMACORT	PER MG	INH	J7684
AZMACORT CONCENTRATED	PER MG	INH	J7683
AZTREONAM	500 MG	IV, IM	S0073
BACLOFEN	50 MCG	IT	J0476
BACLOFEN	10 MG	IT	J0475
BACTOCILL	250 MG	IM, IV	J2700
BACTRIM IV	10 ML	IV	S0039

Drug Name	Unit Per	Route	Code
BAL	100 MG	IM	J0470
BAMLANIVIMAB AND ETESEVIMAB	2100 MG	IV	Q0245
BASILIXIMAB	20 MG	IV	J0480
BAVENCIO	10 MG	INF	J9023
BAXDELA	1 MG	ORAL, IV	C9462
BCG LIVE INTRAVESICAL	1 MG	OTH	J9030
BEBTELOVIMAB	175 MG	IV	Q0222
BEBULIN VH	1 IU	IV	J7194
BECAPLERMIN GEL 0.01%	0.5 G	OTH	S0157
BECLOMETHASONE COMPOUNDED	1 MG	INH	J7622
BECLOVENT COMPOUNDED	1 MG	INH	J7622
BECONASE COMPOUNDED	1 MG	INH	J7622
BELANTAMAB MAFODONTIN-BLMF	0.5 MG	IV	J9037
BELATACEPT	1 MG	IV	J0485
BELEODAQ	10 MG	IV	J9032
BELIMUMAB	10 MG	IV	J0490
BELINOSTAT	10 MG	IV	J9032
BELLACELL HD	SQ CM	OTH	Q4220
BELRAPZO	1 MG	IV	J9036
BENA-D 10	50 MG	IV, IM	J1200
BENA-D 50	50 MG	IV, IM	J1200
BENADRYL	50 MG	IV, IM	J1200
BENAHIST 10	50 MG	IV, IM	J1200
BENAHIST 50	50 MG	IV, IM	J1200
BENDAMUSTINE HCL	1 MG	IV	J9033
BENDAMUSTINE HCL	1 MG	IV	J9034
BENDAMUSTINE HYDROCHLORIDE	1 MG	IV	J9036
BENDEKA	1 MG	IV	J9034
BENLYSTA	10 MG	IV	J0490
BENOJECT-10	50 MG	IV, IM	J1200
BENOJECT-50	50 MG	IV, IM	J1200
BENRALIZUMAB	1 MG	SC	J0517
BENTYL	20 MG	IM	J0500
BENZTROPINE MESYLATE	1 MG	IM, IV	J0515
BEOVU	1 MG	INJ	J0179
BERINERT	10 U	IV	J0597
BERUBIGEN	1,000 MCG	SC, IM	J3420
BESPONSA	0.1 MG	IV	J9229
BETA-2	1 MG	INH	J7648
BETALIN 12	1,000 MCG	SC, IM	J3420
BETAMETHASONE ACETATE AND BETAMETHASONE SODIUM PHOSPHATE	3 MG/3 MG	IM	J0702
BETAMETHASONE COMPOUNDED, UNIT DOSE	1 MG	INH	J7624
BETASERON	0.25 MG	SC	J1830
BETHANECHOL CHLORIDE, MYOTONACHOL OR URECHOLINE	5 MG	SC	J0520
BEVACIZUMAB	10 MG	IV	J9035
BEVACIZUMAB	0.25 MG	IV	C9257
BEVACIZUMAB-AWWB, BIOSIMILAR	10 MG	IV	Q5107
BEVACIZUMAB-BVZR, BIOSIMILAR	10 MG	IV	Q5118
~~BEVACIZUMAB-MALY, BIOSIMILAR~~	~~10 MG~~	~~IV~~	~~C9142~~

4 — Appendixes

© 2022 Optum, Inc.

Drug Name	Unit Per	Route	Code
BEVACIZUMAB-MALY, BIOSIMILAR, (ALYMSYS)	10 MG	IV	Q5126
BEZLOTOXUMAB	10 MG	INF	J0565
BICILLIN CR	100,000 UNITS	IM	J0558
BICILLIN CR 900/300	100,000 UNITS	IM	J0558
BICILLIN CR TUBEX	100,000 UNITS	IM	J0558
BICILLIN LA	100,000 U	IM	J0561
BICNU	100 MG	IV	J9050
BIMATOPROST, INTRACAMERAL IMPLANT	1 MCG	OTH	J7351
BIO-CONNEKT	SQ CM	OTH	Q4161
BIO-CONNEKT WOUND MATRIX	SQ CM	OTH	A2003
BIODEXCEL	SQ CM	OTH	Q4137
BIODFENCE	SQ CM	OTH	Q4140
BIODFENCE DRYFLEX	SQ CM	OTH	Q4138
BIODMATRIX	1 CC	OTH	Q4139
BIOSKIN	SQ CM	OTH	Q4163
BIOSKIN FLOW	SQ CM	OTH	Q4162
BIOTROPIN	1 MG	SC	J2941
BIOVANCE	SQ CM	OTH	Q4154
BIOWOUND, BIOWOUND PLUS, BIOWOUND XPLUS	SQ CM	OTH	Q4217
BIPERIDEN LACTATE	5 MG	IM, IV	J0190
BITOLTEROL MESYLATE, COMPOUNDED CONCENTRATED	PER MG	INH	J7628
BITOLTEROL MESYLATE, COMPOUNDED UNIT DOSE	PER MG	INH	J7629
BIVALIRUDIN	1 MG	IV	J0583
BIVIGAM	500 MG	IV	J1556
BLENOXANE	15 U	IM, IV, SC	J9040
BLENREP	0.5 MG	IV	J9037
BLEOMYCIN LYOPHILLIZED	15 U	IM, IV, SC	J9040
BLEOMYCIN SULFATE	15 U	IM, IV, SC	J9040
BLINATUMOMAB	1 MCG	IV	J9039
BLINCYTO	1 MCG	IV	J9039
BONIVA	1 MG	IV	J1740
BORTEZOMIB	0.1 MG	IV, SC	J9041
BORTEZOMIB (FRESENIUS KABI), NOT THERAPEUTICALLY EQUIVALENT TO J9041	0.1 MG	IV	J9048
BORTEZOMIB (HOSPIRA), NOT THERAPEUTICALLY EQUIVALENT TO J9041	0.1 MG	IV	J9049
BORTEZOMIB, (DR. REDDY'S), NOT THERAPEUTICALLY EQUIVALENT TO J9041	0.1 MG	IV	J9046
BOTOX	1 UNIT	IM, OTH	J0585
BOTOX COSMETIC	1 UNIT	IM, OTH	J0585
BOTULINUM TOXIN TYPE A	1 UNIT	IM, OTH	J0585
BOTULINUM TOXIN TYPE B	100 U	OTH	J0587
BRAVELLE	75 IU	SC, IM	J3355
BRENTUXIMAB VEDOTIN	1 MG	IV	J9042
BRETHINE	PER MG	INH	J7681
BRETHINE CONCENTRATED	PER MG	INH	J7680
BREXANOLONE	1 MG	IV	J1632
BREXUCABTAGENE AUTOLEUCEL	UP TO 200 MILLION CELLS	IV	Q2053
BREYANZI	UP TO 110 MILLION CELLS	IV	Q2054

Drug Name	Unit Per	Route	Code
BRICANYL	PER MG	INH	J7681
BRICANYL CONCENTRATED	PER MG	INH	J7680
BRINEURA	1 MG	OTH	J0567
BROLUCIZUMAB-DBLL	1 MG	INJ	J0179
BROM-A-COT	10 MG	IM, SC, IV	J0945
BROMPHENIRAMINE MALEATE	10 MG	IM, SC, IV	J0945
BUDESONIDE COMPOUNDED, CONCETRATED	0.25 MG	INH	J7634
BUDESONIDE, COMPOUNDED, UNIT DOSE	0.5 MG	INH	J7627
BUDESONIDE, NONCOMPOUNDED, CONCENTRATED	0.25 MG	INH	J7633
BUDESONIDE, NONCOMPOUNDED, UNIT DOSE	0.5 MG	INH	J7626
BUMETANIDE	0.5 MG	IM, IV	S0171
BUNAVAIL	2.1 MG	ORAL	J0572
BUNAVAIL	6.3 MG	ORAL	J0574
BUNAVAIL	4.2 MG	ORAL	J0573
BUPIVACAINE	1 MG	INJ	C9144
BUPIVACAINE AND MELOXICAM	1 MG/0.03 MG	OTH	C9088
BUPIVACAINE HCL	30 ML	VAR	S0020
BUPIVACAINE LIPOSOME	1 MG	VAR	C9290
BUPIVACAINE, COLLAGEN-MATRIX IMPLANT	1 MG	OTH	C9089
BUPRENEX	0.1 MG	IM, IV	J0592
BUPRENORPHIN/NALOXONE	UP TO 3 MG	ORAL	J0572
BUPRENORPHIN/NALOXONE	> 10 MG	ORAL	J0575
BUPRENORPHINE EXTENDED-RELEASE	> 100 MG	SC	Q9992
BUPRENORPHINE EXTENDED-RELEASE	≤ 100 MG	SC	Q9991
BUPRENORPHINE HCL	0.1 MG	IM, IV	J0592
BUPRENORPHINE IMPLANT	74.2 MG	OTH	J0570
BUPRENORPHINE ORAL	1 MG	ORAL	J0571
BUPRENORPHINE/NALOXONE	3.1 TO 6 MG	ORAL	J0573
BUPRENORPHINE/NALOXONE	6.1 TO 10 MG	ORAL	J0574
BUPROPION HCL	150 MG	ORAL	S0106
BUROSUMAB-TWZA	1 MG	SC	J0584
BUSULFAN	1 MG	IV	J0594
BUSULFAN	2 MG	ORAL	J8510
BUSULFEX	2 MG	ORAL	J8510
BUTORPHANOL TARTRATE	2 MG	IM, IV	J0595
BUTORPHANOL TARTRATE	25 MG	OTH	S0012
BYOOVIZ	0.1 MG	INJ	Q5124
C-1 ESTERASE INHIBITOR (HUMAN)	10 UNITS	SC	J0599
C1 ESTERASE INHIBITOR (HUMAN) (BERINERT)	10 UNITS	IV	J0597
C1 ESTERASE INHIBITOR (HUMAN) (CINRYZE)	10 UNITS	IV	J0598
C1 ESTERASE INHIBITOR (RECOMBINANT)	10 UNITS	IV	J0596
CABAZITAXEL	1 MG	IV	J9043
CABENUVA	2 MG/3 MG	IM	J0741
CABERGOLINE	0.25 MG	ORAL	J8515
CABLIVI	1 MG	IV, SC	C9047
CABOTEGRAVIR	1 MG	IM	J0739
CABOTEGRAVIR AND RILPIVIRINE	2 MG/3 MG	IM	J0741

Appendix 1 — Table of Drugs and Biologicals

Drug Name	Unit Per	Route	Code
CAFCIT	5 MG	IV	J0706
CAFFEINE CITRATE	5 MG	IV	J0706
CALASPARGASE PEGOL-MKNL	10 UNITS	IV	J9118
CALCIJEX	0.25 MCG	INJ	S0169
CALCIJEX	0.1 MCG	IM	J0636
CALCIMAR	UP TO 400 U	SC, IM	J0630
CALCITONIN SALMON	400 U	SC, IM	J0630
CALCITRIOL	0.1 MCG	IM	J0636
CALCITROL	0.25 MCG	IM	S0169
CALCIUM DISODIUM VERSENATE	1,000 MG	IV, SC, IM	J0600
CALCIUM GLUCONATE (FRESENIUS KABI)	10 ML	IV	J0610
CALCIUM GLUCONATE (WG CRITICAL CARE)	10 ML	IV	J0611
CALCIUM GLYCEROPHOSPHATE AND CALCIUM LACTATE	10 ML	IM, SC	J0620
CALDOLOR	100 MG	IV	J1741
CAMCEVI	1 MG	SC	J1952
CAMPTOSAR	20 MG	IV	J9206
CANAKINUMAB	1 MG	SC	J0638
CANCIDAS	5 MG	IV	J0637
CAPECITABINE	150 MG	ORAL	J8520
CAPLACIZUMAB-YHDP	1 MG	IV, SC	C9047
CAPROMAB PENDETIDE	STUDY DOSE UP TO 10 MCI	IV	A9507
CAPSAICIN 8% PATCH	1 SQ CM	OTH	J7336
CARBIDOPA/LEVODOPA	5 MG/20 MG	ORAL	J7340
CARBOCAINE	10 ML	VAR	J0670
CARBOPLATIN	50 MG	IV	J9045
CARDIOGEN 82	STUDY DOSE UP TO 60 MCI	IV	A9555
CARDIOLITE	STUDY DOSE	IV	A9500
CAREPATCH	SQ CM	OTH	Q4236
CARFILZOMIB	1 MG	IV	J9047
CARMUSTINE	100 MG	IV	J9050
CARNITOR	1 G	IV	J1955
CARTICEL		OTH	J7330
~~CARVYKTI~~	~~UP TO 100 MILLION CELLS~~	~~IV~~	~~C9098~~
CARVYKTI	UP TO 100 MILLION CELLS	IV	Q2056
CASIMERSEN	10 MG	IV	J1426
CASIRIVIMAB AND IMDEVIMAB	2400 MG	IV	Q0243
CASIRIVIMAB AND IMDEVIMAB	600 MG	IV	Q0240
CASIRIVIMAB AND IMDEVIMAB	1200 MG	IV	Q0244
CASPOFUNGIN ACETATE	5 MG	IV	J0637
CATAPRES	1 MG	OTH	J0735
CATHFLO	1 MG	IV	J2997
CAVERJECT	1.25 MCG	VAR	J0270
CEA SCAN	STUDY DOSE UP TO 45 MCI	IV	A9568
CEENU	10 MG	ORAL	S0178
CEFAZOLIN SODIUM	500 MG	IM, IV	J0690
CEFAZOLIN SODIUM (BAXTER), NOT THERAPEUTICALLY EQUIVALENT TO J0690	500 MG	IV	J0689
CEFEPIME HCL	500 MG	IV	J0692

Drug Name	Unit Per	Route	Code
CEFEPIME HCL (B. BRAUN), NOT THERAPEUTICALLY EQUIVALENT TO MAXIPIME	500 MG	IV	J0703
CEFEPIME HCL (BAXTER), NOT THERAPEUTICALLY EQUIVALENT TO MAXIPIME	500 MG	IV	J0701
CEFIDEROCOL	10 MG	IV	J0699
CEFIZOX	500 MG	IV, IM	J0715
CEFOBID	1 G	IV	S0021
CEFOPERAZONE SODIUM	1 G	IV	S0021
CEFOTAN	500 MG	IM, IV	S0074
CEFOTAXIME SODIUM	1 GM	IV, IM	J0698
CEFOTETAN DISODIUM	500 MG	IM. IV	S0074
CEFOXITIN SODIUM	1 GM	IV, IM	J0694
CEFTAROLINE FOSAMIL	10 MG	IV	J0712
CEFTAZIDIME	500 MG	IM, IV	J0713
CEFTAZIDIME AND AVIBACTAM	0.5 G/0.125 G	IV	J0714
CEFTIZOXIME SODIUM	500 MG	IV, IM	J0715
CEFTOLOZANE AND TAZOBACTAM	50 MG/25 MG	IV	J0695
CEFTRIAXONE SODIUM	250 MG	IV, IM	J0696
CEFUROXIME	750 MG	IM, IV	J0697
CEFUROXIME SODIUM STERILE	750 MG	IM, IV	J0697
CELERA DUAL LAYER/MEMBRANE	SQ CM	OTH	Q4259
CELESTONE SOLUSPAN	3 MG/3 MG	IM	J0702
CELLCEPT	250 MG	ORAL	J7517
CELLESTA CORD	SQ CM	OTH	Q4214
CELLESTA FLOWABLE AMNION	0.5 CC	OTH	Q4185
CELLESTA OR CELLESTA DUO	SQ CM	OTH	Q4184
CEMIPLIMAB-RWLC	1 MG	IV	J9119
CENACORT FORTE	5 MG	IM	J3302
CENTRUROIDES (SCORPION) IMMUNE F(AB)2 (EQUINE)	UP TO 120 MG	IV	J0716
CEPHALOTHIN SODIUM	UP TO 1 G	INJ	J1890
CEPHAPIRIN SODIUM	1 G	IV	J0710
CEPTAZ	500 MG	IM, IV	J0713
CEREBRYX	50 MG	IM, IV	Q2009
CEREBRYX	750 MG	IM, IV	S0078
CEREDASE	10 U	IV	J0205
CERETEC	STUDY DOSE UP TO 25 MCI	IV	A9521
CEREZYME	10 U	IV	J1786
CERIANNA	1 MCI	IV	A9591
CERLIPONASE ALFA	1 MG	OTH	J0567
CERTOLIZUMAB PEGOL	1 MG	SC	J0717
CERUBIDINE	10 MG	IV	J9150
CESAMET	1 MG	ORAL	J8650
CETIRIZINE HCL	0.5 MG	IV	J1201
CETUXIMAB	10 MG	IV	J9055
CHEALAMIDE	150 MG	IV	J3520
CHLORAMBUCIL	2 MG	ORAL	S0172
CHLORAMPHENICOL SODIUM SUCCINATE	1 G	IV	J0720
CHLORDIAZEPOXIDE HCL	100 MG	IM, IV	J1990
CHLOROMYCETIN	1 G	IV	J0720
~~CHLOROPROCAINE HCL~~	~~30 ML~~	~~VAR~~	~~J2400~~
CHLOROPROCAINE HCL	1 MG	INJ	J2401
CHLOROPROCAINE HCL (CLOROTEKAL)	1 MG	INJ	J2402

Drug Name	Unit Per	Route	Code
CHLOROQUINE HCL	UP TO 250 MG	IM, IV	J0390
CHLOROTHIAZIDE SODIUM	500 MG	IV	J1205
CHLORPROMAZINE HCL	5 MG	ORAL	Q0161
CHLORPROMAZINE HCL	50 MG	IM, IV	J3230
CHOLETEC	STUDY DOSE UP TO 15 MCI	IV	A9537
CHOLINE C 11, DIAGNOSTIC, PER STUDY DOSE	UP TO 20 MCI	IV	A9515
CHOREX	1000 USP	IM	J0725
CHORIONIC GONADOTROPIN	1,000 USP U	IM	J0725
CHROMIC PHOSPHATE P32 (THERAPEUTIC)	1 MCI	IV	A9564
CHROMITOPE SODIUM	STUDY DOSE UP TO 250 UCI	IV	A9553
CHROMIUM CR-51 SODIUM IOTHALAMATE, DIAGNOSTIC	STUDY DOSE UP TO 250 UCI	IV	A9553
CIDOFOVIR	375 MG	IV	J0740
CILASTATIN SODIUM	250 MG	IV, IM	J0743
CILTACABTAGENE AUTOLEUCEL	UP TO 100 MILLION CELLS	IV	C9098
CILTACABTAGENE AUTOLEUCEL	UP TO 100 MILLION CELLS	IV	Q2056
CIMETIDINE HCL	300 MG	IM, IV	S0023
CIMZIA	1 MG	SC	J0717
CINACALCET	1 MG	ORAL	J0604
CINQUAIR	1 MG	IV	J2786
CINRZYE	10 UNITS	IV	J0598
CINVANTI	1 MG	IV	J0185
CIPLA	1 MG	SC, INJ	J1932
CIPRO	200 MG	IV	J0744
CIPROFLOXACIN FOR INTRAVENOUS INFUSION	200 MG	IV	J0744
CIPROFLOXACIN OTIC SUSPENSION	6 MG	OTIC	J7342
CIS-MDP	STUDY DOSE UP TO 30 MCI	IV	A9503
CIS-PYRO	STUDY DOSE UP TO 25 MCI	IV	A9538
CISPLATIN	10 MG	IV	J9060
CLADRIBINE	1 MG	IV	J9065
CLAFORAN	1 GM	IV, IM	J0698
CLARIX 100	SQ MC	OTH	Q4156
CLARIX CORD 1K	SQ CM	OTH	Q4148
CLARIXFLO	1 MG	OTH	Q4155
CLEOCIN PHOSPHATE	300 MG	IV	S0077
CLEVIDIPINE BUTYRATE	1 MG	IV	C9248
CLEVIPREX	1 MG	IV	C9248
CLINDAMYCIN PHOSPHATE	300 MG	IV	S0077
CLOFARABINE	1 MG	IV	J9027
CLOLAR	1 MG	IV	J9027
CLONIDINE HCL	1 MG	OTH	J0735
CLOZAPINE	25 MG	ORAL	S0136
CLOZARIL	25 MG	ORAL	S0136
COAGADEX	1 IU	IV	J7175
COAGULATION FACTOR XA (RECOMBINANT), INACTIVATED-ZHZO	10 MG	IV	J7169
COBAL	1,000 MCG	IM, SC	J3420
COBALT CO-57 CYNOCOBALAMIN, DIAGNOSTIC	STUDY DOSE UP TO 1 UCI	ORAL	A9559

Drug Name	Unit Per	Route	Code
COBATOPE 57	STUDY DOSE UP TO 1 UCI	ORAL	A9559
COBEX	1,000 MCG	SC, IM	J3420
COCAINE HYDROCHLORIDE NASAL SOLUTION	1 MG	OTH	C9046
COCAINE HYDROCHLORIDE NASAL SOLUTION (NUMBRINO)	1 MG	OTH	C9143
COCOON MEMBRANE	SQ CM	OTH	Q4264
CODEINE PHOSPHATE	30 MG	IM, IV, SC	J0745
COGENEX AMNIOTIC MEMBRANE	SQ CM	OTH	Q4229
COGENEX FLOWABLE AMNION	0.5 CC	OTH	Q4230
COGENTIN	1 MG	IM, IV	J0515
COGNEX	10 MG	ORAL	S0014
COLCHICINE	1 MG	IV	J0760
COLHIST	10 MG	IM, SC, IV	J0945
COLISTIMETHATE SODIUM	1 MG	INH	S0142
COLISTIMETHATE SODIUM	150 MG	IM, IV	J0770
COLL-E-DERM	SQ CM	OTH	Q4193
COLLAGEN BASED WOUND FILLER DRY FOAM	1 GM	OTH	A6010
COLLAGEN BASED WOUND FILLER, GEL/PASTE	1 GM	OTH	A6011
COLLAGEN MATRIX NERVE WRAP	0.5 CM	OTH	C9361
COLLAGEN NERVE CUFF	0.5 CM LENGTH	OTH	C9355
COLLAGEN WOUND DRESSING	SQ CM	OTH	Q4164
COLLAGENASE, CLOSTRIDIUM HISTOLYTICUM	0.01 MG	OTH	J0775
COLY-MYCIN M	150 MG	IM, IV	J0770
COMPAZINE	10 MG	IM, IV	J0780
COMPAZINE	5 MG	ORAL	S0183
COMPAZINE	5 MG	ORAL	Q0164
CONIVAPTAN HYDROCHLORIDE	1 MG	INJ	C9488
CONTRACEPTIVE SUPPLY, HORMONE CONTAINING PATCH	EACH	OTH	J7304
CONTRAST FOR ECHOCARDIOGRAM	STUDY	IV	A9700
COPANLISIB	1 MG	IV	J9057
COPAXONE	20 MG	SC	J1595
COPPER CU-64, DOTATATE, DIAGNOSTIC	1 MCI	IV	A9592
COPPER T MODEL TCU380A IUD COPPER WIRE/COPPER COLLAR	EA	OTH	J7300
CORDARONE	30 MG	IV	J0282
CORECYTE	0.5 CC	OTH	Q4240
CORETEXT	1 CC	OTH	Q4246
CORIFACT	1 IU	IV	J7180
CORPLEX	SQ CM	OTH	Q4232
CORPLEX P	1 CC	OTH	Q4231
CORTASTAT	1 MG	IM, IV, OTH	J1100
CORTASTAT LA	1 MG	IM	J1094
CORTICORELIN OVINE TRIFLUTATE	1 MCG	IV	J0795
CORTICOTROPIN	40 U	IV, IM, SC	J0800
CORTIMED	80 MG	IM	J1040
CORTROSYN	0.25 MG	IM, IV	J0834
CORVERT	1 MG	IV	J1742
COSELA	1 MG	IV	J1448
COSMEGEN	0.5 MG	IV	J9120
COSYNTROPIN	0.25 MG	IM, IV	J0834
COTOLONE	5 MG	ORAL	J7510

Appendix 1 — Table of Drugs and Biologicals

Drug Name	Unit Per	Route	Code
CRESEMBA	1 MG	IV	J1833
CRIZANLIZUMAB-TMCA	5 MG	IV	J0791
CROFAB	UP TO 1 GM	IV	J0840
CROMOLYN SODIUM COMPOUNDED	PER 10 MG	INH	J7632
CROMOLYN SODIUM NONCOMPOUNDED	10 MG	INH	J7631
CROTALIDAE IMMUNE F(AB')2 (EQUINE)	120 MG	IV	J0841
CROTALIDAE POLYVALENT IMMUNE FAB (OVINE)	UP TO 1 GM	IV	J0840
CRYO-CORD	SQ CM	OTH	Q4237
CRYSTAL B12	1,000 MCG	IM, SC	J3420
CRYSTICILLIN 300 A.S.	600,000 UNITS	IM, IV	J2510
CRYSTICILLIN 600 A.S.	600,000 UNITS	IM, IV	J2510
CRYSVITA	1 MG	SC	J0584
CUBICIN	1 MG	IV	J0878
CUTAQUIG	100 MG	IV	J1551
CUVITRU	100 MG	SC	J1555
CYANO	1,000 MCG	IM, SC	J3420
CYANOCOBALAMIN	1,000 MCG	IM, SC	J3420
CYANOCOBALAMIN COBALT 57/58	STUDY DOSE UP TO 1 UCI	IV	A9546
CYANOCOBALAMIN COBALT CO-57	STUDY DOSE UP TO 1 UCI	ORAL	A9559
CYCLOPHOSPHAMIDE	25 MG	ORAL	J8530
CYCLOPHOSPHAMIDE	10 MG	IV	C9087
CYCLOPHOSPHAMIDE	100 MG	IV	J9070
CYCLOPHOSPHAMIDE, (AUROMEDICS)	5 MG	IV	J9071
CYCLOSPORINE	25 MG	ORAL	J7515
CYCLOSPORINE	100 MG	ORAL	J7502
CYCLOSPORINE	250 MG	IV	J7516
CYGNUS	SQ CM	OTH	Q4170
CYGNUS MATRIX	SQ CM	OTH	Q4199
CYMETRA	1 CC	INJ	Q4112
CYRAMZA	5 MG	IV	J9308
CYSVIEW	STUDY DOSE	OTH	A9589
CYTAL	SQ CM	OTH	Q4166
CYTARABINE	100 MG	SC, IV	J9100
CYTARABINE LIPOSOME	10 MG	IT	J9098
CYTOGAM	VIAL	IV	J0850
CYTOMEGALOVIRUS IMMUNE GLOB	VIAL	IV	J0850
CYTOSAR-U	100 MG	SC, IV	J9100
CYTOTEC	200 MCG	ORAL	S0191
CYTOVENE	500 MG	IV	J1570
CYTOXAN	25 MG	ORAL	J8530
CYTOXAN	100 MG	IV	J9070
D.H.E. 45	1 MG	IM, IV	J1110
DACARBAZINE	100 MG	IV	J9130
DACLIZUMAB	25 MG	OTH	J7513
DACOGEN	1 MG	IV	J0894
DACTINOMYCIN	0.5 MG	IV	J9120
DALALONE	1 MG	IM, IV, OTH	J1100
DALALONE LA	1 MG	IM	J1094
DALBAVANCIN	5 MG	IV	J0875
DALTEPARIN SODIUM	2,500 IU	SC	J1645

Drug Name	Unit Per	Route	Code
DALVANCE	5 MG	IV	J0875
DANYELZA	1 MG	IV	J9348
DAPTOMYCIN	1 MG	IV	J0878
DAPTOMYCIN (HOSPIRA), NOT THERAPEUTICALLY EQUIVALENT TO J0878	1 MG	IV	J0877
DARATUMUMAB	10 MG	IV	J9145
DARATUMUMAB AND HYALURONIDASE-FIHJ	10 MG	SC	J9144
DARBEPOETIN ALFA, ESRD USE	1 MCG	SC, IV	J0882
DARBEPOETIN ALFA, NON-ESRD USE	1 MCG	SC, IV	J0881
DARZALEX	10 MG	IV	J9145
DARZALEX FASPRO	10 MG	SC	J9144
DATSCAN	STUDY DOSE	IV	A9584
DAUNORUBICIN	10 MG	IV	J9150
DAUNORUBICIN CITRATE, LIPOOSOMAL FORMULATION	10 MG	IV	J9151
DAUNOXOME	10 MG	IV	J9151
DDAVP	1 MCG	IV, SC	J2597
DECADRON	0.25 MG	ORAL	J8540
DECAJECT	1 MG	IM, IV, OTH	J1100
DECITABINE	1 MG	IV	J0894
DECITABINE (SUN PHARMA), NOT THERAPEUTICALLY EQUIVALENT TO J0894	1 MG	IV	J0893
DECOLONE-50	50 MG	IM	J2320
DEFEROXAMINE MESYLATE	500 MG	IM, SC, IV	J0895
DEGARELIX	1 MG	SC	J9155
DELAFLOXACIN	1 MG	ORAL, IV	C9462
DELATESTRYL	1 MG	IM	J3121
DELESTROGEN	10 MG	IM	J1380
DELTA-CORTEF	5 MG	ORAL	J7510
DEMADEX	10 MG	IV	J3265
DEMEROL	100 MG	IM, IV, SC	J2175
DENILEUKIN DIFTITOX	300 MCG	IV	J9160
DENOSUMAB	1 MG	SC	J0897
DEOXYCHOLIC ACID	1 MG	SC	J0591
DEPGYNOGEN	UP TO 5 MG	IM	J1000
DEPHENACEN-50	50 MG	IM, IV	J1200
DEPMEDALONE	40 MG	IM	J1030
DEPMEDALONE	80 MG	IM	J1040
DEPO-ESTRADIOL CYPIONATE	UP TO 5 MG	IM	J1000
DEPO-MEDROL	40 MG	IM, OTH	J1030
DEPO-MEDROL	80 MG	IM, OTH	J1040
DEPO-MEDROL	20 MG	IM, OTH	J1020
DEPO-TESTOSTERONE	1 MG	IM	J1071
DEPOCYT	10 MG	IT	J9098
DEPOGEN	UP TO 5 MG	IM	J1000
DERM-MAXX	SQ CM	OTH	Q4238
DERMA-GIDE	SQ CM	OTH	Q4203
DERMACELL, DERMACELL AWM OR DERMACELL AWM POROUS	SQ CM	OTH	Q4122
DERMACYTE AMNIOTIC MEMBRANE ALLOGRAFT	SQ CM	OTH	Q4248
DERMAGRAFT	SQ CM	OTH	Q4106
DERMAL SUBSTITUTE, NATIVE, NONDENATURED COLLAGEN, FETAL	0.5 SQ CM	OTH	C9358

Drug Name	Unit Per	Route	Code
DERMAL SUBSTITUTE, NATIVE, NONDENATURED COLLAGEN, NEONATAL	0.5 SQ CM	OTH	C9360
DERMAPURE	SQ CM	OTH	Q4152
DERMAVEST AND PLURIVEST	SQ CM	OTH	Q4153
DESFERAL	500 MG	IM, SC, IV	J0895
DESMOPRESSIN ACETATE	1 MCG	IV, SC	J2597
DETECTNET	1 MCI	IV	A9592
DEXAMETHASONE	0.25 MG	ORAL	J8540
DEXAMETHASONE 9%	1 MCG	OTH	J1095
DEXAMETHASONE ACETATE	1 MG	IM	J1094
DEXAMETHASONE ACETATE ANHYDROUS	1 MG	IM	J1094
DEXAMETHASONE INTRAVITREAL IMPLANT	0.1 MG	OTH	J7312
DEXAMETHASONE SODIUM PHOSPHATE	1 MG	IM, IV, OTH	J1100
DEXAMETHASONE, COMPOUNDED, CONCENTRATED	1 MG	INH	J7637
DEXAMETHASONE, COMPOUNDED, UNIT DOSE	1 MG	INH	J7638
DEXAMETHASONE, LACRIMAL OPHTHALMIC INSERT	0.1 MG	OTH	J1096
DEXASONE	1 MG	IM, IV, OTH	J1100
DEXEDRINE	5 MG	ORAL	S0160
DEXIM	1 MG	IM, IV, OTH	J1100
DEXONE	0.25 MG	ORAL	J8540
DEXONE	1 MG	IM, IV, OTH	J1100
DEXONE LA	1 MG	IM	J1094
DEXRAZOXANE HCL	250 MG	IV	J1190
DEXTENZA	0.1 MG	OTH	J1096
DEXTRAN 40	500 ML	IV	J7100
DEXTROAMPHETAMINE SULFATE	5 MG	ORAL	S0160
DEXTROSE	500 ML	IV	J7060
DEXTROSE, STERILE WATER, AND/OR DEXTROSE DILUENT/FLUSH	10 ML	VAR	A4216
DEXTROSE/SODIUM CHLORIDE	5%	VAR	J7042
DEXTROSE/THEOPHYLLINE	40 MG	IV	J2810
DEXTROSTAT	5 MG	ORAL	S0160
DEXYCU	1 MCG	OTH	J1095
DI-SPAZ	UP TO 20 MG	IM	J0500
DIALYSIS/STRESS VITAMINS	100 CAPS	ORAL	S0194
DIAMOX	500 MG	IM, IV	J1120
DIASTAT	5 MG	IV, IM	J3360
DIAZEPAM	5 MG	IV, IM	J3360
DIAZOXIDE	300 MG	IV	J1730
DIBENT	UP TO 20 MG	IM	J0500
DICLOFENAC SODIUM	0.5 MG	OTH	J1130
DICYCLOMINE HCL	20 MG	IM	J0500
DIDANOSINE (DDI)	25 MG	ORAL	S0137
DIDRONEL	300 MG	IV	J1436
DIETHYLSTILBESTROL DIPHOSPHATE	250 MG	INJ	J9165
DIFELIKEFALIN	0.1 MCG	IV	J0879
DIFLUCAN	200 MG	IV	J1450
DIGIBIND	VIAL	IV	J1162
DIGIFAB	VIAL	IV	J1162
DIGOXIN	0.5 MG	IM, IV	J1160
DIGOXIN IMMUNE FAB	VIAL	IV	J1162

Drug Name	Unit Per	Route	Code
DIHYDROERGOTAMINE MESYLATE	1 MG	IM, IV	J1110
DILANTIN	50 MG	IM, IV	J1165
DILAUDID	250 MG	OTH	S0092
DILAUDID	4 MG	SC, IM, IV	J1170
DIMENHYDRINATE	50 MG	IM, IV	J1240
DIMERCAPROL	100 MG	IM	J0470
DIMINE	50 MG	IV, IM	J1200
DINATE	50 MG	IM, IV	J1240
DIOVAL	10 MG	IM	J1380
DIOVAL 40	10 MG	IM	J1380
DIOVAL XX	10 MG	IM	J1380
DIPHENHYDRAMINE HCL	50 MG	ORAL	Q0163
DIPHENHYDRAMINE HCL	50 MG	IV, IM	J1200
DIPRIVAN	10 MG	IV	J2704
DIPYRIDAMOLE	10 MG	IV	J1245
DISOTATE	150 MG	IV	J3520
DIURIL	500 MG	IV	J1205
DIURIL SODIUM	500 MG	IV	J1205
DIZAC	5 MG	IV, IM	J3360
DMSO, DIMETHYL SULFOXIDE	50%, 50 ML	OTH	J1212
DOBUTAMINE HCL	250 MG	IV	J1250
DOBUTREX	250 MG	IV	J1250
DOCETAXEL	1 MG	IV	J9171
DOLASETRON MESYLATE	100 MG	ORAL	Q0180
DOLASETRON MESYLATE	10 MG	IV	J1260
DOLASETRON MESYLATE	50 MG	ORAL	S0174
DOLOPHINE	5 MG	ORAL	S0109
DOLOPHINE HCL	10 MG	IM, SC	J1230
DOMMANATE	50 MG	IM, IV	J1240
DOPAMINE HCL	40 MG	IV	J1265
DORIBAX	10 MG	IV	J1267
DORIPENEM	10 MG	IV	J1267
DORNASE ALPHA, NONCOMPOUNDED, UNIT DOSE	1 MG	INH	J7639
DOSTARLIMAB-GXLY	10 MG	IV	J9272
DOSTINEX	0.25 MG	ORAL	J8515
DOTAREM	0.1 ML	IV	A9575
DOXERCALCIFEROL	1 MG	IV	J1270
DOXORUBICIN HCL	10 MG	IV	J9000
DOXORUBICIN HYDROCHLORIDE, LIPOSOMAL, IMPORTED LIPODOX	10 MG	IV	Q2049
DRAMAMINE	50 MG	IM, IV	J1240
DRAMANATE	50 MG	IM, IV	J1240
DRAMILIN	50 MG	IM, IV	J1240
DRAMOCEN	50 MG	IM, IV	J1240
DRAMOJECT	50 MG	IM, IV	J1240
DRAXIMAGE MDP-10	STUDY DOSE UP TO 30 MCI	IV	A9503
DRAXIMAGE MDP-25	STUDY DOSE UP TO 30 MCI	IV	A9503
DRONABINAL	2.5 MG	ORAL	Q0167
DROPERIDOL	5 MG	IM, IV	J1790
DROPERIDOL AND FENTANYL CITRATE	2 ML	IM, IV	J1810
DROXIA	500 MG	ORAL	S0176
DTIC-DOME	100 MG	IV	J9130
DTPA	STUDY DOSE UP TO 25 MCI	IV	A9539

Appendix 1 — Table of Drugs and Biologicals

2023 HCPCS Level II

Drug Name	Unit Per	Route	Code
DTPA	STUDY DOSE UP TO 25 MCI	INH	A9567
DUAL LAYER IMPAX MEMBRANE	SQ CM	OTH	Q4262
DUOPA	5 MG/20 MG	ORAL	J7340
DURACILLIN A.S.	600,000 UNITS	IM, IV	J2510
DURACLON	1 MG	OTH	J0735
DURAGEN-10	10 MG	IM	J1380
DURAGEN-20	10 MG	IM	J1380
DURAGEN-40	10 MG	IM	J1380
DURAMORPH	500 MG	OTH	S0093
DURAMORPH PF	10 MG	OTH	J2274
DURO CORT	80 MG	IM	J1040
DUROLANE	1 MG	INJ	J7318
DURVALUMAB	10 MG	IV	J9173
DURYSTA	1 MCG	OTH	J7351
DYLOJECT	0.5 MG	OTH	J1130
DYMENATE	50 MG	IM, IV	J1240
DYPHYLLINE	500 MG	IM	J1180
DYSPORT	5 UNITS	IM	J0586
E.D.T.A.	150 MG	IV	J3520
ECALLANTIDE	1 MG	SC	J1290
ECHOCARDIOGRAM IMAGE ENHANCER OCTAFLUOROPROPANE	1 ML	IV	Q9956
ECHOCARDIOGRAM IMAGE ENHANCER PERFLEXANE	1 ML	IV	Q9955
ECULIZUMAB	10 MG	IV	J1300
EDARAVONE	1 MG	IV	J1301
EDETATE CALCIUM DISODIUM	1,000 MG	IV, SC, IM	J0600
EDETATE DISODIUM	150 MG	IV	J3520
EDEX	1.25 MCG	VAR	J0270
EFGARTIGIMOD ALFA-FCAB	2 MG	IV	J9332
ELAPRASE	1 MG	IV	J1743
ELAVIL	20 MG	IM	J1320
ELELYSO	10 U	IV	J3060
ELIGARD	7.5 MG	SC	J9217
ELITEK	0.5 MG	IM	J2783
ELLENCE	2 MG	IV	J9178
ELLIOTTS B SOLUTION	1 ML	IV, IT	J9175
ELOCTATE	IU	IV	J7205
ELOSULFASE ALFA	1 MG	IV	J1322
ELOTUZUMAB	1 MG	IV	J9176
ELOXATIN	0.5 MG	IV	J9263
ELSPAR	1,000 IU	IM, IV, SC	J9019
ELZONRIS	10 MCG	IV	J9269
EMAPALUMAB-LZSG	1 MG	IV	J9210
EMEND	5 MG	ORAL	J8501
EMEND	1 MG	IV	J1453
EMICIZUMAB-KXWH	0.5 MG	SC	J7170
EMINASE	30 U	IV	J0350
EMPLICITI	1 MG	IV	J9176
ENBREL	25 MG	IM, IV	J1438
ENDOXAN-ASTA	100 MG	IV	J9070
ENDRATE	150 MG	IV	J3520
ENFORTUMAB VEDOTIN-EJFV	0.25 MG	IV	J9177
ENFUVIRTIDE	1 MG	SC	J1324
ENHERTU	1 MG	IV	J9358

Drug Name	Unit Per	Route	Code
ENJAYMO	~~10 MG~~	~~IV~~	~~C9094~~
ENJAYMO	10 MG	IV	J1302
ENOXAPARIN SODIUM	10 MG	SC	J1650
ENTYVIO	1 MG	IV	J3380
ENVARSUS XR	0.25 MG	ORAL	J7503
ENVERSE	SQ CM	OTH	Q4258
EOVIST	1 ML	IV	A9581
EPICORD	SQ CM	OTH	Q4187
EPIFIX	SQ CM	OTH	Q4186
EPIFIX, INJECTABLE	1 MG	OTH	Q4145
EPINEPHRINE	0.1 MG	IM, IV, SC	J0171
EPINEPHRINE (BELCHER), NOT THERAPEUTICALLY EQUIVALENT TO J0171	0.1 MG	IV	J0173
EPIRUBICIN HCL	2 MG	IV	J9178
EPOETIN ALFA FOR ESRD DIALYSIS	100 U	INJ	Q4081
EPOETIN ALFA, BIOSIMILAR	100 UNITS	INJ, IV	Q5105
EPOETIN ALFA, BIOSIMILAR	1000 UNITS	INJ, IV	Q5106
EPOETIN ALFA, NON-ESRD USE	1,000 U	SC, IV	J0885
EPOETIN BETA FOR ESRD ON DIALYSIS	1 MCG	IV	J0887
EPOETIN BETA FOR NON-ESRD	1 MCG	IV, SC	J0888
EPOGEN/NON-ESRD	1,000 U	SC, IV	J0885
EPOPROSTENOL	0.5 MG	IV	J1325
EPOPROSTENOL STERILE DILUTANT	50 ML	IV	S0155
EPTIFIBATIDE	5 MG	IM, IV	J1327
EPTINEZUMAB-JJMR	1 MG	IV	J3032
ERAVACYCLINE	1 MG	IV	J0122
ERAXIS	1 MG	IV	J0348
ERBITUX	10 MG	IV	J9055
ERGAMISOL	50 MG	ORAL	S0177
ERGONOVINE MALEATE	0.2 MG	IM, IV	J1330
ERIBULIN MESYLATE	0.1 MG	IV	J9179
ERTAPENEM SODIUM	500 MG	IM, IV	J1335
ERYTHROCIN LACTOBIONATE	500 MG	IV	J1364
ESKETAMINE, NASAL SPRAY	1 MG	OTH	S0013
ESPEROCT	1 IU	IV	J7204
ESTONE AQUEOUS	1 MG	IM, IV	J1435
ESTRA-L 20	10 MG	IM	J1380
ESTRA-L 40	10 MG	IM	J1380
ESTRADIOL CYPIONATE	UP TO 5 MG	IM	J1000
ESTRADIOL L.A.	10 MG	IM	J1380
ESTRADIOL L.A. 20	10 MG	IM	J1380
ESTRADIOL L.A. 40	10 MG	IM	J1380
ESTRADIOL VALERATE	10 MG	IM	J1380
ESTRAGYN	1 MG	IV, IM	J1435
ESTRO-A	1 MG	IV, IM	J1435
ESTROGEN CONJUGATED	25 MG	IV, IM	J1410
ESTRONE	1 MG	IV, IM	J1435
ESTRONOL	1 MG	IM, IV	J1435
ETANERCEPT	25 MG	IM, IV	J1438
ETELCALCETIDE	0.1 MG	IV	J0606
ETEPLIRSEN	10 MG	INF	J1428
ETHAMOLIN	100 MG	IV	J1430
ETHANOLAMINE OLEATE	100 MG	IV	J1430
ETHINYL ESTRADIOL AND ETONOGESTREL VAGINAL RING	0.015 MG/ 0.12 MG	OTH	J7295

Drug Name	Unit Per	Route	Code
ETHYOL	500 MG	IV	J0207
ETIDRONATE DISODIUM	300 MG	IV	J1436
ETONOGESTREL	IMPLANT	OTH	J7307
ETOPOSIDE	50 MG	ORAL	J8560
ETOPOSIDE	10 MG	IV	J9181
EUFLEXXA	PER DOSE	INJ	J7323
EULEXIN	125 MG	ORAL	S0175
EVENITY	1 MG	SC	J3111
EVEROLIMUS	0.25 MG	ORAL	J7527
EVINACUMAB-DGNB	5 MG	IV	J1305
EVKEEZA	5 MG	IV	J1305
EVOMELA	1 MG	IV	J9246
EVUSHELD	300 MG	IM	Q0220
EVUSHELD	600 MG	IM	Q0221
EXAMETAZIME LABELED AUTOLOGOUS WHITE BLOOD CELLS, TECHNETIUM TC-99M	STUDY DOSE	IV	A9569
EXCELLAGEN	0.1 CC	OTH	Q4149
EXMESTANE	25 MG	ORAL	S0156
EXONDYS 51	10 MG	INF	J1428
EXPAREL	1 MG	VAR	C9290
EZ-DERM	SQ CM	OTH	Q4136
FABRAZYME	1 MG	IV	J0180
FACTOR IX (ANTIHEMOPHILIC FACTOR, RECOMBINANT), RIXIBUS, PER I.U.	IU	IV	J7200
FACTOR IX NON-RECOMBINANT	1 IU	IV	J7193
FACTOR IX+ COMPLEX	1 IU	IV	J7194
FACTOR IX, (ANTIHEMOPHILIC FACTOR, RECOMBINANT), GLYCOPEGYLATED	1 IU	IV	J7203
FACTOR IX, ALBUMIN FUSION PROTEIN, (RECOMBINANT)	1 IU	IV	J7202
FACTOR IX, FC FUSION PROTEIN (ANTIHEMOPHILIC FACTOR, RECOMBINANT), ALPROLIX	IU	IV	J7201
FACTOR VIIA (ANTIHEMOPHILIC FACTOR, RECOMBINANT)-JNCW	1 MCG	IV	J7212
FACTOR VIIA RECOMBINANT	1 MCG	IV	J7189
FACTOR VIII (ANTIHEMOPHILIC FACTOR, RECOMBINANT)	1 IU	IV	J7209
FACTOR VIII (ANTIHEMOPHILIC FACTOR, RECOMBINANT)	IU	IV	J7188
FACTOR VIII (ANTIHEMOPHILIC FACTOR, RECOMBINANT) (NOVOEIGHT), PER IU	IU	INJ	J7182
FACTOR VIII (ANTIHEMOPHILIC FACTOR, RECOMBINANT) PEGYLATED	1 IU	IV	J7207
FACTOR VIII FC FUSION (RECOMBINANT)	IU	IV	J7205
FACTOR VIII PORCINE	1 IU	IV	J7191
FACTOR VIII, (ANTIHEMOPHILIC FACTOR, RECOMBINANT) (AFSTYLA)	1 I.U.	IV	J7210
FACTOR VIII, (ANTIHEMOPHILIC FACTOR, RECOMBINANT) (KOVALTRY)	1 I.U.	IV	J7211
FACTOR VIII, (ANTIHEMOPHILIC FACTOR, RECOMBINANT), PEGYLATED-AUCL	1 IU	IV	J7208

Drug Name	Unit Per	Route	Code
FACTOR VIII, ANTIHEMOPHILIC FACTOR (RECOMBINANT), GLYCOPEGYLATED-EXEI	1 IU	IV	J7204
FACTOR VIII, HUMAN	1 IU	IV	J7190
FACTOR X (HUMAN)	1 IU	IV	J7175
FACTOR XIII (ANTIHEMOPHILIC FACTOR, HUMAN)	1 IU	IV	J7180
FACTOR XIII A-SUBUNIT (RECOMBINANT)	10 IU	IV	J7181
FACTREL	100 MCG	SC, IV	J1620
FAM-TRASTUZUMAB DERUXTECAN-NXKI	1 MG	IV	J9358
FAMOTIDINE	20 MG	IV	S0028
FARICIMAB-SVOA	0.1 MG	INJ	C9097
FARICIMAB-SVOA	0.1 MG	INJ	J2777
FASENRA	1 MG	SC	J0517
FASLODEX	25 MG	IM	J9395
FDG	STUDY DOSE UP TO 45 MCI	IV	A9552
FEIBA-VH AICC	1 IU	IV	J7198
FENSOLVI	0.25 MG	SC	J1951
FENTANYL CITRATE	0.1 MG	IM, IV	J3010
FERAHEME (FOR ESRD)	1 MG	IV	Q0139
FERAHEME (NON-ESRD)	1 MG	IV	Q0138
FERIDEX IV	1 ML	IV	Q9953
FERRIC CARBOXYMALTOSE	1 MG	IV	J1439
FERRIC DERISOMALTOSE	10 MG	IV	J1437
FERRIC PYROPHOSPHATE CITRATE POWDER	0.1 MG	IV	J1444
FERRIC PYROPHOSPHATE CITRATE SOLUTION	0.1 MG	IV	J1443
FERRIC PYROPHOSPHATE CITRATE SOLUTION	0.1 MG	IV	J1445
FERRLECIT	12.5 MG	IV	J2916
FERTINEX	75 IU	SC	J3355
FERUMOXYTOL (FOR ESRD)	1 MG	IV	Q0139
FERUMOXYTOL (NON-ESRD)	1 MG	IV	Q0138
FETROJA	10 MG	IV	J0699
FIBRIN SEALANT (HUMAN)	2 ML	OTH	C9250
FIBRYGA	1 MG	IV	J7177
FILGRASTIM	1 MCG	SC, IV	J1442
FILGRASTIM-AAFI, BIOSIMILAR	1 MCG	INJ	Q5110
FILGRASTIM-AYOW, BIOSIMILAR	1 MCG	SC	C9096
FILGRASTIM-AYOW, BIOSIMILAR	1 MCG	SC, IV	Q5125
FILGRASTIM-SNDZ, BIOSIMILAR	1 MCG	IV, SC	Q5101
FINASTERIDE	5 MG	ORAL	S0138
FIRAZYR	1 MG	SC	J1744
FIRMAGON	1 MG	SC	J9155
FISH OIL TRIGLYCERIDES	10 G	IV	B4187
FLAGYL	500 MG	IV	S0030
FLEBOGAMMA	500 MG	IV	J1572
FLEXHD	SQ CM	OTH	Q4128
FLEXON	60 MG	IV, IM	J2360
FLOLAN	0.5 MG	IV	J1325
FLORBETABEN F-18, DIAGNOSTIC	STUDY DOSE UP TO 8.1 MCI	IV	Q9983
FLORTAUCIPIR F-18, DIAGNOSTIC	1 MCI	IV	A9601
FLOWERAMNIOFLO	SQ CM	OTH	Q4177
FLOWERAMNIOPATCH	SQ CM	OTH	Q4178

Appendix 1 — Table of Drugs and Biologicals

2023 HCPCS Level II

Drug Name	Unit Per	Route	Code
FLOWERDERM	SQ CM	OTH	Q4179
FLOXIN IV	400 MG	IV	S0034
FLOXURIDINE	500 MG	IV	J9200
FLUCICLOVINE F-18, DIAGNOSTIC	1 MCI	IV	A9588
FLUCONAZOLE	200 MG	IV	J1450
FLUDARA	50 MG	IV	J9185
FLUDARABINE PHOSPHATE	10 MG	ORAL	J8562
FLUDARABINE PHOSPHATE	50 MG	IV	J9185
FLUDEOXYGLUCOSE F18	STUDY DOSE UP TO 45 MCI	IV	A9552
FLUID FLOW, FLUID GF	1 CC	OTH	Q4206
FLULAVAL	EA	IM	Q2036
FLUMADINE (DEMONSTATION PROJECT)	100 MG	ORAL	G9036
FLUNISOLIDE, COMPOUNDED, UNIT DOSE	1 MG	INH	J7641
FLUOCINOLONE ACETONIDE INTRAVITREAL IMPLANT	IMPLANT	OTH	J7311
FLUOCINOLONE ACETONIDE, INTRAVITREAL IMPLANT	0.01 MG	OTH	J7313
FLUOCINOLONE ACETONIDE, INTRAVITREAL IMPLANT	0.01 MG	OTH	J7314
FLUORODEOXYGLUCOSE F-18 FDG, DIAGNOSTIC	STUDY DOSE UP TO 45 MCI	IV	A9552
FLUORODOPA F-18, DIAGNOSTIC	1 MCI	IV	A9602
FLUOROESTRADIOL F 18, DIAGNOSTIC	1 MCI	IV	A9591
FLUOROURACIL	500 MG	IV	J9190
FLUPHENAZINE DECANOATE	25 MG	SC, IM	J2680
FLUTAMIDE	125 MG	ORAL	S0175
FLUTEMETAMOL F18, DIAGNOSTIC	STUDY DOSE UP TO 5 MCI	IV	Q9982
FLUVIRIN	EA	IM	Q2037
FLUZONE	EA	IM	Q2038
FOLEX	5 MG	IV, IM, IT, IA	J9250
FOLEX	50 MG	IV, IM, IT, IA	J9260
FOLEX PFS	5 MG	IV, IM, IT, IA	J9250
FOLEX PFS	50 MG	IV, IM, IT, IA	J9260
FOLLISTIM	75 IU	SC, IM	S0128
FOLLITROPIN ALFA	75 IU	SC	S0126
FOLLITROPIN BETA	75 IU	SC, IM	S0128
FOLOTYN	1 MG	IV	J9307
FOMEPIZOLE	15 MG	IV	J1451
FOMIVIRSEN SODIUM	1.65 MG	OTH	J1452
FONDAPARINUX SODIUM	0.5 MG	SC	J1652
FORMOTEROL FUMERATE NONCOMPOUNDED UNIT DOSE FORM	20 MCG	INH	J7606
FORMOTEROL, COMPOUNDED, UNIT DOSE	12 MCG	INH	J7640
FORTAZ	500 MG	IM, IV	J0713
FORTEO	10 MCG	SC	J3110
FORTOVASE	200 MG	ORAL	S0140
FOSAPREPITANT	1 MG	IV	J1453
FOSAPREPITANT (TEVA), NOT THERAPEUTICALLY EQUIVALENT TO J1453	1 MG	IV	J1456
FOSCARNET SODIUM	1,000 MG	IV	J1455
FOSCAVIR	1,000 MG	IV	J1455

Drug Name	Unit Per	Route	Code
FOSNETUPITANT AND PALONOSETRON	235 MG/ 0.25 MG	IV	J1454
FOSPHENYTOIN	50 MG	IM, IV	Q2009
FOSPHENYTOIN SODIUM	750 MG	IM, IV	S0078
FRAGMIN	2,500 IU	SC	J1645
FREMANEZUMAB-VFRM	1 MG	SC	J3031
FUDR	500 MG	IV	J9200
FULPHILA	0.5 MG	SC	Q5108
FULVESTRANT	25 MG	IM	J9395
FULVESTRANT (FRESENIUS KABI) NOT THERAPEUTICALLY EQUIVALENT TO J9395	25 MG	IM	J9394
FULVESTRANT (TEVA) NOT THERAPEUTICALLY EQUIVALENT TO J9395	25 MG	IM	J9393
FUNGIZONE	50 MG	IV	J0285
FUROSEMIDE	20 MG	IM, IV	J1940
FUZEON	1 MG	SC	J1324
FYARRO	1 MG	IV	J9331
~~FYARRO~~	~~1 MG~~	~~IV~~	~~C9091~~
GABLOFEN	10 MG	IT	J0475
GABLOFEN	50 MCG	IT	J0476
GADAVIST	0.1 ML	IV	A9585
GADOBENATE DIMEGLUMINE (MULTIHANCE MULTIPACK)	1 ML	IV	A9577
GADOBUTROL	0.1 ML	IV	A9585
GADOFOSVESET TRISODIUM	1 ML	IV	A9583
GADOTERATE MEGLUMINE	0.1 ML	IV	A9575
GADOTERIDOL (PROHANCE MULTIPACK)	1 ML	IV	A9576
GADOXETATE DISODIUM	1 ML	IV	A9581
GALLIUM GA-67	1 MCI	IV	A9556
GALLIUM GA-68 GOZETOTIDE, DIAGNOSTIC	1 MCI	IV	A9596
GALLIUM GA-68 GOZETOTIDE, DIAGNOSTIC	1 MCI	IV	A9800
GALLIUM GA-68 PSMA-11, DIAGNOSTIC, (UCLA)	1 MCI	IV	A9594
GALLIUM GA-68 PSMA-11, DIAGNOSTIC, (UCSF)	1 MCI	IV	A9593
GALLIUM GA-68, DOTATATE, DIAGNOSTIC	0.1 MCI	IV	A9587
GALLIUM GA-68, DOTATOC, DIAGNOSTIC	0.01 MCI	IV	C9067
GALLIUM NITRATE	1 MG	IV	J1457
GALSULFASE	1 MG	IV	J1458
GAMASTAN	1 CC	IM	J1460
GAMASTAN	OVER 10 CC	IM	J1560
GAMASTAN SD	1 CC	IM	J1460
GAMASTAN SD	OVER 10 CC	IM	J1560
GAMIFANT	1 MG	IV	J9210
GAMMA GLOBULIN	1 CC	IM	J1460
GAMMA GLOBULIN	OVER 10 CC	IM	J1560
GAMMAGARD	500 MG	IV	J1569
GAMMAGRAFT	SQ CM	OTH	Q4111
GAMMAKED	500 MG	IV, SC	J1561
GAMMAPLEX	500 MG	IV	J1557
GAMUNEX	500 MG	IV, SQ	J1561
GAMUNEX-C	500 MG	IV, SC	J1561

2023 HCPCS Level II — Appendix 1 — Table of Drugs and Biologicals

Drug Name	Unit Per	Route	Code
GANCICLOVIR	4.5 MG	OTH	J7310
GANCICLOVIR SODIUM	500 MG	IV	J1570
GANCICLOVIR SODIUM (EXELA) NOT THERAPEUTICALLY EQUIVALENT TO J1570	1 MG	IV	J1574
GANIRELIX ACETATE	250 MCG	SC	S0132
GANITE	1 MG	IV	J1457
GARAMYCIN	80 MG	IM, IV	J1580
GASTROCROM	10 MG	INH	J7631
GASTROMARK	1 ML	ORAL	Q9954
GATIFLOXACIN	10 MG	IV	J1590
GAZYVA	10 MG	IV	J9301
GEFITINIB	250 MG	ORAL	J8565
GEL-ONE	PER DOSE	INJ	J7326
GELSYN-3	0.1 MG	INJ	J7328
GEMCITABINE HYDROCHLORIDE	100 MG	IV	J9198
GEMTUZUMAB OZOGAMICIN	0.1 MG	INF	J9203
GENESIS AMNIOTIC MEMBRANE	SQ CM	OTH	Q4198
GENGRAF	25 MG	ORAL	J7515
GENGRAF	100 MG	ORAL	J7502
GENOTROPIN	1 MG	SC	J2941
GENOTROPIN MINIQUICK	1 MG	SC	J2941
GENOTROPIN NUTROPIN	1 MG	SC	J2941
GENTAMICIN	80 MG	IM, IV	J1580
GENTRAN	500 ML	IV	J7100
GENTRAN 75	500 ML	IV	J7110
GENVISC 850	1 MG	INJ	J7320
GEODON	10 MG	IM	J3486
GEREF	1 MCG	SC	Q0515
GIVLAARI	0.5 MG	SC	J0223
GIVOSIRAN	0.5 MG	SC	J0223
GLASSIA	10 MG	IV	J0257
GLATIRAMER ACETATE	20 MG	SC	J1595
GLEEVEC	100 MG	ORAL	S0088
GLOFIL-125	STUDY DOSE UP TO 10 UCI	IV	A9554
GLUCAGEN	1 MG	SC, IM, IV	J1610
GLUCAGON	1 MG	SC, IM, IV	J1610
GLUCAGON HCL (FRESENIUS KABI), NOT THERAPEUTICALLY EQUIVALENT TO J1610	1 MG	INJ	J1611
GLUCOTOPE	STUDY DOSE UP TO 45 MCI	IV	A9552
GLYCOPYRROLATE, COMPOUNDED CONCENTRATED	PER MG	INH	J7642
GLYCOPYRROLATE, COMPOUNDED, UNIT DOSE	1 MG	INH	J7643
GOLD SODIUM THIOMALATE	50 MG	IM	J1600
GOLIMUMAB	1 MG	IV	J1602
GOLODIRSEN	10 MG	IV	J1429
GONADORELIN HCL	100 MCG	SC, IV	J1620
GONAL-F	75 IU	SC	S0126
GOPRELTO	1 MG	OTH	C9046
GOSERELIN ACETATE	3.6 MG	SC	J9202
GRAFIX CORE	SQ CM	OTH	Q4132
GRAFIX PRIME	SQ CM	OTH	Q4133
GRAFIXPL CORE	SQ CM	OTH	Q4132
GRAFIXPL PRIME	SQ CM	OTH	Q4133

Drug Name	Unit Per	Route	Code
GRAFTJACKET	SQ CM	OTH	Q4107
GRAFTJACKET EXPRESS	1 CC	INJ	Q4113
GRANISETRON HCL	1 MG	ORAL	Q0166
GRANISETRON HCL	100 MCG	IV	J1626
GRANISETRON HCL	1 MG	IV	S0091
GRANISETRON, EXTENDED-RELEASE	0.1 MG	SC	J1627
GRANIX	1 MCG	IV	J1447
GUARDIAN	SQ CM	OTH	Q4151
GUSELKUMAB	1 MG	SC	J1628
GYNOGEN L.A. 10	10 MG	IM	J1380
GYNOGEN L.A. 20	10 MG	IM	J1380
GYNOGEN L.A. 40	10 MG	IM	J1380
H.P. ACTHAR GEL	UP TO 40 UNITS	OTH	J0800
HAEGARDA	10 UNITS	SC	J0599
HALAVEN	0.1 MG	IV	J9179
HALDOL	5 MG	IM, IV	J1630
HALDOL DECANOATE	50 MG	IM	J1631
HALOPERIDOL	5 MG	IM, IV	J1630
HECTOROL	1 MG	IV	J1270
HELICOLL	SQ CM	OTH	Q4164
HEMIN	1 MG	IV	J1640
HEMLIBRA	0.5 MG	SC	J7170
HEMOFIL-M	1 IU	IV	J7190
HEMOSPRAY	UNKNOWN	OTH	C1052
HEMOSTATIC AGENT, GASTROINTESTINAL	UNKNOWN	OTH	C1052
HEP LOCK	10 U	IV	J1642
HEP-PAK	10 UNITS	IV	J1642
HEPAGAM B	0.5 ML	IM	J1571
HEPAGAM B	0.5 ML	IV	J1573
HEPARIN SODIUM	10 U	IV	J1642
HEPARIN SODIUM	1,000 U	IV, SC	J1644
HEPARIN SODIUM (PFIZER), NOT THERAPEUTICALLY EQUIVALENT TO J1644	1000 UNITS	INJ, IV, SC, OTH	J1643
HEPATITIS B IMMUNE GLOBULIN	0.5 ML	IV	J1573
HEPATOLITE	STUDY DOSE UP TO 15 MCI	IV	A9510
HERCEPTIN HYLECTA	10 MG	SC	J9356
HERCEPTIN, EXCLUDES BIOSIMILAR	10 MG	IV	J9355
HERZUMA	10 MG	IV	Q5113
HEXADROL	0.25 MG	ORAL	J8540
HEXAMINOLEVULINATE HYDROCHLORIDE	STUDY DOSE	OTH	A9589
HIGH OSMOLAR CONTRAST MATERIAL, UP TO 149 MG/ML IODINE CONCENTRATION	1 ML	IV	Q9958
HIGH OSMOLAR CONTRAST MATERIAL, UP TO 150-199 MG/ML IODINE CONCENTRATION	1 ML	IV	Q9959
HIGH OSMOLAR CONTRAST MATERIAL, UP TO 200-249 MG/ML IODINE CONCENTRATION	1 ML	IV	Q9960
HIGH OSMOLAR CONTRAST MATERIAL, UP TO 250-299 MG/ML IODINE CONCENTRATION	1 ML	IV	Q9961

© 2022 Optum, Inc.

Appendix 1 — Table of Drugs and Biologicals

Drug Name	Unit Per	Route	Code
HIGH OSMOLAR CONTRAST MATERIAL, UP TO 300-349 MG/ML IODINE CONCENTRATION	1 ML	IV	Q9962
HIGH OSMOLAR CONTRAST MATERIAL, UP TO 350-399 MG/ML IODINE CONCENTRATION	1 ML	IV	Q9963
HIGH OSMOLAR CONTRAST MATERIAL, UP TO 400 OR GREATER MG/ML IODINE CONCENTRATION	1 ML	IV	Q9964
HISTERLIN IMPLANT (VANTAS)	50 MG	OTH	J9225
HISTRELIN ACETATE	10 MG	INJ	J1675
HISTRELIN IMPLANT (SUPPRELIN LA)	50 MG	OTH	J9226
HIZENTRA	100 MG	SC	J1559
HMATRIX	SQ CM	OTH	Q4134
HUMALOG	5 U	SC	J1815
HUMALOG	50 U	SC	J1817
HUMAN FIBRINOGEN CONCENTRATE	1 MG	IV	J7177
HUMAN HEALTH FACTOR 10 AMNIOTIC PATCH (HHF10-P)	SQ CM	OTH	Q4224
HUMATE-P	1 IU	IV	J7187
HUMATROPE	1 MG	SC	J2941
HUMIRA	20 MG	SC	J0135
HUMULIN	5 U	SC	J1815
HUMULIN	50 U	SC	J1817
HUMULIN R	5 U	SC	J1815
HUMULIN R U-500	5 U	SC	J1815
HYALGAN	PER DOSE	INJ	J7321
HYALOMATRIX	SQ CM	OTH	Q4117
HYALURONAN	0.1 MG	INJ	J7328
HYALURONAN	1 MG	INJ	J7322
HYALURONAN	PER DOSE	INJ	J7324
HYALURONAN	PER DOSE	INJ	J7321
HYALURONAN	1 MG	INJ	J7325
HYALURONAN	PER DOSE	INJ	J7327
HYALURONAN	PER DOSE	INJ	J7326
HYALURONAN	1 MG	INJ	J7320
HYALURONAN	PER DOSE	INJ	J7323
HYALURONAN	1 MG	INJ	J7332
HYALURONAN	1 MG	INJ	J7331
HYALURONAN	1 MG	INJ	J7329
HYALURONAN	1 MG	INJ	J7318
HYALURONIDASE	150 UNITS	VAR	J3470
HYALURONIDASE RECOMBINANT	1 USP UNIT	SC	J3473
HYALURONIDASE, OVINE, PRESERVATIVE FREE	1000 USP	OTH	J3472
HYALURONIDASE, OVINE, PRESERVATIVE FREE	1 USP	OTH	J3471
HYCAMTIN	0.1 MG	IV	J9351
HYCAMTIN	0.25 MG	ORAL	J8705
HYDRALAZINE HCL	20 MG	IV, IM	J0360
HYDRATE	50 MG	IM, IV	J1240
HYDREA	500 MG	ORAL	S0176
HYDROCORTISONE ACETATE	25 MG	IV, IM, SC	J1700
HYDROCORTISONE SODIUM PHOSPHATE	50 MG	IV, IM, SC	J1710
HYDROCORTISONE SODIUM SUCCINATE	100 MG	IV, IM, SC	J1720

Drug Name	Unit Per	Route	Code
HYDROCORTONE PHOSPHATE	50 MG	SC, IM, IV	J1710
HYDROMORPHONE HCL	250 MG	OTH	S0092
HYDROMORPHONE HCL	4 MG	SC, IM, IV	J1170
HYDROXOCOBALAMIN	1,000 MCG	IM, SC	J3420
HYDROXYCOBAL	1,000 MCG	IM, SC	J3420
HYDROXYPROGESTERONE CAPROATE (MAKENA)	10 MG	IM	J1726
HYDROXYUREA	500 MG	ORAL	S0176
HYDROXYZINE HCL	25 MG	IM	J3410
HYDROXYZINE PAMOATE	25 MG	ORAL	Q0177
HYMOVIS	1 MG	INJ	J7322
HYOSCYAMINE SULFATE	0.25 MG	SC, IM, IV	J1980
HYPERRHO S/D	300 MCG	IV	J2790
HYPERTET SD	UP TO 250 MG	IM	J1670
HYPERTONIC SALINE SOLUTION	1 ML	VAR	J7131
HYQVIA	100 MG	IV	J1575
HYREXIN	50 MG	IV, IM	J1200
HYZINE	25 MG	IM	J3410
HYZINE-50	25 MG	IM	J3410
IBALIZUMAB-UIYK	10 MG	IV	J1746
IBANDRONATE SODIUM	1 MG	IV	J1740
IBRITUMOMAB TUXETAN	STUDY DOSE UP TO 5 MCI	IV	A9542
IBUPROFEN	100 MG	IV	J1741
IBUTILIDE FUMARATE	1 MG	IV	J1742
ICATIBANT	1 MG	SC	J1744
IDAMYCIN	5 MG	IV	J9211
IDAMYCIN PFS	5 MG	IV	J9211
IDARUBICIN HCL	5 MG	IV	J9211
IDECABTAGENE VICLEUCEL	UP TO 460 MILLION CELLS	IV	Q2055
IDELVION	1 IU	IV	J7202
IDURSULFASE	1 MG	IV	J1743
IFEX	1 G	IV	J9208
IFOSFAMIDE	1 G	IV	J9208
IL-2	1 VIAL	IV	J9015
ILARIS	1 MG	SC	J0638
ILETIN	5 UNITS	SC	J1815
ILETIN II NPH PORK	50 U	SC	J1817
ILETIN II REGULAR PORK	5 U	SC	J1815
ILLUCCIX	1 MCI	IV	A9596
ILOPROST INHALATION SOLUTION	PER DOSE UP TO 20 MCG	INH	Q4074
ILUMYA	1 MG	SC	J3245
ILUVIEN	0.01 MG	OTH	J7313
IMAGENT	1 ML	IV	Q9955
IMATINIB	100 MG	ORAL	S0088
IMFINZI	10 MG	IV	J9173
IMIGLUCERASE	10 U	IV	J1786
IMIPENEM, CILASTATIN, AND RELEBACTAM	4 MG/4 MG/ 2 MG	IV	J0742
IMITREX	6 MG	SC	J3030
IMLYGIC	1 MILLION	INTRA-LESIONAL	J9325
IMMUNE GLOBULIN	100 MG	IV	J1551
IMMUNE GLOBULIN (ASCENIV)	500 MG	IV	J1554
IMMUNE GLOBULIN (BIVIGAM)	500 MG	IV	J1556
IMMUNE GLOBULIN (CIVITRU)	100 MG	SC	J1555

Drug Name	Unit Per	Route	Code
IMMUNE GLOBULIN (FLEBOGAMMA, FLEBOGAMMA DIF)	500 MG	IV	J1572
IMMUNE GLOBULIN (GAMMAGARD LIQUID)	500 MG	IV	J1569
IMMUNE GLOBULIN (GAMMAPLEX)	500 MG	IV	J1557
IMMUNE GLOBULIN (GAMUNEX)	500 MG	IV	J1561
IMMUNE GLOBULIN (HIZENTRA)	100 MG	SC	J1559
IMMUNE GLOBULIN (OCTAGAM)	500 MG	IV	J1568
IMMUNE GLOBULIN (PRIVIGEN) NONLYOPHILIZED	500 MG	IV	J1459
IMMUNE GLOBULIN (RHOPHYLAC)	100 IU	IM, IV	J2791
IMMUNE GLOBULIN (XEMBIFY)	100 MG	SC	J1558
IMMUNE GLOBULIN SUBCUTANEOUS	100 MG	SC	J1562
IMMUNE GLOBULIN/ HYALURONIDASE	100 MG	IV	J1575
IMPLANON	IMPLANT	OTH	J7307
IMURAN	50 MG	ORAL	J7500
IN-111 SATUMOMAB PENDETIDE	STUDY DOSE UP TO MCI	IV	A4642
INAPSINE	5 MG	IM, IV	J1790
INCLISIRAN	1 MG	SC	J1306
INCOBUTULINUMTOXINA	1 UNIT	IM	J0588
INDERAL	1 MG	IV	J1800
INDIUM IN-111 IBRITUMOMAB TIUXETAN, DIAGNOSTIC	STUDY DOSE UP TO 5 MCI	IV	A9542
INDIUM IN-111 LABELED AUTOLOGOUS PLATELETS	STUDY DOSAGE	IV	A9571
INDIUM IN-111 LABELED AUTOLOGOUS WHITE BLOOD CELLS	STUDY DOSE	IV	A9570
INDIUM IN-111 OXYQUINOLINE	0.5 MCI	IV	A9547
INDIUM IN-111 PENTETREOTIDE	STUDY DOSE UP TO 6 MCI	IV	A9572
INDURSALFASE	1 MG	IV	J1743
INEBILIZUMAB-CDON	1 MG	IV	J1823
INFED	50 MG	IM, IV	J1750
INFERGEN	1 MCG	SC	J9212
INFLECTRA	10 MG	IV	Q5103
INFLIXIMAB	10 MG	IV	J1745
INFLIXIMAB-ABDA, BIOSIMILAR	10 MG	IV	Q5104
INFLIXIMAB-AXXQ, BIOSIMILAR	10 MG	IV	Q5121
INFLIXIMAB-DYYB, BIOSIMILAR	10 MG	IV	Q5103
INFLIXIMAB-QBTX, BIOSIMILAR	10 MG	IV	Q5109
INFLUENZA VACCINE, AGRIFLU	UNKNOWN	IM	Q2034
INFLUENZA VIRUS VACCINE (AFLURIA)	EA	IM	Q2035
INFLUENZA VIRUS VACCINE (FLULAVAL)	EA	IM	Q2036
INFLUENZA VIRUS VACCINE (FLUVIRIN)	EA	IM	Q2037
INFLUENZA VIRUS VACCINE (FLUZONE)	EA	IM	Q2038
INFUGEM	100 MG	IV	J9198
INFUMORPH	10 MG	IM, IV, SC	J2270
INJECTAFER	1 MG	IV	J1439
INNOHEP	1,000 IU	SC	J1655
INNOVAMATRIX AC	SQ CM	OTH	A2001

Drug Name	Unit Per	Route	Code
INNOVAMATRIX FS	SQ CM	OTH	A2013
INOTUZUMAB OZOGAMICIN	0.1 MG	IV	J9229
INSULIN	5 U	SC	J1815
INSULIN	50 U	SC	J1817
INSULIN LISPRO	5 U	SC	S5551
INSULIN LISPRO	5 U	SC	J1815
INSULIN PURIFIED REGULAR PORK	5 U	SC	J1815
INTAL	10 MG	INH	J7631
INTEGRA BILAYER MATRIX DRESSING	SQ CM	OTH	Q4104
INTEGRA DERMAL REGENERATION TEMPLATE	SQ CM	OTH	Q4105
INTEGRA FLOWABLE WOUND MATRIX	1 CC	INJ	Q4114
INTEGRA MATRIX	SQ CM	OTH	Q4108
INTEGRA MESHED BILAYER WOUND MATRIX	SQ CM	OTH	C9363
INTEGRA MOZAIK OSTEOCONDUCTIVE SCAFFOLD PUTTY	0.5 CC	OTH	C9359
INTEGRA MOZAIK OSTEOCONDUCTIVE SCAFFOLD STRIP	0.5 CC	OTH	C9362
INTEGRA OMNIGRAFT DERMAL REGENERATION MATRIX	SQ CM	OTH	Q4105
INTEGRA OS OSTEOCONDUCTIVE SCAFFOLD PUTTY	0.5 CC	OTH	C9359
INTEGRILIN	5 MG	IM, IV	J1327
INTERFERON ALFA-2A	3,000,000 U	SC, IM	J9213
INTERFERON ALFA-2B	1,000,000 U	SC, IM	J9214
INTERFERON ALFA-N3	250,000 IU	IM	J9215
INTERFERON ALFACON-1	1 MCG	SC	J9212
INTERFERON BETA-1A	1 MCG	IM	Q3027
INTERFERON BETA-1A	30 MCG	IM, SC	J1826
INTERFERON BETA-1A	1 MCG	SC	Q3028
INTERFERON BETA-1B	0.25 MG	SC	J1830
INTERFERON, ALFA-2A, RECOMBINANT	3,000,000 U	SC, IM	J9213
INTERFERON, ALFA-2B, RECOMBINANT	1,000,000 U	SC, IM	J9214
INTERFERON, ALFA-N3, (HUMAN LEUKOCYTE DERIVED)	250,000 IU	IM	J9215
INTERFERON, GAMMA 1-B	3,000,000 U	SC	J9216
INTERFYL	1 MG	OTH	Q4171
INTERLUEKIN	1 VIAL	IV	J9015
INTRON A	1,000,000 U	SC, IM	J9214
INVANZ	500 MG	IM, IV	J1335
INVEGA SUSTENNA	1 MG	IM	J2426
INVIRASE	200 MG	ORAL	S0140
IOBENGUANE SULFATE I-131	0.5 MCI	IV	A9508
IOBENGUANE, I-123, DIAGNOSTIC	PER STUDY DOSE UP TO 15 MCI	IV	A9582
IODINE I-123 IOBENGUANE, DIAGNOSTIC	15 MCI	IV	A9582
IODINE I-123 IOFLUPANE	STUDY DOSE UP TO 5 MCI	IV	A9584
IODINE I-123 SODIUM IODIDE CAPSULE(S), DIAGNOSTIC	100-9999 UCI	ORAL	A9516
IODINE I-123 SODIUM IODIDE, DIAGNOSTIC	1 MCI	IV	A9509

Appendix 1 — Table of Drugs and Biologicals 2023 HCPCS Level II

Drug Name	Unit Per	Route	Code
IODINE I-125 SERUM ALBUMIN, DIAGNOSTIC	5 UCI	IV	A9532
IODINE I-125 SODIUM IOTHALAMATE, DIAGNOSTIC	STUDY DOSE UP TO 10 UCI	IV	A9554
IODINE I-125, SODIUM IODIDE SOLUTION, THERAPEUTIC	1 MCI	ORAL	A9527
IODINE I-131 IOBENGUANE SULFATE, DIAGNOSTIC	0.5 MCI	IV	A9508
IODINE I-131 IODINATED SERUM ALBUMIN, DIAGNOSTIC	PER 5 UCI	IV	A9524
IODINE I-131 SODIUM IODIDE CAPSULE(S), DIAGNOSTIC	1 MCI	ORAL	A9528
IODINE I-131 SODIUM IODIDE CAPSULE(S), THERAPEUTIC	1 MCI	ORAL	A9517
IODINE I-131 SODIUM IODIDE SOLUTION, DIAGNOSTIC	1 MCI	ORAL	A9529
IODINE I-131 SODIUM IODIDE SOLUTION, THERAPEUTIC	1 MCI	ORAL	A9530
IODINE I-131 SODIUM IODIDE, DIAGNOSTIC	PER UCI UP TO 100 UCI	IV	A9531
IODINE I-131, IOBENGUANE	1 MCI	IV	A9590
IODOTOPE THERAPEUTIC CAPSULE(S)	1 MCI	ORAL	A9517
IODOTOPE THERAPEUTIC SOLUTION	1 MCI	ORAL	A9530
IOFLUPANE	STUDY DOSE UP TO 5 MCI	IV	A9584
ION-BASED MAGNETIC RESONANCE CONTRAST AGENT	1 ML	IV	Q9953
IOTHALAMATE SODIUM I-125	STUDY DOSE UP TO 10 UCI	IV	A9554
IPILIMUMAB	1 MG	IV	J9228
IPLEX	1 MG	SC	J2170
IPRATROPIUM BROMIDE, NONCOMPOUNDED, UNIT DOSE	1 MG	INH	J7644
IPTRATROPIUM BROMIDE COMPOUNDED, UNIT DOSE	1 MG	INH	J7645
IRESSA	250 MG	ORAL	J8565
IRINOTECAN	20 MG	IV	J9206
IRINOTECAN LIPOSOME	1 MG	IV	J9205
IRON DEXTRAN, 50 MG	50 MG	IM, IV	J1750
IRON SUCROSE	1 MG	IV	J1756
ISATUXIMAB-IRFC	10 MG	IV	J9227
ISAVUCONAZONIUM	1 MG	IV	J1833
ISOCAINE	10 ML	VAR	J0670
ISOETHARINE HCL COMPOUNDED, CONCENTRATED	1 MG	INH	J7647
ISOETHARINE HCL COMPOUNDED, UNIT DOSE	1 MG	INH	J7650
ISOETHARINE HCL, NONCOMPOUNDED CONCENTRATED	PER MG	INH	J7648
ISOETHARINE HCL, NONCOMPOUNDED, UNIT DOSE	1 MG	INH	J7649
ISOJEX	5 UCI	IV	A9532
ISOPROTERENOL HCL COMPOUNDED, CONCENTRATED	1 MG	INH	J7657
ISOPROTERENOL HCL COMPOUNDED, UNIT DOSE	1 MG	INH	J7660
ISOPROTERENOL HCL, NONCOMPOUNDED CONCENTRATED	1 MG	INH	J7658

Drug Name	Unit Per	Route	Code
ISOPROTERNOL HCL, NONCOMPOUNDED, UNIT DOSE	1 MG	INH	J7659
ISOSULFAN BLUE	1 MG	SC	Q9968
ISTODAX	0.1 MG	IV	J9319
ISUPREL	1 MG	INH	J7658
ISUPREL	1 MG	INH	J7659
ITRACONAZOLE	50 MG	IV	J1835
IXABEPILONE	1 MG	IV	J9207
IXEMPRA	1 MG	IV	J9207
IXIFI	10 MG	IV	Q5109
JELMYTO	1 MG	OTH	J9281
JEMPERLI	10 MG	IV	J9272
JETREA	0.125 MG	OTH	J7316
JEVTANA	1 MG	IV	J9043
JIVI	1 IU	IV	J7208
KADCYLA	1 MG	IV	J9354
KALBITOR	1 MG	SC	J1290
KANAMYCIN	500 MG	IM, IV	J1840
KANAMYCIN	75 MG	IM, IV	J1850
KANJINTI	10 MG	IV	Q5117
KANTREX	75 MG	IM, IV	J1850
KANTREX	500 MG	IM, IV	J1840
KANUMA	1 MG	IV	J2840
KCENTRA	PER IU	IV	J7168
KEFZOL	500 MG	IM, IV	J0690
KEPIVANCE	50 MCG	IV	J2425
KEPPRA	10 MG	IV	J1953
KERAMATRIX OR KERASORB	SQ CM	OTH	Q4165
KERECIS OMEGA3	SQ CM	OTH	Q4158
KEROXX	1 CC	OTH	Q4202
KESTRONE	1 MG	IV, IM	J1435
KETOROLAC TROMETHAMINE	15 MG	IM, IV	J1885
KEYTRUDA	1 MG	IV	J9271
KHAPZORY	0.5 MG	IV	J0642
KIMMTRAK	1 MCG	IV	C9095
KIMMTRAK	1 MCG	IV	J9274
KIMYRSA	10 MG	IV	J2406
KINEVAC	5 MCG	IV	J2805
KOATE-DVI	1 IU	IV	J7190
KONAKION	1 MG	SC, IM, IV	J3430
KONYNE 80	1 IU	IV	J7194
KORSUVA	0.1 MCG	IV	J0879
KOVALTRY	1 I.U.	IV	J7211
KRYSTEXXA	1 MG	IV	J2507
KYBELLA	1 MG	SC	J0591
KYLEENA	19.5 MG	OTH	J7296
KYMRIAH	UP TO 600 MILLION CELLS	IV	Q2042
KYPROLIS	1 MG	IV	J9047
KYTRIL	1 MG	IV	S0091
KYTRIL	1 MG	ORAL	Q0166
KYTRIL	100 MCG	IV	J1626
L.A.E. 20	10 MG	IM	J1380
LACOSAMIDE	1 MG	IV	C9254
LAETRILE	VAR	INJ	J3570
LANADELUMAB-FLYO	1 MG	SC	J0593
LANOXIN	0.5 MG	IM, IV	J1160

Appendix 1 — Table of Drugs and Biologicals

Drug Name	Unit Per	Route	Code
LANREOTIDE	1 MG	SC	J1930
LANREOTIDE	1 MG	SC, INJ	J1932
LANTUS	5 U	SC	J1815
LARONIDASE	0.1 MG	IV	J1931
LARTRUVO	10 MG	INF	J9285
LASIX	20 MG	IM, IV	J1940
LEFAMULIN	1 MG	IV	J0691
LEMTRADA	1 MG	IV	J0202
LENTE ILETIN I	5 U	SC	J1815
LEPIRUDIN	50 MG	IV	J1945
LEQVIO	1 MG	SC	J1306
LEUCOVORIN CALCIUM	50 MG	IM, IV	J0640
LEUKERAN	2 MG	ORAL	S0172
LEUKINE	50 MCG	IV	J2820
LEUPROLIDE	1 MG	SC	J1952
LEUPROLIDE ACETATE	7.5 MG	SC	J9217
LEUPROLIDE ACETATE	1 MG	IM	J9218
LEUPROLIDE ACETATE (FOR DEPOT SUSPENSION)	3.75 MG	IM	J1950
LEUPROLIDE ACETATE DEPOT	7.5 MG	SC	J9217
LEUPROLIDE ACETATE FOR DEPOT SUSPENSION	0.25 MG	SC	J1951
LEUPROLIDE ACETATE IMPLANT	65 MG	OTH	J9219
LEUSTATIN	1 MG	IV	J9065
LEVABUTEROL COMPOUNDED, UNIT DOSE	1 MG	INH	J7615
LEVABUTEROL, COMPOUNDED, CONCENTRATED	0.5 MG	INH	J7607
LEVALBUTEROL NONCOMPOUNDED, CONCENTRATED FORM	0.5 MG	INH	J7612
LEVALBUTEROL, NONCOMPOUNDED, UNIT DOSE	0.5 MG	INH	J7614
LEVAMISOLE HCL	50 MG	ORAL	S0177
LEVAQUIN	250 MG	IV	J1956
LEVEMIR	5 U	SC	J1815
LEVETIRACETAM	10 MG	IV	J1953
LEVO-DROMORAN	UP TO 2 MG	IV, IM	J1960
LEVOCARNITINE	1 G	IV	J1955
LEVOFLOXACIN	250 MG	IV	J1956
LEVOLEUCOVORIN	0.5 MG	IV	J0642
LEVONORGESTREL IMPLANT	IMPLANT	OTH	J7306
LEVONORGESTREL-RELEASING INTRAUTERINE CONTRACEPTIVE (MIRENA)	52 MG	OTH	J7298
LEVONORGESTREL-RELEASING INTRAUTERINE CONTRACEPTIVE (LILETTA)	52 MG	OTH	J7297
LEVONORGESTREL-RELEASING INTRAUTERINE CONTRACEPTIVE SYSTEM (KYLEENA)	19.5 MG	OTH	J7296
LEVONORGESTREL-RELEASING INTRAUTERINE CONTRACEPTIVE SYSTEM (SKYLA)	13.5 MG	OTH	J7301
LEVORPHANOL TARTRATE	2 MG	SC, IV, IM	J1960
LEVSIN	0.25 MG	SC, IM, IV	J1980
LEVULAN KERASTICK	354 MG	OTH	J7308
LEXISCAN	0.1 MG	IV	J2785
LIBRIUM	100 MG	IM, IV	J1990
LIBTAYO	1 MG	IV	J9119

Drug Name	Unit Per	Route	Code
LIDOCAINE 70 MG/TETRACAINE 70 MG	PATCH	OTH	C9285
LIDOCAINE HCL	10 MG	IV	J2001
LILETTA	52 MG	OTH	J7297
LINCOCIN HCL	300 MG	IV	J2010
LINCOMYCIN HCL	300 MG	IM, IV	J2010
LINEZOLID	200 MG	IV	J2020
LINEZOLID (HOSPIRA) NOT THERAPEUTICALLY EQUIVALENT TO J2020	200 MG	IV	J2021
LIORESAL	10 MG	IT	J0475
LIORESAL INTRATHECAL REFILL	50 MCG	IT	J0476
LIPODOX	10 MG	IV	Q2049
LIPOSOMAL, DAUNORUBICIN AND CYTARABINE	1 MG/2.27 MG	IV	J9153
LIQUAEMIN SODIUM	1,000 UNITS	SC, IV	J1644
LISOCABTAGENE MARALEUCEL	UP TO 110 MILLION CELLS	IV	Q2054
LISPRO-PFC	50 U	SC	J1817
LOCAMETZ	1 MCI	IV	A9800
LOK-PAK	10 UNITS	IV	J1642
LOMUSTINE	10 MG	ORAL	S0178
LONCASTUXIMAB TESIRINE-LPYL	0.1 MG	IV	C9084
LONCASTUXIMAB TESIRINE-LPYL	1 MG	IV	J9359
LORAZEPAM	2 MG	IM, IV	J2060
LOVENOX	10 MG	SC	J1650
LOW OSMOLAR CONTRAST MATERIAL, 100-199 MG/ML IODINE CONCENTRATIONS	1 ML	IV	Q9965
LOW OSMOLAR CONTRAST MATERIAL, 200-299 MG/ML IODINE CONCENTRATION	1 ML	IV	Q9966
LOW OSMOLAR CONTRAST MATERIAL, 300-399 MG/ML IODINE CONCENTRATION	1 ML	IV	Q9967
LOW OSMOLAR CONTRAST MATERIAL, 400 OR GREATER MG/ML IODINE CONCENTRATION	1 ML	IV	Q9951
LOXAPINE	1 MG	INH	J2062
LUCENTIS	0.1 MG	IV	J2778
LUMASIRAN	0.5 MG	SC	J0224
LUMASON	1 ML	IV	Q9950
LUMIZYME	10 MG	IV	J0221
LUMOXITI	0.01 MG	IV	J9313
LUPRON	1 MG	SC	J9218
LUPRON DEPOT	PER 3.75 MG	IM	J1950
LUPRON DEPOT	7.5 MG	SC	J9217
LUPRON IMPLANT	65 MG	OTH	J9219
LURBINECTEDIN	0.1 MG	IV	J9223
LUSPATERCEPT-AAMT	0.25 MG	SC	J0896
LUTATHERA	1 MCI	IM	A9513
LUTETIUM LU 177 VIPIVOTIDE TETRAXETAN, THERAPEUTIC	1 MCI	IV	A9607
LUTETIUM LU 177, DOTATATE, THERAPEUTIC	1 MCI	IM	A9513
LUTREPULSE	100 MCG	SC, IV	J1620
LUXTURNA	1 BILLION VECTOR GENOMES	OTH	J3398
LYMPHAZURIN	1 MG	SC	Q9968

Appendix 1 — Table of Drugs and Biologicals

Drug Name	Unit Per	Route	Code
LYMPHOCYTE IMMUNE GLOBULIN, ANTITHYMOCYTE GLOBULIN, EQUINE	250 MG	OTH	J7504
LYMPHOCYTE IMMUNE GLOBULIN, ANTITHYMOCYTE GLOBULIN, RABBIT	25 MG	OTH	J7511
LYMPHOSEEK	0.5 MCI	SC, OTH	A9520
MACUGEN	0.3 MG	OTH	J2503
MAGNESIUM SULFATE	500 MG	IV	J3475
MAGNETIC RESONANCE CONTRAST AGENT	1 ML	ORAL	Q9954
MAGROTEC	STUDY DOSE UP TO 10 MCI	IV	A9540
MAKENA	10 MG	IM	J1726
MANNITOL	25% IN 50 ML	IV	J2150
MANNITOL	5 MG	INH	J7665
MARCAINE HCL	30 ML	VAR	S0020
MARGENZA	5 MG	IV	J9353
MARGETUXIMAB-CMKB	5 MG	IV	J9353
MARINOL	2.5 MG	ORAL	Q0167
MARMINE	50 MG	IM, IV	J1240
MARQIBO KIT	5 MG	IV	J9371
MATRION	SQ CM	OTH	Q4201
MATRISTEM MICROMATRIX	1 MG	OTH	Q4118
MATULANE	50 MG	ORAL	S0182
MAXIPIME	500 MG	IV	J0692
MDP-BRACCO	STUDY DOSE UP TO 30 MCI	IV	A9503
MECASERMIN	1 MG	SC	J2170
MECHLORETHAMINE HCL (NITROGEN MUSTARD)	10 MG	IV	J9230
MEDIDEX	1 MG	IM, IV, OTH	J1100
MEDISKIN	SQ CM	OTH	Q4135
MEDROL	4 MG	ORAL	J7509
MEDROXYPROGESTERONE ACETATE	1 MG	IM	J1050
MEFOXIN	1 G	IV	J0694
MEGACE	20 MG	ORAL	S0179
MEGESTROL ACETATE	20 MG	ORAL	S0179
MELOXICAM	1 MG	IV	J1738
MELPHALAN	1 MG	IV	J9246
MELPHALAN FLUFENAMIDE	1 MG	IV	J9247
MELPHALAN HCL	2 MG	ORAL	J8600
MEMBRANE GRAFT OR MEMBRANE WRAP	SQ CM	OTH	Q4205
MEMODERM	SQ CM	OTH	Q4126
MENADIONE	1 MG	IM, SC, IV	J3430
MENOTROPINS	75 IU	SC, IM, IV	S0122
MEPERGAN	50 MG	IM, IV	J2180
MEPERIDINE AND PROMETHAZINE HCL	50 MG	IM, IV	J2180
MEPERIDINE HCL	100 MG	IM, IV, SC	J2175
MEPIVACAINE HCL	10 ML	VAR	J0670
MEPOLIZUMAB	1 MG	SQ	J2182
MEPSEVII	1 MG	IV	J3397
MERCAPTOPURINE	50 MG	ORAL	S0108
MERITATE	150 MG	IV	J3520
MEROPENEM	100 MG	IV	J2185

Drug Name	Unit Per	Route	Code
MEROPENEM (B. BRAUN) NOT THERAPEUTICALLY EQUIVALENT TO J2185	100 MG	IV	J2184
MEROPENEM, VABORBACTAM	10 MG/10 MG	IV	J2186
MERREM	100 MG	IV	J2185
MESNA	200 MG	IV	J9209
MESNEX	200 MG	IV	J9209
METAPROTERENOL SULFATE COMPOUNDED, UNIT DOSE	10 MG	INH	J7670
METAPROTERENOL SULFATE, NONCOMPOUNDED, CONCENTRATED	10 MG	INH	J7668
METAPROTERENOL SULFATE, NONCOMPOUNDED, UNIT DOSE	10 MG	INH	J7669
METARAMINOL BITARTRATE	10 MG	IV, IM, SC	J0380
METASTRON STRONTIUM 89 CHLORIDE	1 MCI	IV	A9600
METATRACE	STUDY DOSE UP TO 45 MCI	IV	A9552
METHACHOLINE CHLORIDE	1 MG	INH	J7674
METHADONE	5 MG	ORAL	S0109
METHADONE HCL	10 MG	IM, SC	J1230
METHAPREL, COMPOUNDED, UNIT DOSE	10 MG	INH	J7670
METHAPREL, NONCOMPOUNDED, CONCENTRATED	10 MG	INH	J7668
METHAPREL, NONCOMPOUNDED, UNIT DOSE	10 MG	INH	J7669
METHERGINE	0.2 MG	IM, IV	J2210
METHOTREXATE	2.5 MG	ORAL	J8610
METHOTREXATE	5 MG	IV, IM, IT, IA	J9250
METHOTREXATE	50 MG	IV, IM, IT, IA	J9260
METHOTREXATE LPF	5 MG	IV, IM, IT, IA	J9250
METHOTREXATE LPF	50 MG	IV, IM, IT, IA	J9260
METHYL AMINOLEVULINATE 16.8%	1 G	OTH	J7309
METHYLCOTOLONE	80 MG	IM	J1040
METHYLDOPA HCL	UP TO 250 MG	IV	J0210
METHYLDOPATE HCL	UP TO 250 MG	IV	J0210
METHYLENE BLUE	1 MG	SC	Q9968
METHYLERGONOVINE MALEATE	0.2 MG	IM, IV	J2210
METHYLNALTREXONE	0.1 MG	SC	J2212
METHYLPRED	4 MG	ORAL	J7509
METHYLPREDNISOLONE	4 MG	ORAL	J7509
METHYLPREDNISOLONE	125 MG	IM, IV	J2930
METHYLPREDNISOLONE	UP TO 40 MG	IM, IV	J2920
METHYLPREDNISOLONE ACETATE	20 MG	IM	J1020
METHYLPREDNISOLONE ACETATE	80 MG	IM	J1040
METHYLPREDNISOLONE ACETATE	40 MG	IM	J1030
METOCLOPRAMIDE	10 MG	IV	J2765
METRONIDAZOLE	500 MG	IV	S0030
METVIXIA 16.8%	1 G	OTH	J7309
MIACALCIN	400 U	SC, IM	J0630
MIBG	0.5 MCI	IV	A9508
MICAFUNGIN SODIUM	1 MG	IV	J2248
MICAFUNGIN SODIUM (PAR PHARM) NOT THERAPEUTICALLY EQUIVALENT TO J2248	1 MG	IV	J2247
MICRHOGAM	50 MCG	IV	J2788
MICROLYTE MATRIX	SQ CM	OTH	A2005

Drug Name	Unit Per	Route	Code
MICROPOROUS COLLAGEN IMPLANTABLE SLIT TUBE	1 CM LENGTH	OTH	C9353
MICROPOROUS COLLAGEN IMPLANTABLE TUBE	1 CM LENGTH	OTH	C9352
MIDAZOLAM HCl	1 MG	IM, IV	J2250
MIDAZOLAM HCL (WG CRITICAL CARE) NOT THERAPEUTICALLY EQUIVALENT TO J2250	1 MG	IV	J2251
MIFEPRISTONE	200 MG	ORAL	S0190
MILRINONE LACTATE	5 MG	IV	J2260
MINOCIN	1 MG	IV	J2265
MINOCYCLINE HCL	1 MG	IV	J2265
MINOXIDIL	10 MG	ORAL	S0139
MIRCERA	1 MCG	IV	J0887
MIRCERA	1 MCG	SC	J0888
MIRENA	52 MG	OTH	J7298
MIRODERM	SQ CM	OTH	Q4175
MIRRAGEN ADVANCED WOUND MATRIX	SQ CM	OTH	A2002
MISOPROSTOL	200 MG	ORAL	S0191
MITHRACIN	2.5 MG	IV	J9270
MITOMYCIN	5 MG	IV	J9280
MITOMYCIN	0.2 MG	OTH	J7315
MITOMYCIN PYELOCALYCEAL INSTILLATION	1 MG	OTH	J9281
MITOSOL	0.2 MG	OTH	J7315
MITOXANA	1 G	IV	J9208
MITOXANTRONE HCL	5 MG	IV	J9293
MLG-COMPLETE	SQ CM	OTH	Q4256
MOGAMULIZUMAB-KPKC	1 MG	IV	J9204
MOMETASONE FUROATE SINUS IMPLANT	10 MCG	OTH	J7402
MONARC-M	1 IU	IV	J7190
MONJUVI	2 MG	IV	J9349
MONOCLATE-P	1 IU	IV	J7190
MONOFERRIC	10 MG	IV	J1437
MONONINE	1 IU	IV	J7193
MONOPUR	75 IU	SC, IM	S0122
MONOVISC	PER DOSE	INJ	J7327
MORPHINE SULFATE	10 MG	IM, IV, SC	J2270
MORPHINE SULFATE	500 MG	OTH	S0093
MORPHINE SULFATE (FRESENIUS KABI) NOT THERAPEUTICALLY EQUIVALENT TO J2270	10 MG	INJ, IV, SC	J2272
MORPHINE SULFATE, PRESERVATIVE-FREE FOR EPIDURAL OR INTRATHECAL USE	10 MG	OTH	J2274
MOXETUMOMAB PASUDOTOX-TDFK	0.01 MG	IV	J9313
MOXIFLOXACIN	100 MG	IV	J2280
MOXIFLOXACIN (FRESENIUS KABI) NOT THERAPEUTICALLY EQUIVALENT TO J2280	100 MG	IV	J2281
MOZOBIL	1 MG	SC	J2562
MPI INDIUM DTPA	0.5 MCI	IV	A9548
MS CONTIN	500 MG	OTH	S0093
MUCOMYST	1 G	INH	J7608
MUCOSIL	1 G	INH	J7608
MULTIHANCE	1 ML	IV	A9577
MULTIHANCE MULTIPACK	1 ML	IV	A9578

Drug Name	Unit Per	Route	Code
MUROMONAB-CD3	5 MG	OTH	J7505
MUSE	EA	OTH	J0275
MUSTARGEN	10 MG	IV	J9230
MUTAMYCIN	5 MG	IV	J9280
MVASI	10 MG	IV	Q5107
MYCAMINE	1 MG	IV	J2248
MYCOPHENOLATE MOFETIL	250 MG	ORAL	J7517
MYCOPHENOLIC ACID	180 MG	ORAL	J7518
MYFORTIC DELAYED RELEASE	180 MG	ORAL	J7518
MYLERAN	2 MG	ORAL	J8510
MYLOCEL	500 MG	ORAL	S0176
MYLOTARG	0.1 MG	INF	J9203
MYOBLOC	100 U	IM	J0587
MYOCHRYSINE	50 MG	IM	J1600
MYOWN SKIN	SQ CM	OTH	Q4226
MYOZYME	10 MG	IV	J0220
NABILONE	1 MG	ORAL	J8650
NAFCILLIN SODIUM	2 GM	IM, IV	S0032
NAGLAZYME	1 MG	IV	J1458
NALBUPHINE HCL	10 MG	IM, IV, SC	J2300
NALLPEN	2 GM	IM, IV	S0032
NALOXONE HCL	1 MG	IM, IV, SC	J2310
NALOXONE HCL (ZIMHI)	1 MG	SC	J2311
NALTREXONE, DEPOT FORM	1 MG	IM	J2315
NANDROLONE DECANOATE	50 MG	IM	J2320
NARCAN	1 MG	IM, IV, SC	J2310
NAROPIN	1 MG	VAR	J2795
NASALCROM	10 MG	INH	J7631
NATALIZUMAB	1 MG	IV	J2323
NATRECOR	0.1 MG	IV	J2325
NATURAL ESTROGENIC SUBSTANCE	1 MG	IM, IV	J1410
NAVELBINE	10 MG	IV	J9390
NAXITAMAB-GQGK	1 MG	IV	J9348
ND-STAT	10 MG	IM, SC, IV	J0945
NEBCIN	80 MG	IM, IV	J3260
NEBUPENT	300 MG	IM, IV	S0080
NEBUPENT	300 MG	INH	J2545
NECITUMUMAB	1 MG	IV	J9295
NELARABINE	50 MG	IV	J9261
NEMBUTAL SODIUM	50 MG	IM, IV, OTH	J2515
NEOPATCH	SQ CM	OTH	Q4176
NEORAL	25 MG	ORAL	J7515
NEORAL	250 MG	ORAL	J7516
NEOSAR	100 MG	IV	J9070
NEOSCAN	1 MCI	IV	A9556
NEOSTIGMINE METHYLSULFATE	0.5 MG	IM, IV	J2710
NEOTECT	STUDY DOSE UP TO 35 MCI	IV	A9536
NEOX 100	SQ CM	OTH	Q4156
NEOX CORD 1K	SQ CM	OTH	Q4148
NEOX CORD RT	SQ EM	OTH	Q4148
NEOXFLO	1 MG	OTH	Q4155
NESACAINE	30 ML	VAR	J2400
NESACAINE-MPF	30 ML	VAR	J2400
NESIRITIDE	0.1 MG	IV	J2325
NETSPOT	0.1 MCI	IV	A9587

Appendix 1 — Table of Drugs and Biologicals

2023 HCPCS Level II

Drug Name	Unit Per	Route	Code
NETUPITANT AND PALONOSETRON	300 MG/ 0.5 MG	ORAL	J8655
NEULASTA	0.5 MG	SC	J2506
NEUMEGA	5 MG	SC	J2355
NEUPOGEN	1 MCG	SC, IV	J1442
NEURAGEN NERVE GUIDE	1 CM LENGTH	OTH	C9352
NEUROLITE	STUDY DOSE UP TO 25 MCI	IV	A9557
NEUROMATRIX	0.5 CM LENGTH	OTH	C9355
NEUROMEND NERVE WRAP	0.5 CM	OTH	C9361
NEUROWRAP NERVE PROTECTOR	1 CM LENGTH	OTH	C9353
NEUTREXIN	25 MG	IV	J3305
NEUTROSPEC	STUDY DOSE UP TO 25 MCI	IV	A9566
NEXPLANON	IMPLANT	OTH	J7307
NEXTERONE	30 MG	IV	J0283
NEXVIAZYME	4 MG	IV	C9085
NEXVIAZYME	4 MG	IV	J0219
NIPENT	10 MG	IV	J9268
NITROGEN MUSTARD	10 MG	IV	J9230
NITROGEN N-13 AMMONIA, DIAGNOSTIC	STUDY DOSE UP TO 40 MCI	INJ	A9526
NIVESTYM	1 MCG	INJ	Q5110
NIVOLUMAB	1 MG	IV	J9299
NIVOLUMAB AND RELATLIMAB-RMBW	3 MG/1 MG	IV	J9298
NOLVADEX	10 MG	ORAL	S0187
NORDITROPIN	1 MG	SC	J2941
NORDYL	50 MG	IV, IM	J1200
NORFLEX	60 MG	IV, IM	J2360
NORMAL SALINE SOLUTION	1000 CC	IV	J7030
NORMAL SALINE SOLUTION	250 CC	IV	J7050
NORMAL SALINE SOLUTION	500 ML	IV	J7040
NOVACHOR	SQ CM	OTH	Q4194
NOVAFIX	SQ CM	OTH	Q4208
NOVAFIX DL	SQ CM	OTH	Q4254
NOVANTRONE	5 MG	IV	J9293
NOVAREL	1,000 USP U	IM	J0725
NOVOEIGHT	IU	IV	J7182
NOVOLIN	50 U	SC	J1817
NOVOLIN R	5 U	SC	J1815
NOVOLOG	50 U	SC	J1817
NOVOSEVEN	1 MCG	IV	J7189
NOVOSORB SYNPATH DERMAL MATRIX	SQ CM	OTH	A2006
NPH	5 UNITS	SC	J1815
NPLATE	10 MCG	SC	J2796
NUBAIN	10 MG	IM, IV, SC	J2300
NUCALA	1 MG	SQ	J2182
NUDYN	0.5 CC	OTH	Q4233
NULOJIX	1 MG	IV	J0485
NUMBRINO	1 MG	OTH	C9143
NUMORPHAN	1 MG	IV, SC, IM	J2410
NUSHIELD	SQ CM	OTH	Q4160
NUSINERSEN	0.1 MG	INJ	J2326
NUTRI-TWELVE	1,000 MCG	IM, SC	J3420
NUTROPIN	1 MG	SC	J2941
NUTROPIN A.Q.	1 MG	SC	J2941

Drug Name	Unit Per	Route	Code
NUVARING VAGINAL RING	0.015 MG/ 0.12 MG	OTH	J7295
NUWIQ	1 IU	IV	J7209
NUZYRA	1 MG	IV	J0121
NYVEPRIA	0.5 MG	SC	Q5122
OASIS BURN MATRIX	SQ CM	OTH	Q4103
OASIS ULTRA TRI-LAYER WOUND MATRIX	SQ CM	OTH	Q4124
OASIS WOUND MATRIX	SQ CM	OTH	Q4102
OBINUTUZUMAB	10 MG	IV	J9301
OBIZUR	IU	IV	J7188
OCRELIZUMAB	1 MG	INJ	J2350
OCREVUS	1 MG	INJ	J2350
OCRIPLASMIN	0.125 MG	OTH	J7316
OCTAFLUOROPROPANE UCISPHERES	1 ML	IV	Q9956
OCTAGAM	500 MG	IV	J1568
OCTREOSCAN	STUDY DOSE UP TO 6 MCI	IV	A9572
OCTREOTIDE ACETATE DEPOT	1 MG	IM	J2353
OCTREOTIDE, NON-DEPOT FORM	25 MCG	SC, IV	J2354
OFATUMUMAB	10 MG	IV	J9302
OFIRMEV	10 MG	IV	J0131
OFLOXACIN	400 MG	IV	S0034
OFORTA	10 MG	ORAL	J8562
OGIVRI	10 MG	IV	Q5114
OLANZAPINE	2.5 MG	IM	S0166
OLANZAPINE LONG ACTING	1 MG	IM	J2358
OLARATUMAB	10 MG	INF	J9285
OLICERIDINE	0.1 MG	IV	C9101
OLINVYK	0.1 MG	IV	C9101
OMACETAXINE MEPESUCCINATE	0.01 MG	SC	J9262
OMADACYCLINE	1 MG	IV	J0121
OMALIZUMAB	5 MG	SC	J2357
OMEGAVEN	10 G	IV	B4187
OMEZA COLLAGEN MATRIX	100 MG	OTH	A2014
OMIDRIA	1 ML	OTH	J1097
OMNIPAQUE 140	PER ML	IV	Q9965
OMNIPAQUE 180	PER ML	IV	Q9965
OMNIPAQUE 240	PER ML	IV	Q9966
OMNIPAQUE 300	PER ML	IV	Q9967
OMNIPAQUE 350	PER ML	IV	Q9967
OMONTYS (FOR ESRD ON DIALYSIS)	0.1 MG	SC, IV	J0890
ONABOTULINUMTOXINA	1 UNIT	IM, OTH	J0585
ONASEMNOGENE ABEPARVOVEC-XIOI	UP TO 5×10^{15} VECTOR GENOMES	IV	J3399
ONCASPAR	VIAL	IM, IV	J9266
ONCOSCINT	STUDY DOSE, UP TO 6 MCI	IV	A4642
ONDANSETRON	1 MG	ORAL	Q0162
ONDANSETRON	4 MG	ORAL	S0119
ONDANSETRON HYDROCHLORIDE	1 MG	IV	J2405
ONIVYDE	1 MG	IV	J9205
ONPATTRO	0.1 MG	IV	J0222
ONTAK	300 MCG	IV	J9160
ONTRUZANT	10 MG	IV	Q5112

2023 HCPCS Level II — Appendix 1 — Table of Drugs and Biologicals

Drug Name	Unit Per	Route	Code
OPDIVO	1 MG	IV	J9299
OPDUALAG	3 MG/1 MG	IV	J9298
OPRELVEKIN	5 MG	SC	J2355
OPTIRAY	PER ML	IV	Q9967
OPTIRAY 160	PER ML	IV	Q9965
OPTIRAY 240	PER ML	IV	Q9966
OPTIRAY 300	PER ML	IV	Q9967
OPTIRAY 320	PER ML	IV	Q9967
OPTISON	1 ML	IV	Q9956
ORAL MAGNETIC RESONANCE CONTRAST AGENT, PER 100 ML	100 ML	ORAL	Q9954
ORBACTIV	10 MG	IV	J2407
ORENCIA	10 MG	IV	J0129
ORITAVANCIN	10 MG	IV	J2407
ORITAVANCIN	10 MG	IV	J2406
ORPHENADRINE CITRATE	60 MG	IV, IM	J2360
ORTHADAPT BIOIMPLANT	SQ CM	OTH	C1781
ORTHOCLONE OKT3	5 MG	OTH	J7505
ORTHOVISC	PER DOSE	INJ	J7324
OSELTAMIVIR PHOSPHATE (BRAND NAME) (DEMONSTRATION PROJECT)	75 MG	ORAL	G9035
OSELTAMIVIR PHOSPHATE (GENERIC) (DEMONSTRATION PROJECT)	75 MG	ORAL	G9019
OSMITROL	25% IN 50 ML	IV	J2150
OTIPRIO	6 MG	OTIC	J7342
OXACILLIN SODIUM	250 MG	IM, IV	J2700
OXALIPLATIN	0.5 MG	IV	J9263
OXILAN 300	PER ML	IV	Q9967
OXILAN 350	PER ML	IV	Q9967
OXLUMO	0.5 MG	SC	J0224
OXYMORPHONE HCL	1 MG	IV, SC, IM	J2410
OXYTETRACYCLINE HCL	50 MG	IM	J2460
OXYTOCIN	10 U	IV, IM	J2590
OZURDEX	0.1 MG	OTH	J7312
PACIS BCG	1 MG	OTH	J9030
PACLITAXEL	1 MG	IV	J9267
PACLITAXEL PROTEIN-BOUND PARTICLES	1 MG	IV	J9264
PADCEV	0.25 MG	IV	J9177
PALIFERMIN	50 MCG	IV	J2425
PALINGEN OR PALINGEN XPLU	SQ CM	OTH	Q4173
PALINGEN OR PROMATRX	0.36 MG/ 0.25 CC	OTH	Q4174
PALIPERIDONE PALMITATE EXTENDED RELEASED	1 MG	IM	J2426
PALONOSETRON HCL	25 MCG	IV	J2469
PAMIDRONATE DISODIUM	30 MG	IV	J2430
PANHEMATIN	1 MG	IV	J1640
PANITUMUMAB	10 MG	IV	J9303
PANTOPRAZOLE SODIUM	VIAL	IV	C9113
PANTOPRAZOLE SODIUM	40 MG	IV	S0164
PAPAVERINE HCL	60 MG	IV, IM	J2440
PARAGARD T380A	EA	OTH	J7300
PARAPLANTIN	50 MG	IV	J9045
PARICALCITOL	1 MCG	IV, IM	J2501
PARSABIV	0.1 MG	IV	J0606

Drug Name	Unit Per	Route	Code
PASIREOTIDE LONG ACTING	1 MG	IV	J2502
PATISIRAN	0.1 MG	IV	J0222
PEDIAPRED	5 MG	ORAL	J7510
PEG-INTRON	180 MCG	SC	S0145
PEGADEMASE BOVINE	25 IU	IM	J2504
PEGAPTANIB SODIUM	0.3 MG	OTH	J2503
PEGASPARGASE	VIAL	IM, IV	J9266
PEGFILGRASTIM, EXCLUDES BIOSIMILAR	0.5 MG	SC	J2506
PEGFILGRASTIM-APGF, BIOSIMILAR	0.5 MG	SC	Q5122
PEGFILGRASTIM-BMEZ, BIOSIMILAR	0.5 MG	SC	Q5120
PEGFILGRASTIM-CBQV, BIOSIMILAR	0.5 MG	SC	Q5111
PEGFILGRASTIM-JMDB, BIOSIMILAR	0.5 MG	SC	Q5108
PEGINESATIDE (FOR ESRD ON DIALYSIS)	0.1 MG	SC, IV	J0890
PEGINTERFERON ALFA-2A	180 MCG	SC	S0145
PEGLOTICASE	1 MG	IV	J2507
PEGYLATED INTERFERON ALFA-2A	180 MCG	SC	S0145
PEGYLATED INTERFERON ALFA-2B	10 MCG	SC	S0148
PEMBROLIZUMAB	1 MG	IV	J9271
PEMETREXED	10 MG	IV	J9304
PEMFEXY	10 MG	IV	J9304
PENICILLIN G BENZATHINE	100,000 U	IM	J0561
PENICILLIN G BENZATHINE AND PENICILLIN G PROCAINE	100,000 UNITS	IM	J0558
PENICILLIN G POTASSIUM	600,000 U	IM, IV	J2540
PENICILLIN G PROCAINE	600,000 U	IM, IV	J2510
PENTACARINAT	300 MG	INH	S0080
PENTAM	300 MG	IM, IV	J2545
PENTAM 300	300 MG	IM, IV	S0080
PENTAMIDINE ISETHIONATE	300 MG	IM, IV	S0080
PENTAMIDINE ISETHIONATE COMPOUNDED	PER 300 MG	INH	J7676
PENTAMIDINE ISETHIONATE NONCOMPOUNDED	300 MG	INH	J2545
PENTASPAN	100 ML	IV	J2513
PENTASTARCH 10% SOLUTION	100 ML	IV	J2513
PENTATE CALCIUM TRISODIUM	STUDY DOSE UP TO 75 MCI	INH	A9567
PENTATE CALCIUM TRISODIUM	STUDY DOSE UP TO 25 MCI	IV	A9539
PENTATE ZINC TRISODIUM	STUDY DOSE UP TO 25 MCI	IV	A9539
PENTATE ZINC TRISODIUM	STUDY DOSE UP TO 75 MCI	INH	A9567
PENTAZOCINE	30 MG	IM, SC, IV	J3070
PENTOBARBITAL SODIUM	50 MG	IM, IV, OTH	J2515
PENTOSTATIN	10 MG	IV	J9268
PEPAXTO	1 MG	IV	J9247
PEPCID	20 MG	IV	S0028
PERAMIVIR	1 MG	IV	J2547
PERFLEXANE LIPID MICROSPHERE	1 ML	IV	Q9955
PERFLUTREN LIPID MICROSPHERE	1 ML	IV	Q9957
PERFOROMIST	20 MCG	INH	J7606
PERJETA	1 MG	IV	J9306

Appendix 1 — Table of Drugs and Biologicals

2023 HCPCS Level II

Drug Name	Unit Per	Route	Code
PERMACOL	SQ CM	OTH	C9364
PERMEADERM B	SQ CM	OTH	A2016
PERMEADERM C	SQ CM	OTH	A2018
PERMEADERM GLOVE	EA	OTH	A2017
PERPHENAZINE	5 MG	IM, IV	J3310
PERPHENAZINE	4 MG	ORAL	Q0175
PERSANTINE	10 MG	IV	J1245
PERSERIS	0.5 MG	SC	J2798
PERTUZUMAB	1 MG	IV	J9306
PERTUZUMAB, TRASTUZUMAB, AND HYALURONIDASE-ZZXF	10 MG	SC	J9316
PFIZERPEN A.S.	600,000 U	IM, IV	J2510
PHENERGAN	50 MG	IM, IV	J2550
PHENERGAN	12.5 MG	ORAL	Q0169
PHENOBARBITAL SODIUM	120 MG	IM, IV	J2560
PHENTOLAMINE MESYLATE	5 MG	IM, IV	J2760
PHENYLEPHRINE 10.16 MG/ML AND KETOROLAC 2.88 MG/ML OPHTHALMIC IRRIGATION SOLUTION	1 ML	OTH	J1097
PHENYLEPHRINE HCL	1 ML	SC, IM, IV	J2370
PHENYTOIN SODIUM	50 MG	IM, IV	J1165
PHESGO	10 MG	SC	J9316
PHOENIX WOUND MATRIX	SQ CM	OTH	A2015
PHOSPHOCOL	1 MCI	IV	A9563
PHOSPHOTEC	STUDY DOSE UP TO 25 MCI	IV	A9538
PHOTOFRIN	75 MG	IV	J9600
PHOTREXA VISCOUS	UP TO 3 ML	OTH	J2787
PHYTONADIONE	1 MG	IM, SC, IV	J3430
PIFLUFOLASTAT F-18, DIAGNOSTIC	1 MCI	IV	A9595
PIPERACILLIN SODIUM	500 MG	IM, IV	S0081
PIPERACILLIN SODIUM/ TAZOBACTAM SODIUM	1 G/1.125 GM	IV	J2543
PITOCIN	10 U	IV, IM	J2590
PLASMINOGEN, HUMAN-TVMH	1 MG	IV	C9090
PLASMINOGEN, HUMAN-TVMH	1 MG	IV	J2998
PLATINOL AQ	10 MG	IV	J9060
PLAZOMICIN	5 MG	IV	J0291
PLERIXAFOR	1 MG	SC	J2562
PLICAMYCIN	2.5 MG	IV	J9270
PLUVICTO	1 MCI	IV	A9607
PNEUMOCOCCAL CONJUGATE	EA	IM	S0195
PNEUMOVAX II	EA	IM	S0195
POLATUZUMAB VEDOTIN-PIIQ	1 MG	IV	J9309
POLIVY	1 MG	IV	J9309
POLOCAINE	10 ML	VAR	J0670
POLYCYTE	0.5 CC	OTH	Q4241
PORCINE IMPLANT, PERMACOL	SQ CM	OTH	C9364
PORFIMER SODIUM	75 MG	IV	J9600
PORK INSULIN	5 U	SC	J1815
POROUS PURIFIED COLLAGEN MATRIX BONE VOID FILLER	0.5 CC	OTH	C9362
POROUS PURIFIED COLLAGEN MATRIX BONE VOID FILLER, PUTTY	0.5 CC	OTH	C9359
PORTRAZZA.	1 MG	IV	J9295
POSIMIR	1 MG	INJ	C9144

Drug Name	Unit Per	Route	Code
POTASSIUM CHLORIDE	2 MEQ	IV	J3480
POTELIGEO	1 MG	IV	J9204
PRALATREXATE	1 MG	IV	J9307
PRALIDOXIME CHLORIDE	1 MG	IV, IM, SC	J2730
PREDNISOLONE	5 MG	ORAL	J7510
PREDNISOLONE ACETATE	1 ML	IM	J2650
PREDNISONE, IMMEDIATE RELEASE OR DELAYED RELEASE	1 MG	ORAL	J7512
PREDNORAL	5 MG	ORAL	J7510
PREGNYL	1,000 USP U	IM	J0725
PRELONE	5 MG	ORAL	J7510
PREMARIN	25 MG	IV, IM	J1410
PRENATAL VITAMINS	30 TABS	ORAL	S0197
PRI-METHYLATE	80 MG	IM	J1040
PRIALT	1 MCG	OTH	J2278
PRIMACOR	5 MG	IV	J2260
PRIMATRIX	SQ CM	OTH	Q4110
PRIMAXIN	250 MG	IV, IM	J0743
PRIMESTRIN AQUEOUS	1 MG	IM, IV	J1410
PRIMETHASONE	1 MG	IM, IV, OTH	J1100
PRIVIGEN	500 MG	IV	J1459
PROBUPHINE IMPLANT	74.2 MG	OTH	J0570
PROCAINAMIDE HCL	1 G	IM, IV	J2690
PROCARBAZINE HCL	50 MG	ORAL	S0182
PROCENTA	200 MG	OTH	Q4244
PROCHLOPERAZINE MALEATE	5 MG	ORAL	S0183
PROCHLORPERAZINE	10 MG	IM, IV	J0780
PROCHLORPERAZINE MALEATE	5 MG	ORAL	Q0164
PROCRIT, NON-ESRD USE	1,000 U	SC, IV	J0885
PROFILNINE HEAT-TREATED	1 IU	IV	J7194
PROFILNINE SD	1 IU	IV	J7194
PROFONIX	VIAL	INJ	C9113
PROGENAMATRIX	SQ CM	OTH	Q4222
PROGESTERONE	50 MG	IM	J2675
PROGRAF	5 MG	OTH	J7525
PROGRAF	1 MG	ORAL	J7507
PROLEUKIN	1 VIAL	VAR	J9015
PROLIA	1 MG	SC	J0897
PROLIXIN DECANOATE	25 MG	SC, IM	J2680
PROMAZINE HCL	25 MG	IM	J2950
PROMETHAZINE HCL	12.5 MG	ORAL	Q0169
PROMETHAZINE HCL	50 MG	IM, IV	J2550
PRONESTYL	1 G	IM, IV	J2690
PROPECIA	5 MG	ORAL	S0138
PROPLEX SX-T	1 IU	IV	J7194
PROPLEX T	1 IU	IV	J7194
PROPOFOL	10 MG	IV	J2704
PROPRANOLOL HCL	1 MG	IV	J1800
PROREX	50 MG	IM, IV	J2550
PROSCAR	5 MG	ORAL	S0138
PROSTASCINT	STUDY DOSE UP TO 10 MCI	IV	A9507
PROSTIGMIN	0.5 MG	IM, IV	J2710
PROSTIN VR	1.25 MCG	INJ	J0270
PROTAMINE SULFATE	10 MG	IV	J2720
PROTEIN C CONCENTRATE	10 IU	IV	J2724
PROTEXT	1 CC	OTH	Q4246

22 — Appendixes

© 2022 Optum, Inc.

Drug Name	Unit Per	Route	Code
PROTHROMBIN COMPLEX CONCENTRATE (HUMAN)	PER IU	IV	J7168
PROTIRELIN	250 MCG	IV	J2725
PROTONIX IV	40 MG	IV	S0164
PROTONIX IV	VIAL	IV	C9113
PROTOPAM CHLORIDE	1 G	SC, IM, IV	J2730
PROTROPIN	1 MG	SC, IM	J2940
PROVENGE	INFUSION	IV	Q2043
PROVENTIL NONCOMPOUNDED, CONCENTRATED	1 MG	INH	J7611
PROVENTIL NONCOMPOUNDED, UNIT DOSE	1 MG	INH	J7613
PROVOCHOLINE POWDER	1 MG	INH	J7674
PROZINE-50	25 MG	IM	J2950
PULMICORT	0.25 MG	INH	J7633
PULMICORT RESPULES	0.5 MG	INH	J7627
PULMICORT RESPULES NONCOMPOUNDED, CONCETRATED	0.25 MG	INH	J7626
PULMOZYME	1 MG	INH	J7639
PURAPLY	SQ CM	OTH	Q4195
PURAPLY AM	SQ CM	OTH	Q4196
PURAPLY XT	SQ CM	OTH	Q4197
PURINETHOL	50 MG	ORAL	S0108
PYLARIFY	1 MCI	IV	A9595
PYRIDOXINE HCL	100 MG	IM, IV	J3415
QUADRAMET	PER DOSE UP TO 150 MCI	IV	A9604
QUELICIN	20 MG	IM, IV	J0330
QUINUPRISTIN/DALFOPRISTIN	500 MG	IV	J2770
QUTENZA	1 SQ CM	OTH	J7336
QUZYTIIR	0.5 MG	IV	J1201
RADICAVA	1 MG	IV	J1301
RADIESSE	0.1 ML	OTH	Q2026
RADIUM (RA) 223 DICHLORIDE THERAPEUTIC	PER MICROCURIE	IV	A9606
RAMUCIRUMAB	5 MG	IV	J9308
RANIBIZUMAB	0.1 MG	OTH	J2778
RANIBIZUMAB	0.1 MG	OTH	J2779
RANIBIZUMAB, VIA SUSTAINED RELEASE INTRAVITREAL IMPLANT	0.1 MG	OTH	C9093
RANIBIZUMAB-NUNA	0.1 MG	INJ	Q5124
RANITIDINE HCL	25 MG	INJ	J2780
RAPAMUNE	1 MG	ORAL	J7520
RAPIVAB	1 MG	IV	J2547
RASBURICASE	0.5 MG	IM	J2783
RAVULIZUMAB-CWVZ	10 MG	IV	J1303
REBETRON KIT	1,000,000 U	SC, IM	J9214
REBIF	30 MCG	SC	J1826
REBIF	1 MCG	SC	Q3028
REBINYN	1 IU	IV	J7203
REBLOZYL	0.25 MG	SC	J0896
RECARBRIO	4 MG/4 MG/2 MG	IV	J0742
RECLAST	1 MG	IV	J3489
REDISOL	1,000 MCG	SC. IM	J3420
REFLUDAN	50 MG	IM, IV	J1945
REGADENOSON	0.1 MG	IV	J2785

Drug Name	Unit Per	Route	Code
REGEN-COV	1200 MG	IV	Q0244
REGITINE	5 MG	IM, IV	J2760
REGLAN	10 MG	IV	J2765
REGRANEX GEL	0.5 G	OTH	S0157
REGUARD	SQ CM	OTH	Q4255
REGULAR INSULIN	5 UNITS	SC	J1815
RELAXIN	10 ML	IV, IM	J2800
RELENZA (DEMONSTRATION PROJECT)	10 MG	INH	G9034
RELESE	SQ CM	OTH	Q4257
RELEUKO	1 MCG	SC	C9096
RELEUKO	1 MCG	SC, IV	Q5125
RELION	5 U	SC	J1815
RELION NOVOLIN	50 U	SC	J1817
RELISTOR	0.1 MG	SC	J2212
REMDESIVIR	1 MG	IV	J0248
REMICADE	10 MG	IV	J1745
REMODULIN	1 MG	SC	J3285
RENFLEXIS	10 MG	IV	Q5104
REODULIN	1 MG	SC	J3285
REOPRO	10 MG	IV	J0130
REPRIZA	SQ CM	OTH	Q4143
REPRONEX	75 IU	SC, IM, IV	S0122
RESLIZUMAB	1 MG	IV	J2786
RESPIROL NONCOMPOUNDED, CONCENTRATED	1 MG	INH	J7611
RESPIROL NONCOMPOUNDED, UNIT DOSE	1 MG	INH	J7613
RESTORIGIN	1 CC	INJ	Q4192
RESTORIGIN	SQ CM	OTH	Q4191
RESTRATA	SQ CM	OTH	A2007
RETACRIT	100 UNITS	INJ, IV	Q5105
RETACRIT	1000 UNITS	INJ, IV	Q5106
RETAVASE	18.1 MG	IV	J2993
RETEPLASE	18.1 MG	IV	J2993
RETISERT	IMPLANT	OTH	J7311
RETROVIR	10 MG	IV	J3485
RETROVIR	100 MG	ORAL	S0104
REVEFENACIN INHALATION	1 MCG	INH	J7677
REVITA	SQ CM	OTH	Q4180
REVITALON	SQ CM	OTH	Q4157
RHEOMACRODEX	500 ML	IV	J7100
RHEUMATREX	2.5 MG	ORAL	J8610
RHEUMATREX DOSE PACK	2.5 MG	ORAL	J8610
RHO D IMMUNE GLOBULIN	300 MCG	IV	J2790
RHO D IMMUNE GLOBULIN (RHOPHYLAC)	100 IU	IM, IV	J2791
RHO D IMMUNE GLOBULIN MINIDOSE	50 MCG	IM	J2788
RHO D IMMUNE GLOBULIN SOLVENT DETERGENT	100 IU	IV	J2792
RHOGAM	50 MCG	IM	J2788
RHOGAM	300 MCG	IM	J2790
RHOPHYLAC	100 IU	IM, IV	J2791
RIABNI	10 MG	IV	Q5123
RIBOFLAVIN 5'-PHOSPHATE, OPHTHALMIC SOLUTION	UP TO 3 ML	OTH	J2787
RILONACEPT	1 MG	SC	J2793

Appendix 1 — Table of Drugs and Biologicals

Drug Name	Unit Per	Route	Code
RIMANTADINE HCL (DEMONSTRATION PROJECT)	100 MG	ORAL	G9020
RIMANTADINE HCL (DEMONSTRATION PROJECT)	100 MG	ORAL	G9036
RIMSO 50	50 ML	IV	J1212
RINGERS LACTATE INFUSION	UP TO 1000 CC	IV	J7120
RISANKIZUMAB-RZAA	1 MG	IV	J2327
RISPERDAL CONSTA	0.5 MG	IM	J2794
RISPERIDONE	0.5 MG	SC	J2798
RISPERIDONE	0.5 MG	IM	J2794
RITUXAN	10 MG	IV	J9312
RITUXAN HYCELA	10 MG	SC	J9311
RITUXIMAB	10 MG	IV	J9312
RITUXIMAB 10 MG AND HYALURONIDASE	10 MG	SC	J9311
RITUXIMAB-ABBS, BIOSIMILAR	10 MG	IV	Q5115
RITUXIMAB-ARRX, BIOSIMILAR	10 MG	IV	Q5123
RITUXIMAB-PVVR, BIOSIMILAR	10 MG	IV	Q5119
RIXUBIS	IU	IV	J7200
ROBAXIN	10 ML	IV, IM	J2800
ROCEPHIN	250 MG	IV, IM	J0696
ROFERON-A	3,000,000 U	SC, IM	J9213
ROLAPITANT	1 MG	ORAL	J8670
ROLAPITANT	0.5 MG	ORAL, IV	J2797
ROMIDEPSIN, LYOPHILIZED	0.1 MG	IV	J9319
ROMIDEPSIN, NONLYOPHILIZED	0.1 MG	IV	J9318
ROMIPLOSTIM	10 MCG	SC	J2796
ROMOSOZUMAB-AQQG	1 MG	SC	J3111
ROPIVACAINE HYDROCHLORIDE	1 MG	VAR	J2795
RUBEX	10 MG	IV	J9000
RUBIDIUM RB-82	STUDY DOSE UP TO 60 MCI	IV	A9555
RUBRAMIN PC	1,000 MCG	SC, IM	J3420
RUBRATOPE 57	STUDY DOSE UP TO 1 UCI	ORAL	A9559
RUCONEST	10 UNITS	IV	J0596
RUXIENCE	10 MG	IV	Q5119
RYBREVANT	2 MG	IV	J9061
RYLAZE	0.1 MG	IM	J9021
~~RYPLAZIM~~	~~1 MG~~	~~IV~~	~~C9090~~
RYPLAZIM	1 MG	IV	J2998
SACITUZUMAB GOVITECAN-HZIY	2.5 MG	IV	J9317
SAIZEN	1 MG	SC	J2941
SAIZEN SOMATROPIN RDNA ORIGIN	1 MG	SC	J2941
SALINE OR STERILE WATER, METERED DOSE DISPENSER	10 ML	INH	A4218
SALINE, STERILE WATER, AND/OR DEXTROSE DILUENT/FLUSH	10 ML	VAR	A4216
SALINE/STERILE WATER	500 ML	VAR	A4217
SAMARIUM LEXIDRONAM	PER DOSE UP TO 150 MCI	IV	A9604
SANDIMMUNE	100 MG	ORAL	J7502
SANDIMMUNE	250 MG	IV	J7516
SANDIMMUNE	25 MG	ORAL	J7515
SANDOSTATIN	25 MCG	SC, IV	J2354
SANDOSTATIN LAR	1 MG	IM	J2353
SANGCYA	100 MG	ORAL	J7502

Drug Name	Unit Per	Route	Code
SANO-DROL	40 MG	IM	J1030
SANO-DROL	80 MG	IM	J1040
SAPHNELLO	1 MG	IV	J0491
~~SAPHNELO~~	~~1 MG~~	~~IV~~	~~C9086~~
SAQUINAVIR	200 MG	ORAL	S0140
SARCLISA	10 MG	IV	J9227
SARGRAMOSTIM (GM-CSF)	50 MCG	IV	J2820
SCANDONEST	PER 10 ML	IV	J0670
SCENESSE	1 MG	OTH	J7352
SCULPTRA	0.5 ML	OTH	Q2028
SEBELIPASE ALFA	1 MG	IV	J2840
SECREFLO	1 MCG	IV	J2850
SECRETIN, SYNTHETIC, HUMAN	1 MCG	IV	J2850
SEGESTERONE ACETATE AND ETHINYL ESTRADIOL VAGINAL RING	0.15 MG/ 0.013 MG	OTH	J7294
SENSIPAR	1 MG	ORAL	J0604
SENSORCAINE	30 ML	VAR	S0020
SEPTRA IV	10 ML	IV	S0039
SERMORELIN ACETATE	1 MCG	IV	Q0515
SEROSTIM	1 MG	SC	J2941
SEROSTIM RDNA ORIGIN	1 MG	SC	J2941
SEVENFACT	1 MCG	IV	J7212
SIGNATURE APATCH	SQ CM	OTH	Q4260
SIGNIFOR LAR	1 MG	IV	J2502
SILDENAFIL CITRATE	25 MG	ORAL	S0090
SILTUXIMAB	10 MG	IV	J2860
SIMPONI	1 MG	IV	J1602
SIMULECT	20 MG	IV	J0480
SINCALIDE	5 MCG	IV	J2805
SINUVA	10 MCG	OTH	J7402
SIPULEUCEL-T	INFUSION	IV	Q2043
SIROLIMUS	1 MG	ORAL	J7520
~~SIROLIMUS PROTEIN-BOUND PARTICLES~~	~~1 MG~~	~~IV~~	~~C9091~~
SIROLIMUS PROTEIN-BOUND PARTICLES	1 MG	IV	J9331
SIVEXTRO	1 MG	IV	J3090
~~SKIN SUBSTITUTE, SYNTHETIC, RESORBABLE~~	~~SQ CM~~	~~OTH~~	~~C1849~~
SKINTE	SQ CM	OTH	Q4200
SKYLA	13.5 MG	OTH	J7301
SKYRIZI	1 MG	IV	J2327
SMZ-TMP	10 ML	IV	S0039
SODIUM FERRIC GLUCONATE COMPLEX IN SUCROSE	12.5 MG	IV	J2916
SODIUM FLUORIDE F-18, DIAGNOSTIC	STUDY DOSE UP TO 30 MCI	IV	A9580
SODIUM IODIDE I-131 CAPSULE DIAGNOSTIC	1 MCI	ORAL	A9528
SODIUM IODIDE I-131 CAPSULE THERAPEUTIC	1 MCI	ORAL	A9517
SODIUM IODIDE I-131 SOLUTION THERAPEUTIC	1 MCI	ORAL	A9530
SODIUM PHOSPHATE P32	1 MCI	IV	A9563
SOLGANAL	50 MG	IM	J2910
SOLIRIS	10 MG	IV	J1300
SOLTAMOX	10 MG	ORAL	S0187
SOLU-CORTEF	100 MG	IV, IM, SC	J1720

Drug Name	Unit Per	Route	Code
SOLU-MEDROL	40 MG	IM, IV	J2920
SOLU-MEDROL	125 MG	IM, IV	J2930
SOLUREX	1 MG	IM, IV, OTH	J1100
SOMATREM	1 MG	SC, IM	J2940
SOMATROPIN	1 MG	SC	J2941
SOMATULINE	1 MG	SC	J1930
SOTALOL HYDROCHLORIDE	1 MG	IV	C9482
SOTROVIMAB	500 MG	IV	Q0247
SPECTINOMYCIN DIHYDROCHLORIDE	2 G	IM	J3320
SPECTRO-DEX	1 MG	IM, IV, OTH	J1100
SPINRAZA	0.1 MG	INJ	J2326
SPORANOX	50 MG	IV	J1835
SPRAVATO	1 MG	OTH	S0013
STADOL	1 MG	IM, IV	J0595
STADOL NS	25 MG	OTH	S0012
STELARA	1 MG	SC	J3357
STELARA	1 MG	SC, IV	J3358
STERILE WATER OR SALINE, METERED DOSE DISPENSER	10 ML	INH	A4218
STERILE WATER, SALINE, AND/OR DEXTROSE DILUENT/FLUSH	10 ML	VAR	A4216
STERILE WATER/SALINE	500 ML	VAR	A4217
STRATTICE TM	SQ CM	OTH	Q4130
STRAVIX	SQ CM	OTH	Q4133
STRAVIXPL	SQ CM	OTH	Q4133
STREPTASE	250,000 IU	IV	J2995
STREPTOKINASE	250,000 IU	IV	J2995
STREPTOMYCIN	1 G	IM	J3000
STREPTOZOCIN	1 G	IV	J9320
STRONTIUM 89 CHLORIDE	1 MCI	IV	A9600
SUBLIMAZE	0.1 MG	IM, IV	J3010
SUBLOCADE	≤ 100 MG	SC	Q9991
SUBLOCADE	> 100 MG	SC	Q9992
SUBOXONE	4 MG	ORAL	J0573
SUBOXONE	2 MG	ORAL	J0572
SUBOXONE	12 MG	ORAL	J0575
SUBOXONE	8 MG	ORAL	J0574
SUBUTEX	1 MG	ORAL	J0571
SUCCINYLCHOLINE CHLORIDE	20 MG	IM, IV	J0330
SULFAMETHOXAZOLE AND TRIMETHOPRIM	10 ML	IV	S0039
SULFUR HEXAFLUORIDE LIPID MICROSPHERES	1 ML	IV	Q9950
SULFUTRIM	10 ML	IV	S0039
SUMATRIPTAN SUCCINATE	6 MG	SC	J3030
SUPARTZ	PER DOSE	INJ	J7321
SUPPRELIN LA	10 MCG	OTH	J1675
SUPRA SDRM	SQ CM	OTH	A2011
SUPRATHEL	SQ CM	OTH	A2012
SUREDERM	SQ CM	OTH	Q4220
SURFACTOR	0.5 CC	OTH	Q4233
SURGICORD	SQ CM	OTH	Q4218
SURGIGRAFT	SQ CM	OTH	Q4183
SURGIGRAFT-DUAL	SQ CM	OTH	Q4219
SURGIMEND COLLAGEN MATRIX, FETAL	0.5 SQ CM	OTH	C9358
SURGIMEND COLLAGEN MATRIX, NEONATAL	0.5 SQ CM	OTH	C9360
SURGRAFT	SQ CM	OTH	Q4209
SURGRAFT TL	SQ CM	OTH	Q4263
SUSTOL	0.1 MG	SC	J1627
~~SUSVIMO~~	~~0.1 MG~~	~~OTH~~	~~C9093~~
SUSVIMO	0.1 MG	OTH	J2779
~~SUTIMLIMAB-JOME~~	~~10 MG~~	~~IV~~	~~C9094~~
SUTIMLIMAB-JOME	10 MG	IV	J1302
SYLVANT	10 MG	IV	J2860
SYMMETREL (DEMONSTRATION PROJECT)	100 MG	ORAL	G9033
SYMPHONY	SQ CM	OTH	A2009
SYNERA	70 MG/70 MG	OTH	C9285
SYNERCID	500 MG	IV	J2770
SYNOJOYNT	1 MG	INJ	J7331
SYNRIBO	0.01 MG	SC	J9262
SYNTOCINON	10 UNITS	IV	J2590
SYNVISC/SYNVISC-ONE	1 MG	INJ	J7325
SYTOBEX	1,000 MCG	SC, IM	J3420
T-GEN	250 MG	ORAL	Q0173
TACRINE HCL	10 MG	ORAL	S0014
TACROLIMUS	1 MG	ORAL	J7507
TACROLIMUS	5 MG	OTH	J7525
TACROLIMUS, EXTENDED RELEASE	0.25 MG	ORAL	J7503
TACROLIMUS, EXTENDED RELEASE	0.1 MG	ORAL	J7508
TAFASITAMAB-CXIX	2 MG	IV	J9349
TAG	SQ CM	OTH	Q4261
TAGAMET HCL	300 MG	IM, IV	S0023
TAGRAXOFUSP-ERZS	10 MCG	IV	J9269
TAKHZYRO	1 MG	SC	J0593
TALIGLUCERASE ALFA	10 U	IV	J3060
TALIMOGENE LAHERPAREPVEC	1 MILLION	INTRA-LESIONAL	J9325
TALWIN	30 MG	IM, SC, IV	J3070
TALYMED	SQ CM	OTH	Q4127
TAMIFLU (DEMONSTRATION PROJECT)	75 MG	ORAL	G9019
TAMIFLU (DEMONSTRATION PROJECT)	75 MG	ORAL	G9035
TAMOXIFEN CITRATE	10 MG	ORAL	S0187
TAUVID	1 MCI	IV	A9601
TAXOL	1 MG	IV	J9267
TAXOTERE	1 MG	IV	J9171
TAZICEF	500 MG	IM, IV	J0713
TBO-FILGRASTIM	1 MCG	IV	J1447
TC 99M TILOMANOCEPT	0.5 MCI	SC, OTH	A9520
TEBAMIDE	250 MG	ORAL	Q0173
~~TEBENTAFUSP-TEBN~~	~~1 MCG~~	~~IV~~	~~C9095~~
TEBENTAFUSP-TEBN	1 MCG	IV	J9274
TEBOROXIME TECHNETIUM TC 99M	STUDY DOSE	IV	A9501
TEBOROXIME, TECHNETIUM	STUDY DOSE	IV	A9501
TECARTUS	UP TO 200 MILLION CELLS	IV	Q2053
TECENTRIQ	10 MG	INF	J9022
TECHNEPLEX	STUDY DOSE UP TO 25 MCI	IV	A9539

Appendix 1 — Table of Drugs and Biologicals

2023 HCPCS Level II

Drug Name	Unit Per	Route	Code
TECHNESCAN	STUDY DOSE UP TO 30 MCI	IV	A9561
TECHNESCAN FANOLESOMAB	STUDY DOSE UP TO 25 MCI	IV	A9566
TECHNESCAN MAA	STUDY DOSE UP TO 10 MCI	IV	A9540
TECHNESCAN MAG3	STUDY DOSE UP TO 15 MCI	IV	A9562
TECHNESCAN PYP	STUDY DOSE UP TO 25 MCI	IV	A9538
TECHNESCAN PYP KIT	STUDY DOSE UP TO 25 MCI	IV	A9538
TECHNETIUM SESTAMBI	STUDY DOSE	IV	A9500
TECHNETIUM TC 99M APCITIDE	STUDY DOSE UP TO 20 MCI	IV	A9504
TECHNETIUM TC 99M ARCITUMOMAB, DIAGNOSTIC	STUDY DOSE UP TO 45 MCI	IV	A9568
TECHNETIUM TC 99M BICISATE	STUDY DOSE UP TO 25 MCI	IV	A9557
TECHNETIUM TC 99M DEPREOTIDE	STUDY DOSE UP TO 35 MCI	IV	A9536
TECHNETIUM TC 99M EXAMETAZIME	STUDY DOSE UP TO 25 MCI	IV	A9521
TECHNETIUM TC 99M FANOLESOMAB	STUDY DOSE UP TO 25 MCI	IV	A9566
TECHNETIUM TC 99M LABELED RED BLOOD CELLS	STUDY DOSE UP TO 30 MCI	IV	A9560
TECHNETIUM TC 99M MACROAGGREGATED ALBUMIN	STUDY DOSE UP TO 10 MCI	IV	A9540
TECHNETIUM TC 99M MDI-MDP	STUDY DOSE UP TO 30 MCI	IV	A9503
TECHNETIUM TC 99M MEBROFENIN	STUDY DOSE UP TO 15 MCI	IV	A9537
TECHNETIUM TC 99M MEDRONATE	STUDY DOSE UP TO 30 MCI	IV	A9503
TECHNETIUM TC 99M MERTIATIDE	STUDY DOSE UP TO 15 MCI	IV	A9562
TECHNETIUM TC 99M OXIDRONATE	STUDY DOSE UP TO 30 MCI	IV	A9561
TECHNETIUM TC 99M PENTETATE	STUDY DOSE UP TO 25 MCI	IV	A9539
TECHNETIUM TC 99M PYROPHOSPHATE	STUDY DOSE UP TO 25 MCI	IV	A9538
TECHNETIUM TC 99M SODIUM GLUCEPATATE	STUDY DOSE UP TO 25 MCI	IV	A9550
TECHNETIUM TC 99M SUCCIMER	STUDY DOSE UP TO 10 MCI	IV	A9551
TECHNETIUM TC 99M SULFUR COLLOID	STUDY DOSE UP TO 20 MCI	IV	A9541
TECHNETIUM TC 99M TETROFOSMIN, DIAGNOSTIC	STUDY DOSE	IV	A9502
TECHNETIUM TC-99M EXAMETAZIME LABELED AUTOLOGOUS WHITE BLOOD CELLS	STUDY DOSE	IV	A9569
TECHNETIUM TC-99M TEBOROXIME	STUDY DOSE	IV	A9501
TECHNILITE	1 MCI	IV	A9512
TEDIZOLID PHOSPHATE	1 MG	IV	J3090
TEFLARO	10 MG	IV	J0712
TELAVANCIN	10 MG	IV	J3095
TEMODAR	5 MG	ORAL	J8700
TEMODAR	1 MG	IV	J9328

Drug Name	Unit Per	Route	Code
TEMOZOLOMIDE	5 MG	ORAL	J8700
TEMOZOLOMIDE	1 MG	IV	J9328
TEMSIROLIMUS	1 MG	IV	J9330
TENDON, POROUS MATRIX	SQ CM	OTH	C9356
TENDON, POROUS MATRIX CROSS-LINKED AND GLYCOSAMINOGLYCAN MATRIX	SQ CM	OTH	C9356
TENECTEPLASE	1 MG	IV	J3101
TENIPOSIDE	50 MG	IV	Q2017
TENOGLIDE TENDON PROTECTOR	SQ CM	OTH	C9356
TENOGLIDE TENDON PROTECTOR SHEET	SQ CM	OTH	C9356
TENSIX	SQ CM	OTH	Q4146
TEPEZZA	10 MG	IV	J3241
TEPROTUMUMAB-TRBW	10 MG	IV	J3241
TEQUIN	10 MG	IV	J1590
TERBUTALINE SULFATE	1 MG	SC, IV	J3105
TERBUTALINE SULFATE, COMPOUNDED, CONCENTRATED	1 MG	INH	J7680
TERBUTALINE SULFATE, COMPOUNDED, UNIT DOSE	1 MG	INH	J7681
TERIPARATIDE	10 MCG	SC	J3110
TERRAMYCIN	50 MG	IM	J2460
TESTOSTERONE CYPIONATE	1 MG	IM	J1071
TESTOSTERONE ENANTHATE	1 MG	IM	J3121
TESTOSTERONE PELLET	75 MG	OTH	S0189
TESTOSTERONE UNDECANOATE	1 MG	IM	J3145
TETANUS IMMUNE GLOBULIN	250 U	IM	J1670
TETRACYCLINE HCL	250 MG	IV	J0120
TEZEPELUMAB-EKKO	1 MG	SC	J2356
TEZSPIRE	1 MG	SC	J2356
THALLOUS CHLORIDE	1 MCI	IV	A9505
THALLOUS CHLORIDE TL-201	1 MCI	IV	A9505
THALLOUS CHLORIDE USP	1 MCI	IV	A9505
THEELIN AQUEOUS	1 MG	IM, IV	J1435
THEOPHYLLINE	40 MG	IV	J2810
THERACYS	1 MG	OTH	J9030
THERAGENESIS	SQ CM	OTH	A2008
THERASKIN	SQ CM	OTH	Q4121
THERION	SQ CM	OTH	Q4176
THIAMINE HCL	100 MG	INJ	J3411
THIETHYLPERAZINE MALEATE	10 MG	IM	J3280
THIETHYLPERAZINE MALEATE	10 MG	ORAL	Q0174
THIMAZIDE	250 MG	ORAL	Q0173
THIOTEPA	15 MG	IV	J9340
THORAZINE	50 MG	IM, IV	J3230
THROMBATE III	1 IU	IV	J7197
THYMOGLOBULIN	25 MG	OTH	J7511
THYROGEN	0.9 MG	IM, SC	J3240
THYROTROPIN ALPHA	0.9 MG	IM, SC	J3240
TICARCILLIN DISODIUM AND CLAVULANATE	3.1 G	IV	S0040
TICE BCG	1 MG	OTH	J9030
TICON	250 MG	IM	Q0173
TIGAN	200 MG	IM	J3250
TIGECYCLINE	1 MG	IV	J3243

Drug Name	Unit Per	Route	Code
TIGECYCLINE (ACCORD) NOT THERAPEUTICALLY EQUIVALENT TO J3243	1 MG	IV	J3244
TIJECT-20	200 MG	IM	J3250
TILDRAKIZUMAB	1 MG	SC	J3245
TIMENTIN	3.1 G	IV	S0040
TINZAPARIN	1,000 IU	SC	J1655
TIROFIBAN HCL	0.25 MG	IM, IV	J3246
TISAGENLECLEUCEL	UP TO 600 MILLION CELLS	IV	Q2042
TISOTUMAB VEDOTIN-TFTV	1 MG	IV	J9273
TIVDAK	1 MG	IV	J9273
TIXAGEVIMAB AND CILGAVIMAB	300 MG	IM	Q0220
TIXAGEVIMAB AND CILGAVIMAB	600 MG	IM	Q0221
TNKASE	1 MG	IV	J3101
TOBI	300 MG	INH	J7682
TOBRAMYCIN COMPOUNDED, UNIT DOSE	300 MG	INH	J7685
TOBRAMYCIN SULFATE	80 MG	IM, IV	J3260
TOBRAMYCIN, NONCOMPOUNDED, UNIT DOSE	300 MG	INH	J7682
TOCILIZUMAB	1 MG	IV	J3262
TOCILIZUMAB	1 MG	IV	Q0249
TOLAZOLINE HCL	25 MG	IV	J2670
TOPOSAR	10 MG	IV	J9181
TOPOTECAN	0.25 MG	ORAL	J8705
TOPOTECAN	0.1 MG	IV	J9351
TORADOL	15 MG	IV	J1885
TORISEL	1 MG	IV	J9330
TORNALATE	PER MG	INH	J7629
TORNALATE CONCENTRATE	PER MG	INH	J7628
TORSEMIDE	10 MG	IV	J3265
TOSITUMOMAB	450 MG	IV	G3001
TOTECT	PER 250 MG	IV	J1190
TRABECTEDIN	0.1 MG	IV	J9352
TRANSCYTE	SQ CM	OTH	Q4182
TRASTUZUMAB AND HYALURONIDASE-OYSK	10 MG	SC	J9356
TRASTUZUMAB, EXCLUDES BIOSIMILAR	10 MG	IV	J9355
TRASTUZUMAB-ANNS, BIOSIMILAR	10 MG	IV	Q5117
TRASTUZUMAB-DKST, BIOSIMILAR	10 MG	IV	Q5114
TRASTUZUMAB-DTTB, BIOSIMILAR	10 MG	IV	Q5112
TRASTUZUMAB-PKRB, BIOSIMILAR	10 MG	IV	Q5113
TRASTUZUMAB-QYYP, BIOSIMILAR	10 MG	IV	Q5116
TRASYLOL	10,000 KIU	IV	J0365
TRAZIMERA	10 MG	IV	Q5116
TREANDA	1 MG	IV	J9033
TRELSTAR DEPOT	3.75 MG	IM	J3315
TRELSTAR DEPOT PLUS DEBIOCLIP KIT	3.75 MG	IM	J3315
TRELSTAR LA	3.75 MG	IM	J3315
TREMFYA	1 MG	SC	J1628
TREPROSTINIL	1 MG	SC	J3285

Drug Name	Unit Per	Route	Code
TREPROSTINIL, INHALATION SOLUTION	1.74 MG	INH	J7686
TRETINOIN	5 G	OTH	S0117
TRETTEN	10 IU	IV	J7181
TRIAMCINOLONE ACETONIDE	1 MG	INJ	J3299
TRIAMCINOLONE ACETONIDE, PRESERVATIVE FREE	1 MG	INJ	J3300
TRIAMCINOLONE ACETONIDE, PRESERVATIVE-FREE, EXTENDED-RELEASE, MICROSPHERE FORMULATION	1 MG	OTH	J3304
TRIAMCINOLONE ACETONIDE, SUPRACHOROIDAL	1 MG	INJ	C9092
TRIAMCINOLONE DIACETATE	5 MG	IM	J3302
TRIAMCINOLONE HEXACETONIDE	5 MG	VAR	J3303
TRIAMCINOLONE, COMPOUNDED, CONCENTRATED	1 MG	INH	J7683
TRIAMCINOLONE, COMPOUNDED, UNIT DOSE	1 MG	INH	J7684
TRIBAN	250 MG	ORAL	Q0173
TRIESENCE	1 MG	OTH	J3300
TRIFERIC AVNU	0.1 MG	IV	J1445
TRIFERIC POWDER	0.1 MG	IV	J1444
TRIFERIC SOLUTION	0.1 MG	IV	J1443
TRIFLUPROMAZINE HCL	UP TO 20 MG	INJ	J3400
TRILACICLIB	1 MG	IV	J1448
TRILIFON	4 MG	ORAL	Q0175
TRILONE	5 MG	IM	J3302
TRILURON	1 MG	INJ	J7332
TRIMETHOBENZAMIDE HCL	200 MG	IM	J3250
TRIMETHOBENZAMIDE HCL	250 MG	ORAL	Q0173
TRIMETREXATE GLUCURONATE	25 MG	IV	J3305
TRIPTODUR	3.75 MG	IM	J3316
TRIPTORELIN PAMOATE	3.75 MG	IM	J3315
TRIPTORELIN, EXTENDED-RELEASE	3.75 MG	IM	J3316
TRISENOX	1 MG	IV	J9017
TRIVARIS	1 MG	VAR	J3300
TRIVISC	1 MG	INJ	J7329
TROBICIN	2 G	IM	J3320
TRODELVY	2.5 MG	IV	J9317
TROGARZO	10 MG	IV	J1746
TRUSKIN	SQ CM	OTH	Q4167
TRUXADRYL	50 MG	IV, IM	J1200
TRUXIMA	10 MG	IV	Q5115
TYGACIL	1 MG	IV	J3243
TYPE A BOTOX	1 UNIT	IM, OTH	J0585
TYSABRI	1 MG	IV	J2323
TYVASO	1.74 MG	INH	J7686
UDENYCA	0.5 MG	SC	Q5111
ULTOMIRIS	10 MG	IV	J1303
ULTRA-TECHNEKOW	1 MCI	IV	A9512
ULTRALENTE	5 U	SC	J1815
ULTRATAG	STUDY DOSE UP TO 30 MCI	IV	A9560
ULTRAVIST 150	1 ML	IV	Q9965
ULTRAVIST 240	1 ML	IV	Q9966
ULTRAVIST 300	1 ML	IV	Q9967
ULTRAVIST 370	1 ML	IV	Q9967

Appendix 1 — Table of Drugs and Biologicals

Drug Name	Unit Per	Route	Code
UNASYN	1.5 G	IM, IV	J0295
UPLIZNA	1 MG	IV	J1823
UREA	40 G	IV	J3350
URECHOLINE	UP TO 5 MG	SC	J0520
UROFOLLITROPIN	75 IU	SC, IM	J3355
UROKINASE	5,000 IU	IV	J3364
UROKINASE	250,000 IU	IV	J3365
USTEKINUMAB	1 MG	SC	J3357
USTEKINUMAB	1 MG	SC, IV	J3358
VABOMERE	10 MG/10 MG	IV	J2186
VABYSMO	0.1 MG	INJ	C9097
VABYSMO	0.1 MG	INJ	J2777
VALERGEN	10 MG	IM	J1380
VALIUM	5 MG	IV, IM	J3360
VALRUBICIN INTRAVESICAL	200 MG	OTH	J9357
VALSTAR	200 MG	OTH	J9357
VANCOCIN	500 MG	IM, IV	J3370
VANCOMYCIN HCL	500 MG	IV, IM	J3370
VANCOMYCIN HCL (MYLAN) NOT THERAPEUTICALLY EQUIVALENT TO J3370	500 MG	IV	J3371
VANCOMYCIN HCL (XELLIA) NOT THERAPEUTICALLY EQUIVALENT TO J3370	500 MG	IV	J3372
VANTAS	50 MG	OTH	J9225
VAPRISOL	1 MG	INJ	C9488
VARUBI	1 MG	ORAL	J8670
VARUBI	0.5 MG	ORAL, IV	J2797
VECTIBIX	10 MG	IV	J9303
VEDOLIZUMAB	1 MG	IV	J3380
VEKLURY	1 MG	IV	J0248
VELAGLUCERASE ALFA	100 U	IV	J3385
VELBAN	I MG	IV	J9360
VELCADE	0.1 MG	IV, SC	J9041
VELETRI	0.5 MG	IV	J1325
VELOSULIN	5 U	SC	J1815
VELOSULIN BR	5 U	SC	J1815
VENDAJE	SQ CM	OTH	Q4252
VENOFER	1 MG	IV	J1756
VENTOLIN NONCOMPOUNDED, CONCENTRATED	1 MG	INH	J7611
VENTOLIN NONCOMPOUNDED, UNIT DOSE	1 MG	INH	J7613
VEPESID	50 MG	ORAL	J8560
VEPESID	10 MG	IV	J9181
VERITAS	SQ CM	OTH	C9354
VERSED	1 MG	IM, IV	J2250
VERTEPORFIN	0.1 MG	IV	J3396
VESTRONIDASE ALFA-VJBK	1 MG	IV	J3397
VFEND	200 MG	IV	J3465
VIAGRA	25 MG	ORAL	S0090
VIBATIV	10 MG	IV	J3095
VIDAZA	1 MG	SC	J9025
VIDEX	25 MG	ORAL	S0137
VILTEPSO	10 MG	IV	J1427
VILTOLARSEN	10 MG	IV	J1427
VIM	SQ CM	OTH	Q4251
VIMIZIM	1 MG	IV	J1322

Drug Name	Unit Per	Route	Code
VIMPAT	1 MG	IV, ORAL	C9254
VINBLASTINE SULFATE	1 MG	IV	J9360
VINCASCAR	1 MG	IV	J9370
VINCRISTINE SULFATE	1 MG	IV	J9370
VINCRISTINE SULFATE LIPOSOME	5 MG	IV	J9371
VINORELBINE TARTRATE	10 MG	IV	J9390
VIRILON	1 CC, 200 MG	IM	J1080
VISCO-3	PER DOSE	INJ	J7321
VISTAJECT-25	25 MG	IM	J3410
VISTARIL	25 MG	IM	J3410
VISTARIL	25 MG	ORAL	Q0177
VISTIDE	375 MG	IV	J0740
VISUDYNE	0.1 MG	IV	J3396
VITAMIN B-12 CYANOCOBALAMIN	1,000 MCG	IM, SC	J3420
VITAMIN B-17	VAR	INJ	J3570
VITRASE	1 USP	OTH	J3471
VITRASE	1,000 USP	OTH	J3472
VITRASERT	4.5 MG	OTH	J7310
VITRAVENE	1.65 MG	OTH	J1452
VIVITROL	1 MG	IM	J2315
VON WILLEBRAND FACTOR (RECOMBINANT)	1 IU	IV	J7179
VON WILLEBRAND FACTOR COMPLEX (HUMAN) (WILATE)	1 IU	IV	J7183
VON WILLEBRAND FACTOR COMPLEX, HUMATE-P	1 IU	IV	J7187
VON WILLEBRAND FACTOR VIII COMPLEX, HUMAN	PER FACTOR VIII IU	IV	J7186
VONVENDI	1 IU	IV	J7179
VORAXAZE	10 UNITS	IV	C9293
VORETIGENE NEPARVOVEC-RZYL	1 BILLION VECTOR GENOMES	OTH	J3398
VORICONAZOLE	200 MG	IV	J3465
VPRIV	100 U	IV	J3385
VUMON	50 MG	IV	Q2017
VUTRISIRAN	1 MG	SC	J0225
VYEPTI	1 MG	IV	J3032
VYONDYS 53	10 MG	IV	J1429
VYVGART	2 MG	IV	J9332
VYXEOS	1 MG/2.27 MG	IV	J9153
WEHAMINE	50 MG	IM, IV	J1240
WEHDRYL	50 MG	IM, IV	J1200
WELBUTRIN SR	150 MG	ORAL	S0106
WILATE	1 IU	IV	J7183
WINRHO SDF	100 IU	IV	J2792
WOUNDEX	SQ CM	OTH	Q4163
WOUNDEX FLOW	0.5 CC	OTH	Q4162
WOUNDFIX, WOUNDFIX PLUS, WOUNDFIX XPLUS	SQ CM	OTH	Q4217
WYCILLIN	600,000 U	IM, IV	J2510
XARACOLL	1 MG	OTH	C9089
XCELLERATE	SQ CM	OTH	Q4234
XCELLISTEM	1 MG	OTH	A2004
XCM BIOLOGIC TISSUE MATRIX	SQ CM	OTH	Q4142
XELODA	150 MG	ORAL	J8520
XELODA	500 MG	ORAL	J8521
XEMBIFY	100 MG	SC	J1558

Drug Name	Unit Per	Route	Code
XENLETA	1 MG	IV	J0691
XENON XE-133	10 MCI	INH	A9558
XEOMIN	1 UNIT	IM	J0588
XERAVA	1 MG	IV	J0122
XGEVA	1 MG	SC	J0897
XIAFLEX	0.01 MG	OTH	J0775
~~XIPERE~~	~~1 MG~~	~~INJ~~	~~C9092~~
XIPERE	1 MG	INJ	J3299
XOFIGO	PER MICROCURIE	IV	A9606
XOLAIR	5 MG	SC	J2357
XWRAP	SQ CM	OTH	Q4204
XYLOCAINE	10 MG	IV	J2001
XYNTHA	1 IU	IV	J7185
YERVOY	1 MG	IV	J9228
YESCARTA	UP TO 200 MILLION CELLS	IV	Q2041
YONDELIS	0.1 MG	IV	J9352
YTTRIUM 90 IBRITUMOMAB TIUXETAN	TX DOSE UP TO 40 MCI	IV	A9543
YUPELRI	1 MCG	INH	J7677
YUTIQ	0.01 MG	OTH	J7314
ZALTRAP	1 MG	IV	J9400
ZANAMIVIR (BRAND) (DEMONSTRATION PROJECT)	10 MG	INH	G9034
ZANAMIVIR (GENERIC) (DEMONSTRATION PROJECT)	10 MG	INH	G9018
ZANOSAR	1 GM	IV	J9320
ZANTAC	25 MG	INJ	J2780
ZARXIO	1 MCG	IV, SC	Q5101
ZEMDRI	5 MG	IV	J0291
ZEMPLAR	1 MCG	IV, IM	J2501
ZENAPAX	25 MG	OTH	J7513
ZENITH AMNIOTIC MEMBRANE	SQ CM	OTH	Q4253
ZEPZELCA	0.1 MG	IV	J9223
ZERBAXA	50 MG/25 MG	IV	J0695
ZEVALIN	STUDY DOSE UP TO 5 MCI	IV	A9542
ZEVALIN DIAGNOSTIC	STUDY DOSE UP TO 5 MCI	IV	A9542
ZEVALIN THERAPEUTIC	TX DOSE UP TO 40 MCI	IV	A9543
ZICONOTIDE	1 MCG	IT	J2278
ZIDOVUDINE	100 MG	ORAL	S0104
ZIDOVUDINE	10 MG	IV	J3485
ZIEXTENZO	0.5 MG	SC	Q5120
ZILRETTA	1 MG	OTH	J3304
ZIMHI	1 MG	SC	J2311
ZINACEFT	PER 750 MG	IM, IV	J0697
ZINECARD	250 MG	IV	J1190
ZINPLAVA	10 MG	INF	J0565
ZIPRASIDONE MESYLATE	10 MG	IM	J3486
ZIRABEV	10 MG	IV	Q5118
ZITHROMAX	500 MG	IV	J0456
ZITHROMAX	1 G	ORAL	Q0144
ZIV-AFLIBERCEPT	1 MG	IV	J9400
ZOFRAN	1 MG	IV	J2405
ZOFRAN	4 MG	ORAL	S0119

Drug Name	Unit Per	Route	Code
ZOFRAN	1 MG	ORAL	Q0162
ZOLADEX	3.6 MG	SC	J9202
ZOLEDRONIC ACID	1 MG	IV	J3489
ZOLGENSMA	UP TO 5X10^{15} VECTOR GENOMES	IV	J3399
ZOMETA	1 MG	IV	J3489
ZORBTIVE	1 MG	SC	J2941
ZORTRESS	0.25 MG	ORAL	J7527
ZOSYN	1 G/1.125 GM	IV	J2543
ZOVIRAX	5 MG	IV	J0133
ZUBSOLV	1.4 MG	ORAL	J0572
ZUBSOLV	5.7 MG	ORAL	J0573
ZULRESSO	1 MG	IV	J1632
ZUPLENZ	4 MG	ORAL	S0119
ZUPLENZ	1 MG	ORAL	Q0162
ZYLONTA	1 MG	IV	J9359
~~ZYNLONTA~~	~~0.1 MG~~	~~IV~~	~~C9084~~
ZYNRELEF	1 MG/0.03 MG	OTH	C9088
ZYPREXA	2.5 MG	IM	S0166
ZYPREXA RELPREVV	1 MG	IM	J2358
ZYVOX	200 MG	IV	J2020

NOT OTHERWISE CLASSIFIED DRUGS

Drug Name	Unit Per	Route	Code
ALFENTANIL	500 MCG	IV	J3490
ALGLUCOSIDASE ALFA NOS	10 MG	IV	J0220
ALIMTA	10 MG	IV	J9305
ALKERAN	50 MG	IV	J9245
ALLOPURINOL SODIUM	500 MG	IV	J3490
ALPHA 1 - PROTEINASE INHIBITOR (HUMAN) NOS	10 MG	IV	J0256
AMINOCAPROIC ACID	250 MG	IV	J3490
ANTIEMETIC NOC	VAR	ORAL	Q0181
ANTIEMETIC DRUG NOC	VAR	OTH	J8498
ANTIEMETIC DRUG, ORAL, NOS	VAR	ORAL	J8597
ANTIEMETIC DRUG, RECTAL/ SUPPOSITORY, NOS	1 EA	OTH	J8498
ANTIHEMOPHILIC FACTOR HUMAN METHOD M MONOCLONAL PURIFIED	1 IU	IV	J7192
ANTITHROMBIN III	1 IU	IV	J7195
ASPARAGINASE	10,000 U	IM, IV, SC	J9020
AZTREONAM	500 MG	IM, IV	J3490
BENEFIX	1 IU	IV	J7195
BIOCLATE	1 IU	IV	J7192
~~BORTEZOMIB, NOT OTHERWISE SPECIFIED~~	~~0.1 MG~~	~~IV, SC~~	~~J9044~~
BUMETANIDE	0.25 MG	IM, IV	J3490
BUPIVACAINE, 0.25%	1 ML	OTH	J3490
BUPIVACAINE, 0.50%	1 ML	OTH	J3490
BUPIVACAINE, 0.75%	1 ML	OTH	J3490
CALCIUM CHLORIDE	100 MG	IV	J3490
CARIMUNE	500 MG	IV	J1566
CENACORT A-40	10 MG	IM	J3301
CLAVULANTE POTASSIUM/ TICARCILLIN DISODIUM	0.1-3 GM	IV	J3490
CLEVIDIPINE BUTYRATE	1 MG	IV	J3490

Appendix 1 — Table of Drugs and Biologicals

Drug Name	Unit Per	Route	Code
CLINDAMYCIN PHOSPHATE	150 MG	IV	J3490
COMPOUNDED DRUG, NOT OTHERWISE CLASSIFIED	VAR	VAR	J7999
COPPER SULFATE	0.4 MG	INJ	J3490
DILTIAZEM HCL	5 MG	IV	J3490
DOXAPRAM HCL	20 MG	IV	J3490
DOXORUBICIN HYDROCHLORIDE, LIPOSOMAL, NOT OTHERWISE SPECIFIED, 10 MG	10 MG	IV	Q2050
DOXYCYCLINE HYCLATE	100 MG	INJ	J3490
DRUG OR BIOLOGICAL, PART B DRUG COMPETITIVE ACQUISITION PROGRAM (CAP)	VAR	VAR	Q4082
ELSPAR	10,000 U	IM, IV, SC	J9020
ENALAPRILAT	1.25 MG	IV	J3490
ESMOLOL HYDROCHLORIDE	10 MG	IV	J3490
ESOMEPRAZOLE SODIUM	20 MG	IV	J3490
ETOMIDATE	2 MG	IV	J3490
FACTOR IX RECOMBINANT	1 IU	IV	J7195
FACTOR VIII RECOMBINANT	1 IU	IV	J7192
FAMOTIDINE	10 MG	IV	J3490
FLUMAZENIL	0.1 MG	IV	J3490
FOLIC ACID	5 MG	SC, IM, IV	J3490
FOSPROPOFOL DISODIUM	35 MG	IV	J3490
GADOLINIUM -BASED CONTRAST NOS	1 ML	IV	A9579
GAMMAGARD S/D	500 MG	IV	J1566
GEMCITABINE HCL	200 MG	IV	J9201
GEMZAR	200 MG	IV	J9201
GLUCARPIDASE	10 U	IV	J3490
GLYCOPYRROLATE	0.2 MG	IM, IV	J3490
HEMOFIL-M	1 IU	IV	J7192
HEMOPHILIA CLOTTING FACTOR, NOC	VAR	INJ	J7199
HEXAMINOLEVULINATE HCL	100 MG PER STUDY DOSE	IV	J3490
HUMAN FIBRINOGEN CONCENTRATE, NOT OTHERWISE SPECIFIED	1 MG	IV	J7178
HYDROXYPROGESTERONE CAPROATE, NOT OTHERWISE SPECIFIED	10 MG	IM	J1729
IMMUNE GLOBULIN LYOPHILIZED	500 MG	IV	J1566
IMMUNE GLOBULIN, NONLYOPHILIZED (NOS)	500 MG	IV	J1599
IMMUNOSUPPRESSIVE DRUG, NOC	VAR	VAR	J7599
INFLUENZA VIRUS VACCINE, NOT OTHERWISE SPECIFIED	EA	IM	Q2039
IVEEGAM	500 MG	IV	J1566
KENAJECT-40	10 MG	IM	J3301
KENALOG-10	10 MG	IM	J3301
KENALOG-40	10 MG	IM	J3301
KOGENATE FS	1 IU	IV	J7192
L-PHENYLALANINE MUSTARD	50 MG	IV	J9245
LABETALOL HCL	5 MG	INJ	J3490
LEVOLEUCOVORIN, NOS	0.5 MG	IV	J0641
MAGNEVIST	1 ML	IV	A9579
MELPHALAN HCL, NOS	50 MG	IV	J9245
METOPROLOL TARTRATE	1 MG	IV	J3490

Drug Name	Unit Per	Route	Code
METRONIDAZOLE INJ	500 MG	IV	J3490
MORRHUATE SODIUM	50 MG	OTH	J3490
MULTIPLE VITAMINS, WITH OR WITHOUT MINERALS AND TRACE ELEMENTS	VAR	ORAL	A9153
NITROGLYCERIN	5 MG	IV	J3490
NOC DRUGS, INHALATION SOLUTION ADMINISTERED THROUGH DME	1 EA	OTH	J7699
NOC DRUGS, OTHER THAN INHALATION DRUGS, ADMINISTERED THROUGH DME	1 EA	OTH	J7799
NONRADIOACTIVE CONTRACT IMAGING MATERIAL	STUDY DOSE	IV	A9698
NOT OTHERWISE CLASSIFIED, ANTINEOPLASTIC DRUGS	VAR	VAR	J9999
OLANZAPINE SHORT ACTING INTRAMUSCULAR INJECTION	0.5 MG	IM	J3490
OMNISCAN	1 ML	IV	A9579
PEMETREXED NOS	10 MG	IV	J9305
PHENYLEPHRINE KETOROLAC	4 ML	IRR	J3490
POLYGAM	500 MG	IV	J1566
POLYGAM S/D	500 MG	IV	J1566
POSITRON EMISSION TOMOGRAPHY RADIOPHARMACEUTICAL, DIAGNOSTIC, FOR NON-TUMOR IDENTIFICATION	STUDY DOSE	IV	A9598
POSITRON EMISSION TOMOGRAPHY RADIOPHARMACEUTICAL, DIAGNOSTIC, FOR TUMOR IDENTIFICATION	STUDY DOSE	IV	A9597
PRESCRIPTION DRUG, ORAL, CHEMOTHERAPEUTIC, NOS	VAR	ORAL	J8999
PRESCRIPTION DRUG, ORAL, NONCHEMOTHERAPEUTIC, NOS	VAR	ORAL	J8499
PROLASTIN	10 MG	IV	J0256
PROTEINASE INHIBITOR (HUMAN)	10 MG	IV	J0256
RADIOPHARMACEUTICAL, DIAGNOSTIC, NOC	VAR	VAR	A4641
RADIOPHARMACEUTICAL, THERAPEUTIC	STUDY DOSE	IV	A9699
RECOMBINATE	1 IU	IV	J7192
REFACTO	1 IU	IV	J7192
RIFAMPIN	600 MG	IV	J3490
SINGLE VITAMIN/MINERAL/TRACE ELEMENT	VAR	ORAL	A9152
SKIN SUBSTITUTE, FDA-CLEARED AS A DEVICE, NOT OTHERWISE SPECIFIED	SQ CM	OTH	A4100
SKIN SUBSTITUTE, NOS	VAR	OTH	Q4100
SODIUM ACETATE	2 MEQ	IV	J3490
SODIUM CHLORIDE, HYPERTONIC (3%-5% INFUSION)	250 CC	IV	J3490
SULFAMETHOXAZOLE-TRIMETHOPRIM	80 MG/16 MG	IV	J3490
SURGIMEND	0.5 SQ CM	OTH	J3490
THROMBATE III	1 IU	IV	J7195
TRI-KORT	10 MG	IM	J3301
TRIAM-A	10 MG	IM	J3301
TRIAMCINOLONE ACETONIDE	10 MG	IM	J3301

Drug Name	Unit Per	Route	Code
TRILOG	10 MG	IM	J3301
UNCLASSIFIED BIOLOGICS	VAR	VAR	J3590
UNCLASSIFIED DRUG OR BIOLOGICAL USED FOR ESRD ON DIALYSIS	VAR	VAR	J3591
UNCLASSIFIED DRUGS OR BIOLOGICALS	VAR	VAR	C9399
VASOPRESSIN	20 UNITS	SC, IM	J3490
VECURONIUM BROMIDE	1 MG	IV	J3490
WOUND FILLER, DRY FORM, PER G, NOS	1 G	OTH	A6262
WOUND FILLER, GEL/PASTE, PER FL OZ, NOS	1 OZ	OTH	A6261
ZEMAIRA	10 MG	IV	J0256

Appendix 2 — Modifiers

A modifier is a two-position code that is added to the end of a code to clarify the services being billed. Modifiers provide a means by which a service can be altered without changing the procedure code. They add more information, such as the anatomical site, to the code. In addition, they help to eliminate the appearance of duplicate billing and unbundling. Modifiers are used to increase accuracy in reimbursement, coding consistency, editing, and to capture payment data.

A1	Dressing for one wound
A2	Dressing for two wounds
A3	Dressing for three wounds
A4	Dressing for four wounds
A5	Dressing for five wounds
A6	Dressing for six wounds
A7	Dressing for seven wounds
A8	Dressing for eight wounds
A9	Dressing for nine or more wounds
AA	Anesthesia services performed personally by anesthesiologist
AB	Audiology service furnished personally by an audiologist without a physician/NPP order for nonacute hearing assessment unrelated to disequilibrium, or hearing aids, or examinations for the purpose of prescribing, fitting, or changing hearing aids; service may be performed once every 12 months, per beneficiary
AD	Medical supervision by a physician: more than four concurrent anesthesia procedures
AE	Registered dietician
AF	Specialty physician
AG	Primary physician
AH	Clinical psychologist
AI	Principal physician of record
AJ	Clinical social worker
AK	Nonparticipating physician
AM	Physician, team member service
AO	Alternate payment method declined by provider of service
AP	Determination of refractive state was not performed in the course of diagnostic ophthalmological examination
AQ	Physician providing a service in an unlisted health professional shortage area (HPSA)
AR	Physician provider services in a physician scarcity area
AS	Physician assistant, nurse practitioner, or clinical nurse specialist services for assistant at surgery
AT	Acute treatment (this modifier should be used when reporting service 98940, 98941, 98942)
AU	Item furnished in conjunction with a urological, ostomy, or tracheostomy supply
AV	Item furnished in conjunction with a prosthetic device, prosthetic or orthotic
AW	Item furnished in conjunction with a surgical dressing
AX	Item furnished in conjunction with dialysis services
AY	Item or service furnished to an ESRD patient that is not for the treatment of ESRD
AZ	Physician providing a service in a dental health professional shortage area for the purpose of an electronic health record incentive payment
BA	Item furnished in conjunction with parenteral enteral nutrition (PEN) services
BL	Special acquisition of blood and blood products
BO	Orally administered nutrition, not by feeding tube
BP	The beneficiary has been informed of the purchase and rental options and has elected to purchase the item
BR	The beneficiary has been informed of the purchase and rental options and has elected to rent the item
BU	The beneficiary has been informed of the purchase and rental options and after 30 days has not informed the supplier of his/her decision
CA	Procedure payable only in the inpatient setting when performed emergently on an outpatient who expires prior to admission
CB	Service ordered by a renal dialysis facility (RDF) physician as part of the ESRD beneficiary's dialysis benefit, is not part of the composite rate, and is separately reimbursable
CC	Procedure code change (use CC when the procedure code submitted was changed either for administrative reasons or because an incorrect code was filed)
CD	AMCC test has been ordered by an ESRD facility or MCP physician that is part of the composite rate and is not separately billable
CE	AMCC test has been ordered by an ESRD facility or MCP physician that is a composite rate test but is beyond the normal frequency covered under the rate and is separately reimbursable based on medical necessity
CF	AMCC test has been ordered by an ESRD facility or MCP physician that is not part of the composite rate and is separately billable
CG	Policy criteria applied
CH	Zero percent impaired, limited or restricted
CI	At least 1 percent but less than 20 percent impaired, limited or restricted
CJ	At least 20 percent but less than 40 percent impaired, limited or restricted
CK	At least 40 percent but less than 60 percent impaired, limited or restricted
CL	At least 60 percent but less than 80 percent impaired, limited or restricted
CM	At least 80 percent but less than 100 percent impaired, limited or restricted
CN	100 percent impaired, limited or restricted
CO	Outpatient occupational therapy services furnished in whole or in part by an occupational therapy assistant
CQ	Outpatient physical therapy services furnished in whole or in part by a physical therapist assistant
CR	Catastrophe/disaster related
CS	Cost-sharing waived for specified COVID-19 testing-related services that result in an order for or administration of a COVID-19 test and/or used for cost-sharing waived preventive services furnished via telehealth in rural health clinics and federally qualified health centers during the COVID-19 public health emergency
CT	Computed tomography services furnished using equipment that does not meet each of the attributes of the national electrical manufacturers association (NEMA) XR-29-2013 standard

Appendix 2 — Modifiers

Code	Description
DA	Oral health assessment by a licensed health professional other than a dentist
E1	Upper left, eyelid
E2	Lower left, eyelid
E3	Upper right, eyelid
E4	Lower right, eyelid
EA	Erythropoetic stimulating agent (ESA) administered to treat anemia due to anticancer chemotherapy
EB	Erythropoetic stimulating agent (ESA) administered to treat anemia due to anticancer radiotherapy
EC	Erythropoetic stimulating agent (ESA) administered to treat anemia not due to anticancer radiotherapy or anticancer chemotherapy
ED	Hematocrit level has exceeded 39 percent (or hemoglobin level has exceeded 13.0 G/dl) for three or more consecutive billing cycles immediately prior to and including the current cycle
EE	Hematocrit level has not exceeded 39 percent (or hemoglobin level has not exceeded 13.0 G/dl) for three or more consecutive billing cycles immediately prior to and including the current cycle
EJ	Subsequent claims for a defined course of therapy, e.g., EPO, sodium hyaluronate, infliximab
EM	Emergency reserve supply (for ESRD benefit only)
EP	Service provided as part of Medicaid early periodic screening diagnosis and treatment (EPSDT) program
ER	Items and services furnished by a provider-based, off-campus emergency department
ET	Emergency services
EX	Expatriate beneficiary
EY	No physician or other licensed health care provider order for this item or service
F1	Left hand, second digit
F2	Left hand, third digit
F3	Left hand, fourth digit
F4	Left hand, fifth digit
F5	Right hand, thumb
F6	Right hand, second digit
F7	Right hand, third digit
F8	Right hand, fourth digit
F9	Right hand, fifth digit
FA	Left hand, thumb
FB	Item provided without cost to provider, supplier or practitioner, or full credit received for replaced device (examples, but not limited to, covered under warranty, replaced due to defect, free samples)
FC	Partial credit received for replaced device
FP	Service provided as part of family planning program
FQ	The service was furnished using audio-only communication technology
FR	The supervising practitioner was present through two-way, audio/video communication technology
FS	Split (or shared) evaluation and management visit
▲ FT	Unrelated evaluation and management (E/M) visit during a postoperative period, or on the same day as a procedure or another E/M visit. (Report when an E/M visit is furnished within the global period but is unrelated, or when one or more additional E/M visits furnished on the same day are unrelated)
FX	X-ray taken using film
FY	X-ray taken using computed radiography technology/cassette-based imaging
G0	Telehealth services for diagnosis, evaluation, or treatment, of symptoms of an acute stroke
G1	Most recent URR reading of less than 60
G2	Most recent URR reading of 60 to 64.9
G3	Most recent URR reading of 65 to 69.9
G4	Most recent URR reading of 70 to 74.9
G5	Most recent URR reading of 75 or greater
G6	ESRD patient for whom less than six dialysis sessions have been provided in a month
G7	Pregnancy resulted from rape or incest or pregnancy certified by physician as life threatening
G8	Monitored anesthesia care (MAC) for deep complex, complicated, or markedly invasive surgical procedure
G9	Monitored anesthesia care for patient who has history of severe cardiopulmonary condition
GA	Waiver of liability statement issued as required by payer policy, individual case
GB	Claim being resubmitted for payment because it is no longer covered under a global payment demonstration
GC	This service has been performed in part by a resident under the direction of a teaching physician
GE	This service has been performed by a resident without the presence of a teaching physician under the primary care exception
GF	Nonphysician (e.g., nurse practitioner (NP), certified registered nurse anesthetist (CRNA), certified registered nurse (CRN), clinical nurse specialist (CNS), physician assistant (PA)) services in a critical access hospital
GG	Performance and payment of a screening mammogram and diagnostic mammogram on the same patient, same day
GH	Diagnostic mammogram converted from screening mammogram on same day
GJ	"Opt out" physician or practitioner emergency or urgent service
GK	Reasonable and necessary item/service associated with a GA or GZ modifier
GL	Medically unnecessary upgrade provided instead of nonupgraded item, no charge, no advance beneficiary notice (ABN)
GM	Multiple patients on one ambulance trip
GN	Services delivered under an outpatient speech language pathology plan of care
GO	Services delivered under an outpatient occupational therapy plan of care
GP	Services delivered under an outpatient physical therapy plan of care
GQ	Via asynchronous telecommunications system
GR	This service was performed in whole or in part by a resident in a Department of Veterans Affairs medical center or clinic, supervised in accordance with VA policy
GS	Dosage of erythropoietin stimulating agent has been reduced and maintained in response to hematocrit or hemoglobin level
GT	Via interactive audio and video telecommunication systems
GU	Waiver of liability statement issued as required by payer policy, routine notice
GV	Attending physician not employed or paid under arrangement by the patient's hospice provider
GW	Service not related to the hospice patient's terminal condition
GX	Notice of liability issued, voluntary under payer policy

Code	Description
GY	Item or service statutorily excluded, does not meet the definition of any Medicare benefit or, for non-Medicare insurers, is not a contract benefit
GZ	Item or service expected to be denied as not reasonable and necessary
H9	Court-ordered
HA	Child/adolescent program
HB	Adult program, nongeriatric
HC	Adult program, geriatric
HD	Pregnant/parenting women's program
HE	Mental health program
HF	Substance abuse program
HG	Opioid addiction treatment program
HH	Integrated mental health/substance abuse program
HI	Integrated mental health and intellectual disability/developmental disabilities program
HJ	Employee assistance program
HK	Specialized mental health programs for high-risk populations
HL	Intern
HM	Less than bachelor degree level
HN	Bachelors degree level
HO	Masters degree level
HP	Doctoral level
HQ	Group setting
HR	Family/couple with client present
HS	Family/couple without client present
HT	Multidisciplinary team
HU	Funded by child welfare agency
HV	Funded state addictions agency
HW	Funded by state mental health agency
HX	Funded by county/local agency
HY	Funded by juvenile justice agency
HZ	Funded by criminal justice agency
J1	Competitive acquisition program no-pay submission for a prescription number
J2	Competitive acquisition program, restocking of emergency drugs after emergency administration
J3	Competitive acquisition program (CAP), drug not available through CAP as written, reimbursed under average sales price methodology
J4	DMEPOS item subject to DMEPOS competitive bidding program that is furnished by a hospital upon discharge
J5	Off-the-shelf orthotic subject to DMEPOS competitive bidding program that is furnished as part of a physical therapist or occupational therapist professional service
JA	Administered intravenously
JB	Administered subcutaneously
JC	Skin substitute used as a graft
JD	Skin substitute not used as a graft
JE	Administered via dialysate
JF	Compounded drug
▲ JG	Drug or biological acquired with 340B drug pricing program discount, reported for informational purposes
JW	Drug amount discarded/not administered to any patient
● JZ	Zero drug amount discarded/not administered to any patient
K0	Lower extremity prosthesis functional level 0 - does not have the ability or potential to ambulate or transfer safely with or without assistance and a prosthesis does not enhance their quality of life or mobility.
K1	Lower extremity prosthesis functional level 1 - has the ability or potential to use a prosthesis for transfers or ambulation on level surfaces at fixed cadence, typical of the limited and unlimited household ambulator
K2	Lower extremity prosthesis functional level 2 - has the ability or potential for ambulation with the ability to traverse low level environmental barriers such as curbs, stairs or uneven surfaces, typical of the limited community ambulator
K3	Lower extremity prosthesis functional level 3 - has the ability or potential for ambulation with variable cadence, typical of the community ambulator who has the ability to transverse most environmental barriers and may have vocational, therapeutic, or exercise activity that demands prosthetic utilization beyond simple locomotion
K4	Lower extremity prosthesis functional level 4 - has the ability or potential for prosthetic ambulation that exceeds the basic ambulation skills, exhibiting high impact, stress, or energy levels, typical of the prosthetic demands of the child, active adult, or athlete
KA	Add on option/accessory for wheelchair
KB	Beneficiary requested upgrade for ABN, more than four modifiers identified on claim
KC	Replacement of special power wheelchair interface
KD	Drug or biological infused through DME
KE	Bid under round one of the DMEPOS competitive bidding program for use with noncompetitive bid base equipment
KF	Item designated by FDA as Class III device
KG	DMEPOS item subject to DMEPOS competitive bidding program number 1
KH	DMEPOS item, initial claim, purchase or first month rental
KI	DMEPOS item, second or third month rental
KJ	DMEPOS item, parenteral enteral nutrition (PEN) pump or capped rental, months four to fifteen
KK	DMEPOS item subject to DMEPOS competitive bidding program number 2
KL	DMEPOS item delivered via mail
KM	Replacement of facial prosthesis including new impression/moulage
KN	Replacement of facial prosthesis using previous master model
KO	Single drug unit dose formulation
KP	First drug of a multiple drug unit dose formulation
KQ	Second or subsequent drug of a multiple drug unit dose formulation
KR	Rental item, billing for partial month
KS	Glucose monitor supply for diabetic beneficiary not treated with insulin
KT	Beneficiary resides in a competitive bidding area and travels outside that competitive bidding area and receives a competitive bid item
KU	DMEPOS item subject to DMEPOS competitive bidding program number 3
KV	DMEPOS item subject to DMEPOS competitive bidding program that is furnished as part of a professional service
KW	DMEPOS item subject to DMEPOS competitive bidding program number 4
KX	Requirements specified in the medical policy have been met
KY	DMEPOS item subject to DMEPOS competitive bidding program number 5
KZ	New coverage not implemented by managed care

LC	Left circumflex coronary artery		PI	Positron emission tomography (PET) or pet/computed tomography (CT) to inform the initial treatment strategy of tumors that are biopsy proven or strongly suspected of being cancerous based on other diagnostic testing
LD	Left anterior descending coronary artery			
LL	Lease/rental (use the LL modifier when DME equipment rental is to be applied against the purchase price)			
LM	Left main coronary artery		PL	Progressive addition lenses
LR	Laboratory round trip		PM	Post mortem
LS	FDA-monitored intraocular lens implant		PN	Nonexcepted service provided at an off-campus, outpatient, provider-based department of a hospital
LT	Left side (used to identify procedures performed on the left side of the body)		PO	Excepted service provided at an off-campus, outpatient, provider-based department of a hospital
• LU	Fractionated payment of CAR-T therapy		PS	Positron emission tomography (PET) or pet/computed tomography (CT) to inform the subsequent treatment strategy of cancerous tumors when the beneficiary's treating physician determines that the PET study is needed to inform subsequent antitumor strategy
M2	Medicare secondary payer (MSP)			
MA	Ordering professional is not required to consult a Clinical Decision Support Mechanism due to service being rendered to a patient with a suspected or confirmed emergency medical condition			
MB	Ordering professional is not required to consult a Clinical Decision Support Mechanism due to the significant hardship exception of insufficient internet access		PT	Colorectal cancer screening test; converted to diagnostic test or other procedure
			Q0	Investigational clinical service provided in a clinical research study that is in an approved clinical research study
MC	Ordering professional is not required to consult a Clinical Decision Support Mechanism due to the significant hardship exception of electronic health record or Clinical Decision Support Mechanism vendor issues		Q1	Routine clinical service provided in a clinical research study that is in an approved clinical research study
			Q2	Demonstration procedure/service
			Q3	Live kidney donor surgery and related services
MD	Ordering professional is not required to consult a Clinical Decision Support Mechanism due to the significant hardship exception of extreme and uncontrollable circumstances		Q4	Service for ordering/referring physician qualifies as a service exemption
			Q5	Service furnished under a reciprocal billing arrangement by a substitute physician or by a substitute physical therapist furnishing outpatient physical therapy services in a health professional shortage area, a medically underserved area, or a rural area
ME	The order for this service adheres to Appropriate Use Criteria in the Clinical Decision Support Mechanism consulted by the ordering professional			
MF	The order for this service does not adhere to the Appropriate Use Criteria in the Clinical Decision Support Mechanism consulted by the ordering professional		Q6	Service furnished under a fee-for-time compensation arrangement by a substitute physician or by a substitute physical therapist furnishing outpatient physical therapy services in a health professional shortage area, a medically underserved area, or a rural area
MG	The order for this service does not have applicable Appropriate Use Criteria in the qualified Clinical Decision Support Mechanism consulted by the ordering professional			
MH	Unknown if ordering professional consulted a Clinical Decision Support Mechanism for this service, related information was not provided to the furnishing professional or provider		Q7	One Class A finding
			Q8	Two Class B findings
			Q9	One Class B and two Class C findings
MS	Six month maintenance and servicing fee for reasonable and necessary parts and labor which are not covered under any manufacturer or supplier warranty		QA	Prescribed amounts of stationary oxygen for daytime use while at rest and nighttime use differ and the average of the two amounts is less than 1 liter per minute (LPM)
NB	Nebulizer system, any type, FDA-cleared for use with specific drug		QB	Prescribed amounts of stationary oxygen for daytime use while at rest and nighttime use differ and the average of the two amounts exceeds 4 liters per minute (LPM) and portable oxygen is prescribed
NR	New when rented (use the NR modifier when DME which was new at the time of rental is subsequently purchased)			
NU	New equipment		QC	Single channel monitoring
P1	A normal healthy patient		QD	Recording and storage in solid state memory by a digital recorder
P2	A patient with mild systemic disease			
P3	A patient with severe systemic disease		QE	Prescribed amount of stationary oxygen while at rest is less than 1 liter per minute (LPM)
P4	A patient with severe systemic disease that is a constant threat to life		QF	Prescribed amount of stationary oxygen while at rest exceeds 4 liters per minute (LPM) and portable oxygen is prescribed
P5	A moribund patient who is not expected to survive without the operation		QG	Prescribed amount of stationary oxygen while at rest is greater than 4 liters per minute (LPM)
P6	A declared brain-dead patient whose organs are being removed for donor purposes		QH	Oxygen conserving device is being used with an oxygen delivery system
PA	Surgical or other invasive procedure on wrong body part		QJ	Services/items provided to a prisoner or patient in state or local custody; however, the state or local government, as applicable, meets the requirements in 42 CFR 411.4 (B)
PB	Surgical or other invasive procedure on wrong patient			
PC	Wrong surgery or other invasive procedure on patient		QK	Medical direction of two, three, or four concurrent anesthesia procedures involving qualified individuals
PD	Diagnostic or related nondiagnostic item or service provided in a wholly owned or operated entity to a patient who is admitted as an inpatient within three days			
			QL	Patient pronounced dead after ambulance called
			QM	Ambulance service provided under arrangement by a provider of services

Code	Description
QN	Ambulance service furnished directly by a provider of services
QP	Documentation is on file showing that the laboratory test(s) was ordered individually or ordered as a CPT-recognized panel other than automated profile codes 80002-80019, G0058, G0059, and G0060.
QQ	Ordering professional consulted a qualified clinical decision support mechanism for this service and the related data was provided to the furnishing professional
QR	Prescribed amounts of stationary oxygen for daytime use while at rest and nighttime use differ and the average of the two amounts is greater than 4 liters per minute (LPM)
QS	Monitored anesthesiology care service
QT	Recording and storage on tape by an analog tape recorder
QW	CLIA waived test
QX	CRNA service: with medical direction by a physician
QY	Medical direction of one certified registered nurse anesthetist (CRNA) by an anesthesiologist
QZ	CRNA service: without medical direction by a physician
RA	Replacement of a DME, orthotic or prosthetic item
RB	Replacement of a part of a DME, orthotic or prosthetic item furnished as part of a repair
RC	Right coronary artery
RD	Drug provided to beneficiary, but not administered "incident-to"
RE	Furnished in full compliance with FDA-mandated risk evaluation and mitigation strategy (REMS)
RI	Ramus intermedius coronary artery
RR	Rental (use the RR modifier when DME is to be rented)
RT	Right side (used to identify procedures performed on the right side of the body)
SA	Nurse practitioner rendering service in collaboration with a physician
SB	Nurse midwife
SC	Medically necessary service or supply
SD	Services provided by registered nurse with specialized, highly technical home infusion training
SE	State and/or federally-funded programs/services
SF	Second opinion ordered by a professional review organization (PRO) per section 9401, p.l. 99-272 (100 percent reimbursement - no Medicare deductible or coinsurance)
SG	Ambulatory surgical center (ASC) facility service
SH	Second concurrently administered infusion therapy
SJ	Third or more concurrently administered infusion therapy
SK	Member of high risk population (use only with codes for immunization)
SL	State supplied vaccine
SM	Second surgical opinion
SN	Third surgical opinion
SQ	Item ordered by home health
SS	Home infusion services provided in the infusion suite of the IV therapy provider
ST	Related to trauma or injury
SU	Procedure performed in physician's office (to denote use of facility and equipment)
SV	Pharmaceuticals delivered to patient's home but not utilized
SW	Services provided by a certified diabetic educator
SY	Persons who are in close contact with member of high-risk population (use only with codes for immunization)
SZ	Habilitative services
T1	Left foot, second digit
T2	Left foot, third digit
T3	Left foot, fourth digit
T4	Left foot, fifth digit
T5	Right foot, great toe
T6	Right foot, second digit
T7	Right foot, third digit
T8	Right foot, fourth digit
T9	Right foot, fifth digit
TA	Left foot, great toe
▲ TB	Drug or biological acquired with 340B drug pricing program discount, reported for informational purposes for select entities
TC	Technical component; under certain circumstances, a charge may be made for the technical component alone; under those circumstances the technical component charge is identified by adding modifier TC to the usual procedure number; technical component charges are institutional charges and not billed separately by physicians; however, portable x-ray suppliers only bill for technical component and should utilize modifier TC; the charge data from portable x-ray suppliers will then be used to build customary and prevailing profiles
TD	RN
TE	LPN/LVN
TF	Intermediate level of care
TG	Complex/high tech level of care
TH	Obstetrical treatment/services, prenatal or postpartum
TJ	Program group, child and/or adolescent
TK	Extra patient or passenger, nonambulance
TL	Early intervention/individualized family service plan (IFSP)
TM	Individualized education program (IEP)
TN	Rural/outside providers' customary service area
TP	Medical transport, unloaded vehicle
TQ	Basic life support transport by a volunteer ambulance provider
TR	School-based individualized education program (IEP) services provided outside the public school district responsible for the student
TS	Follow-up service
TT	Individualized service provided to more than one patient in same setting
TU	Special payment rate, overtime
TV	Special payment rates, holidays/weekends
TW	Back-up equipment
U1	Medicaid level of care 1, as defined by each state
U2	Medicaid level of care 2, as defined by each state
U3	Medicaid level of care 3, as defined by each state
U4	Medicaid level of care 4, as defined by each state
U5	Medicaid level of care 5, as defined by each state
U6	Medicaid level of care 6, as defined by each state
U7	Medicaid level of care 7, as defined by each state
U8	Medicaid level of care 8, as defined by each state
U9	Medicaid level of care 9, as defined by each state
UA	Medicaid level of care 10, as defined by each state
UB	Medicaid level of care 11, as defined by each state
UC	Medicaid level of care 12, as defined by each state

Code	Description
UD	Medicaid level of care 13, as defined by each state
UE	Used durable medical equipment
UF	Services provided in the morning
UG	Services provided in the afternoon
UH	Services provided in the evening
UJ	Services provided at night
UK	Services provided on behalf of the client to someone other than the client (collateral relationship)
UN	Two patients served
UP	Three patients served
UQ	Four patients served
UR	Five patients served
US	Six or more patients served
V1	Demonstration modifier 1
V2	Demonstration modifier 2
V3	Demonstration modifier 3
V4	Demonstration modifier 4
V5	Vascular catheter (alone or with any other vascular access)
V6	Arteriovenous graft (or other vascular access not including a vascular catheter)
V7	Arteriovenous fistula only (in use with two needles)
V8	Infection present
V9	No infection present
VM	Medicare Diabetes Prevention Program (MDPP) virtual make-up session
VP	Aphakic patient
X1	Continuous/broad services: for reporting services by clinicians, who provide the principal care for a patient, with no planned endpoint of the relationship; services in this category represent comprehensive care, dealing with the entire scope of patient problems, either directly or in a care coordination role; reporting clinician service examples include, but are not limited to, primary care, and clinicians providing comprehensive care to patients in addition to specialty care
X2	Continuous/focused services: for reporting services by clinicians whose expertise is needed for the ongoing management of a chronic disease or a condition that needs to be managed and followed with no planned endpoint to the relationship; reporting clinician service examples include, but are not limited to, a rheumatologist taking care of the patient's rheumatoid arthritis longitudinally but not providing general primary care services
X3	Episodic/broad servies: for reporting services by clinicians who have broad responsibility for the comprehensive needs of the patient that is limited to a defined period and circumstance such as a hospitalization; reporting clinician service examples include, but are not limited to, the hospitalist's services rendered providing comprehensive and general care to a patient while admitted to the hospital
X4	Episodic/focused services: for reporting services by clinicians who provide focused care on particular types of treatment limited to a defined period and circumstance; the patient has a problem, acute or chronic, that will be treated with surgery, radiation, or some other type of generally time-limited intervention; reporting clinician service examples include, but are not limited to, the orthopedic surgeon performing a knee replacement and seeing the patient through the postoperative period
X5	Diagnostic services requested by another clinician: for reporting services by a clinician who furnishes care to the patient only as requested by another clinician or subsequent and related services requested by another clinician; this modifier is reported for patient relationships that may not be adequately captured by the above alternative categories; reporting clinician service examples include, but are not limited to, the radiologist's interpretation of an imaging study requested by another clinician
XE	Separate encounter, a service that is distinct because it occurred during a separate encounter
XP	Separate practitioner, a service that is distinct because it was performed by a different practitioner
XS	Separate structure, a service that is distinct because it was performed on a separate organ/structure
XU	Unusual nonoverlapping service, the use of a service that is distinct because it does not overlap usual components of the main service

Appendix 3 — Abbreviations and Acronyms

HCPCS Abbreviations and Acronyms
The following abbreviations and acronyms are used in the HCPCS descriptions:

/	or
<	less than
<=	less than equal to
>	greater than
>=	greater than equal to
AC	alternating current
ACE/ACEI	angiotensin-converting enzyme inhibitor
AFO	ankle-foot orthosis
AHI	apnea hypopnea index
AICC	anti-inhibitor coagulant complex
AK	above the knee
AKA	above knee amputation
ALS	advanced life support
AMP	ampule
AO	ankle orthosis
ARB	angiotensin receptor blocker
ART	artery
ART	arterial
ASC	ambulatory surgery center
ATT	attached
A-V	arteriovenous
AVF	arteriovenous fistula
BICROS	bilateral routing of signals
BK	below the knee
BLS	basic life support
BMI	body mass index
BP	blood pressure
BTE	behind the ear (hearing aid)
CAPD	continuous ambulatory peritoneal dialysis
Carb	carbohydrate
CBC	complete blood count
cc	cubic centimeter
CCPD	continuous cycling peritoneal analysis
CGM	continuous glucose monitoring
CHF	congestive heart failure
CIC	completely in the canal (hearing aid)
CIM	Coverage Issue Manual
CKD	chronic kidney disease
Clsd	closed
cm	centimeter
CMN	certificate of medical necessity
CMS	Centers for Medicare and Medicaid Services
CMV	cytomegalovirus
Conc	concentrate
Conc	concentrated
Cont	continuous
CP	clinical psychologist
CPAP	continuous positive airway pressure
CPT	Current Procedural Terminology
CRF	chronic renal failure
CRNA	certified registered nurse anesthetist
CROS	contralateral routing of signals
CSW	clinical social worker
CT	computed tomography
CTLSO	cervical-thoracic-lumbar-sacral orthosis
cu	cubic
DC	direct current
DI	diurnal rhythm
Dx	diagnosis
DLI	donor leukocyte infusion
DME	durable medical equipment
DME MAC	durable medical equipment Medicare administrative contractor
DMEPOS	durable medical equipment, prosthetics, orthotics and other supplies
DMERC	durable medical equipment regional carrier
DR	diagnostic radiology
DX	diagnostic
e.g.	for example
Ea	each
ECF	extended care facility
EEG	electroencephalogram
EGFR	estimated glomerular filtration rate
EKG	electrocardiogram
EMG	electromyography
EO	elbow orthosis
EP	electrophysiologic
EPO	epoetin alfa
EPSDT	early periodic screening, diagnosis and treatment
ERCP	endoscopic retrograde cholangiopancreatography
ESRD	end-stage renal disease
EWHO	elbow-wrist-hand orthotic
Ex	extended
Exper	experimental
Ext	external
F	french
FDA	Food and Drug Administration
FDG-PET	positron emission with tomography with 18 fluorodeoxyglucose
Fem	female
FO	finger orthosis
FPD	fixed partial denture
Fr	french
ft	foot
G-CSF	filgrastim (granulocyte colony-stimulating factor)
gm	gram (g)
H2O	water
HCl	hydrochloric acid, hydrochloride
HCPCS	Healthcare Common Procedural Coding System
HCT	hematocrit
HFO	hand-finger orthosis
HHA	home health agency
HI	high
HI-LO	high-low
HIT	home infusion therapy
HKAFO	hip-knee-ankle foot orthosis
HLA	human leukocyte antigen
HMES	heat and moisture exchange system
HNPCC	hereditary non-polyposis colorectal cancer
HO	hip orthosis
HPSA	health professional shortage area
HST	home sleep test
IA	intra-arterial administration
ip	interphalangeal
I-131	Iodine 131
ICF	intermediate care facility
ICU	intensive care unit
IM	intramuscular
in	inch

Appendix 3 — Abbreviations and Acronyms

INF	infusion	PET	positron emission tomography
INH	inhalation solution	PHP	pre-paid health plan
INJ	injection	PHP	physician hospital plan
IOL	intraocular lens	PI	paramedic intercept
IPD	intermittent peritoneal dialysis	PICC	peripherally inserted central venous catheter
IPPB	intermittent positive pressure breathing	PKR	photorefractive keratotomy
IT	intrathecal administration	Pow	powder
ITC	in the canal (hearing aid)	PRK	photoreactive keratectomy
ITE	in the ear (hearing aid)	PRO	peer review organization
IU	international units	PSA	prostate specific antigen
IV	intravenous	PTB	patellar tendon bearing
IVF	in vitro fertilization	PTK	phototherapeutic keratectomy
KAFO	knee-ankle-foot orthosis	PVC	polyvinyl chloride
KO	knee orthosis	QPP	Quality Payment Program
KOH	potassium hydroxide	R	right
L	left	RDI	respiratory disturbance index
LASIK	laser in situ keratomileusis	REI	respiratory event index
LAUP	laser assisted uvulopalatoplasty	Repl	replace
lbs	pounds	RN	registered nurse
LDL	low density lipoprotein	RP	retrograde pyelogram
LDS	lipodystrophy syndrome	Rx	prescription
Lo	low	SACH	solid ankle, cushion heel
LO	lumbar orthosis	SC	subcutaneous
LPM	liters per minute	SCT	specialty care transport
LPN/LVN	Licensed Practical Nurse/Licensed Vocational Nurse	SEO	shoulder-elbow orthosis
LSO	lumbar-sacral orthosis	SEWHO	shoulder-elbow-wrist-hand orthosis
lvad	left ventricular assist device	SEXA	single energy x-ray absorptiometry
lvef	left ventricular ejection fraction	SGD	speech generating device
MAC	Medicare administrative contractor	SGD	sinus rhythm
mp	metacarpophalangeal	SM	samarium
mcg	microgram	SNCT	sensory nerve conduction test
mCi	millicurie	SNF	skilled nursing facility
MCM	Medicare Carriers Manual	SO	sacroilliac othrosis
MCP	metacarparpophalangeal joint	SO	shoulder orthosis
MCP	monthly capitation payment	Sol	solution
mEq	milliequivalent	SQ	square
MESA	microsurgical epididymal sperm aspiration	SR	screen
mg	milligram	ST	standard
mgs	milligrams	ST	sustained release
MHT	megahertz	Syr	syrup
ml	milliliter	TABS	tablets
mm	millimeter	Tc	technetium
mmHg	millimeters of Mercury	Tc 99m	technetium isotope
MRA	magnetic resonance angiography	TENS	transcutaneous electrical nerve stimulator
MRI	magnetic resonance imaging	THKAO	thoracic-hip-knee-ankle orthosis
NA	sodium	TLSO	thoracic-lumbar-sacral-orthosis
NCI	National Cancer Institute	TM	temporomandibular
NEC	not elsewhere classified	TMJ	temporomandibular joint
NG	nasogastric	TPN	total parenteral nutrition
NH	nursing home	U	unit
NMES	neuromuscular electrical stimulation	UACR	urine albumin-creatinine ratio
NOC	not otherwise classified	uCi	microcurie
NOS	not otherwise specified	VAR	various routes of administration
NRS	numeric rating scale	VAS	visual analog scale
O2	oxygen	VRS	visual rating scale
OBRA	Omnibus Budget Reconciliation Act	w	with
OMT	osteopathic manipulation therapy	w/	with
OPPS	outpatient prospective payment system	w/o	without
ORAL	oral administration	WAK	wearable artificial kidney
OSA	obstructive sleep apnea	wc	wheelchair
Ost	ostomy	WHFO	wrist-hand-finger orthotic
OTH	other routes of administration	WHO	wrist-hand orthotic
oz	ounce	Wk	week
PA	physician's assistant	w/o	without
PAR	parenteral	Xe	xenon (isotope mass of xenon 133)
PCA	patient controlled analgesia		
PCH	pouch		
PEN	parenberal and enteral nutrition		
PENS	percutaneous electrical nerve stimulation		

Appendix 4 — Medicare Internet-only Manuals (IOMs)

The Centers for Medicare and Medicaid Services (CMS) restructured its paper-based manual system as a web-based system on October 1, 2003. Called the online CMS manual system, it combines all of the various program instructions into Internet-only Manuals (IOMs), which are used by all CMS programs and contractors. In many instances, the references from the online manuals in appendix 4 contain a mention of the old paper manuals from which the current information was obtained when the manuals were converted. This information is shown in the header of the text, in the following format, when applicable, as A3-3101, HO-210, and B3-2049.

Effective with implementation of the IOMs, the former method of publishing program memoranda (PMs) to communicate program instructions was replaced by the following four templates:

- One-time notification
- Manual revisions
- Business requirements
- Confidential requirements

The web-based system has been organized by functional area (e.g., eligibility, entitlement, claims processing, benefit policy, program integrity) in an effort to eliminate redundancy within the manuals, simplify updating, and make CMS program instructions available more quickly. The web-based system contains the functional areas included below:

Pub. 100	Introduction
Pub. 100-01	Medicare General Information, Eligibility, and Entitlement Manual
Pub. 100-02	Medicare Benefit Policy Manual
Pub. 100-03	Medicare National Coverage Determinations (NCD) Manual
Pub. 100-04	Medicare Claims Processing Manual
Pub. 100-05	Medicare Secondary Payer Manual
Pub. 100-06	Medicare Financial Management Manual
Pub. 100-07	State Operations Manual
Pub. 100-08	Medicare Program Integrity Manual
Pub. 100-09	Medicare Contractor Beneficiary and Provider Communications Manual
Pub. 100-10	Quality Improvement Organization Manual
Pub. 100-11	Programs of All-Inclusive Care for the Elderly (PACE) Manual
Pub. 100-12	State Medicaid Manual (under development)
Pub. 100-13	Medicaid State Children's Health Insurance Program (under development)
Pub. 100-15	Medicaid Integrity Program (MIP)
Pub. 100-16	Medicare Managed Care Manual
Pub. 100-17	CMS/Business Partners Systems Security Manual
Pub. 100-18	Medicare Prescription Drug Benefit Manual
Pub. 100-19	Demonstrations
Pub. 100-20	One-Time Notification
Pub. 100-21	Reserved
Pub. 100-22	Medicare Quality Reporting Incentive Programs Manual
Pub. 100-23	Payment Error Rate Measurement (under development)
Pub. 100-24	State Payment of Medicare Premiums
Pub. 100-25	Information Security Acceptable Risk Safeguards Manual

A brief description of the Medicare manuals primarily used for *HCPCS Level II* follows:

The **National Coverage Determinations Manual** (NCD), is organized according to categories such as diagnostic services, supplies, and medical procedures. The table of contents lists each category and subject within that category. Revision transmittals identify any new or background material, recap the changes, and provide an effective date for the change. The manual contains four sections and is organized in accordance with CPT category sequence and contains a list of HCPCS codes related to coverage determinations, where appropriate.

The **Medicare Benefit Policy Manual** contains Medicare general coverage instructions that are not national coverage determinations. As a general rule, in the past these instructions have been found in chapter II of the **Medicare Carriers Manual**, the **Medicare Intermediary Manual**, other provider manuals, and program memoranda.

The **Medicare Claims Processing Manual** contains instructions for processing claims for contractors and providers.

The **Medicare Program Integrity Manual** communicates the priorities and standards for the Medicare integrity programs.

Medicare IOM References

A printed version of the Medicare IOM references will no longer be published in Optum's *HCPCS Level II* product. Complete versions of all the manuals can be found online at https://www.cms.gov/ Regulations-and-Guidance/Guidance/Manuals/Internet-Only-Manuals-IOMs.

[Source: https://www.cms.gov/Regulations-and-Guidance/Guidance/Manuals/Internet-Only-Manuals-IOMs]

Appendix 5 — New, Revised, and Deleted Codes for 2023

NEW CODES

Code	Description
A2011	Supra SDRM, per sq cm
A2012	SUPRATHEL, per sq cm
A2013	Innovamatrix FS, per sq cm
A2014	Omeza Collagen Matrix, per 100 mg
A2015	Phoenix Wound Matrix, per sq cm
A2016	PermeaDerm B, per sq cm
A2017	PermeaDerm Glove, each
A2018	PermeaDerm C, per sq cm
A4100	Skin substitute, FDA-cleared as a device, not otherwise specified
A4238	Supply allowance for adjunctive continuous glucose monitor (CGM), includes all supplies and accessories, 1 month supply = 1 unit of service
A4239	Supply allowance for nonadjunctive, nonimplanted continuous glucose monitor (CGM), includes all supplies and accessories, 1 month supply = 1 unit of service
A4596	Cranial electrotherapy stimulation (CES) system supplies and accessories, per month
A9291	Prescription digital behavioral therapy, FDA-cleared, per course of treatment
A9596	Gallium Ga-68 gozetotide, diagnostic, (Illuccix), 1 mCi
A9601	Flortaucipir F-18 injection, diagnostic, 1 mCi
A9602	Fluorodopa F-18, diagnostic, per mCi
A9607	Lutetium Lu 177 vipivotide tetraxetan, therapeutic, 1 mCi
A9800	Gallium Ga-68 gozetotide, diagnostic, (Locametz), 1 mCi
C1747	Endoscope, single-use (i.e., disposable), urinary tract, imaging/illumination device (insertable)
C1826	Generator, neurostimulator (implantable), includes closed feedback loop leads and all implantable components, with rechargeable battery and charging system
C1827	Generator, neurostimulator (implantable), nonrechargeable, with implantable stimulation lead and external paired stimulation controller
C1834	Pressure sensor system, includes all components (e.g., introducer, sensor), intramuscular (implantable), excludes mobile (wireless) software application
C7500	Debridement, bone including epidermis, dermis, subcutaneous tissue, muscle and/or fascia, if performed, first 20 sq cm or less with manual preparation and insertion of deep (e.g., subfascial) drug-delivery device(s)
C7501	Percutaneous breast biopsies using stereotactic guidance, with placement of breast localization device(s) (e.g., clip, metallic pellet), when performed, and imaging of the biopsy specimen, when performed, all lesions unilateral and bilateral (for single lesion biopsy, use appropriate code)
C7502	Percutaneous breast biopsies using magnetic resonance guidance, with placement of breast localization device(s) (e.g., clip, metallic pellet), when performed, and imaging of the biopsy specimen, when performed, all lesions unilateral or bilateral (for single lesion biopsy, use appropriate code)
C7503	Open biopsy or excision of deep cervical node(s) with intraoperative identification (e.g., mapping) of sentinel lymph node(s) including injection of nonradioactive dye when performed
C7504	Percutaneous vertebroplasties (bone biopsies included when performed), first cervicothoracic and any additional cervicothoracic or lumbosacral vertebral bodies, unilateral or bilateral injection, inclusive of all imaging guidance
C7505	Percutaneous vertebroplasties (bone biopsies included when performed), first lumbosacral and any additional cervicothoracic or lumbosacral vertebral bodies, unilateral or bilateral injection, inclusive of all imaging guidance
C7506	Arthrodesis, interphalangeal joints, with or without internal fixation
C7507	Percutaneous vertebral augmentations, first thoracic and any additional thoracic or lumbar vertebral bodies, including cavity creations (fracture reductions and bone biopsies included when performed) using mechanical device (e.g., kyphoplasty), unilateral or bilateral cannulations, inclusive of all imaging guidance
C7508	Percutaneous vertebral augmentations, first lumbar and any additional thoracic or lumbar vertebral bodies, including cavity creations (fracture reductions and bone biopsies included when performed) using mechanical device (e.g., kyphoplasty), unilateral or bilateral cannulations, inclusive of all imaging guidance
C7509	Bronchoscopy, rigid or flexible, diagnostic with cell washing(s) when performed, with computer-assisted image-guided navigation, including fluoroscopic guidance when performed
C7510	Bronchoscopy, rigid or flexible, with bronchial alveolar lavage(s), with computer-assisted image-guided navigation, including fluoroscopic guidance when performed
C7511	Bronchoscopy, rigid or flexible, with single or multiple bronchial or endobronchial biopsy(ies), single or multiple sites, with computer-assisted image-guided navigation, including fluoroscopic guidance when performed
C7512	Bronchoscopy, rigid or flexible, with single or multiple bronchial or endobronchial biopsy(ies), single or multiple sites, with transendoscopic endobronchial ultrasound (EBUS) during bronchoscopic diagnostic or therapeutic intervention(s) for peripheral lesion(s), including fluoroscopic guidance when performed
C7513	Dialysis circuit, introduction of needle(s) and/or catheter(s), with diagnostic angiography of the dialysis circuit, including all direct puncture(s) and catheter placement(s), injection(s) of contrast, all necessary imaging from the arterial anastomosis and adjacent artery through entire venous outflow including the inferior or superior vena cava, fluoroscopic guidance, with transluminal balloon angioplasty of central dialysis segment, performed through dialysis circuit, including all required imaging, radiological supervision and interpretation, image documentation and report
C7514	Dialysis circuit, introduction of needle(s) and/or catheter(s), with diagnostic angiography of the dialysis circuit, including all direct puncture(s) and catheter placement(s), injection(s) of contrast, all necessary imaging from the arterial anastomosis and adjacent artery through entire venous outflow including the inferior or superior vena cava, fluoroscopic guidance, with all angioplasty in the central dialysis segment, and transcatheter placement of intravascular stent(s), central dialysis segment, performed through dialysis circuit, including all required imaging, radiological supervision and interpretation, image documentation and report
C7515	Dialysis circuit, introduction of needle(s) and/or catheter(s), with diagnostic angiography of the dialysis circuit, including all direct puncture(s) and catheter placement(s), injection(s) of contrast, all necessary imaging from the arterial anastomosis and adjacent artery through entire venous outflow including the inferior or superior vena cava, fluoroscopic guidance, with dialysis circuit permanent endovascular embolization or occlusion of main circuit or any accessory veins, including all required imaging, radiological supervision and interpretation, image documentation and report
C7516	Catheter placement in coronary artery(s) for coronary angiography, including intraprocedural injection(s) for coronary angiography, with endoluminal imaging of initial coronary vessel or graft using intravascular ultrasound (IVUS) or optical coherence tomography (OCT) during diagnostic evaluation and/or therapeutic intervention including imaging supervision, interpretation and report

NEW CODES (continued)

C7517 Catheter placement in coronary artery(s) for coronary angiography, including intraprocedural injection(s) for coronary angiography, with iliac and/or femoral artery angiography, nonselective, bilateral or ipsilateral to catheter insertion, performed at the same time as cardiac catheterization and/or coronary angiography, includes positioning or placement of the catheter in the distal aorta or ipsilateral femoral or iliac artery, injection of dye, production of permanent images, and radiologic supervision and interpretation

C7518 Catheter placement in coronary artery(ies) for coronary angiography, including intraprocedural injection(s) for coronary angiography, imaging supervision and interpretation, with catheter placement(s) in bypass graft(s) (internal mammary, free arterial, venous grafts) including intraprocedural injection(s) for bypass graft angiography with endoluminal imaging of initial coronary vessel or graft using intravascular ultrasound (IVUS) or optical coherence tomography (OCT) during diagnostic evaluation and/or therapeutic intervention including imaging, supervision, interpretation and report

C7519 Catheter placement in coronary artery(ies) for coronary angiography, including intraprocedural injection(s) for coronary angiography, imaging supervision and interpretation, with catheter placement(s) in bypass graft(s) (internal mammary, free arterial, venous grafts) including intraprocedural injection(s) for bypass graft angiography with intravascular doppler velocity and/or pressure derived coronary flow reserve measurement (initial coronary vessel or graft) during coronary angiography including pharmacologically induced stress

C7520 Catheter placement in coronary artery(ies) for coronary angiography, including intraprocedural injection(s) for coronary angiography, imaging supervision and interpretation, with catheter placement(s) in bypass graft(s) (internal mammary, free arterial, venous grafts) includes intraprocedural injection(s) for bypass graft angiography with iliac and/or femoral artery angiography, nonselective, bilateral or ipsilateral to catheter insertion, performed at the same time as cardiac catheterization and/or coronary angiography, includes positioning or placement of the catheter in the distal aorta or ipsilateral femoral or iliac artery, injection of dye, production of permanent images, and radiologic supervision and interpretation

C7521 Catheter placement in coronary artery(ies) for coronary angiography, including intraprocedural injection(s) for coronary angiography with right heart catheterization with endoluminal imaging of initial coronary vessel or graft using intravascular ultrasound (IVUS) or optical coherence tomography (OCT) during diagnostic evaluation and/or therapeutic intervention including imaging supervision, interpretation and report

C7522 Catheter placement in coronary artery(ies) for coronary angiography, including intraprocedural injection(s) for coronary angiography, imaging supervision and interpretation with right heart catheterization, with intravascular doppler velocity and/or pressure derived coronary flow reserve measurement (initial coronary vessel or graft) during coronary angiography including pharmacologically induced stress

C7523 Catheter placement in coronary artery(ies) for coronary angiography, including intraprocedural injection(s) for coronary angiography, imaging supervision and interpretation, with left heart catheterization including intraprocedural injection(s) for left ventriculography, when performed, with endoluminal imaging of initial coronary vessel or graft using intravascular ultrasound (IVUS) or optical coherence tomography (OCT) during diagnostic evaluation and/or therapeutic intervention including imaging supervision, interpretation and report

C7524 Catheter placement in coronary artery(ies) for coronary angiography, including intraprocedural injection(s) for coronary angiography, imaging supervision and interpretation, with left heart catheterization including intraprocedural injection(s) for left ventriculography, when performed, with intravascular doppler velocity and/or pressure derived coronary flow reserve measurement (initial coronary vessel or graft) during coronary angiography including pharmacologically induced stress

C7525 Catheter placement in coronary artery(ies) for coronary angiography, including intraprocedural injection(s) for coronary angiography, imaging supervision and interpretation, with left heart catheterization including intraprocedural injection(s) for left ventriculography, when performed, catheter placement(s) in bypass graft(s) (internal mammary, free arterial, venous grafts) with bypass graft angiography with endoluminal imaging of initial coronary vessel or graft using intravascular ultrasound (IVUS) or optical coherence tomography (OCT) during diagnostic evaluation and/or therapeutic intervention including imaging supervision, interpretation and report

C7526 Catheter placement in coronary artery(ies) for coronary angiography, including intraprocedural injection(s) for coronary angiography, imaging supervision and interpretation, with left heart catheterization including intraprocedural injection(s) for left ventriculography, when performed, catheter placement(s) in bypass graft(s) (internal mammary, free arterial, venous grafts) with bypass graft angiography with intravascular doppler velocity and/or pressure derived coronary flow reserve measurement (initial coronary vessel or graft) during coronary angiography including pharmacologically induced stress

C7527 Catheter placement in coronary artery(ies) for coronary angiography, including intraprocedural injection(s) for coronary angiography, imaging supervision and interpretation, with right and left heart catheterization including intraprocedural injection(s) for left ventriculography, when performed, with endoluminal imaging of initial coronary vessel or graft using intravascular ultrasound (IVUS) or optical coherence tomography (OCT) during diagnostic evaluation and/or therapeutic intervention including imaging supervision, interpretation and report

C7528 Catheter placement in coronary artery(ies) for coronary angiography, including intraprocedural injection(s) for coronary angiography, imaging supervision and interpretation, with right and left heart catheterization including intraprocedural injection(s) for left ventriculography, when performed, with intravascular doppler velocity and/or pressure derived coronary flow reserve measurement (initial coronary vessel or graft) during coronary angiography including pharmacologically induced stress

C7529 Catheter placement in coronary artery(ies) for coronary angiography, including intraprocedural injection(s) for coronary angiography, imaging supervision and interpretation, with right and left heart catheterization including intraprocedural injection(s) for left ventriculography, when performed, catheter placement(s) in bypass graft(s) (internal mammary, free arterial, venous grafts) with bypass graft angiography with intravascular doppler velocity and/or pressure derived coronary flow reserve measurement (initial coronary vessel or graft) during coronary angiography including pharmacologically induced stress

C7530 Dialysis circuit, introduction of needle(s) and/or catheter(s), with diagnostic angiography of the dialysis circuit, including all direct puncture(s) and catheter placement(s), injection(s) of contrast, all necessary imaging from the arterial anastomosis and adjacent artery through entire venous outflow including the inferior or superior vena cava, fluoroscopic guidance, with transluminal balloon angioplasty, peripheral dialysis segment, including all imaging and radiological supervision and interpretation necessary to perform the angioplasty and all angioplasty in the central dialysis segment, with transcatheter placement of intravascular stent(s), central dialysis segment, performed through dialysis circuit, including all imaging, radiological supervision and interpretation, documentation and report

C7531 Revascularization, endovascular, open or percutaneous, femoral, popliteal artery(ies), unilateral, with transluminal angioplasty with intravascular ultrasound (initial noncoronary vessel) during diagnostic evaluation and/or therapeutic intervention, including radiological supervision and interpretation

C7532 Transluminal balloon angioplasty (except lower extremity artery(ies) for occlusive disease, intracranial, coronary, pulmonary, or dialysis circuit), initial artery, open or percutaneous, including all imaging and radiological supervision and interpretation necessary to perform the angioplasty within the same artery, with intravascular ultrasound (initial noncoronary vessel) during diagnostic evaluation and/or therapeutic intervention, including radiological supervision and interpretation

C7533 Percutaneous transluminal coronary angioplasty, single major coronary artery or branch with transcatheter placement of radiation delivery device for subsequent coronary intravascular brachytherapy

NEW CODES (continued)

- **C7534** Revascularization, endovascular, open or percutaneous, femoral, popliteal artery(ies), unilateral, with atherectomy, includes angioplasty within the same vessel, when performed with intravascular ultrasound (initial noncoronary vessel) during diagnostic evaluation and/or therapeutic intervention, including radiological supervision and interpretation
- **C7535** Revascularization, endovascular, open or percutaneous, femoral, popliteal artery(ies), unilateral, with transluminal stent placement(s), includes angioplasty within the same vessel, when performed, with intravascular ultrasound (initial noncoronary vessel) during diagnostic evaluation and/or therapeutic intervention, including radiological supervision and interpretation
- **C7537** Insertion of new or replacement of permanent pacemaker with atrial transvenous electrode(s), with insertion of pacing electrode, cardiac venous system, for left ventricular pacing, at time of insertion of implantable defibrillator or pacemaker pulse generator (e.g., for upgrade to dual chamber system)
- **C7538** Insertion of new or replacement of permanent pacemaker with ventricular transvenous electrode(s), with insertion of pacing electrode, cardiac venous system, for left ventricular pacing, at time of insertion of implantable defibrillator or pacemaker pulse generator (e.g., for upgrade to dual chamber system)
- **C7539** Insertion of new or replacement of permanent pacemaker with atrial and ventricular transvenous electrode(s), with insertion of pacing electrode, cardiac venous system, for left ventricular pacing, at time of insertion of implantable defibrillator or pacemaker pulse generator (e.g., for upgrade to dual chamber system)
- **C7540** Removal of permanent pacemaker pulse generator with replacement of pacemaker pulse generator, dual lead system, with insertion of pacing electrode, cardiac venous system, for left ventricular pacing, at time of insertion of implantable defibrillator or pacemaker pulse generator (e.g., for upgrade to dual chamber system)
- **C7541** Diagnostic endoscopic retrograde cholangiopancreatography (ERCP), including collection of specimen(s) by brushing or washing, when performed, with endoscopic cannulation of papilla with direct visualization of pancreatic/common bile ducts(s)
- **C7542** Endoscopic retrograde cholangiopancreatography (ERCP) with biopsy, single or multiple, with endoscopic cannulation of papilla with direct visualization of pancreatic/common bile ducts(s)
- **C7543** Endoscopic retrograde cholangiopancreatography (ERCP) with sphincterotomy/papillotomy, with endoscopic cannulation of papilla with direct visualization of pancreatic/common bile ducts(s)
- **C7544** Endoscopic retrograde cholangiopancreatography (ERCP) with removal of calculi/debris from biliary/pancreatic duct(s), with endoscopic cannulation of papilla with direct visualization of pancreatic/common bile ducts(s)
- **C7545** Percutaneous exchange of biliary drainage catheter (e.g., external, internal-external, or conversion of internal-external to external only), with removal of calculi/debris from biliary duct(s) and/or gallbladder, including destruction of calculi by any method (e.g., mechanical, electrohydraulic, lithotripsy) when performed, including diagnostic cholangiography(ies) when performed, imaging guidance (e.g., fluoroscopy), and all associated radiological supervision and interpretation
- **C7546** Removal and replacement of externally accessible nephroureteral catheter (e.g., external/internal stent) requiring fluoroscopic guidance, with ureteral stricture balloon dilation, including imaging guidance and all associated radiological supervision and interpretation
- **C7547** Convert nephrostomy catheter to nephroureteral catheter, percutaneous via pre-existing nephrostomy tract, with ureteral stricture balloon dilation, including diagnostic nephrostogram and/or ureterogram when performed, imaging guidance (e.g., ultrasound and/or fluoroscopy) and all associated radiological supervision and interpretation
- **C7548** Exchange nephrostomy catheter, percutaneous, with ureteral stricture balloon dilation, including diagnostic nephrostogram and/or ureterogram when performed, imaging guidance (e.g., ultrasound and/or fluoroscopy) and all associated radiological supervision and interpretation
- **C7549** Change of ureterostomy tube or externally accessible ureteral stent via ileal conduit with ureteral stricture balloon dilation, including imaging guidance (e.g., ultrasound and/or fluoroscopy) and all associated radiological supervision and interpretation
- **C7550** Cystourethroscopy, with biopsy(ies) with adjunctive blue light cystoscopy with fluorescent imaging agent
- **C7551** Excision of major peripheral nerve neuroma, except sciatic, with implantation of nerve end into bone or muscle
- **C7552** Catheter placement in coronary artery(s) for coronary angiography, including intraprocedural injection(s) for coronary angiography, imaging supervision and interpretation; with catheter placement(s) in bypass graft(s) (internal mammary, free arterial, venous grafts) including intraprocedural injection(s) for bypass graft angiography and right heart catheterization with intravascular doppler velocity and/or pressure derived coronary flow reserve measurement (coronary vessel or graft) during coronary angiography including pharmacologically induced stress, initial vessel
- **C7553** Catheter placement in coronary artery(s) for coronary angiography, including intraprocedural injection(s) for coronary angiography, imaging supervision and interpretation; with right and left heart catheterization including intraprocedural injection(s) for left ventriculography, when performed, catheter placement(s) in bypass graft(s) (internal mammary, free arterial, venous grafts) with bypass graft angiography with pharmacologic agent administration (e.g., inhaled nitric oxide, intravenous infusion of nitroprusside, dobutamine, milrinone, or other agent) including assessing hemodynamic measurements before, during, after and repeat pharmacologic agent administration, when performed
- **C7554** Cystourethroscopy with adjunctive blue light cystoscopy with fluorescent imaging agent
- **C7555** Thyroidectomy, total or complete with parathyroid autotransplantation
- **C7900** Service for diagnosis, evaluation, or treatment of a mental health or substance use disorder, initial 15-29 minutes, provided remotely by hospital staff who are licensed to provide mental health services under applicable state law(s), when the patient is in their home, and there is no associated professional service
- **C7901** Service for diagnosis, evaluation, or treatment of a mental health or substance use disorder, initial 30-60 minutes, provided remotely by hospital staff who are licensed to provided mental health services under applicable state law(s), when the patient is in their home, and there is no associated professional service
- **C7902** Service for diagnosis, evaluation, or treatment of a mental health or substance use disorder, each additional 15 minutes, provided remotely by hospital staff who are licensed to provide mental health services under applicable state law(s), when the patient is in their home, and there is no associated professional service (list separately in addition to code for primary service)
- **C9101** Injection, oliceridine, 0.1 mg
- **C9142** Injection, bevacizumab-maly, biosimilar, (Alymsys), 10 mg
- **C9143** Cocaine HCl nasal solution (Numbrino), 1 mg
- **C9144** Injection, bupivacaine (Posimir), 1 mg
- **C9781** Arthroscopy, shoulder, surgical; with implantation of subacromial spacer (e.g., balloon), includes debridement (e.g., limited or extensive), subacromial decompression, acromioplasty, and biceps tenodesis when performed
- **C9782** Blinded procedure for New York Heart Association (NYHA) Class II or III heart failure, or Canadian Cardiovascular Society (CCS) Class III or IV chronic refractory angina; transcatheter intramyocardial transplantation of autologous bone marrow cells (e.g., mononuclear) or placebo control, autologous bone marrow harvesting and preparation for transplantation, left heart catheterization including ventriculography, all laboratory services, and all imaging with or without guidance (e.g., transthoracic echocardiography, ultrasound, fluoroscopy), performed in an approved investigational device exemption (IDE) study
- **C9783** Blinded procedure for transcatheter implantation of coronary sinus reduction device or placebo control, including vascular access and closure, right heart catherization, venous and coronary sinus angiography, imaging guidance and supervision and interpretation when performed in an approved investigational device exemption (IDE) study

Appendix 5 — New, Revised, and Deleted Codes for 2023

NEW CODES (continued)

Code	Description
E0183	Powered pressure reducing underlay/pad, alternating, with pump, includes heavy duty
E2102	Adjunctive continuous glucose monitor or receiver
E2103	Nonadjunctive, nonimplanted continuous glucose monitor (CGM) or receiver
G0310	Immunization counseling by a physician or other qualified health care professional when the vaccine(s) is not administered on the same date of service, 5-15 minutes time (This code is used for Medicaid billing purposes)
G0311	Immunization counseling by a physician or other qualified health care professional when the vaccine(s) is not administered on the same date of service, 16-30 minutes time (This code is used for Medicaid billing purposes)
G0312	Immunization counseling by a physician or other qualified health care professional when the vaccine(s) is not administered on the same date of service for ages under 21, 5-15 minutes time (This code is used for Medicaid billing purposes)
G0313	Immunization counseling by a physician or other qualified health care professional when the vaccine(s) is not administered on the same date of service for ages under 21, 16-30 minutes time (This code is used for Medicaid billing purposes)
G0314	Immunization counseling by a physician or other qualified health care professional for COVID-19, ages under 21, 16-30 minutes time (This code is used for the Medicaid Early and Periodic Screening, Diagnostic, and Treatment Benefit [EPSDT])
G0315	Immunization counseling by a physician or other qualified health care professional for COVID-19, ages under 21, 5-15 minutes time (This code is used for the Medicaid Early and Periodic Screening, Diagnostic, and Treatment Benefit [EPSDT])
G0316	Prolonged hospital inpatient or observation care evaluation and management service(s) beyond the total time for the primary service (when the primary service has been selected using time on the date of the primary service); each additional 15 minutes by the physician or qualified healthcare professional, with or without direct patient contact (list separately in addition to CPT codes 99223, 99233, and 99236 for hospital inpatient or observation care evaluation and management services). (Do not report G0316 on the same date of service as other prolonged services for evaluation and management codes 99358, 99359, 99418, 99415, 99416). (Do not report G0316 for any time unit less than 15 minutes)
G0317	Prolonged nursing facility evaluation and management service(s) beyond the total time for the primary service (when the primary service has been selected using time on the date of the primary service); each additional 15 minutes by the physician or qualified healthcare professional, with or without direct patient contact (list separately in addition to CPT codes 99306, 99310 for nursing facility evaluation and management services). (Do not report G0317 on the same date of service as other prolonged services for evaluation and management codes 99358, 99359, 99418). (Do not report G0317 for any time unit less than 15 minutes)
G0318	Prolonged home or residence evaluation and management service(s) beyond the total time for the primary service (when the primary service has been selected using time on the date of the primary service); each additional 15 minutes by the physician or qualified healthcare professional, with or without direct patient contact (list separately in addition to CPT codes 99345, 99350 for home or residence evaluation and management services). (Do not report G0318 on the same date of service as other prolonged services for evaluation and management codes 99358, 99359, 99417). (Do not report G0318 for any time unit less than 15 minutes)
G0320	Home health services furnished using synchronous telemedicine rendered via a real-time two-way audio and video telecommunications system
G0321	Home health services furnished using synchronous telemedicine rendered via telephone or other real-time interactive audio-only telecommunications system
G0322	The collection of physiologic data digitally stored and/or transmitted by the patient to the home health agency (i.e., remote patient monitoring)
G0323	Care management services for behavioral health conditions, at least 20 minutes of clinical psychologist or clinical social worker time, per calendar month. (These services include the following required elements: initial assessment or follow-up monitoring, including the use of applicable validated rating scales; behavioral health care planning in relation to behavioral/psychiatric health problems, including revision for patients who are not progressing or whose status changes; facilitating and coordinating treatment such as psychotherapy, coordination with and/or referral to physicians and practitioners who are authorized by Medicare to prescribe medications and furnish E/M services, counseling and/or psychiatric consultation; and continuity of care with a designated member of the care team)
G0330	Facility services for dental rehabilitation procedure(s) performed on a patient who requires monitored anesthesia (e.g., general, intravenous sedation (monitored anesthesia care) and use of an operating room
G3002	Chronic pain management and treatment, monthly bundle including, diagnosis; assessment and monitoring; administration of a validated pain rating scale or tool; the development, implementation, revision, and/or maintenance of a person-centered care plan that includes strengths, goals, clinical needs, and desired outcomes; overall treatment management; facilitation and coordination of any necessary behavioral health treatment; medication management; pain and health literacy counseling; any necessary chronic pain related crisis care; and ongoing communication and care coordination between relevant practitioners furnishing care e.g., physical therapy and occupational therapy, complementary and integrative approaches, and community-based care, as appropriate. Requires initial face-to-face visit at least 30 minutes provided by a physician or other qualified health professional; first 30 minutes personally provided by physician or other qualified health care professional, per calendar month. (When using G3002, 30 minutes must be met or exceeded)
G3003	Each additional 15 minutes of chronic pain management and treatment by a physician or other qualified health care professional, per calendar month. (List separately in addition to code for G3002. When using G3003, 15 minutes must be met or exceeded)
H2038	Skills training and development, per diem
J0134	Injection, acetaminophen (Fresenius Kabi) not therapeutically equivalent to J0131, 10 mg
J0136	Injection, acetaminophen (B. Braun) not therapeutically equivalent to J0131, 10 mg
J0173	Injection, epinephrine (Belcher) not therapeutically equivalent to J0171, 0.1 mg
J0219	Injection, avalglucosidase alfa-ngpt, 4 mg
J0225	Injection, vutrisiran, 1 mg
J0283	Injection, amiodarone HCl (Nexterone), 30 mg
J0491	Injection, anifrolumab-fnia, 1 mg
J0611	Injection, calcium gluconate (WG Critical Care), per 10 ml
J0689	Injection, cefazolin sodium (Baxter), not therapeutically equivalent to J0690, 500 mg
J0701	Injection, cefepime HCl (Baxter), not therapeutically equivalent to Maxipime, 500 mg
J0703	Injection, cefepime HCl (B. Braun), not therapeutically equivalent to Maxipime, 500 mg
J0739	Injection, cabotegravir, 1 mg
J0877	Injection, daptomycin (Hospira), not therapeutically equivalent to J0878, 1 mg
J0879	Injection, difelikefalin, 0.1 mcg, (for ESRD on dialysis)
J0891	Injection, argatroban (Accord), not therapeutically equivalent to J0883, 1 mg (for non-ESRD use)
J0892	Injection, argatroban (Accord), not therapeutically equivalent to J0884, 1 mg (for ESRD on dialysis)
J0893	Injection, decitabine (Sun Pharma) not therapeutically equivalent to J0894, 1 mg
J0898	Injection, argatroban (Auromedics), not therapeutically equivalent to J0883, 1 mg (for non-ESRD use)
J0899	Injection, argatroban (Auromedics), not therapeutically equivalent to J0884, 1 mg (for ESRD on dialysis)
J1302	Injection, sutimlimab-jome, 10 mg
J1306	Injection, inclisiran, 1 mg

NEW CODES (continued)

Code	Description
J1456	Injection, fosaprepitant (Teva), not therapeutically equivalent to J1453, 1 mg
J1551	Injection, immune globulin (Cutaquig), 100 mg
J1574	Injection, ganciclovir sodium (Exela) not therapeutically equivalent to J1570, 500 mg
J1611	Injection, glucagon HCl (Fresenius Kabi), not therapeutically equivalent to J1610, per 1 mg
J1643	Injection, heparin sodium (Pfizer), not therapeutically equivalent to J1644, per 1000 units
J1932	Injection, lanreotide, (Cipla), 1 mg
J2021	Injection, linezolid (Hospira) not therapeutically equivalent to J2020, 200 mg
J2184	Injection, meropenem (B. Braun) not therapeutically equivalent to J2185, 100 mg
J2247	Injection, micafungin sodium (Par pharmaceutical) not therapeutically equivalent to J2248, 1 mg
J2251	Injection, midazolam HCl (WG Critical Care) not therapeutically equivalent to J2250, per 1 mg
J2272	Injection, morphine sulfate (Fresenius Kabi) not therapeutically equivalent to J2270, up to 10 mg
J2281	Injection, moxifloxacin (Fresenius Kabi) not therapeutically equivalent to J2280, 100 mg
J2311	Injection, naloxone HCl (Zimhi), 1 mg
J2327	Injection, risankizumab-rzaa, intravenous, 1 mg
J2356	Injection, tezepelumab-ekko, 1 mg
J2401	Injection, chloroprocaine HCl, per 1 mg
J2402	Injection, chloroprocaine HCl (Clorotekal), per 1 mg
J2777	Injection, faricimab-svoa, 0.1 mg
J2779	Injection, ranibizumab, via intravitreal implant (Susvimo), 0.1 mg
J2998	Injection, plasminogen, human-tvmh, 1 mg
J3244	Injection, tigecycline (Accord) not therapeutically equivalent to J3243, 1 mg
J3299	Injection, triamcinolone acetonide (Xipere), 1 mg
J3371	Injection, vancomycin HCl (Mylan) not therapeutically equivalent to J3370, 500 mg
J3372	Injection, vancomycin HCl (Xellia) not therapeutically equivalent to J3370, 500 mg
J9046	Injection, bortezomib, (Dr. Reddy's), not therapeutically equivalent to J9041, 0.1 mg
J9048	Injection, bortezomib (Fresenius Kabi), not therapeutically equivalent to J9041, 0.1 mg
J9049	Injection, bortezomib (Hospira), not therapeutically equivalent to J9041, 0.1 mg
J9071	Injection, cyclophosphamide, (AuroMedics), 5 mg
J9273	Injection, tisotumab vedotin-tftv, 1 mg
J9274	Injection, tebentafusp-tebn, 1 mcg
J9298	Injection, nivolumab and relatlimab-rmbw, 3 mg/1 mg
J9331	Injection, sirolimus protein-bound particles, 1 mg
J9332	Injection, efgartigimod alfa-fcab, 2 mg
J9359	Injection, loncastuximab tesirine-lpyl, 0.075 mg
J9393	Injection, fulvestrant (Teva) not therapeutically equivalent to J9395, 25 mg
J9394	Injection, fulvestrant (Fresenius Kabi) not therapeutically equivalent to J9395, 25 mg
K1028	Power source and control electronics unit for oral device/appliance for neuromuscular electrical stimulation of the tongue muscle for the reduction of snoring and obstructive sleep apnea, controlled by phone application
K1029	Oral device/appliance for neuromuscular electrical stimulation of the tongue muscle, used in conjunction with the power source and control electronics unit, controlled by phone application, 90-day supply
K1030	External recharging system for battery (internal) for use with implanted cardiac contractility modulation generator, replacement only
K1031	Nonpneumatic compression controller without calibrated gradient pressure
K1032	Nonpneumatic sequential compression garment, full leg
K1033	Nonpneumatic sequential compression garment, half leg
K1034	Provision of COVID-19 test, nonprescription self-administered and self-collected use, FDA approved, authorized or cleared, one test count
M0001	Advancing Cancer Care MIPS Value Pathways
M0002	Optimal Care for Kidney Health MIPS Value Pathways
M0003	Optimal Care for Patients with Episodic Neurological Conditions MIPS Value Pathways
M0004	Supportive Care for Neurodegenerative Conditions MIPS Value Pathways
M0005	Promoting Wellness MIPS Value Pathways
M0222	Intravenous injection, bebtelovimab, includes injection and post administration monitoring
M0223	Intravenous injection, bebtelovimab, includes injection and post administration monitoring in the home or residence; this includes a beneficiary's home that has been made provider-based to the hospital during the COVID-19 public health emergency
M1150	Left ventricular ejection fraction (LVEF) less than or equal to 40% or documentation of moderately or severely depressed left ventricular systolic function
M1151	Patients with a history of heart transplant or with a left ventricular assist device (LVAD)
M1152	Patients with a history of heart transplant or with a left ventricular assist device (LVAD)
M1153	Patient with diagnosis of osteoporosis on date of encounter
M1154	Hospice services provided to patient any time during the measurement period
M1155	Patient had anaphylaxis due to the pneumococcal vaccine any time during or before the measurement period
M1156	Patient received active chemotherapy any time during the measurement period
M1157	Patient received bone marrow transplant any time during the measurement period
M1158	Patient had history of immunocompromising conditions prior to or during the measurement period
M1159	Hospice services provided to patient any time during the measurement period
M1160	Patient had anaphylaxis due to the meningococcal vaccine any time on or before the patient's 13th birthday
M1161	Patient had anaphylaxis due to the tetanus, diphtheria or pertussis vaccine any time on or before the patient's 13th birthday
M1162	Patient had encephalitis due to the tetanus, diphtheria or pertussis vaccine any time on or before the patient's 13th birthday
M1163	Patient had anaphylaxis due to the HPV vaccine any time on or before the patient's 13th birthday
M1164	Patients with dementia any time during the patient's history through the end of the measurement period
M1165	Patients who use hospice services any time during the measurement period
M1166	Pathology report for tissue specimens produced from wide local excisions or re-excisions
M1167	In hospice or using hospice services during the measurement period
M1168	Patient received an influenza vaccine on or between July 1 of the year prior to the measurement period and June 30 of the measurement period
M1169	Documentation of medical reason(s) for not administering influenza vaccine (e.g., prior anaphylaxis due to the influenza vaccine)
M1170	Patient did not receive an influenza vaccine on or between July 1 of the year prior to the measurement period and June 30 of the measurement period
M1171	Patient received at least 1 TD vaccine or one TDaP vaccine between 9 years prior to the encounter and the end of the measurement period

NEW CODES (continued)

Code	Description
M1172	Documentation of medical reason(s) for not administering TD or TDaP vaccine (e.g., prior anaphylaxis due to the TD or TDaP vaccine or history of encephalopathy within 7 days after a previous dose of a TD-containing vaccine)
M1173	Patient did not receive at least 1 TD vaccine or one TDaP vaccine between 9 years prior to the encounter and the end of the measurement period
M1174	Patient received at least 1 dose of the herpes zoster live vaccine or 2 doses of the herpes zoster recombinant vaccine (at least 28 days apart) anytime on or after the patient's 50th birthday before or during the measurement period
M1175	Documentation of medical reason(s) for not administering zoster vaccine (e.g., prior anaphylaxis due to the zoster vaccine)
M1176	Patient did not receive at least 1 dose of the herpes zoster live vaccine or 2 doses of the herpes zoster recombinant vaccine (at least 28 days apart) anytime on or after the patient's 50th birthday before or during the measurement period
M1177	Patient received any pneumococcal conjugate or polysaccharide vaccine on or after their 60th birthday and before the end of the measurement period
M1178	Documentation of medical reason(s) for not administering pneumococcal vaccine (e.g., prior anaphylaxis due to the pneumococcal vaccine)
M1179	Patient did not receive any pneumococcal conjugate or polysaccharide vaccine, on or after their 60th birthday and before or during measurement period
M1180	Patients on immune checkpoint inhibitor therapy
M1181	Grade 2 or above diarrhea and/or Grade 2 or above colitis
M1182	Patients not eligible due to pre-existing inflammatory bowel disease (IBD) (e.g., ulcerative colitis, Crohn's disease)
M1183	Documentation of immune checkpoint inhibitor therapy held and corticosteroids or immunosuppressants prescribed or administered
M1184	Documentation of medical reason(s) for not prescribing or administering corticosteroid or immunosuppressant treatment (e.g., allergy, intolerance, infectious etiology, pancreatic insufficiency, hyperthyroidism, prior bowel surgical interventions, celiac disease, receiving other medication, awaiting diagnostic workup results for alternative etiologies, other medical reasons/contraindication)
M1185	Documentation of immune checkpoint inhibitor therapy not held and/or corticosteroids or immunosuppressants prescribed or administered was not performed, reason not given
M1186	Patients who have an order for or are receiving hospice or palliative care
M1187	Patients with a diagnosis of end stage renal disease (ESRD)
M1188	Patients with a diagnosis of chronic kidney disease (CKD) Stage 5
M1189	Documentation of a kidney health evaluation defined by an estimated glomerular filtration rate (EGFR) and urine albumin-creatinine ratio (UACR) performed
M1190	Documentation of a kidney health evaluation was not performed or defined by an estimated glomerular filtration rate (EGFR) and urine albumin-creatinine ratio (UACR)
M1191	Hospice services provided to patient any time during the measurement period
M1192	Patients with an existing diagnosis of squamous cell carcinoma of the esophagus
M1193	Surgical pathology reports that contain impression or conclusion of or recommendation for testing of MMR by immunohistochemistry, MSI by DNA-based testing status, or both
M1194	Documentation of medical reason(s) surgical pathology reports did not contain impression or conclusion of or recommendation for testing of MMR by immunohistochemistry, MSI by DNA-based testing status, or both tests were not included (e.g., patient will not be treated with checkpoint inhibitor therapy, no residual carcinoma is present in the sample [tissue exhausted or status post neoadjuvant treatment], insufficient tumor for testing)
M1195	Surgical pathology reports that do not contain impression or conclusion of or recommendation for testing of MMR by immunohistochemistry, MSI by DNA-based testing status, or both, reason not given
M1196	Initial (index visit) numeric rating scale (NRS), visual rating scale (VRS), or ItchyQuant assessment score of greater than or equal to 4
M1197	Itch severity assessment score is reduced by 2 or more points from the initial (index) assessment score to the follow-up visit score
M1198	Itch severity assessment score was not reduced by at least 2 points from initial (index) score to the follow-up visit score or assessment was not completed during the follow-up encounter
M1199	Patients receiving RRT
M1200	Ace inhibitor (ACE-I) or ARB therapy prescribed during the measurement period
M1201	Documentation of medical reason(s) for not prescribing ACE inhibitor (ACE-I) or ARB therapy during the measurement period (e.g., pregnancy, history of angioedema to ACE-I, other allergy to ACE-I and ARB, hyperkalemia or history of hyperkalemia while on ACE-I or ARB therapy, acute kidney injury due to ACE-I or ARB therapy), other medical reasons)
M1202	Documentation of patient reason(s) for not prescribing ACE inhibitor or ARB therapy during the measurement period, (e.g., patient declined, other patient reasons)
M1203	Ace inhibitor or ARB therapy not prescribed during the measurement period, reason not given
M1204	Initial (index visit) numeric rating scale (NRS), visual rating scale (VRS), or ItchyQuant assessment score of greater than or equal to 4
M1205	Itch severity assessment score is reduced by 2 or more points from the initial (index) assessment score to the follow-up visit score
M1206	Itch severity assessment score was not reduced by at least 2 points from initial (index) score to the follow-up visit score or assessment was not completed during the follow-up encounter
M1207	Number of patients screened for food insecurity, housing instability, transportation needs, utility difficulties, and interpersonal safety
M1208	Number of patients not screened for food insecurity, housing instability, transportation needs, utility difficulties, and interpersonal safety
M1209	At least two orders for high-risk medications from the same drug class, (Table 4), not ordered
M1210	At least two orders for high-risk medications from the same drug class, (Table 4), not ordered
Q0221	Injection, tixagevimab and cilgavimab, for the pre-exposure prophylaxis only, for certain adults and pediatric individuals (12 years of age and older weighing at least 40kg) with no known sars-cov-2 exposure, who either have moderate to severely compromised immune systems or for whom vaccination with any available covid-19 vaccine is not recommended due to a history of severe adverse reaction to a covid-19 vaccine(s) and/or covid-19 vaccine component(s), 600 mg
Q0222	Injection, bebtelovimab, 175 mg
Q2056	Ciltacabtagene autoleucel, up to 100 million autologous B-cell maturation antigen (BCMA) directed CAR-positive T cells, including leukapheresis and dose preparation procedures, per therapeutic dose
Q4224	Human Health Factor 10 Amniotic Patch (HHF10-P), per sq cm
Q4225	AmnioBind, per sq cm
Q4236	carePATCH, per sq cm
Q4256	MLG-Complete, per sq cm
Q4257	Relese, per sq cm
Q4258	Enverse, per sq cm
Q4259	Celera Dual Layer or Celera Dual Membrane, per sq cm
Q4260	Signature APatch, per sq cm
Q4261	TAG, per sq cm
Q4262	Dual Layer Impax Membrane, per sq cm
Q4263	SurGraft TL, per sq cm
Q4264	Cocoon Membrane, per sq cm
Q5124	Injection, ranibizumab-nuna, biosimilar, (Byooviz), 0.1 mg

NEW CODES (continued)

Code	Description
Q5125	Injection, filgrastim-ayow, biosimilar, (Releuko), 1 mcg
Q5126	Injection, bevacizumab-maly, biosimilar, (Alymsys), 10 mg
T1032	Services performed by a doula birth worker, per 15 minutes
T1033	Services performed by a doula birth worker, per diem
T2050	Financial management, self-directed, waiver; per diem
T2051	Supports brokerage, self-directed, waiver; per diem
V2525	Contact lens, hydrophilic, dual focus, per lens

REVISED CODES

Code	Description
A2004	XCelliStem, 1 mg
A4238	Supply allowance for adjunctive, nonimplanted continuous glucose monitor (CGM), includes all supplies and accessories, 1 month supply = 1 unit of service
A9276	Sensor; invasive (e.g., subcutaneous), disposable, for use with nondurable medical equipment interstitial continuous glucose monitoring system (CGM), one unit = 1 day supply
A9277	Transmitter; external, for use with nondurable medical equipment interstitial continuous glucose monitoring system (CGM)
A9278	Receiver (monitor); external, for use with nondurable medical equipment interstitial continuous glucose monitoring system (CGM)
A9291	Prescription digital cognitive and/or behavioral therapy, FDA-cleared, per course of treatment
C1831	Interbody cage, anterior, lateral or posterior, personalized (implantable)
C9761	Cystourethroscopy, with ureteroscopy and/or pyeloscopy, with lithotripsy, and ureteral catheterization for steerable vacuum aspiration of the kidney, collecting system, ureter, bladder, and urethra if applicable (must use a steerable ureteral catheter)
E0483	High frequency chest wall oscillation system, with full anterior and/or posterior thoracic region receiving simultaneous external oscillation, includes all accessories and supplies, each
E2102	Adjunctive, nonimplanted continuous glucose monitor (CGM) or receiver
G0029	Tobacco screening not performed or tobacco cessation intervention not provided during the measurement period or in the six months prior to the measurement period
G0030	Patient screened for tobacco use and received tobacco cessation intervention during the measurement period or in the six months prior to the measurement period (counseling, pharmacotherapy, or both), if identified as a tobacco user
G0442	Annual alcohol misuse screening, 5 to 15 minutes
G0444	Annual depression screening, 5 to 15 minutes
G0917	Patient care survey was not completed by patient
G2136	Back pain measured by the visual analog scale (VAS) or numeric pain scale at three months (6 to 20 weeks) postoperatively was less than or equal to 3.0 or back pain measured by the visual analog scale (VAS) or numeric pain scale within three months preoperatively and at three months (6 to 20 weeks) postoperatively demonstrated an improvement of 5.0 points or greater
G2137	Back pain measured by the visual analog scale (VAS) or numeric pain scale at three months (6 to 20 weeks) postoperatively was greater than 3.0 and back pain measured by the visual analog scale (VAS) or numeric pain scale within three months preoperatively and at three months (6 to 20 weeks) postoperatively demonstrated less than an improvement of 5.0 points
G2138	Back pain as measured by the visual analog scale (VAS) or numeric pain scale at one year (9 to 15 months) postoperatively was less than or equal to 3.0 or back pain measured by the visual analog scale (VAS) or numeric pain scale within three months preoperatively and at one year (9 to 15 months) postoperatively demonstrated an improvement of 5.0 points or greater
G2139	Back pain measured by the visual analog scale (VAS) or numeric pain scale at one year (9 to 15 months) postoperatively was greater than 3.0 and back pain measured by the visual analog scale (VAS) or numeric pain scale within three months preoperatively and at one year (9 to 15 months) postoperatively demonstrated less than an improvement of 5.0 points
G2140	Leg pain measured by the visual analog scale (VAS) or numeric pain scale at three months (6 to 20 weeks) postoperatively was less than or equal to 3.0 or leg pain measured by the visual analog scale (VAS) or numeric pain scale within three months preoperatively and at three months (6 to 20 weeks) postoperatively demonstrated an improvement of 5.0 points or greater
G2141	Leg pain measured by the visual analog scale (VAS) or numeric pain scale at three months (6 to 20 weeks) postoperatively was greater than 3.0 and leg pain measured by the visual analog scale (VAS) or numeric pain scale within three months preoperatively and at three months (6 to 20 weeks) postoperatively demonstrated less than an improvement of 5.0 points
G2146	Leg pain as measured by the visual analog scale (VAS) or numeric pain scale at one year (9 to 15 months) postoperatively was less than or equal to 3.0 or leg pain measured by the visual analog scale (VAS) or numeric pain scale within three months preoperatively and at one year (9 to 15 months) postoperatively demonstrated an improvement of 5.0 points or greater
G2147	Leg pain measured by the visual analog scale (VAS) or numeric pain scale at one year (9 to 15 months) postoperatively was greater than 3.0 and leg pain measured by the visual analog scale (VAS) or numeric pain scale within three months preoperatively and at one year (9 to 15 months) postoperatively demonstrated less than an improvement of 5.0 points
G2152	Residual score for the neck impairment successfully calculated and the score was equal to zero (0) or greater than zero (> 0)
G2167	Residual score for the neck impairment successfully calculated and the score was less than zero (< 0)
G2174	URI episodes when the patient had an active prescription of antibiotics in the 30 days prior to the episode date or is still active the same day of the encounter
G2182	Patient receiving first-time biologic and/or immune response modifier therapy
G2199	Patient not screened for unhealthy alcohol use using a systematic screening method
G2202	Patient did not receive brief counseling if identified as an unhealthy alcohol user
G2204	Patients between 45 and 85 years of age who received a screening colonoscopy during the performance period
G2207	Reason for not administering adjuvant treatment course including both chemotherapy and HER2-targeted therapy (e.g., poor performance status (ECOG 3-4; Karnofsky <=50), cardiac contraindications, insufficient renal function, insufficient hepatic function, other active or secondary cancer diagnoses, other medical contraindications, patients who died during initial treatment course or transferred during or after initial treatment course)
G2210	Residual score for the neck impairment not measured because the patient did not complete the neck FS PROM at initial evaluation and/or near discharge, reason not given
G2212	Prolonged office or other outpatient evaluation and management service(s) beyond the maximum required time of the primary procedure which has been selected using total time on the date of the primary service; each additional 15 minutes by the physician or qualified healthcare professional, with or without direct patient contact (list separately in addition to CPT codes 99205, 99215, 99483 for office or other outpatient evaluation and management services.) (Do not report G2212 on the same date of service as codes 99358, 99359, 99415, 99416). (Do not report G2212 for any time unit less than 15 minutes)
G4013	Mental/behavioral and Psychiatry MIPS specialty set
G4020	Ophthalmology/Optometry MIPS specialty set
G8451	Beta-blocker therapy for LVEF <=40% not prescribed for reasons documented by the clinician (e.g., low blood pressure, fluid overload, asthma, patients recently treated with an intravenous positive inotropic agent, allergy, intolerance, other medical reasons, patient declined, other patient reasons)
G8539	Functional outcome assessment documented as positive using a standardized tool and a care plan based on identified deficiencies is documented within two days of the functional outcome assessment

REVISED CODES (continued)

- **G8543** Documentation of a positive functional outcome assessment using a standardized tool; care plan not documented within two days of assessment, reason not given
- **G8600** IV thrombolytic therapy initiated within 4.5 hours (<= 270 minutes) of time last known well
- **G8601** IV thrombolytic therapy not initiated within 4.5 hours (= 270 minutes) of time last known well for reasons documented by clinician (e.g., patient enrolled in clinical trial for stroke, patient admitted for elective carotid intervention, patient received tenecteplase (TNK))
- **G8602** IV thrombolytic therapy not initiated within 4.5 hours (<= 270 minutes) of time last known well, reason not given
- **G8647** Residual score for the knee impairment successfully calculated and the score was equal to zero (0) or greater than zero (> 0)
- **G8648** Residual score for the knee impairment successfully calculated and the score was less than zero (< 0)
- **G8650** Residual score for the knee impairment not measured because the patient did not complete the LEPF PROM at initial evaluation and/or near discharge, reason not given
- **G8651** Residual score for the hip impairment successfully calculated and the score was equal to zero (0) or greater than zero (> 0)
- **G8652** Residual score for the hip impairment successfully calculated and the score was less than zero (< 0)
- **G8654** Residual score for the hip impairment not measured because the patient did not complete the LEPF PROM at initial evaluation and/or near discharge, reason not given
- **G8655** Residual score for the lower leg, foot or ankle impairment successfully calculated and the score was equal to zero (0) or greater than zero (> 0)
- **G8656** Residual score for the lower leg, foot or ankle impairment successfully calculated and the score was less than zero (< 0)
- **G8658** Residual score for the lower leg, foot or ankle impairment not measured because the patient did not complete the LEPF PROM at initial evaluation and/or near discharge, reason not given
- **G8659** Residual score for the low back impairment successfully calculated and the score was equal to zero (0) or greater than zero (> 0)
- **G8660** Residual score for the low back impairment successfully calculated and the score was less than zero (< 0)
- **G8662** Residual score for the low back impairment not measured because the patient did not complete the low back FS PROM at initial evaluation and/or near discharge, reason not given
- **G8663** Residual score for the shoulder impairment successfully calculated and the score was equal to zero (0) or greater than zero (> 0)
- **G8664** Residual score for the shoulder impairment successfully calculated and the score was less than zero (< 0)
- **G8666** Residual score for the shoulder impairment not measured because the patient did not complete the shoulder FS PROM at initial evaluation and/or near discharge, reason not given
- **G8667** Residual score for the elbow, wrist or hand impairment successfully calculated and the score was equal to zero (0) or greater than zero (> 0)
- **G8668** Residual score for the elbow, wrist or hand impairment successfully calculated and the score was less than zero (< 0)
- **G8670** Residual score for the elbow, wrist or hand impairment not measured because the patient did not complete the elbow/wrist/hand FS PROM at initial evaluation and/or near discharge, reason not given
- **G8694** Left ventricular ejection fraction (LVEF) < = 40% or documentation of moderate or severe LVSD
- **G8708** Patient not prescribed antibiotic
- **G8710** Patient prescribed antibiotic
- **G8711** Prescribed antibiotic on or within 3 days after the episode date
- **G8734** Elder maltreatment screen documented as negative, follow-up is not required
- **G8842** Apnea hypopnea index (AHI), respiratory disturbance index (RDI) or respiratory event index (REI) documented or measured within 2 months of initial evaluation for suspected obstructive sleep apnea
- **G8843** Documentation of reason(s) for not measuring an apnea hypopnea index (AHI), a respiratory disturbance index (RDI), or a respiratory event index (REI) within 2 months of initial evaluation for suspected obstructive sleep apnea (e.g., medical, neurological, or psychiatric disease that prohibits successful completion of a sleep study, patients for whom a sleep study would present a bigger risk than benefit or would pose an undue burden, dementia, patients who decline AHI/RDI/REI measurement, patients who had a financial reason for not completing testing, test was ordered but not completed, patients decline because their insurance (payer) does not cover the expense))
- **G8844** Apnea hypopnea index (AHI), respiratory disturbance index (RDI), or respiratory event index (REI) not documented or measured within 2 months of initial evaluation for suspected obstructive sleep apnea, reason not given
- **G8852** Positive airway pressure therapy was prescribed
- **G8854** Documentation of reason(s) for not objectively measuring adherence to positive airway pressure therapy (e.g., patient didn't bring data from continuous positive airway pressure [CPAP], therapy not yet initiated, not available on machine)
- **G8923** Left ventricular ejection fraction (LVEF) <= 40% or documentation of moderately or severely depressed left ventricular systolic function
- **G8934** Left ventricular ejection fraction (LVEF) <=40% or documentation of moderately or severely depressed left ventricular systolic function
- **G8942** Functional outcomes assessment using a standardized tool is documented within the previous 30 days and care plan, based on identified deficiencies is documented within two days of the functional outcome assessment
- **G8968** Documentation of medical reason(s) for not prescribing an FDA-approved anticoagulant (e.g., present or planned atrial appendage occlusion or ligation)
- **G9315** Amoxicillin, with or without clavulanate, prescribed as a first line antibiotic at the time of diagnosis
- **G9404** Patient did not receive follow-up within 30 days after discharge
- **G9407** Patient did not receive follow-up within 7 days after discharge
- **G9418** Primary nonsmall cell lung cancer lung biopsy and cytology specimen report documents classification into specific histologic type following IASLC guidance or classified as NSCLC-NOS with an explanation
- **G9500** Radiation exposure indices documented in final report for procedure using fluoroscopy
- **G9501** Radiation exposure indices not documented in final report for procedure using fluoroscopy, reason not given
- **G9624** Patient not screened for unhealthy alcohol use using a systematic screening method or patient did not receive brief counseling if identified as an unhealthy alcohol user
- **G9662** Previously diagnosed or have a diagnosis of clinical ASCVD, including ASCVD procedure
- **G9663** Any LDL-C laboratory result >= 190 mg/dl
- **G9781** Documentation of medical reason(s) for not currently being a statin therapy user or receiving an order (prescription) for statin therapy (e.g., patients with statin-associated muscle symptoms or an allergy to statin medication therapy, patients who are receiving palliative or hospice care, patients with active liver disease or hepatic disease or insufficiency, patients with end stage renal disease [ESRD], or other medical reasons)
- **G9789** Blood pressure recorded during inpatient stays, emergency room visits, or urgent care visits
- **G9847** Patient received systemic cancer-directed therapy in the last 14 days of life
- **G9848** Patient did not receive systemic cancer-directed therapy in the last 14 days of life
- **G9905** Patient not screened for tobacco use
- **G9906** Patient identified as a tobacco user received tobacco cessation intervention during the measurement period or in the six months prior to the measurement period (counseling and/or pharmacotherapy)

REVISED CODES (continued)

Code	Description
G9908	Patient identified as tobacco user did not receive tobacco cessation intervention during the measurement period or in the six months prior to the measurement period (counseling and/or pharmacotherapy)
G9913	Hepatitis B virus (HBV) status not assessed and results interpreted prior to initiating anti-TNF (tumor necrosis factor) therapy, reason not otherwise specified
G9943	Back pain was not measured by the visual analog scale (VAS) or numeric pain scale at three months (6 to 20 weeks) postoperatively
G9946	Back pain was not measured by the visual analog scale (VAS) or numeric pain scale at one year (9 to 15 months) postoperatively
G9949	Leg pain was not measured by the visual analog scale (VAS) or numeric pain scale at three months (6 to 20 weeks) postoperatively
G9968	Patient was referred to another clinician or specialist during the measurement period
G9969	Clinician who referred the patient to another clinician received a report from the clinician to whom the patient was referred
G9970	Clinician who referred the patient to another clinician did not receive a report from the clinician to whom the patient was referred
G9990	Patient did not receive any pneumococcal conjugate or polysaccharide vaccine on or after their 60th birthday and before the end of the measurement period
G9991	Patient received any pneumococcal conjugate or polysaccharide vaccine on or after their 60th birthday and before the end of the measurement period
G9993	Patient was provided palliative care services any time during the measurement period
J0131	Injection, acetaminophen, not otherwise specified, 10 mg
J0610	Injection, calcium gluconate (Fresenius Kabi), per 10 ml
J9041	Injection, bortezomib, 0.1 mg
K1002	Cranial electrotherapy stimulation (CES) system, any type
K1019	Replacement supplies and accessories for external upper limb tremor stimulator of the peripheral nerves of the wrist
M1003	TB screening performed and results interpreted within twelve months prior to initiation of first-time biologic and/or immune response modifier therapy
M1052	Leg pain was not measured by the visual analog scale (VAS) or numeric pain scale at one year (9 to 15 months) postoperatively
Q4128	FlexHD, or AllopatchHD, per sq cm
Q9001	Assessment by chaplain services
Q9002	Counseling, individual, by chaplain services
Q9003	Counseling, group, by chaplain services

DELETED CODES

C1841	C1842	C1849	C9084	C9085	C9086	C9087
C9090	C9091	C9092	C9093	C9094	C9095	C9096
C9097	C9098	C9142	G0028	G0308	G0309	G1009
G2095	G2170	G2171	G2198	G2201	G2203	G9196
G9197	G9198	G9250	G9251	G9359	G9360	G9506
G9618	G9620	G9623	G9631	G9632	G9633	G9678
G9718	G9774	G9778	G9808	G9809	G9810	G9811
G9904	G9907	G9909	G9932	G9942	G9948	G9989
J2400	J9044	K0553	K0554	M1017	M1071	M1145

Appendix 6 — Place of Service and Type of Service

Place-of-Service Codes for Professional Claims

Listed below are place of service codes and descriptions. These codes should be used on professional claims to specify the entity where service(s) were rendered. Check with individual payers (e.g., Medicare, Medicaid, other private insurance) for reimbursement policies regarding these codes. To comment on a code(s) or description(s), please send your request to posinfo@cms.gov.

01	Pharmacy	A facility or location where drugs and other medically related items and services are sold, dispensed, or otherwise provided directly to patients.
02	Telehealth Provided Other than in Patient's Home	The location where health services and health related services are provided or received, through telecommunication technology. Patient is not located in their home when receiving health services or health related services through telecommunication technology.
03	School	A facility whose primary purpose is education.
04	Homeless Shelter	A facility or location whose primary purpose is to provide temporary housing to homeless individuals (e.g., emergency shelters, individual or family shelters).
05	Indian Health Service Free-standing Facility	A facility or location, owned and operated by the Indian Health Service, which provides diagnostic, therapeutic (surgical and nonsurgical), and rehabilitation services to American Indians and Alaska Natives who do not require hospitalization.
06	Indian Health Service Provider-based Facility	A facility or location, owned and operated by the Indian Health Service, which provides diagnostic, therapeutic (surgical and nonsurgical), and rehabilitation services rendered by, or under the supervision of, physicians to American Indians and Alaska Natives admitted as inpatients or outpatients.
07	Tribal 638 Free-standing Facility	A facility or location owned and operated by a federally recognized American Indian or Alaska Native tribe or tribal organization under a 638 agreement, which provides diagnostic, therapeutic (surgical and nonsurgical), and rehabilitation services to tribal members who do not require hospitalization.
08	Tribal 638 Provider-based Facility	A facility or location owned and operated by a federally recognized American Indian or Alaska Native tribe or tribal organization under a 638 agreement, which provides diagnostic, therapeutic (surgical and nonsurgical), and rehabilitation services to tribal members admitted as inpatients or outpatients.
09	Prison/Correctional Facility	A prison, jail, reformatory, work farm, detention center, or any other similar facility maintained by either Federal, State or local authorities for the purpose of confinement or rehabilitation of adult or juvenile criminal offenders.
10	Telehealth Provided in Patient's Home	The location where health services and health related services are provided or received, through telecommunication technology. Patient is located in their home (which is a location other than a hospital or other facility where the patient receives care in a private residence) when receiving health services or health related services through telecommunication technology.
11	Office	Location, other than a hospital, skilled nursing facility (SNF), military treatment facility, community health center, State or local public health clinic, or intermediate care facility (ICF), where the health professional routinely provides health examinations, diagnosis, and treatment of illness or injury on an ambulatory basis.
12	Home	Location, other than a hospital or other facility, where the patient receives care in a private residence.
13	Assisted Living Facility	Congregate residential facility with self-contained living units providing assessment of each resident's needs and on-site support 24 hours a day, 7 days a week, with the capacity to deliver or arrange for services including some health care and other services.
14	Group home	A residence, with shared living areas, where clients receive supervision and other services such as social and/or behavioral services, custodial service, and minimal services (e.g., medication administration).
15	Mobile Unit	A facility/unit that moves from place-to-place equipped to provide preventive, screening, diagnostic, and/or treatment services.
16	Temporary Lodging	A short-term accommodation such as a hotel, campground, hostel, cruise ship or resort where the patient receives care, and which is not identified by any other POS code.
17	Walk-in Retail Health Clinic	A walk-in health clinic, other than an office, urgent care facility, pharmacy, or independent clinic and not described by any other place of service code, that is located within a retail operation and provides, on an ambulatory basis, preventive and primary care services.
18	Place of Employment-Worksite	A location, not described by any other POS code, owned or operated by a public or private entity where the patient is employed, and where a health professional provides on-going or episodic occupational medical, therapeutic or rehabilitative services to the individual.

© 2022 Optum, Inc.

Appendixes — 53

Appendix 6 — Place of Service and Type of Service

19	Off Campus-Outpatient Hospital	A portion of an off-campus hospital provider based department which provides diagnostic, therapeutic (both surgical and nonsurgical), and rehabilitation services to sick or injured persons who do not require hospitalization or institutionalization.
20	Urgent Care Facility	Location, distinct from a hospital emergency room, an office, or a clinic, whose purpose is to diagnose and treat illness or injury for unscheduled, ambulatory patients seeking immediate medical attention.
21	Inpatient Hospital	A facility, other than psychiatric, which primarily provides diagnostic, therapeutic (both surgical and nonsurgical), and rehabilitation services by, or under, the supervision of physicians to patients admitted for a variety of medical conditions.
22	On Campus-Outpatient Hospital	A portion of a hospital's main campus which provides diagnostic, therapeutic (both surgical and nonsurgical), and rehabilitation services to sick or injured persons who do not require hospitalization or institutionalization.
23	Emergency Room—Hospital	A portion of a hospital where emergency diagnosis and treatment of illness or injury is provided.
24	Ambulatory Surgical Center	A freestanding facility, other than a physician's office, where surgical and diagnostic services are provided on an ambulatory basis.
25	Birthing center	A facility, other than a hospital's maternity facilities or a physician's office, which provides a setting for labor, delivery, and immediate post-partum care as well as immediate care of new born infants.
26	Military Treatment Facility	A medical facility operated by one or more of the Uniformed services. Military Treatment Facility (MTF) also refers to certain former US Public Health Service (USPHS) facilities now designated as Uniformed Service Treatment Facilities (USTF).
27-30	Unassigned	N/A
31	Skilled Nursing Facility	A facility which primarily provides inpatient skilled nursing care and related services to patients who require medical, nursing, or rehabilitative services but does not provide the level of care or treatment available in a hospital.
32	Nursing Facility	A facility which primarily provides to residents skilled nursing care and related services for the rehabilitation of injured, disabled, or sick persons, or, on a regular basis, health-related care services above the level of custodial care to individuals other than those with intellectual disabilities.
33	Custodial Care Facility	A facility which provides room, board, and other personal assistance services, generally on a long-term basis, and which does not include a medical component.
34	Hospice	A facility, other than a patient's home, in which palliative and supportive care for terminally ill patients and their families are provided.
35-40	Unassigned	N/A
41	Ambulance—Land	A land vehicle specifically designed, equipped and staffed for lifesaving and transporting the sick or injured.
42	Ambulance—Air or Water	An air or water vehicle specifically designed, equipped and staffed for lifesaving and transporting the sick or injured.
43-48	Unassigned	N/A
49	Independent Clinic	A location, not part of a hospital and not described by any other Place-of-Service code, that is organized and operated to provide preventive, diagnostic, therapeutic, rehabilitative, or palliative services to outpatients only.
50	Federally Qualified Health Center	A facility located in a medically underserved area that provides Medicare beneficiaries preventive primary medical care under the general direction of a physician.
51	Inpatient Psychiatric Facility	A facility that provides inpatient psychiatric services for the diagnosis and treatment of mental illness on a 24-hour basis, by or under the supervision of a physician.
52	Psychiatric Facility-Partial Hospitalization	A facility for the diagnosis and treatment of mental illness that provides a planned therapeutic program for patients who do not require full time hospitalization, but who need broader programs than are possible from outpatient visits to a hospital-based or hospital-affiliated facility.
53	Community Mental Health Center	A facility that provides the following services: outpatient services, including specialized outpatient services for children, the elderly, individuals who are chronically ill, and residents of the CMHC's mental health services area who have been discharged from inpatient treatment at a mental health facility; 24 hour a day emergency care services; day treatment, other partial hospitalization services, or psychosocial rehabilitation services; screening for patients being considered for admission to State mental health facilities to determine the appropriateness of such admission; and consultation and education services.
54	Intermediate Care Facility/Individuals with Intellectual Disabilities	A facility which primarily provides health-related care and services above the level of custodial care to individuals but does not provide the level of care or treatment available in a hospital or SNF.
55	Residential Substance Abuse Treatment Facility	A facility which provides treatment for substance (alcohol and drug) abuse to live-in residents who do not require acute medical care. Services include individual and group therapy and counseling, family counseling, laboratory tests, drugs and supplies, psychological testing, and room and board.
56	Psychiatric Residential Treatment Center	A facility or distinct part of a facility for psychiatric care which provides a total 24-hour therapeutically planned and professionally staffed group living and learning environment.
57	Non-residential Substance Abuse Treatment Facility	A location which provides treatment for substance (alcohol and drug) abuse on an ambulatory basis. Services include individual and group therapy and counseling, family counseling, laboratory tests, drugs and supplies, and psychological testing.

58	Non-residential Opioid Treatment Facility	A location that provides treatment for opioid use disorder on an ambulatory basis. Services include methadone and other forms of Medication Assisted Treatment (MAT).
59	Unassigned	N/A
60	Mass Immunization Center	A location where providers administer pneumococcal pneumonia and influenza virus vaccinations and submit these services as electronic media claims, paper claims, or using the roster billing method. This generally takes place in a mass immunization setting, such as, a public health center, pharmacy, or mall but may include a physician office setting.
61	Comprehensive Inpatient Rehabilitation Facility	A facility that provides comprehensive rehabilitation services under the supervision of a physician to inpatients with physical disabilities. Services include physical therapy, occupational therapy, speech pathology, social or psychological services, and orthotics and prosthetics services.
62	Comprehensive Outpatient Rehabilitation Facility	A facility that provides comprehensive rehabilitation services under the supervision of a physician to outpatients with physical disabilities. Services include physical therapy, occupational therapy, and speech pathology services.
63-64	Unassigned	N/A
65	End-Stage Renal Disease Treatment Facility	A facility other than a hospital, which provides dialysis treatment, maintenance, and/or training to patients or caregivers on an ambulatory or home-care basis.
66-70	Unassigned	N/A
71	Public Health Clinic	A facility maintained by either State or local health departments that provides ambulatory primary medical care under the general direction of a physician.
72	Rural Health Clinic	A certified facility which is located in a rural medically underserved area that provides ambulatory primary medical care under the general direction of a physician.
73-80	Unassigned	N/A
81	Independent Laboratory	A laboratory certified to perform diagnostic and/or clinical tests independent of an institution or a physician's office.
82-98	Unassigned	N/A
99	Other Place of Service	Other place of service not identified above.

Type of Service

Common Working File Type of Service (TOS) Indicators

For submitting a claim to the Common Working File (CWF), use the following table to assign the proper TOS. Some procedures may have more than one applicable TOS. CWF will reject codes with incorrect TOS designations. CWF will produce alerts on codes with incorrect TOS designations.

The only exceptions to this annual update are:

- Surgical services billed for dates of service through December 31, 2007, containing the ASC facility service modifier SG must be reported as TOS F. Effective for services on or after January 1, 2008, the SG modifier is no longer applicable for Medicare services. ASC providers should discontinue applying the SG modifier on ASC facility claims. The indicator F does not appear in the TOS table because its use depends upon claims submitted with POS 24 (ASC facility) from an ASC (specialty 49). This became effective for dates of service January 1, 2008, or after.
- Surgical services billed with an assistant-at-surgery modifier (80-82, AS,) must be reported with TOS 8. The 8 indicator does not appear on the TOS table because its use is dependent upon the use of the appropriate modifier. (See Pub. 100-04 *Medicare Claims Processing Manual,* chapter 12, "Physician/Practitioner Billing," for instructions on when assistant-at-surgery is allowable.)
- TOS H appears in the list of descriptors. However, it does not appear in the table. In CWF, "H" is used only as an indicator for hospice. The contractor should not submit TOS H to CWF at this time.
- For outpatient services, when a transfusion medicine code appears on a claim that also contains a blood product, the service is paid under reasonable charge at 80 percent; coinsurance and deductible apply. When transfusion medicine codes are paid under the clinical laboratory fee schedule they are paid at 100 percent; coinsurance and deductible do not apply.

Note: For injection codes with more than one possible TOS designation, use the following guidelines when assigning the TOS:

When the choice is L or 1:

- Use TOS L when the drug is used related to ESRD; or
- Use TOS 1 when the drug is not related to ESRD and is administered in the office.

When the choice is G or 1:

- Use TOS G when the drug is an immunosuppressive drug; or
- Use TOS 1 when the drug is used for other than immunosuppression.

When the choice is P or 1:

- Use TOS P if the drug is administered through durable medical equipment (DME); or
- Use TOS 1 if the drug is administered in the office.

The place of service or diagnosis may be considered when determining the appropriate TOS. The descriptors for each of the TOS codes listed in the annual HCPCS update are:

0	Whole blood only
1	Medical care
2	Surgery
3	Consultation
4	Diagnostic radiology
5	Diagnostic laboratory
6	Therapeutic radiology
7	Anesthesia
8	Assistant at surgery
9	Other medical items or services
A	Used durable medical equipment (DME)
D	Ambulance
E	Enteral/parenteral nutrients/supplies
F	Ambulatory surgical center (facility usage for surgical services)
G	Immunosuppressive drugs
J	Diabetic shoes
K	Hearing items and services
L	ESRD supplies
M	Monthly capitation payment for dialysis
N	Kidney donor
P	Lump sum purchase of DME, prosthetics, orthotics
Q	Vision items or services
R	Rental of DME
S	Surgical dressings or other medical supplies
T	Outpatient mental health limitation
U	Occupational therapy
V	Pneumococcal/flu vaccine
W	Physical therapy

Appendix 7 — Deleted Code Crosswalk

Code	Cross Reference
C9084	To report, see J9359
C9085	To report, see J0219
C9086	To report, see J0491
C9087	To report, see J9071
C9090	To report, see J2998
C9091	To report, see J9331
C9092	To report, see J3299
C9093	To report, see J2779
C9142	To report, see Q5126
G0424	To report, see 94626
G2064	To report, see 99424–99425
G2065	To report, see 99426–99427
G2170	To report, see 36836
G2171	To report, see 36837
J2400	To report, see J2401, J2402
J9044	To report, see J9041, J9046, J9048, J9049

Appendix 8 — Glossary

accession. Process of identifying a specimen and entering a unique specimen identifier into laboratory records.

alveoplasty. Procedure in which the physician alters the contours of the alveolus by removing sharp areas or undercuts of alveolar bone.

angiography. Radiographic imaging of the arteries. Imaging may be performed to study the vasculature of any given organ, body system, or area of circulation such as the brain, heart, chest, kidneys, limbs, gastrointestinal tract, aorta, and pulmonary circulation to visualize the formation and the function of the blood vessels to detect problems such as a blockage or stricture. A catheter is inserted through an accessible blood vessel and the artery is injected with a radiopaque contrast material after which x-rays are taken.

apnea. Absence of breathing or breath.

apnea monitor. Device used to monitor breathing during sleep that sounds an alarm if breathing stops for more than the specified amount of time.

aqueous shunt. Silicone tube inserted into the anterior chamber of the eye and connected to a reservoir plate behind the pars plana to enhance drainage in the eye's anterior chamber and improve aqueous flow.

arthroscopy. Use of an endoscope to examine the interior of a joint (diagnostic) or to perform surgery on joint structures (therapeutic).

auditory osseointegrated implant. Surgically placed titanium bone-anchored implant that delivers sound to the inner ear via direct bone conduction.

ballistocardiogram. Graphic recording of the movements of the body caused by cardiac contractions and blood flow, used to evaluate cardiac function.

BMI. Body mass index. Tool for calculating weight appropriateness in adults. The Centers for Disease Control and Prevention places adult BMIs in the following categories: below 18.5, underweight; 18.5 to 24.9, normal; 25.0 to 29.9 overweight; 30.0 and above, obese. BMI may be a factor in determining medical necessity for bariatric procedures.

brace. Orthotic device that supports, in correct position, any moveable body part, and allows for limited movement. Medicare has a strict definition of a brace that includes only rigid or semirigid devices.

brachytherapy. Form of radiation therapy in which radioactive pellets or seeds are implanted directly into the tissue being treated to deliver their dose of radiation in a more directed fashion. Brachytherapy provides radiation to the prescribed body area while minimizing exposure to normal tissue.

cardiointegram. Experimental, noninvasive analysis of electrical signals of the heart. Cardiointegram converts analog EKG signals to digital and performs a computer analysis that considers the time element.

cardiokymography. Noninvasive test that measures left anterior ventricle segmental wall motion.

cardioverter-defibrillator. Device that uses both low energy cardioversion or defibrillating shocks and antitachycardia pacing to treat ventricular tachycardia or ventricular fibrillation.

cast. *1)* Rigid encasement or dressing molded to the body from a substance that hardens upon drying to hold a body part immobile during the healing period; a model or reproduction made from an impression or mold. Generally, the supply of a cast is included in the codes describing the reduction. *2)* In dentistry and some other specialties, model or reproduction made from taking an impression or mold.

catheter. Flexible tube inserted into an area of the body for introducing or withdrawing fluid.

cervical cap. Contraceptive device similar in form and function to the diaphragm but that can be left in place for 48 hours.

chemotherapy. Treatment of disease, especially cancerous conditions, using chemical agents.

CMS. Centers for Medicare and Medicaid Services. Federal agency that administers the public health programs.

CMV. *1)* Controlled mechanical ventilation. *2)* Cytomegalovirus.

collagen. Protein based substance of strength and flexibility that is the major component of connective tissue, found in cartilage, bone, tendons, and skin.

colorectal cancer screening test. One of the following procedures performed for the purpose of detecting colorectal cancer: screening barium enema, screening fecal-occult blood test, screening flexible sigmoidoscopy, screening colonography, and screening colonoscopy.

compression sleeve. Fitted wrap that accelerates recovery in patients with vein disease, lymphedema, or diabetes. Compression sleeves increase circulation and decrease swelling and fluid buildup following surgery.

contrast material. Radiopaque substance placed into the body to enable a system or body structure to be visualized, such as nonionic and low osmolar contrast media (LOCM), ionic and high osmolar contrast media (HOCM), barium, and gadolinium.

covered osteoporosis drug. Injectable drug approved for treating post-menopausal osteoporosis provided to an individual that has suffered a bone fracture related to post-menopausal osteoporosis.

dermis. Skin layer found under the epidermis that contains a papillary upper layer and the deep reticular layer of collagen, vascular bed, and nerves.

dermis graft. Skin graft that has been separated from the epidermal tissue and the underlying subcutaneous fat, used primarily as a substitute for fascia grafts in plastic surgery.

dialysis. Artificial filtering of the blood to remove contaminating waste elements and restore normal balance.

disarticulation. Removal of a limb through a joint.

diskectomy. Surgical excision of an intervertebral disk.

DME MAC. Durable medical equipment Medicare administrative contractor. Entity where claims for specific DMEPOS must be submitted for processing and reimbursement.

DME PDAC. Durable Medical Equipment Pricing Data Analysis and Coding. Medicare contractor responsible for maintaining the durable medical equipment classification system (DMECS), including HCPCS coding determinations, and providing durable medical equipment, prosthetics, orthotics, and supplies (DMEPOS) allowables.

drug eluting stent. Specialized device placed inside blood vessels for intraluminal support that is coated with a controlled time-release drug that enters the surrounding tissue and helps prevent or slow the growth of plaque or stenotic tissue.

drug formulary. List of prescription medications preferred for use by a health plan and dispensed through participating pharmacies to covered persons.

drugs and biologicals. Drugs and biologicals included - or approved for inclusion - in the United States Pharmacopoeia, the National Formulary, the United States Homeopathic Pharmacopoeia, in New Drugs or Accepted Dental Remedies, or approved by the pharmacy and drug therapeutics committee of the medical staff of the hospital. Also included are medically accepted and FDA approved drugs used in an anticancer chemotherapeutic regimen. The carrier determines medical acceptance based on supportive clinical evidence.

dual-lead device. Implantable cardiac device (pacemaker or implantable cardioverter-defibrillator [ICD]) in which pacing and sensing components are placed in only two chambers of the heart.

durable medical equipment. Medical equipment that can withstand repeated use, is not disposable, is used to serve a medical purpose, is generally not useful to a person in the absence of a sickness or injury, and is appropriate for use in the home. Examples of durable medical equipment include hospital beds, wheelchairs, and oxygen equipment.

Dx. Diagnosis.

electrocardiogram. Recording of the electrical activity of the heart on a moving strip of paper that detects and records the electrical potential of the heart during contraction.

electroencephalography. Testing involving amplification, recording, and analysis of the electrical activity of the brain.

electromyography. Test that measures muscle response to nerve stimulation determining if muscle weakness is present and if it is related to the muscles themselves or a problem with the nerves that supply the muscles.

enteral. Pertaining to the intestines; enteral is often used in the context of nutrition management: formulas, jejunostomy tubes, nasogastric devices, etc.

epidermis. Outermost, nonvascular layer of skin that contains four to five differentiated layers depending on its body location: stratum corneum, lucidum, granulosum, spinosum, and basale.

EPO. *1)* Epoetin alpha. *2)* Exclusive provider organization. In health care contracting, an organization similar to an HMO, but the member must remain within the provider network to receive benefits. EPOs are regulated under insurance statutes rather than HMO legislation.

ESRD. End stage renal disease. Progression of chronic renal failure to lasting and irreparable kidney damage that requires dialysis or renal transplant for survival.

EVAR. Endovascular aortic repair. Deployment of a prosthetic stent via a catheter into the site of an abdominal aortic aneurysm (AAA). The stent provides a safe conduit for blood flow to relieve pressure on the aneurysm as the blood flows through the stent instead of continuing to bulge the sac formed by the aorta wall dilation.

event recorder. Portable, ambulatory heart monitor worn by the patient that makes electrocardiographic recordings of the length and frequency of aberrant cardiac rhythm to help diagnose heart conditions and to assess pacemaker functioning or programming.

fecal microbiota transplant (FMT). Procedure in which healthy bacteria (microbiota) is extracted from the feces of a screened donor and transferred to the colon of the recipient via colonoscopy or upper endoscopy, most often to treat persistent *C. difficile* infections.

Food and Drug Administration (FDA). Federal agency responsible for protecting public health by substantiating the safety, efficacy, and security of human and veterinary drugs, biological products, medical devices, national food supply, cosmetics, and items that give off radiation.

FOTO. Focus on therapeutic outcomes.

gait. Manner in which a person walks.

gene. Basic unit of heredity that contains nucleic acid. Genes are arranged in different and unique sequences or strings that determine the gene's function. Human genes usually include multiple protein coding regions such as exons separated by introns which are nonprotein coding sections.

genetic test. Test that is able to detect a gene mutation, either inherited or caused by the environment.

gingivoplasty. Repair or reconstruction of the gum tissue, altering the gingival contours by excising areas of gum tissue or making incisions through the gingiva to create a gingival flap.

glaucoma. Rise in intraocular pressure, restricting blood flow and decreasing vision.

habilitative services. Procedures or services provided to assist a patient in learning, keeping, and improving new skills needed to perform daily living activities. Habilitative services assist patients in acquiring a skill for the first time.

halo. Tool for stabilizing the head and spine.

health care provider. Entity that administers diagnostic and therapeutic services.

hemodialysis. Cleansing of wastes and contaminating elements from the blood by virtue of different diffusion rates through a semipermeable membrane, which separates blood from a filtration solution that diffuses other elements out of the blood.

home health services. Services furnished to patients in their homes under the care of physicians. These services include part-time or intermittent skilled nursing care, physical therapy, medical social services, medical supplies, and some rehabilitation equipment. Home health supplies and services must be prescribed by a physician, and the beneficiary must be confined at home in order for Medicare to pay the benefits in full.

hospice. Organization that furnishes inpatient, outpatient, and home health care for the terminally ill. Hospices emphasize support and counseling services for terminally ill people and their families, pain relief, and symptom management. When the Medicare beneficiary chooses hospice benefits, all other Medicare benefits are discontinued, except physician services and treatment of conditions not related to the terminal illness.

hypertrophic. Enlarged or overgrown from an increase in cell size of the affected tissue.

implant. Material or device inserted or placed within the body for therapeutic, reconstructive, or diagnostic purposes.

implantable cardioverter-defibrillator. Implantable electronic cardiac device used to control rhythm abnormalities such as tachycardia, fibrillation, or bradycardia by producing high- or low-energy stimulation and pacemaker functions. It may also have the capability to provide the functions of an implantable loop recorder or implantable cardiovascular monitor.

in situ. Located in the natural position or contained within the origin site, not spread into neighboring tissue.

incontinence. Inability to control urination or defecation.

infusion. Introduction of a therapeutic fluid, other than blood, into the bloodstream.

infusion pump. Device that delivers a measured amount of drug or intravenous solution through injection over a period of time.

intra-arterial. Within an artery or arteries.

intramuscular. Within a muscle.

intraocular lens. Artificial lens implanted into the eye to replace a damaged natural lens or cataract.

intravenous. Within a vein or veins.

introducer. Instrument, such as a catheter, needle, or tube, through which another instrument or device is introduced into the body.

keratoprosthesis. Surgical procedure in which the physician creates a new anterior chamber with a plastic optical implant to replace a severely damaged cornea that cannot be repaired.

LDS. Lipodystrophy syndrome. Syndrome which involves the partial or total absence of fat and/or the abnormal deposition and distribution of fat in the body due to a disturbance of the lipid metabolism.

magnetic resonance angiography. Diagnostic technique utilizing magnetic fields and radio waves rather than radiation to produce detailed, cross-sectional images of internal body structures.

multiple-lead device. Implantable cardiac device (pacemaker or implantable cardioverter-defibrillator [ICD]) in which pacing and sensing components are placed in at least three chambers of the heart.

mutation. Alteration in gene function that results in changes to a gene or chromosome. Can cause deficits or disease that can be inherited, can have beneficial effects, or result in no noticeable change.

nasogastric tube. Long, hollow, cylindrical catheter made of soft rubber or plastic that is inserted through the nose down into the stomach, and is used for feeding, instilling medication, or withdrawing gastric contents.

nebulizer. Latin for mist, a device that converts liquid into a fine spray and is commonly used to deliver medicine to the upper respiratory, bronchial, and lung areas.

negative pressure dressing. Adjunctive therapy used to speed wound healing in skin grafts or large wounds. It has been shown to increase blood flow, decrease bacterial count, and increase formation of granulation tissues. A foam pad is placed on the defect and covered with an occlusive drape. A small tube that is non-collapsible is placed into the foam and attached to a disposable pump that provides negative pressure up to -125 mmHg.

NMES. Neuromuscular electrical stimulation. Technology that uses percutaneous stimulation to deliver electrical impulses for muscle flexion to trigger action. NMES can, in some cases, create an ability to ambulate among paraplegic patients.

obturator. Prosthesis used to close an acquired or congenital opening in the palate that aids in speech and chewing.

occult blood test. Chemical or microscopic test to determine the presence of blood in a specimen.

occupational therapy. Training, education, and assistance intended to assist a person who is recovering from a serious illness or injury perform the activities of daily life.

ocular implant. Implant inside muscular cone.

omnicardiogram. Method of mathematically interpreting the usual linear form of the electrocardiogram in a different, roughly circular shape. This interpretation is then compared to a normal template and an analysis is performed on two randomly selected cycles from leads I, II, V4, V, and/or V6.

oral. Pertaining to the mouth.

ordering physician. Physician who orders nonphysician services (e.g., laboratory services, pharmaceutical services, imaging services, or durable medical equipment) for a patient.

orphan drugs. Drugs that treat diseases that affect fewer than 200,000 people in the United States, as designated by the FDA. Orphan drugs follow a varied process from other drugs regulated by the FDA.

orthosis. Derived from a Greek word meaning "to make straight," it is an artificial appliance that supports, aligns, or corrects an anatomical deformity or improves the use of a moveable body part. Unlike a prosthesis, an orthotic device is always functional in nature.

orthotic. Associated with the making and fitting of an orthosis(es).

osteo-. Having to do with bone.

osteogenesis stimulator. Device used to stimulate the growth of bone by electrical impulses or ultrasound.

ostomy. Artificial (surgical) opening in the body used for drainage or for delivery of medications or nutrients.

pacemaker. Implantable cardiac device that controls the heart's rhythm and maintains regular beats by artificial electric discharges. This device consists of the pulse generator with a battery and the electrodes, or leads, which are placed in single or dual chambers of the heart, usually transvenously.

parenteral. Other than the alimentary canal and is usually used in a method of delivery context: total parenteral nutrition (TPN) and parenteral nutrition therapy (PNT) formulas, kits, and devices.

parenteral nutrition. Nutrients provided subcutaneously, intravenously, intramuscularly, or intradermally for patients during the postoperative period and in other conditions, such as shock, coma, and renal failure.

partial hospitalization. Situation in which the patient only stays part of each day over a long period. Cardiac, rehabilitation, and chronic pain patients, for example, could use this service.

passive mobilization. Pressure, movement, or pulling of a limb or body part utilizing an apparatus or device.

periradicular. Surrounding part of the tooth's root.

peritoneal. Space between the lining of the abdominal wall, or parietal peritoneum, and the surface layer of the abdominal organs, or visceral peritoneum. It contains a thin, watery fluid that keeps the peritoneal surfaces moist.

peritoneal dialysis. Dialysis that filters waste from blood inside the body using the peritoneum, the natural lining of the abdomen, as the semipermeable membrane across which ultrafiltration is accomplished. A special catheter is inserted into the abdomen and a dialysis solution is drained into the abdomen. This solution extracts fluids and wastes, which are then discarded when the fluid is drained. Various forms of peritoneal dialysis include CAPD, CCPD, and NIDP.

peritoneal effusion. Persistent escape of fluid within the peritoneal cavity.

pessary. Device placed in the vagina to support and reposition a prolapsing or retropositioned uterus, rectum, or vagina.

photocoagulation. Application of an intense laser beam of light to disrupt tissue and condense protein material to a residual mass, used especially for treating ocular conditions.

physician. Legally authorized practitioners including a doctor of medicine or osteopathy, a doctor of dental surgery or of dental medicine, a doctor of podiatric medicine, a doctor of optometry, and a chiropractor only with respect to treatment by means of manual manipulation of the spine (to correct a subluxation).

PICC. Peripherally inserted central catheter. PICC is inserted into one of the large veins of the arm and threaded through the vein until the tip sits in a large vein just above the heart.

prehensile. Ability to grasp, seize, or hold.

prodrug. Inactive drug that goes through a metabolic process when given resulting in a chemical conversion that changes the drug into an active pharmacological agent.

prophylaxis. Intervention or protective therapy intended to prevent a disease.

prostate cancer screening tests. Test that consists of any (or all) of the procedures provided for the early detection of prostate cancer to a man 50 years of age or older who has not had a test during the preceding year. The procedures are as follows: A digital rectal examination; A prostate-specific antigen blood test. After 2002, the list of procedures may be expanded as appropriate for the early detection of prostate cancer, taking into account changes in technology and standards of medical practice, availability, effectiveness, costs, and other factors.

prosthetic. Device that replaces all or part of an internal body organ or body part, or that replaces part of the function of a permanently inoperable or malfunctioning internal body organ or body part.

pulse generator. Component of a pacemaker or an implantable cardioverter defibrillator that contains the battery and the electronics for producing the electrical discharge sent to the heart to control cardiac rhythm. Insertion or replacement of the pulse generator may be done alone, not in conjunction with insertion or replacement of the entire pacemaker system.

qualitative. To determine the nature or characteristics of the components of a substance.

quantitative. To determine the number or amount of the components of a substance.

rehabilitation services. Therapy services provided primarily for assisting in a rehabilitation program of evaluation and service including cardiac rehabilitation, medical social services, occupational therapy, physical therapy, respiratory therapy, skilled nursing, speech therapy, psychiatric rehabilitation, and alcohol and substance abuse rehabilitation.

residual limb. Portion of an arm or leg that remains attached to the body after an amputation.

screening mammography. Radiologic images taken of the female breast for the early detection of breast cancer.

screening pap smear. Diagnostic laboratory test consisting of a routine exfoliative cytology test (Papanicolaou test) provided to a woman for the early detection of cervical or vaginal cancer. The exam includes a clinical breast examination and a physician's interpretation of the results.

sialodochoplasty. Surgical repair of a salivary gland duct.

single-lead device. Implantable cardiac device (pacemaker or implantable cardioverter-defibrillator [ICD]) in which pacing and sensing components are placed in only one chamber of the heart.

skin substitute. Non-autologous human or non-human skin that forms a base for skin growth, often considered a graft dressing.

speech prosthetic. Electronic speech aid device for patient who has had a laryngectomy. One operates by placing a vibrating head against the throat;

the other amplifies sound waves through a tube which is inserted into the user's mouth.

splint. Brace or support. *1)* dynamic splint: brace that permits movement of an anatomical structure such as a hand, wrist, foot, or other part of the body after surgery or injury. *2)* static splint: brace that prevents movement and maintains support and position for an anatomical structure after surgery or injury.

stent. Tube to provide support in a body cavity or lumen.

stereotactic radiosurgery. Delivery of externally-generated ionizing radiation to specific targets for destruction or inactivation. Most often utilized in the treatment of brain or spinal tumors, high-resolution stereotactic imaging is used to identify the target and then deliver the treatment. Computer-assisted planning may also be employed. Simple and complex cranial lesions and spinal lesions are typically treated in a single planning and treatment session, although a maximum of five sessions may be required. No incision is made for stereotactic radiosurgery procedures.

subcutaneous. Below the skin.

TENS. Transcutaneous electrical nerve stimulator. TENS is applied by placing electrode pads over the area to be stimulated and connecting the electrodes to a transmitter box, which sends a current through the skin to sensory nerve fibers to help decrease pain in that nerve distribution.

terminal device. Addition to an upper limb prosthesis that replaces the function and/or appearance of a missing hand.

tracheostomy. Formation of a tracheal opening on the neck surface with tube insertion to allow for respiration in cases of obstruction or decreased patency. A tracheostomy may be planned or performed on an emergency basis for temporary or long-term use.

traction. Drawing out or holding tension on an area by applying a direct therapeutic pulling force.

transcutaneous electrical nerve stimulator. Device that delivers a controlled amount of electricity to an area of the body to stimulate healing and/or to mitigate post-surgical or post-traumatic pain.

transesophageal echocardiography. Guidance of a small probe into the esophagus under sedation to closely evaluate the heart and blood vessels within the chest.

type A emergency department. Emergency department licensed and advertised to be available to provide emergent care 24 hours a day, seven days a week. Type A emergency departments must meet both the CPT book definition of an emergency department and the EMTALA definition of a dedicated emergency department.

type B emergency department. Emergency department licensed and advertised to provide emergent care less than 24 hours a day, seven days a week. Type B emergency departments must meet the EMTALA definition of a dedicated emergency department.

vascular closure device. vascular closure devices seal femoral artery punctures caused by invasive or interventional procedures. The closure or seal is achieved by percutaneous delivery of the device's two primary structures, which are usually an anchor and a suture, clip or biologic substance (e.g., collagen, bioabsorbable polymer) or suture through the tissue tract.

Appendix 9 — Quality Payment Program

In 2015, Congress passed the Medicare Access and CHIP Reauthorization Act (MACRA), which included sweeping changes for practitioners who provide services reimbursed under the Medicare physician fee schedule (MPFS). The act focused on repealing the faulty Medicare sustainable growth rate, focusing on quality of patient outcomes, and controlling Medicare spending.

A MACRA final rule in October 2016 established the Quality Payment Program (QPP), which was effective January 1, 2017. This value-based payment model rewards eligible clinicians (ECs) who provide high-quality care and reduce the payments for those who fail to meet specific performance standards.

ECs can receive incentives under the QPP. Once the performance threshold is established, all ECs who score above that threshold are eligible to receive a positive payment adjustment. Keep in mind that the key requirement is that an EC **submit data** to avoid the negative payment adjustment and receive the incentives. The Centers for Medicare and Medicaid Services (CMS) has redesigned the scoring so that clinicians are able to know how well they are doing in the program, as benchmarks are known in advance of participating.

The QPP consists of two tracks that clinicians may choose from based on their practice size, location, specialty, or patient population:

- The merit-based incentive payment system (MIPS)
- Alternative payment models (APMs)

The 2017 QPP final rule established regulations for MIPS and APMs as well as related policies applicable to eligible clinicians who participate in the Shared Savings Program. These policies included requirements for Shared Savings Program accountable care organizations (ACOs) regarding reporting for the MIPS Quality performance category and a policy that gave ACOs full credit for the MIPS Improvement Activities performance category based on their participation in the Shared Savings Program. Since that time, revisions and modifications have been made to allow more focus on measurement efforts and to reduce barriers to entry into advanced APMs. Refinements will continue in order to reduce reporting burden and focus on patient outcomes.

MIPS provides specified performance categories under which payment adjustments may be earned for Part B covered professional services. Eligible clinicians can obtain a composite performance score (CPS) of up to 100 points from these weighted performance categories, which focus on patient care quality and cost, improvements in patient engagement and clinical care processes, and use of certified electronic health record technology (CEHRT). This performance score then defines the payment adjustments in the second calendar year after the year the score is obtained. For instance, the score obtained for the 2020 performance year is linked to payment for Medicare Part B services in 2022.

ECs currently have three available reporting frameworks, depending on individual needs and eligibility—traditional MIPS, MIPS Value Pathways (MVPs), and the alternative payment model (APM) performance pathway (APP).

Traditional MIPS currently consists of the following performance categories:

- Quality
- Improvement Activities
- Promoting Interoperability (PI)
- Cost

MVPs, which were added as a result of complaints by some physicians of confusing quality measures, allow clinicians to report only on those measures that apply to their specialty. The CY 2023 proposed rule continues refinement and focus on subgroups for MVP reporting that will provide more granularity in reporting and improve patient care. Additional MVPs will gradually be implemented for more specialties and subspecialties that participate in the program.

The APP is intended for MIPS-eligible ECs who also participate in MIPS APMs. Performance is measured across three areas (Quality, Improvement Activities, and Promoting Interoperability) in this reporting and scoring pathway, which aims to decrease reporting burden, encourage APM participation, and create new opportunities for scoring for existing MIPS APM participants. For performance year 2022, the APP Quality performance category accounted for 50 percent of the MIPS final score; the PI performance category weight was 30 percent; and the Improvement Activities performance category weight was 20 percent.

Proposed 2023 Changes

As noted earlier, the majority of the proposed updates for CY 2023 focus on MVP refinement. In addition to the MVPs proposed for the 2023 performance year, other proposals in the CY 2023 proposed rule include:

- Requesting input on proposed increase in conversion factor in lieu of lump sum payment, noting that there is currently no incentive authorized for performance year 2023
- Increasing the number of measures related to health equity
- Developing measures focused on amputation avoidance in diabetic patients, especially for underserved populations
- Exploring vendor ability to select which MVPs to support
- Seeking feedback regarding continuing medical education (CME) or accreditation entities acting as third-party intermediaries to reduce clinician reporting burden
- Advancing trusted exchange framework and common agreement (TEFCA) information regarding participation and submission of clinical documentation
- Continuing the transition to digital quality measurement and using fast healthcare interoperability resources (FHIR) with data standardization and approaches to transition
- Transitioning to individual QP determinations to encourage specialists' participation in Advanced APMs

Evaluation continues regarding an incremental timeline to transition to mandatory MVP reporting that will coincide with the sunset of traditional MIPS. The timeline currently being considered is the end of the CY 2027 performance period/2029 MIPS payment year, although this is not an official proposal at this time.

Detailed information regarding the Quality Payment Program may be found at https://qpp.cms.gov/. This website will also announce the final CMS determinations of MVPs, advanced APMs, and MIPS APMs for the 2023 performance period.

Appendix 7 — Deleted Code Crosswalk

Code	Cross Reference
C9084	To report, see J9359
C9085	To report, see J0219
C9086	To report, see J0491
C9087	To report, see J9071
C9090	To report, see J2998
C9091	To report, see J9331
C9092	To report, see J3299
C9093	To report, see J2779
C9142	To report, see Q5126
G0424	To report, see 94626
G2064	To report, see 99424–99425
G2065	To report, see 99426–99427
G2170	To report, see 36836
G2171	To report, see 36837
J2400	To report, see J2401, J2402
J9044	To report, see J9041, J9046, J9048, J9049

Appendix 8 — Glossary

accession. Process of identifying a specimen and entering a unique specimen identifier into laboratory records.

alveoplasty. Procedure in which the physician alters the contours of the alveolus by removing sharp areas or undercuts of alveolar bone.

angiography. Radiographic imaging of the arteries. Imaging may be performed to study the vasculature of any given organ, body system, or area of circulation such as the brain, heart, chest, kidneys, limbs, gastrointestinal tract, aorta, and pulmonary circulation to visualize the formation and the function of the blood vessels to detect problems such as a blockage or stricture. A catheter is inserted through an accessible blood vessel and the artery is injected with a radiopaque contrast material after which x-rays are taken.

apnea. Absence of breathing or breath.

apnea monitor. Device used to monitor breathing during sleep that sounds an alarm if breathing stops for more than the specified amount of time.

aqueous shunt. Silicone tube inserted into the anterior chamber of the eye and connected to a reservoir plate behind the pars plana to enhance drainage in the eye's anterior chamber and improve aqueous flow.

arthroscopy. Use of an endoscope to examine the interior of a joint (diagnostic) or to perform surgery on joint structures (therapeutic).

auditory osseointegrated implant. Surgically placed titanium bone-anchored implant that delivers sound to the inner ear via direct bone conduction.

ballistocardiogram. Graphic recording of the movements of the body caused by cardiac contractions and blood flow, used to evaluate cardiac function.

BMI. Body mass index. Tool for calculating weight appropriateness in adults. The Centers for Disease Control and Prevention places adult BMIs in the following categories: below 18.5, underweight; 18.5 to 24.9, normal; 25.0 to 29.9 overweight; 30.0 and above, obese. BMI may be a factor in determining medical necessity for bariatric procedures.

brace. Orthotic device that supports, in correct position, any moveable body part, and allows for limited movement. Medicare has a strict definition of a brace that includes only rigid or semirigid devices.

brachytherapy. Form of radiation therapy in which radioactive pellets or seeds are implanted directly into the tissue being treated to deliver their dose of radiation in a more directed fashion. Brachytherapy provides radiation to the prescribed body area while minimizing exposure to normal tissue.

cardiointegram. Experimental, noninvasive analysis of electrical signals of the heart. Cardiointegram converts analog EKG signals to digital and performs a computer analysis that considers the time element.

cardiokymography. Noninvasive test that measures left anterior ventricle segmental wall motion.

cardioverter-defibrillator. Device that uses both low energy cardioversion or defibrillating shocks and antitachycardia pacing to treat ventricular tachycardia or ventricular fibrillation.

cast. *1)* Rigid encasement or dressing molded to the body from a substance that hardens upon drying to hold a body part immobile during the healing period; a model or reproduction made from an impression or mold. Generally, the supply of a cast is included in the codes describing the reduction. *2)* In dentistry and some other specialties, model or reproduction made from taking an impression or mold.

catheter. Flexible tube inserted into an area of the body for introducing or withdrawing fluid.

cervical cap. Contraceptive device similar in form and function to the diaphragm but that can be left in place for 48 hours.

chemotherapy. Treatment of disease, especially cancerous conditions, using chemical agents.

CMS. Centers for Medicare and Medicaid Services. Federal agency that administers the public health programs.

CMV. *1)* Controlled mechanical ventilation. *2)* Cytomegalovirus.

collagen. Protein based substance of strength and flexibility that is the major component of connective tissue, found in cartilage, bone, tendons, and skin.

colorectal cancer screening test. One of the following procedures performed for the purpose of detecting colorectal cancer: screening barium enema, screening fecal-occult blood test, screening flexible sigmoidoscopy, screening colonography, and screening colonoscopy.

compression sleeve. Fitted wrap that accelerates recovery in patients with vein disease, lymphedema, or diabetes. Compression sleeves increase circulation and decrease swelling and fluid buildup following surgery.

contrast material. Radiopaque substance placed into the body to enable a system or body structure to be visualized, such as nonionic and low osmolar contrast media (LOCM), ionic and high osmolar contrast media (HOCM), barium, and gadolinium.

covered osteoporosis drug. Injectable drug approved for treating post-menopausal osteoporosis provided to an individual that has suffered a bone fracture related to post-menopausal osteoporosis.

dermis. Skin layer found under the epidermis that contains a papillary upper layer and the deep reticular layer of collagen, vascular bed, and nerves.

dermis graft. Skin graft that has been separated from the epidermal tissue and the underlying subcutaneous fat, used primarily as a substitute for fascia grafts in plastic surgery.

dialysis. Artificial filtering of the blood to remove contaminating waste elements and restore normal balance.

disarticulation. Removal of a limb through a joint.

diskectomy. Surgical excision of an intervertebral disk.

DME MAC. Durable medical equipment Medicare administrative contractor. Entity where claims for specific DMEPOS must be submitted for processing and reimbursement.

DME PDAC. Durable Medical Equipment Pricing Data Analysis and Coding. Medicare contractor responsible for maintaining the durable medical equipment classification system (DMECS), including HCPCS coding determinations, and providing durable medical equipment, prosthetics, orthotics, and supplies (DMEPOS) allowables.

drug eluting stent. Specialized device placed inside blood vessels for intraluminal support that is coated with a controlled time-release drug that enters the surrounding tissue and helps prevent or slow the growth of plaque or stenotic tissue.

drug formulary. List of prescription medications preferred for use by a health plan and dispensed through participating pharmacies to covered persons.

drugs and biologicals. Drugs and biologicals included - or approved for inclusion - in the United States Pharmacopoeia, the National Formulary, the United States Homeopathic Pharmacopoeia, in New Drugs or Accepted Dental Remedies, or approved by the pharmacy and drug therapeutics committee of the medical staff of the hospital. Also included are medically accepted and FDA approved drugs used in an anticancer chemotherapeutic regimen. The carrier determines medical acceptance based on supportive clinical evidence.

dual-lead device. Implantable cardiac device (pacemaker or implantable cardioverter-defibrillator [ICD]) in which pacing and sensing components are placed in only two chambers of the heart.

durable medical equipment. Medical equipment that can withstand repeated use, is not disposable, is used to serve a medical purpose, is generally not useful to a person in the absence of a sickness or injury, and is appropriate for use in the home. Examples of durable medical equipment include hospital beds, wheelchairs, and oxygen equipment.

Dx. Diagnosis.

electrocardiogram. Recording of the electrical activity of the heart on a moving strip of paper that detects and records the electrical potential of the heart during contraction.

electroencephalography. Testing involving amplification, recording, and analysis of the electrical activity of the brain.

electromyography. Test that measures muscle response to nerve stimulation determining if muscle weakness is present and if it is related to the muscles themselves or a problem with the nerves that supply the muscles.

enteral. Pertaining to the intestines; enteral is often used in the context of nutrition management: formulas, jejunostomy tubes, nasogastric devices, etc.

epidermis. Outermost, nonvascular layer of skin that contains four to five differentiated layers depending on its body location: stratum corneum, lucidum, granulosum, spinosum, and basale.

EPO. 1) Epoetin alpha. 2) Exclusive provider organization. In health care contracting, an organization similar to an HMO, but the member must remain within the provider network to receive benefits. EPOs are regulated under insurance statutes rather than HMO legislation.

ESRD. End stage renal disease. Progression of chronic renal failure to lasting and irreparable kidney damage that requires dialysis or renal transplant for survival.

EVAR. Endovascular aortic repair. Deployment of a prosthetic stent via a catheter into the site of an abdominal aortic aneurysm (AAA). The stent provides a safe conduit for blood flow to relieve pressure on the aneurysm as the blood flows through the stent instead of continuing to bulge the sac formed by the aorta wall dilation.

event recorder. Portable, ambulatory heart monitor worn by the patient that makes electrocardiographic recordings of the length and frequency of aberrant cardiac rhythm to help diagnose heart conditions and to assess pacemaker functioning or programming.

fecal microbiota transplant (FMT). Procedure in which healthy bacteria (microbiota) is extracted from the feces of a screened donor and transferred to the colon of the recipient via colonoscopy or upper endoscopy, most often to treat persistent *C. difficile* infections.

Food and Drug Administration (FDA). Federal agency responsible for protecting public health by substantiating the safety, efficacy, and security of human and veterinary drugs, biological products, medical devices, national food supply, cosmetics, and items that give off radiation.

FOTO. Focus on therapeutic outcomes.

gait. Manner in which a person walks.

gene. Basic unit of heredity that contains nucleic acid. Genes are arranged in different and unique sequences or strings that determine the gene's function. Human genes usually include multiple protein coding regions such as exons separated by introns which are nonprotein coding sections.

genetic test. Test that is able to detect a gene mutation, either inherited or caused by the environment.

gingivoplasty. Repair or reconstruction of the gum tissue, altering the gingival contours by excising areas of gum tissue or making incisions through the gingiva to create a gingival flap.

glaucoma. Rise in intraocular pressure, restricting blood flow and decreasing vision.

habilitative services. Procedures or services provided to assist a patient in learning, keeping, and improving new skills needed to perform daily living activities. Habilitative services assist patients in acquiring a skill for the first time.

halo. Tool for stabilizing the head and spine.

health care provider. Entity that administers diagnostic and therapeutic services.

hemodialysis. Cleansing of wastes and contaminating elements from the blood by virtue of different diffusion rates through a semipermeable membrane, which separates blood from a filtration solution that diffuses other elements out of the blood.

home health services. Services furnished to patients in their homes under the care of physicians. These services include part-time or intermittent skilled nursing care, physical therapy, medical social services, medical supplies, and some rehabilitation equipment. Home health supplies and services must be prescribed by a physician, and the beneficiary must be confined at home in order for Medicare to pay the benefits in full.

hospice. Organization that furnishes inpatient, outpatient, and home health care for the terminally ill. Hospices emphasize support and counseling services for terminally ill people and their families, pain relief, and symptom management. When the Medicare beneficiary chooses hospice benefits, all other Medicare benefits are discontinued, except physician services and treatment of conditions not related to the terminal illness.

hypertrophic. Enlarged or overgrown from an increase in cell size of the affected tissue.

implant. Material or device inserted or placed within the body for therapeutic, reconstructive, or diagnostic purposes.

implantable cardioverter-defibrillator. Implantable electronic cardiac device used to control rhythm abnormalities such as tachycardia, fibrillation, or bradycardia by producing high- or low-energy stimulation and pacemaker functions. It may also have the capability to provide the functions of an implantable loop recorder or implantable cardiovascular monitor.

in situ. Located in the natural position or contained within the origin site, not spread into neighboring tissue.

incontinence. Inability to control urination or defecation.

infusion. Introduction of a therapeutic fluid, other than blood, into the bloodstream.

infusion pump. Device that delivers a measured amount of drug or intravenous solution through injection over a period of time.

intra-arterial. Within an artery or arteries.

intramuscular. Within a muscle.

intraocular lens. Artificial lens implanted into the eye to replace a damaged natural lens or cataract.

intravenous. Within a vein or veins.

introducer. Instrument, such as a catheter, needle, or tube, through which another instrument or device is introduced into the body.

keratoprosthesis. Surgical procedure in which the physician creates a new anterior chamber with a plastic optical implant to replace a severely damaged cornea that cannot be repaired.

LDS. Lipodystrophy syndrome. Syndrome which involves the partial or total absence of fat and/or the abnormal deposition and distribution of fat in the body due to a disturbance of the lipid metabolism.

magnetic resonance angiography. Diagnostic technique utilizing magnetic fields and radio waves rather than radiation to produce detailed, cross-sectional images of internal body structures.

multiple-lead device. Implantable cardiac device (pacemaker or implantable cardioverter-defibrillator [ICD]) in which pacing and sensing components are placed in at least three chambers of the heart.

mutation. Alteration in gene function that results in changes to a gene or chromosome. Can cause deficits or disease that can be inherited, can have beneficial effects, or result in no noticeable change.

nasogastric tube. Long, hollow, cylindrical catheter made of soft rubber or plastic that is inserted through the nose down into the stomach, and is used for feeding, instilling medication, or withdrawing gastric contents.

nebulizer. Latin for mist, a device that converts liquid into a fine spray and is commonly used to deliver medicine to the upper respiratory, bronchial, and lung areas.

negative pressure dressing. Adjunctive therapy used to speed wound healing in skin grafts or large wounds. It has been shown to increase blood flow, decrease bacterial count, and increase formation of granulation tissues. A foam pad is placed on the defect and covered with an occlusive drape. A small tube that is non-collapsible is placed into the foam and attached to a disposable pump that provides negative pressure up to -125 mmHg.

NMES. Neuromuscular electrical stimulation. Technology that uses percutaneous stimulation to deliver electrical impulses for muscle flexion to trigger action. NMES can, in some cases, create an ability to ambulate among paraplegic patients.

obturator. Prosthesis used to close an acquired or congenital opening in the palate that aids in speech and chewing.

occult blood test. Chemical or microscopic test to determine the presence of blood in a specimen.

occupational therapy. Training, education, and assistance intended to assist a person who is recovering from a serious illness or injury perform the activities of daily life.

ocular implant. Implant inside muscular cone.

omnicardiogram. Method of mathematically interpreting the usual linear form of the electrocardiogram in a different, roughly circular shape. This interpretation is then compared to a normal template and an analysis is performed on two randomly selected cycles from leads I, II, V4, V, and/or V6.

oral. Pertaining to the mouth.

ordering physician. Physician who orders nonphysician services (e.g., laboratory services, pharmaceutical services, imaging services, or durable medical equipment) for a patient.

orphan drugs. Drugs that treat diseases that affect fewer than 200,000 people in the United States, as designated by the FDA. Orphan drugs follow a varied process from other drugs regulated by the FDA.

orthosis. Derived from a Greek word meaning "to make straight," it is an artificial appliance that supports, aligns, or corrects an anatomical deformity or improves the use of a moveable body part. Unlike a prosthesis, an orthotic device is always functional in nature.

orthotic. Associated with the making and fitting of an orthosis(es).

osteo-. Having to do with bone.

osteogenesis stimulator. Device used to stimulate the growth of bone by electrical impulses or ultrasound.

ostomy. Artificial (surgical) opening in the body used for drainage or for delivery of medications or nutrients.

pacemaker. Implantable cardiac device that controls the heart's rhythm and maintains regular beats by artificial electric discharges. This device consists of the pulse generator with a battery and the electrodes, or leads, which are placed in single or dual chambers of the heart, usually transvenously.

parenteral. Other than the alimentary canal and is usually used in a method of delivery context: total parenteral nutrition (TPN) and parenteral nutrition therapy (PNT) formulas, kits, and devices.

parenteral nutrition. Nutrients provided subcutaneously, intravenously, intramuscularly, or intradermally for patients during the postoperative period and in other conditions, such as shock, coma, and renal failure.

partial hospitalization. Situation in which the patient only stays part of each day over a long period. Cardiac, rehabilitation, and chronic pain patients, for example, could use this service.

passive mobilization. Pressure, movement, or pulling of a limb or body part utilizing an apparatus or device.

periradicular. Surrounding part of the tooth's root.

peritoneal. Space between the lining of the abdominal wall, or parietal peritoneum, and the surface layer of the abdominal organs, or visceral peritoneum. It contains a thin, watery fluid that keeps the peritoneal surfaces moist.

peritoneal dialysis. Dialysis that filters waste from blood inside the body using the peritoneum, the natural lining of the abdomen, as the semipermeable membrane across which ultrafiltration is accomplished. A special catheter is inserted into the abdomen and a dialysis solution is drained into the abdomen. This solution extracts fluids and wastes, which are then discarded when the fluid is drained. Various forms of peritoneal dialysis include CAPD, CCPD, and NIDP.

peritoneal effusion. Persistent escape of fluid within the peritoneal cavity.

pessary. Device placed in the vagina to support and reposition a prolapsing or retropositioned uterus, rectum, or vagina.

photocoagulation. Application of an intense laser beam of light to disrupt tissue and condense protein material to a residual mass, used especially for treating ocular conditions.

physician. Legally authorized practitioners including a doctor of medicine or osteopathy, a doctor of dental surgery or of dental medicine, a doctor of podiatric medicine, a doctor of optometry, and a chiropractor only with respect to treatment by means of manual manipulation of the spine (to correct a subluxation).

PICC. Peripherally inserted central catheter. PICC is inserted into one of the large veins of the arm and threaded through the vein until the tip sits in a large vein just above the heart.

prehensile. Ability to grasp, seize, or hold.

prodrug. Inactive drug that goes through a metabolic process when given resulting in a chemical conversion that changes the drug into an active pharmacological agent.

prophylaxis. Intervention or protective therapy intended to prevent a disease.

prostate cancer screening tests. Test that consists of any (or all) of the procedures provided for the early detection of prostate cancer to a man 50 years of age or older who has not had a test during the preceding year. The procedures are as follows: A digital rectal examination; A prostate-specific antigen blood test. After 2002, the list of procedures may be expanded as appropriate for the early detection of prostate cancer, taking into account changes in technology and standards of medical practice, availability, effectiveness, costs, and other factors.

prosthetic. Device that replaces all or part of an internal body organ or body part, or that replaces part of the function of a permanently inoperable or malfunctioning internal body organ or body part.

pulse generator. Component of a pacemaker or an implantable cardioverter defibrillator that contains the battery and the electronics for producing the electrical discharge sent to the heart to control cardiac rhythm. Insertion or replacement of the pulse generator may be done alone, not in conjunction with insertion or replacement of the entire pacemaker system.

qualitative. To determine the nature or characteristics of the components of a substance.

quantitative. To determine the number or amount of the components of a substance.

rehabilitation services. Therapy services provided primarily for assisting in a rehabilitation program of evaluation and service including cardiac rehabilitation, medical social services, occupational therapy, physical therapy, respiratory therapy, skilled nursing, speech therapy, psychiatric rehabilitation, and alcohol and substance abuse rehabilitation.

residual limb. Portion of an arm or leg that remains attached to the body after an amputation.

screening mammography. Radiologic images taken of the female breast for the early detection of breast cancer.

screening pap smear. Diagnostic laboratory test consisting of a routine exfoliative cytology test (Papanicolaou test) provided to a woman for the early detection of cervical or vaginal cancer. The exam includes a clinical breast examination and a physician's interpretation of the results.

sialodochoplasty. Surgical repair of a salivary gland duct.

single-lead device. Implantable cardiac device (pacemaker or implantable cardioverter-defibrillator [ICD]) in which pacing and sensing components are placed in only one chamber of the heart.

skin substitute. Non-autologous human or non-human skin that forms a base for skin growth, often considered a graft dressing.

speech prosthetic. Electronic speech aid device for patient who has had a laryngectomy. One operates by placing a vibrating head against the throat;

the other amplifies sound waves through a tube which is inserted into the user's mouth.

splint. Brace or support. *1)* dynamic splint: brace that permits movement of an anatomical structure such as a hand, wrist, foot, or other part of the body after surgery or injury. *2)* static splint: brace that prevents movement and maintains support and position for an anatomical structure after surgery or injury.

stent. Tube to provide support in a body cavity or lumen.

stereotactic radiosurgery. Delivery of externally-generated ionizing radiation to specific targets for destruction or inactivation. Most often utilized in the treatment of brain or spinal tumors, high-resolution stereotactic imaging is used to identify the target and then deliver the treatment. Computer-assisted planning may also be employed. Simple and complex cranial lesions and spinal lesions are typically treated in a single planning and treatment session, although a maximum of five sessions may be required. No incision is made for stereotactic radiosurgery procedures.

subcutaneous. Below the skin.

TENS. Transcutaneous electrical nerve stimulator. TENS is applied by placing electrode pads over the area to be stimulated and connecting the electrodes to a transmitter box, which sends a current through the skin to sensory nerve fibers to help decrease pain in that nerve distribution.

terminal device. Addition to an upper limb prosthesis that replaces the function and/or appearance of a missing hand.

tracheostomy. Formation of a tracheal opening on the neck surface with tube insertion to allow for respiration in cases of obstruction or decreased patency. A tracheostomy may be planned or performed on an emergency basis for temporary or long-term use.

traction. Drawing out or holding tension on an area by applying a direct therapeutic pulling force.

transcutaneous electrical nerve stimulator. Device that delivers a controlled amount of electricity to an area of the body to stimulate healing and/or to mitigate post-surgical or post-traumatic pain.

transesophageal echocardiography. Guidance of a small probe into the esophagus under sedation to closely evaluate the heart and blood vessels within the chest.

type A emergency department. Emergency department licensed and advertised to be available to provide emergent care 24 hours a day, seven days a week. Type A emergency departments must meet both the CPT book definition of an emergency department and the EMTALA definition of a dedicated emergency department.

type B emergency department. Emergency department licensed and advertised to provide emergent care less than 24 hours a day, seven days a week. Type B emergency departments must meet the EMTALA definition of a dedicated emergency department.

vascular closure device. vascular closure devices seal femoral artery punctures caused by invasive or interventional procedures. The closure or seal is achieved by percutaneous delivery of the device's two primary structures, which are usually an anchor and a suture, clip or biologic substance (e.g., collagen, bioabsorbable polymer) or suture through the tissue tract.

Appendix 9 — Quality Payment Program

In 2015, Congress passed the Medicare Access and CHIP Reauthorization Act (MACRA), which included sweeping changes for practitioners who provide services reimbursed under the Medicare physician fee schedule (MPFS). The act focused on repealing the faulty Medicare sustainable growth rate, focusing on quality of patient outcomes, and controlling Medicare spending.

A MACRA final rule in October 2016 established the Quality Payment Program (QPP), which was effective January 1, 2017. This value-based payment model rewards eligible clinicians (ECs) who provide high-quality care and reduce the payments for those who fail to meet specific performance standards.

ECs can receive incentives under the QPP. Once the performance threshold is established, all ECs who score above that threshold are eligible to receive a positive payment adjustment. Keep in mind that the key requirement is that an EC **submit data** to avoid the negative payment adjustment and receive the incentives. The Centers for Medicare and Medicaid Services (CMS) has redesigned the scoring so that clinicians are able to know how well they are doing in the program, as benchmarks are known in advance of participating.

The QPP consists of two tracks that clinicians may choose from based on their practice size, location, specialty, or patient population:

- The merit-based incentive payment system (MIPS)
- Alternative payment models (APMs)

The 2017 QPP final rule established regulations for MIPS and APMs as well as related policies applicable to eligible clinicians who participate in the Shared Savings Program. These policies included requirements for Shared Savings Program accountable care organizations (ACOs) regarding reporting for the MIPS Quality performance category and a policy that gave ACOs full credit for the MIPS Improvement Activities performance category based on their participation in the Shared Savings Program. Since that time, revisions and modifications have been made to allow more focus on measurement efforts and to reduce barriers to entry into advanced APMs. Refinements will continue in order to reduce reporting burden and focus on patient outcomes.

MIPS provides specified performance categories under which payment adjustments may be earned for Part B covered professional services. Eligible clinicians can obtain a composite performance score (CPS) of up to 100 points from these weighted performance categories, which focus on patient care quality and cost, improvements in patient engagement and clinical care processes, and use of certified electronic health record technology (CEHRT). This performance score then defines the payment adjustments in the second calendar year after the year the score is obtained. For instance, the score obtained for the 2020 performance year is linked to payment for Medicare Part B services in 2022.

ECs currently have three available reporting frameworks, depending on individual needs and eligibility—traditional MIPS, MIPS Value Pathways (MVPs), and the alternative payment model (APM) performance pathway (APP).

Traditional MIPS currently consists of the following performance categories:

- Quality
- Improvement Activities
- Promoting Interoperability (PI)
- Cost

MVPs, which were added as a result of complaints by some physicians of confusing quality measures, allow clinicians to report only on those measures that apply to their specialty. The CY 2023 proposed rule continues refinement and focus on subgroups for MVP reporting that will provide more granularity in reporting and improve patient care. Additional MVPs will gradually be implemented for more specialties and subspecialties that participate in the program.

The APP is intended for MIPS-eligible ECs who also participate in MIPS APMs. Performance is measured across three areas (Quality, Improvement Activities, and Promoting Interoperability) in this reporting and scoring pathway, which aims to decrease reporting burden, encourage APM participation, and create new opportunities for scoring for existing MIPS APM participants. For performance year 2022, the APP Quality performance category accounted for 50 percent of the MIPS final score; the PI performance category weight was 30 percent; and the Improvement Activities performance category weight was 20 percent.

Proposed 2023 Changes

As noted earlier, the majority of the proposed updates for CY 2023 focus on MVP refinement. In addition to the MVPs proposed for the 2023 performance year, other proposals in the CY 2023 proposed rule include:

- Requesting input on proposed increase in conversion factor in lieu of lump sum payment, noting that there is currently no incentive authorized for performance year 2023
- Increasing the number of measures related to health equity
- Developing measures focused on amputation avoidance in diabetic patients, especially for underserved populations
- Exploring vendor ability to select which MVPs to support
- Seeking feedback regarding continuing medical education (CME) or accreditation entities acting as third-party intermediaries to reduce clinician reporting burden
- Advancing trusted exchange framework and common agreement (TEFCA) information regarding participation and submission of clinical documentation
- Continuing the transition to digital quality measurement and using fast healthcare interoperability resources (FHIR) with data standardization and approaches to transition
- Transitioning to individual QP determinations to encourage specialists' participation in Advanced APMs

Evaluation continues regarding an incremental timeline to transition to mandatory MVP reporting that will coincide with the sunset of traditional MIPS. The timeline currently being considered is the end of the CY 2027 performance period/2029 MIPS payment year, although this is not an official proposal at this time.

Detailed information regarding the Quality Payment Program may be found at https://qpp.cms.gov/. This website will also announce the final CMS determinations of MVPs, advanced APMs, and MIPS APMs for the 2023 performance period.